Ali Dabbagh • Fardad Esmailian
Sary Aranki
Editors

Postoperative Critical Care for Adult Cardiac Surgical Patients

Second Edition

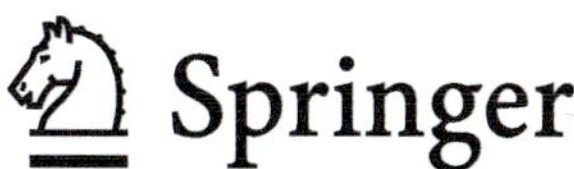

Springer

Editors
Ali Dabbagh
Faculty of Medicine
Cardiac Anesthesiology Department
Anesthesiology Research Center
Shahid Beheshti University
of Medical Sciences
Tehran
Iran

Fardad Esmailian
Department of Surgery
Cedars-Sinai Heart Institute
Los Angeles, CA
USA

Sary Aranki
Brigham and Women's Hospital
Boston, MA
USA

ISBN 978-3-319-75746-9 ISBN 978-3-319-75747-6 (eBook)
https://doi.org/10.1007/978-3-319-75747-6

Library of Congress Control Number: 2018941109

Printed on acid-free paper

This Springer imprint is published by the registered company Springer International Publishing AG part of Springer Nature.
The registered company address is: Gewerbestrasse 11, 6330 Cham, Switzerland

To my wife Samira and to my parents

Ali Dabbagh

To my family: Yvonne, Gabriel and Aaron, and to my parents

Fardad Esmailian

To Nadia, Alex, Heather, and Abla

Sary Aranki

Foreword to the First Edition

Postoperative Critical Care for Cardiac Surgical Patients is a superb amalgamation of a wide variety of clinical expertise in the perioperative and postoperative care of cardiac surgical patients edited by three very fine academicians from three outstanding medical centers and who are in the position of being able to judge the best perioperative and postoperative cardiac surgical care. The three editors have a wide variety of cardiac surgical interest. Dr. Dabbagh is a cardiac anesthesiologist, who is intimately involved in the intraoperative and postoperative care of cardiac surgery patients; Dr. Esmailian is an expert in the care of patients receiving cardiac assist devices and cardiac transplantation, which are some of the most challenging postoperative patients; and Dr. Aranki is an extremely talented surgeon in all aspects of cardiac surgery, especially coronary artery bypass grafting and valve repair and replacement.

This book brings the entire spectrum of cardiac surgical perioperative treatment and postoperative care under one cover. Postoperative critical care in cardiac surgery is extremely important and I believe this book has the potential to be the gold standard in postoperative care for cardiac surgical patients. The key to good surgical results is the combination of an excellent operation and meticulous perioperative and postoperative care, the essence of this book.

The authors are to be complimented for providing up-to-date, accurate, and intellectual contributions for this most important area of cardiac surgery. This book is an excellent effort in advancing the art and science of perioperative and postoperative surgical care.

Boston, MA, USA — Lawrence H. Cohn, M.D.

Foreword to the Second Edition

Postoperative Critical Care for Adult Cardiac Surgical Patients is a successful and succinct guide to this challenging phase of perioperative adult cardiac practice. The three editors from around the world have continued their excellent organized approach to postoperative care in the adult cardiac arena in this second edition. Dr. Ali Dabbagh is a distinguished cardiac anesthesiologist who is an expert in the perioperative care of adult cardiac surgical patients. Dr. Fardad Esmailian is a recognized authority in mechanical circulatory support and heart transplantation that both often have very challenging postoperative care considerations. Dr. Sary Aranki is a renowned and talented cardiac surgeon with special interests in coronary artery bypass grafting, valve repairs, and valve replacements. These three expert editors have combined their expertise and unique perspectives with a select group of contributors to present a comprehensive handbook of adult postoperative cardiac care in 22 chapters.

The second edition has an expanded scope with an additional 11 chapters. The trio of expert editors have taken advantage of this expanded reach to cover in detail additional aspects such as nutrition, safety, economics, transplantation, extracorporeal membrane oxygenation, fluid and acid-base management, infectious and inflammatory complications, as well as organ-based complications in the respiratory, renal, and gastrointestinal systems. This expanded coverage of the specialty has kept the entire spectrum of contemporary postoperative care for the adult cardiac surgical patient under one cover. As Dr. Lawrence Cohn pointed out in his foreword to the first edition, the editors have to be congratulated for developing an excellent postoperative handbook that could become the gold standard in the field.

The essence of excellence in adult cardiac surgery remains the combination of an expert operation with meticulous care throughout the postoperative period. The editors and their selected authors have to be thanked for their combined effort to present the practitioner with a concise and clear approach to postoperative management of the adult cardiac surgical patient with respect to both the art and the science. The second edition of *Postoperative Critical Care for Adult Cardiac Surgical Patients* advances the quality of care in the field in a significant fashion and will very likely be a valuable bedside reference for all of us.

Philadelphia, PA, USA
Jacob T. Gutsche, M.D., F.A.S.E.
John G. Augoustides, M.D., F.A.S.E., F.A.H.A.

Preface to the Second Edition

As many people especially those working in health care know, a patient undergoes a journey during the perioperative pod; in almost all patients the journey is a stress provoking one, both for the patients and their families. The same happens for cardiac surgical patients undergoing procedures in the operating room or in cardiac catheterization lab, which includes a whole process, not merely an event. Surgery is not, therefore, an end, but rather a "chapter" of the whole process.

Nowadays cardiac procedures rank among the most common type of all procedures, both due to the prevalence of cardiac diseases and improvements in quality of care in this field. At the same time, they are one of the most challenging and most complicated groups of therapeutic modalities, leading to a great and vast field of instructive issues upon students and faculty alike.

Postoperative care plays a crucial role in determining the clinical result for the patient; the success of postoperative care is also directly affected by the quality of the pre- and intraoperative experiences. So, the second edition of *Postoperative Critical Care for Adult Cardiac Surgical Patients* covers the entire postoperative cardiac surgical care, starting from risk assessment models, basic physiologic and pharmacologic knowledge organ based monitoring related to these patients, leading to postoperative clinical care in different major systems; a separate chapter titled "Infectious Diseases and Management After Cardiac Surgery" is added to this part. The next chapters deal with fluid, electrolyte, acid base and pain management and also postoperative considerations related to cardiopulmonary bypass. In this edition, four new chapters complete the book dealing with Postoperative Critical Care in "transplant, ECMO, patient safety, and nutrition." We have to highly appreciate the very impressive and invaluable contribution of all the authors, both in the first and in this edition of the book.

The first edition of this book was welcomed by cardiac surgeons, cardiac anesthesiologists, intensivists, and cardiac intensive care nurses, as well as the students, interns, and residents learning in these environments. Some of the book audiences sent us their fruitful critics regarding potential chapters to be added; the echo of their feedbacks helped us a lot to improve the book and add the new chapters or revise many of the previous ones.

We as the editors would have to acknowledge the very committed and compassionate teamwork of Springer Company, which helped us with the second edition of the book.

And finally, we have to acknowledge our families who have inspired us with accompaniment, empathy, sacrifice, and endless love in such a way that we could promote this effort.

Tehran, Iran Ali Dabbagh, M.D.
Los Angeles, CA, USA Fardad Esmailian, M.D.
Boston, MA, USA Sary Aranki, M.D.

Contents

Contributors

Felice Eugenio Agrò, M.D. Postgraduate School of Anesthesia and Intensive Care, Anesthesia, Intensive Care and Pain Management Department, University School of Medicine Campus Bio-Medico of Rome, Rome, Italy

Elizabeth Behringer, M.D. Department of Anesthesiology, Southern California Permanente Medical Group, Kaiser Permanente Los Angeles Medical Center, Los Angeles, CA, USA

Maria Benedetto, M.D. Postgraduate School of Anesthesia and Intensive Care, Anesthesia, Intensive Care and Pain Management Department, University School of Medicine Campus Bio-Medico of Rome, Rome, Italy

Edward A. Bittner, M.D., Ph.D., M.S.Ed., F.C.C.M. Critical Care-Anesthesiology Fellowship, Massachusetts General Hospital, Harvard Medical School, Boston, MA, USA

Surgical Intensive Care Unit, Massachusetts General Hospital, Harvard Medical School, Boston, MA, USA

Department of Anesthesia, Critical Care and Pain Medicine, Massachusetts General Hospital, Harvard Medical School, Boston, MA, USA

Manuel Caceres, M.D. Department of Thoracic Surgery, UCLA Medical Center, Los Angeles, CA, USA

Alice Chan, R.N., M.N., C.N.S., C.C.R.N. Cedars-Sinai Medical Center, Los Angeles, CA, USA

Antosnio Hernandez Conte, M.D., M.B.A. University of California, Irvine School of Medicine, Orange, CA, USA

Kaiser Permanente Los Angeles Medical Center, Los Angeles, CA, USA

Gaston Cudemus, M.D. Cardiothoracic Anesthesiology and Critical Care, Department of Anesthesia, Critical Care and Pain Medicine, Corrigan Minehan Heart Center, Boston, MA, USA

Division of Cardiac Surgery, Massachusetts General Hospital, Harvard Medical School, Boston, MA, USA

Ali Dabbagh, M.D. Faculty of Medicine, Cardiac Anesthesiology Department, Anesthesiology Research Center, Shahid Beheshti University of Medical Sciences, Tehran, Iran

Cardiac Anesthesiology Fellowship Program, Shahid Beheshti University of Medical Sciences, Tehran, Iran

Erik R. Dong, D.O., M.D. Critical Care Cardiology, Heart Institute, Cedars-Sinai Medical Center, Los Angeles, CA, USA

Dominic Emerson, M.D. Department of Surgery, Cedars Sinai Medical Center, Los Angeles, CA, USA

Fardad Esmailian, M.D. Department of Surgery, Cedars-Sinai Heart Institute, Los Angeles, CA, USA

Heart Transplantation, Cedars-Sinai Heart Institute, Los Angeles, CA, USA

Mahnoosh Foroughi, M.D. Cardiovascular Research Center, Shahid Beheshti University of Medical Sciences, Tehran, Iran

Oren Friedman, M.D. Critical Care Medicine, Pulmonary Medicine, Cardiothoracic Surgery and Transplant Team, Cedars-Sinai Medical Center, Los Angeles, CA, USA

Majid Haghjoo, M.D. Department of Cardiac Electrophysiology, Rajaie Cardiovascular Medical and Research Center, Cardiac Electrophysiology Research Center, Iran University of Medical Sciences, Tehran, Iran

Alireza Imani, Ph.D. Department of Physiology, School of Medicine, Tehran University of Medical Science, Tehran, Islamic Republic of Iran

Kevin Kommalsingh, M.D. Department of Cardiothoracic Surgery, University of Washington, Seattle, WA, USA

Abdolreza Norouzy, M.D., Ph.D. Department of Nutrition, School of Medicine, Mashhad University of Medical Sciences, Mashhad, Iran

Michael Nurok, M.D. Cardiac Surgery Intensive Care Unit, Cedars-Sinai Medical Center, Los Angeles, CA, USA

Jamel Ortoleva, M.D. Adult Cardiothoracic Anesthesiology Program, Yale-New Haven Hospital, New Haven, CT, USA

Juan M. Perrone, M.D. Department of Anesthesiology, Critical Care and Pain Medicine, Massachusetts General Hospital, Harvard Medical School, Boston, MA, USA

Paul A. Perry, M.D. Department of Surgery, University of California, Davis, CA, USA

Samira Rajaei, M.D., Ph.D. Department of Immunology, School of Medicine, Tehran University of Medical Science, Tehran, Islamic Republic of Iran

Andrew G. Rudikoff, M.D. Kaiser Permanente Los Angeles Medical Center, Los Angeles, CA, USA

Mehdi Shadnoush, M.D., Ph.D. Department of Clinical Nutrition, School of Nutrition Sciences and Food Technology, Shahid Beheshti University of Medical Sciences, Tehran, Iran

Ardeshir Tajbakhsh, M.D. Anesthesiology Department, Anesthesiology Research Center, Shahid Beheshti University of Medical Sciences, Tehran, Iran

Zahra Talebi, Pharm. D. Anesthesiology Research Center, Shahid Beheshti University of Medical Sciences, Tehran, Iran

Marialuisa Vennari, M.D. Postgraduate School of Anesthesia and Intensive Care, Anesthesia, Intensive Care and Pain Management Department, University School of Medicine Campus Bio-Medico of Rome, Rome, Italy

Introduction and History of Postoperative Care for Adult Cardiac Surgical Patients

1

Mahnoosh Foroughi

Abstract

There is about seven decades that cardiac surgery began to take shape as we know it.

Cardiopulmonary bypass (CPB) is one of the most important advances in medicine and essential milestone of cardiac surgery to maintain tissue oxygenation, myocardial protection, and systemic circulation during cardioplegic cardiac arrest with suspension of ventilatory support. During this period, both CPB machine and protocols have been changed frequently. Despite the steady progress in CPB techniques, it is not a perfect model, and optimal design to reduce its complication is a great challenge.

The concept of critical care unit was first introduced in the late 1950s for life-threatened patients. The progressive technologic advances let the care units as multidisciplinary organization with continuous bedside rather than remote monitoring for old patients with multiple comorbidities who should tolerate the deleterious effects of CPB too.

Keyword

History · Cardiac surgery · Cardiac anesthesia · Postoperative care

M. Foroughi, M.D.
Cardiovascular Research Center, Shahid Beheshti University of Medical Sciences, Tehran, Iran
e-mail: m_foroughi@sbmu.ac.ir

A. Dabbagh et al. (eds.), *Postoperative Critical Care for Adult Cardiac Surgical Patients*, https://doi.org/10.1007/978-3-319-75747-6_1

1.1 History of Cardiac Surgery in Brief

In spite of improvement in many fields of surgery, cardiac surgery was absent for long periods due to technical difficulties of this untouchable structure. The heart was recognized as a forbidden area for surgery till 1882, as Theodor Billroth who was the pioneer of abdominal surgery believed any effort to stitch on a heart was equal to losing surgeon's respect between his colleagues. The real need requirements for cardiac surgery were determining of anticoagulant property of heparin, blood types and transfusion, silicone antifoam and development of oxygenator in the early nineteenth century. Indeed, combination of surgery, physiology, and research triggered to create heart-lung machine.

John Gibbon was the pioneer to use heart-lung machine and successfully operated an ASD patient in 1953. Lillehi et al. reported the success of controlled cross-circulation technique in a series of patients in 1955. They cannulated and connected femoral artery and vein of the patient to the donor and used a pump to regulate the rate of flow exchange between them.

During its short existence, cardiopulmonary bypass (CPB) has evolved significantly from the concept of extracorporeal circulation to the present trend of minimal extracorporeal circulation, assist devices, and total artificial hearts. At the begining, the bubble oxygenator was used, but it was changed several times to improve oxygenation, lessen blood element trauma, and have more biocompatible hollow fiber membranous oxygenator. The well-known damaging effects of extracorporeal circulation have been reduced significantly by improvement in CPB techniques.

It has become the standard part of cardiac operation to permit the safe and effective surgical correction of intracardiac disease while maintaining oxygenated blood flow to all other organs. The cardiac operation is a good example of multidisciplinary team working (surgeon, perfusionist, and anesthesiologist) (Stephenson 2008; Braile and Godoy 2012; Punjabi and Taylor 2013; Hessel 2015).

1.2 History of Cardiac Anesthesia in Brief

Over the recent century, accumulative basic knowledge in physiology and pharmacology fields was the foundation for development of cardiac anesthesia. Numerous anesthetic agents have ever been invented and used with extensive range of efficacy and side effects in the history of cardiac anesthesia. Today, it is a safe daily practice for patients undergoing cardiac surgery.

The general anesthetic agents (ether and chloroform) were developed in the middle of the nineteenth century. Inhalational agents were introduced in 1956, morphine anesthesia in 1969, and total intravenous anesthetics in 1989. The concern about safety of anesthetic agents had changed from inflammable effect of ether to bradycardia and hypotension with morphine; prolonged respiratory depression with fentanyl; hypoxia with nitrous oxide; myocardial depression, arrhythmias, and hepatitis with halothane; and prolonged sedation and increased need for inotropic support with thiopentone, and the story has continued.

Historically sucking stab wound in the chest was incompatible with life. In 1899, the effective solution was found by tracheal intubation with intermittent positive pressure ventilation. After the discovery of anticoagulation property of heparin, more experimental studies with CPB had been done. In 1957, systemic hypothermia was introduced to decrease metabolic rate and organ protection during hypoperfusion state of CPB. In 1972, IABP was made as mechanical circulatory tool to support low cardiac output and CPB weaning.

The two most important monitoring instruments for cardiovascular system are pulmonary artery catheter (PAC) and transesophageal echocardiography (TEE). PAC was introduced to measure pulmonary arterial pressure, cardiac output, and systemic vascular resistance in 1979. Currently, PAC is not used routinely and has no important impression on patients' survival in many patients. Also, a considerable number of Central Nervous System monitoring devices have been developed; hoping to decrease potential neurologic drawbacks of the perioperative period with an emphasis on the operation time period. Other sophisticated monitoring devices including but not limited to coagulation pathway monitoring has been incorporated to patient care in adult cardiac surgery.

TEE was introduced in the 1980s and, in contrast to PAC, is the essential part of clinical practice in cardiac operation rooms to monitor diagnosis of cardiac dysfunction and change the plan of operation and reevaluation. It improves outcome after cardiac surgery.

In addition to surgeons, cardiac anesthesiologists should evaluate patients completely before operation to prevent or reduce preventable complications and also, should be involved as a core member of the care provider team throughout the perioperative period (Alexander 2015; Alston et al. 2015; Szelkowski et al. 2015). Also, during the last decades, in many anesthesiology departments, Cardiac Anesthesiology Fellowship programs have been well developed; both for adult and pediatric cardiac anesthesia; targeting improved quality of education and improved patient care.

1.3 History of Postoperative Critical Care for Adult Cardiac Surgical Patients

The concept of critical care unit was first introduced in the late 1950s for life-threatened patients by continuous monitoring of hemodynamic and respiratory parameters at the centralized nursing station.

During the period of experimental studies for CPB, mechanical ventilation, hemodialysis, defibrillation, and pacemaker insertion were designed. Increasing knowledge on cardiovascular physiology aid to measure central venous arterial pressure and cardiac output, and to guide proper treatment as volume repletion and administration of inotropic agents. The engineers and technicians with understanding of life-support biology introduced bedsides rather than remote monitors and measurements to have the ability for appropriate intervention (like electrocardiogram, pulse oximetry, blood gas assessment, end-tidal CO2, chest radiography, near-infrared spectroscopy, transcranial cerebral oximetry). Today all necessary functions are performed locally at the bedside and independently of the central nursing station associated with computerized patient charting. However, this development could not be substituted by time-consuming medical history taking and accurate physical examination.

The postoperative management in ICU needs to have multidisciplinary team, including cardiac surgeons, anesthesiologists, and nurse specialists for elderly patients with more comorbidity. The major difference with general ICU is the management of patients who undergo CPB that are associated with extensive and predictable physiologic and pathologic sequelae secondary to CPB. The significant changes are due to dilutional anemia, coagulopathy, and systemic inflammatory response.

The most important concerns after cardiac surgery in ICU include bleeding and coagulopathy, the need for mediastinal exploration, mechanical circulatory support, vasoactive medication, arrhythmias, pulmonary complication (prolonged intubation, pneumonia, pulmonary embolism, atelectasis, and pleural effusions), neurologic events (stroke, cognitive disorder), renal injury, thrombocytopenia, and wound infection.

Shortening length of ICU stay is another important issue. Prolonged ICU stay in addition to increase cost and the use of resources, significantly has an important impact on long-term prognosis. Some defined factors are associated with prolonged ICU stay: preoperative anemia, emergency operation, heart failure, neurologic and renal dysfunction, prolonged aortic clamp time, postoperative hyperglycemic state, and type of surgery. There is consensus to decrease intubation time (fast-track) for cardiac surgery patients if the hemodynamic condition is acceptable with minimal use of inotropic agents, no major bleeding, and no neurologic and renal failure (Gullo and Lumb 2009; Parnell and Massey 2009; Szelkowski et al. 2015; Kapadohos et al. 2017; Yapıcı 2017).

1.4 Current Aspects and Future Perspectives of Postoperative Critical Care for Adult Cardiac Surgical Patients

CPB technology has advanced greatly during this century. It permits to have safe cardiac surgery with minimal mortality and morbidity. Such innovative system was not without challenge, as it is effective but not ideal and perfect. This fact leads to discard some accepted policies during this period, many changes were made, and uncertainty about optimal design continues.

The challenge remains to reduce the deleterious side effects to have secure operation. Some of unresolved issues include concern about optimal hematocrit during CPB, temperature management, biocompatibility of surface coating, hemolysis, minimized circuit and venous drainage, pulsatile or continuous flow, pump designs, anticoagulation, bleeding and blood product transfusion, perfect myocardial protection (cardioplegic solution), modifying systemic inflammatory response, minimal invasive cardiac surgery, use of simulation for education, percutaneous valve repair and replacement, total artificial heart, and ventricular assist devices.

Rapid advances in measurement technology field are another attractive and interesting subject, which provide to use less invasive and expensive instruments (such as tissue capnometry) to evaluate hemodynamic condition and differential diagnosis of hypotension and ischemia state during postoperative cardiac surgery (Punjabi and Taylor 2013; Szelkowski et al. 2015; Kapadohos et al. 2017).

References

Alexander D. Principles of cardiac anaesthesia. Anaesth Intensive Care. 2015;16:479–83.

Alston RP, Ranucci M, Myles PS. Oxford textbook of cardiothoracic anaesthesia. Oxford: Oxford University Press; 2015.

Braile DM, Godoy MF. History of heart surgery in the world, 1996. Rev Bras Cir Cardiovasc. 2012;27:125–36.

Gullo A, Lumb PD. Intensive and critical care medicine. Milan: Springer; 2009.

Hessel EA 2nd. History of cardiopulmonary bypass (CPB). Best Pract Res Clin Anaesthesiol. 2015;29:99–111.

Kapadohos T, Angelopoulos E, Vasileiadis I, Nanas S, Kotanidou A, Karabinis A, Marathias K, Routsi C. Determinants of prolonged intensive care unit stay in patients after cardiac surgery: a prospective observational study. J Thorac Dis. 2017;9:70.

Parnell AD, Massey NJ. Postoperative care of the adult cardiac surgical patient. Anaesth Intensive Care. 2009;10:430–6.

Punjabi PP, Taylor KM. The science and practice of cardiopulmonary bypass: from cross circulation to ECMO and SIRS. Glob Cardiol Sci Pract. 2013;2013:249–60.

Stephenson LW. History of cardiac surgery. Surgery. 2008:1471–9.

Szelkowski LA, Puri NK, Singh R, Massimiano PS. Current trends in preoperative, intraoperative, and postoperative care of the adult cardiac surgery patient. Curr Probl Surg. 2015;52:531–69.

Yapıcı N. Who should be responsible from cardiac surgery intensive care? From the perspective of a cardiac anesthesiologist/intensive care specialist. Turkish J Thorac Cardiovasc Surg. 2017;25:314–8.

Risk and Outcome Assessments

2

Manuel Caceres

Abstract

The assessment of outcomes in medicine at an institutional and practitioner level has become target of intense scrutiny in the current practice of organized medicine. Comparison of outcomes among providers and against established benchmarks has become commonplace for the purpose of hospital accreditation and as an essential tool in the selection of providers by the consumer. Therefore, the establishment of valid metrics in the assessment of outcomes and the accurate risk-adjusted comparison of them is critical in the modern practice of medicine.

The reporting of outcomes in cardiac surgery has evolved from the release of raw mortality rates to the risk-adjusted assessment of various endpoints following an index intervention. With the advent of less invasive interventions as options for the treatment of coronary and valve pathology, there has been a significant increase in the risk profile of patients undergoing cardiac surgery and thus a wide variability in the risk profile of patients presenting to various institutions. Consequently, the establishment of accurate risk models with periodic calibration is essential to adjust for an ever-changing patient risk profile.

With the heightened scrutiny on quality measures among institutions and practitioners, it is imperative to establish effective methods of risk assessment and outcome comparison. The reporting of outcomes, initially limited to raw mortality rates, has evolved over the last three decades into the calculation of risk-adjusted metrics of a variety of quality indicators. With the intricate evolution in the complexity of organized medicine, practitioners face increasing oversight by private- and government-based regulatory entities; therefore, it is incumbent to the medical community to be knowledgeable on the various strategies in the assessment of the quality of care provided.

M. Caceres, M.D.
Department of Thoracic Surgery, UCLA Medical Center, Los Angeles, CA, USA

A. Dabbagh et al. (eds.), *Postoperative Critical Care for Adult Cardiac Surgical Patients*, https://doi.org/10.1007/978-3-319-75747-6_2

The current chapter intends to describe the essentials in the process of risk adjustment and to present some of the most commonly utilized registries pertinent to the practice of cardiac surgery.

Keywords
Risk · Outcome · Risk modeling · Goodness of fit · Model validation · Risk-adjusted comparison metrics · Observed-to-Expected ratio · Propensity score analysis · The Medicare Provider Analysis and Review (MedPAR) · California Discharge Database · National inpatient sample (NIS) · New York State Department of Health (NYS DOH) · Veterans Administration Database · Society of Thoracic Surgeons (STS) · Adult Cardiac Surgery Database (ACSD) · New York Heart Association (NYHA) · STS cardiac surgery risk calculator · EuroSCORE

2.1 Historical Background

The assessment of outcomes in healthcare was initially addressed in the middle of the nineteenth century by Florence Nightingale, the founder of modern nursing, who advocated for the reporting of hospital mortality rates and, notably, anticipated the need of proper methods for risk adjustment to accurately compare outcomes among all of London's Hospitals. Despite her efforts for the systematic collection and analysis of data, this implementation was not welcomed by the medical society and was eventually interrupted by the British Medical Association; thus, this practice remained sporadic for over a century (Ellis 2008; https://plus.maths.org/content/florence-nightingale-compassionate-statistician n.d.).

In 1972, the Veterans Affairs Administration initiated the systematic collection of patient-specific data, highlighting the inception of multi-institutional databases. Interest in a structured system of data collection and outcome comparison remained sporadic until the late 1980s. In 1986, the Health Care Financing Administration (HCFA), currently known as the Centers for Medicare and Medicaid Services (CMS), as a result of the Freedom of Information Act was compelled to release hospital mortality rates for Medicare participants; such requirement spurred controversy regarding the significance of raw mortality rates for the comparison of outcomes in the setting of clear disparate patient risk profiles and fueled the interest to implement robust risk-adjustment strategies (Anderson 1994). Subsequent to these events, the monitoring of quality measures and public reporting in healthcare has progressively become commonplace, stimulating the implementation of various initiatives for the purpose of quality improvement.

2.2 Risk-Adjustment Methodology

Randomized controlled trials (RCTs) are the gold standard for the comparison of various treatment strategies; however, they are onerous and costly undertakings, limiting their applicability. Furthermore, RCTs generally follow rigorous inclusion criteria, which restrict the analysis to a small patient sample, not necessarily reproducible to the various risk categories.

Observational studies are capable to encompass a much larger patient population, therefore representing a versatile tool for risk-adjusted comparisons. Various iterations of risk-adjustment methods have been reported; however, two have emerged as primary strategies: logistic regression and propensity score analysis.

2.2.1 Logistic Regression

Logistic regression measures the effect of various factors on a binary outcome variable. The majority of outcomes measured in healthcare conform to the pattern of a binary dependent variable, e.g., mortality and various morbidities; therefore, logistic regression has become the predominant tool to determine the effects of multiple clinically relevant elements on a specific measured outcome.

2.2.1.1 Risk Modeling

Linear regression models a continuous dependent variable as a function of one (simple linear regression) or several (multivariable linear regression) continuous explanatory variables, e.g., length of hospital stay, days in the intensive care unit, etc. Alternatively, logistic regression models a dichotomous outcome variable, e.g., operative mortality, postoperative morbidity, etc., as a function of one or several continuous or categorical explanatory variables (Bewick et al. 2005).

Logistic regression models the natural logarithm of the odds of the outcome variable under investigation, the dependent variable, as a function of relevant explanatory variables that may have an effect on the outcome variable. As opposed to the probability of an event, which indicates the likelihood of an event to occur, the odds of an event indicates the probability of an event to occur divided by the probability of the same event to "not to occur." With this transformation, a probability ranges from 0 to 1, while the odds range from 0 to infinite.

Consider "p" as the probability of an event.

The odds will be defined as $p/(1 - p)$.

The logistic regression model will be constructed according to the following equation:

$$\text{Ln}\left[p/(1-p)\right] = A_0 + A_1^* X_1 + A_2^* X_2 + A_3^* X_3 \ldots A_n^* X_n$$

in which X_n are the relevant explanatory variables selected, A_0 is a constant, and A_n are the coefficients of determination that define the logistic regression equation. The X_n explanatory variables can be continuous (absolute values or any specific variable transformation) or categorical (value, 0 or 1).

The effect of each explanatory variable on the dependent variable is measured by the odds ratios (ORs), which indicates the increased probability of the dependent variable to occur with each unit increase of a continuous explanatory variable or with the presence or absence of a categorical explanatory variable. The OR of an explanatory variable X_n is defined as

$$\text{OR}\left[\text{CI},p-\text{value}\right]=\text{e}^{\text{An}}$$

The CI (confidence interval) and the *p*-value determine the significance of the OR; namely, a statistically significant *p*-value indicates that a variation in the explanatory variable is associated with an effect in the dependent variable, provided the remaining variables remain constant.

2.2.1.2 Variable Selection

Various methodologies exist to select the variables in a risk model, with the end result to include those statistically relevant as predictors of the outcome variable. It is common practice to create a pool of candidate variables and conduct a univariable analysis to select those with a relaxed *p*-value of significance under a specific threshold, generally between 0.1 and 0.2. The selected variables are subsequently entered in a multivariable logistic regression equation one by one in a forward stepwise fashion, retaining those statistically significant; or alternatively, all the variables are entered in the logistic regression equation and excluded one by one in a backward stepwise fashion if they fail to show statistical significance.

Although there are no specific power analysis calculations in logistic regression to determine the maximum number of variables to be included, the model has to be balanced to carry adequate predictive strength. Too few variables can limit the predictive power by ignoring the effect of relevant unmeasured variables; alternatively, an excessive number of variables can create random error or noise, also called over-fitting, which prevents a model from being reproducible. The "rule of ten" in logistic regression suggests that the absolute number of the outcome events should be at least ten times the number of variables initially considered in a model, i.e., with 100 mortality events in a study sample, the model should not consider more than 10 explanatory variables to avoid over-fitting (Peduzzi et al. 1996). Although many institutional studies present risk-adjusted results, the majority lack the necessary power to meet this requirement; therefore, registry data is often necessary to generate more reliable ORs, particularly in low-frequency outcome variables such as operative mortality in cardiac surgery.

2.2.1.3 Risk Model Assessment

There are three major methods to assess the suitability of a risk model in logistic regression: calibration or goodness of fit, discrimination, and validation. Calibration tests the performance of the model across a spectrum of predicted probabilities of the outcome variable. Discrimination tests the ability of the risk model to differentiate between positive and negative outcomes. Validation tests the reproducibility of the risk model by testing calibration and discrimination in a separate dataset comparable to the one used to create the model.

Goodness of Fit

The calibration or goodness of fit of a model is most commonly measured by the Hosmer–Lemeshow test, which divides the study population into ten equal-sized groups arranged from the lowest to the highest predicted probability of the outcome

Table 2.1 Sample structure of the Hosmer–Lemeshow contingency table: The corresponding test statistic determines if there is a significant difference between the observed and expected values

Decile group		Outcome event = 0		Outcome event = 1	
	Total events	Observed events	Expected events	Observed events	Expected events
1	100	95	92.1	5	7.9
2	100	93	90.3	7	9.7
3	100	93	93.1	7	6.9
4	100	91	92.5	9	7.5
5	100	90	88.3	10	11.7
6	100	89	87.8	11	12.2
7	100	87	90.3	13	9.7
8	100	85	81.6	15	18.4
9	100	84	83.2	16	16.8
10	100	82	84.1	18	15.9

The value of expected events is calculated as the average of the predicted risks of the outcome event of all participants within each decile. A $p > 0.05$ for the test statistic suggests that the expected outcomes do not differ from the observed outcomes, consistent with an adequate goodness of fit

event. The observed and predicted values for each of the two outcomes (e.g., death or survival) are entered into a contingency table, and the test statistic is used to determine whether there is a significant difference between the observed and expected values within each decile (Table 2.1). A p-value >0.05 is generally accepted to indicate that the observed frequencies are similar to those predicted by the model, thus reflecting an adequate goodness of fit (Hosmer and Lemeshow 2000).

Model Discrimination

The model discrimination determines the ability to distinguish between the results of a binary outcome, e.g., survival or death. It is calculated with the area under the receiver-operating-characteristic (ROC) curve and is measured by the c-statistic, also known as the concordance statistic, which ranges from "0" to "1" and measures the predictive accuracy of the logistic regression model.

As in any other diagnostic test, as the diagnostic thresholds are adjusted, the sensitivity may increase at the expense of a decrease in the specificity. For example, if using the size of a mass to diagnose a malignant tumor, as the threshold of size decreases, the sensitivity increases; consequently, it will mislabel a large group of negative tumors as positive, decreasing the specificity. Conversely, increasing the threshold of size will miss a large number of malignant tumors and decrease the sensitivity, though identifying most of the negative tumors and increasing the specificity.

The ROC curve plots the true-positive rate (sensitivity) against the false-positive rate (1-specificity). For a logistic regression risk model, the predicted probability of the outcome ranges from "0.0" to "1.0." For each threshold of predicted probability of the outcome, there is a corresponding true-positive rate (sensitivity) and false-positive rate (1-specificity). For example, for a threshold of a predicted probability of 0.2, every observation with a predicted probability higher than 0.2 will be

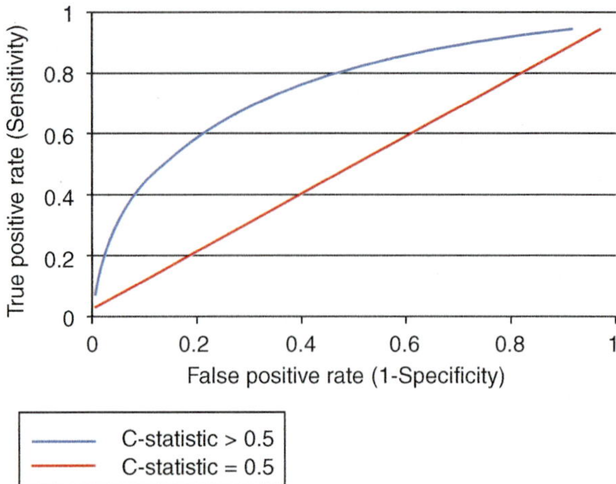

Fig. 2.1 Receiver-operating-characteristic curve: The c-statistic [range (0.0–1.0)] is calculated as the area under the receiver-operating-characteristic curve

considered a positive outcome; therefore, the sensitivity of this threshold will be calculated as the observations that were accurately predicted as positive (true positives), divided by all the positive results. This calculation is conducted for every threshold from 0.0 to 1.0, which generates corresponding sensitivity and specificity pairs. The plotting of the paired "sensitivity" and "1-specificity" values generates the ROC curve, and the c-statistic corresponds to the area under this curve. The c-statistic represents the probability that given two outcomes, e.g., a survivor and a non-survivor, the survivor will have a higher predicted probability of surviving than the non-survivor. A useless diagnostic test corresponds to a c-statistic of 0.5, reflecting the chance to discriminate a positive from a negative result as the flip of a coin. Such test will correspond to the diagonal line drawn in Fig. 2.1. As the ROC curve shifts toward the left upper quadrant of the diagram, the area under the curve increases, corresponding to a parallel increase in the c-statistic (Fig. 2.1). A c-statistic of 0.7–0.9 is generally reported in most models as carrying adequate predicted power (Bewick et al. 2004; Grunkemeier and Jin 2001; Zou et al. 2007).

Model Validation

Validating a risk model with the same dataset that was used to create it will likely confirm an accurate predictive power. The original dataset can be partitioned into a training set (sample used to develop the model) and a testing set (sample used to validate the model). Training and testing datasets are not required to be of the same size, but each one must be representative of the study population. The validation of a risk model is conducted by determining the goodness of fit (p-value) and discrimination (c-statistic) after applying the risk model on the testing dataset (Bewick et al. 2005).

2.2.1.4 Risk-Adjusted Comparison Metrics

Risk models generate ORs for baseline variables under investigation, which indicate the associated risk to a specific outcome with the presence or absence of a categorical variable or with each unit increase in a continuous variable. To assess the effect of a specific treatment, a variable for such intervention is added in the logistic model, and the corresponding OR is calculated; however, these metrics only indicate the effect of specific explanatory variables on the response variable. Alternatively, to illustrate the differences in institution-specific or surgeon-specific outcomes, different metrics are employed to adjust for a dissimilar case-mix or risk profile. The following are common indexes used for these comparisons.

Observed-to-Expected (O/E) Ratio

The logistic regression model calculates the risk of an outcome event to occur, i.e., the individual predicted risk. A random effects variable may also be entered in the model to adjust for the random variation among institutions.

Consider two institutions or providers, group A and group B; the outcomes of both groups can be compared using O/E ratios.

Observed rate: Absolute number of outcome events/total number of subjects, in a specific group

Expected rate = Average of the individual predicted risks of the participating subjects in a specific group

O/E ratio: Observed rate/expected rate

The O/E ratio of a specific group can be compared to the O/E ratio of the entire population, which is regularly in close proximity to the neutral value of 1.0, or it can be compared to the O/E ratio of an alternative institution, provider, etc. A significant difference in this comparison reflects a deviation of the outcome event for a particular group under comparison.

Risk-Adjusted Rates

The outcomes of institutions or providers can also be compared with the risk-adjusted rates of the outcome event (e.g., risk-adjusted mortality):

Risk-adjusted rate = [Observed rate/Expected rate, for a specific group] * Observed rate of the event in the entire population.

While this value does not represent the actual rate of an event, it uses the collective rate of the outcome event as a reference to compare the observed rates among groups of interest.

2.2.2 Propensity Score Analysis

As opposed to logistic regression analysis, propensity score calculations attempt to balance the differences between groups exposed to different treatments. Propensity score methods compare two different treatment groups by balancing the distribution of baseline covariates. This strategy creates two comparable treatment groups subjected to two different treatments under investigation, thus attempting to reproduce the comparison of a RCT.

The foundation of the propensity score methods hinges on the calculation of a propensity score, which is defined as the probability of a patient to be assigned to a specific treatment, conditional on a set of observed covariates. Each patient will have a calculated propensity score according to the set of baseline covariates; therefore, patients with similar propensity scores will have a comparable distribution of baseline covariates. Following the calculation of propensity scores in all the participants in the study population, various methods are utilized to determine the effect of the treatment strategy under investigation.

2.2.2.1 Calculation of the Propensity Score

The propensity score is a number from 0 to 1 and represents the probability that such patient will be assigned to a treatment arm based on the covariates measured prior to treatment selection, e.g., demographic data, comorbidities, etc. Multivariate logistic regression is used to create a model that calculates the propensity score for each patient by using the "treatment category" as the dependent variable: "treated" = 1 and "non-treated" = 0. Relevant covariates are used as the explanatory variables, and the coefficients of determination and constant are calculated following the standard multivariable regression formula previously described:

$$\mathrm{Ln}\left[\mathrm{PS}/\left(1-\mathrm{PS}\right)\right] = A_0 + A_1{}^*X_1 + A_2{}^*X_2 + A_3{}^*X_3 \ldots A_n{}^*X_n$$

PS = Propensity score
A_0 = Constant
n = Number of explanatory variables
A_n = Coefficients of determination
X_n = Explanatory variables, which can be categorical (entry values, 0 or 1) or continuous

Once the risk model is created after determining A_0 and A_n, the PS of each participating patient can be calculated according to the specific explanatory variables (Deb et al. 2016).

2.2.2.2 Assessment of Model Accuracy

Based on the propensity scores calculated, a "treated" group is matched to a "non-treated" group with similar distribution of propensity scores. Once these groups are established, statistical comparisons are conducted between the "treated" and "non-treated" groups to validate that a balanced distribution of patients exists. There is controversy on which statistical tests are appropriate in this setting. Statistical significance testing, e.g., student's t-test, chi-square analysis, etc., is commonly employed to confirm adequate balance; however, this approach has been challenged because it is applied to a sample, the "propensity score-matched sample," which is generally much smaller than the original study population. Testing the null hypothesis of no difference between treated and non-treated groups with traditional significance testing in a preemptively selected sample may be inaccurate. It is suggested that the standardized difference of each covariate between treatment groups is a more accurate approach in determining the balance of the propensity score matching, with a standardized difference < 1 indicating an insignificant difference (Austin 2011).

2.2.2.3 Propensity Score Methods

Four major methods have been described for the propensity score comparison of treatment arms in observational studies: matching, stratification, covariate adjustment, and inverse probability of treatment weighting (IPTW) (Deb et al. 2016).

Propensity Score Matching

Once the propensity scores are calculated, patients in the treated group are matched with patients in the non-treated group. Various algorithms can be used to conduct the matching process, but in essence, they are intended to minimize the propensity score difference in each match. Nearest neighbor matching within a specified caliper distance searches for a match to each treated subject within a propensity score difference; if no match is found, the treated subject is excluded from subsequent analyses. Matching can also be conducted according to a specified number of digits; for a propensity score such as 0.1234567, a match is selected if the score matches the first, for example, five digits; if no match is found, a match on the first four digits is searched and so forth.

Another consideration in propensity matching refers to the ratio of non-treated to treated subjects. This ratio can be 1:1, in which one treated subject is matched to one non-treated subject. The matching ratio could also be 2:1, 3:1, and so forth. Once the matched treated and non-treated subjects are selected, appropriate standard statistical tests are used to compare the outcomes of a specific intervention on the treated and non-treated groups (Austin 2007).

Propensity Score Stratification

Once propensity scores are calculated for the entire study group, they are arranged in strata of similar values. A common strategy is to divide the study group in quintiles of increasing propensity scores, which generally eliminate 90% of the bias from confounding variables. The outcomes of interest are compared between the treated and non-treated subjects within each quintile, by using proper statistical tests. Stratification has the advantage of using the entire study group for the outcome comparison, although it may be less precise than other methods in reducing bias (D'Agostino 2007).

Covariate Adjustment

This method follows three steps. In the first step, the propensity score of receiving the treatment under investigation is calculated using a logistic regression model. The second step creates another logistic regression model to determine the effect of the treatment on the measured outcome. The third step incorporates the propensity score of receiving a specific treatment into this logistic regression model. The OR of the treatment under investigation in this final logistic regression model is adjusted for the propensity to receive such treatment, therefore balancing for all relevant covariates in the model and for the preference of a specific subject to be allocated in the treated or non-treated group. Although this method allows the inclusion of the entire study population, it also carries several disadvantages; the relationship between the propensity score and the outcome cannot be assumed to be linear and needs to be specified, ORs of the treatment effect have been found to have greater bias as compared to other propensity score methods, and the assessment of balance between treatment groups can be quite challenging with this method (D'Agostino 2007).

Inverse Probability of Treatment Weighting

The propensity score of receiving a specific treatment is calculated as previously described. A weight equivalent to the inverse of the probability of receiving a treatment (propensity score) is assigned to the treated subjects, and a weight equivalent to the inverse of the probability of not receiving a treatment (1 – propensity score) is assigned to the non-treated subjects.

Subject	Weight
Treated	$1/P$
Non-treated	$1/(1-P)$

P = Propensity score

Therefore, if a treated "participant A" has a higher probability of receiving the treatment (higher propensity score) than a "participant B," the weight assigned to "participant A" will be lower than the weight assigned to "participant B." Likewise, if a non-treated "participant X" has a higher probability of not receiving the treatment (lower probability of receiving the treatment, i.e., a lower propensity score) than a "participant Y," the weight assigned to "participant X" will be higher than the weight assigned to "participant Y."

This novel method assigns weights to each participant subject according to the inverse of the probability to be assigned to a specific treatment category. Those subjects with a lower probability of receiving a treatment are assigned a higher representation, and those with a higher probability of receiving a treatment are assigned a lower representation. By creating this synthetic balanced study group, the distribution of covariates becomes independent of the treatment assignment. Subsequently, the outcomes under investigation are compared between the arms of treated and non-treated subjects by standard statistical tests (Weintraub et al. 2012; Austin and Stuart 2015).

2.3 Cardiac Surgery Registries

With the increased scrutiny in the quality of cardiac surgery programs and providers, cardiac surgery registries have emerged as versatile tools to generate novel risk models and provide risk-adjusted outcomes.

Two broad categories of registries are commonplace in the assessment of surgical outcomes, clinical and administrative. Data managers with various levels of clinical background generally collect and enter patient-specific data into clinical databases, whereas administrative databases rely largely on the International Classification of Diseases (ICD) codes assigned by coding personnel without specific clinical background. Clinical databases can be voluntary (e.g., the Society of

Thoracic Surgeons National Cardiac Database) or mandatory (e.g., the New York State Cardiac Registry), and administrative databases are generally mandatory according to state or national requirements.

Because of the inherent errors in data collection using ICD code information, the accuracy and detail are generally higher with clinical as opposed to administrative databases. Missing information varies widely among databases, and various imputation techniques are established for adjustment. Intra-variable and inter-variable safe-checks are present in some clinical databases (not available in administrative databases) to assure consistency of the data entered, e.g., a record positive for cardiogenic shock and labeled as an elective admission is inconsistent and is rejected in databases with safe-checks in place. Auditing is an additional measure to ensure data quality and is enforced in some of the clinical registries. Below we describe some of the major cardiac surgery registries in the United States (Murphy et al. 2013).

2.3.1 Administrative Databases

2.3.1.1 The Medicare Provider Analysis and Review (MedPAR) Data Files

The Centers for Medicare and Medicaid Services (CMS) administrative data files contain data from nearly 98% of adults 65 years of age or older. Of these, the MedPAR data files reflect claims that correspond to admissions to CMS-certified hospitals and skilled nursing facilities for Medicare beneficiaries (https://www.cms.gov/research-statistics-data-and-systems/files-for-order/limiteddatasets/medparldshospitalnational.html n.d.). Each record corresponds to a hospital admission, and the data entered originates from the Uniform Billing-92 (UB-92) discharge summary found in all hospital charts. The primary diagnosis, comorbidities, and procedures from each record are identified using ICD codes. The data in this database corresponds to Medicare beneficiaries from Medicare-certified hospitals; thus, it only represents patients older than 65 years using Medicare benefits (Welke et al. 2007).

Clinical and administrative files from various databases, such as the Surveillance, Epidemiology, and End Results (SEER) program, the American Hospital Association (AHA) data files, and the American Medical Association (AMA) masterfile, have been linked to the MedPAR data files. Recently, the Society of Thoracic Surgeons Adult Cardiac Surgery Database established collaboration with CMS to successfully link the files of patients older than 65 years with the MedPAR data files (http://www.sts.org/news/sts-national-database-establishes-important-link-cms-data n.d.). The linkages between these databases expand the versatility of the analysis of clinical and administrative data.

Access to CMS data files is requested to the Research Data Assistance Center (ResDAC). A data request proposal is prepared with the assistance of the ResDAC and presented to CMS once the review is completed. A charge for access to the data files is generated commensurate to the complexity of the data requested (https://www.resdac.org/cms-data/request/cms-data-request-center n.d.).

2.3.1.2 California Discharge Database

All nonfederal hospitals licensed in the State of California are mandated to report discharge data from each hospital admission. These facilities report their discharge data via the Medical Information Reporting for California System (MIRCal). Demographic data, comorbidities, diagnoses, and procedures performed are identified through ICD codes and included in the summary report. Unlike other administrative databases, the California discharge database discriminates between primary and secondary diagnoses and identifies the procedure dates, thus allowing the inclusion of timing of specific interventions as one of the components of the risk models (Weiss et al. 2008). A data subset corresponds to the Coronary Artery Bypass Graft (CABG) file which is a research database created for the purpose of studying outcomes in the surgical treatment of coronary artery disease. The data is analyzed for quality and available for research purposes, subject to review and approval by the Office of Statewide Health Planning and Development (https://www.oshpd.ca.gov/HID/Data_Request_Center/Types_of_Data.html n.d.).

2.3.1.3 National Inpatient Sample (NIS)

Formerly known as the Nationwide Inpatient Sample, it changed the name in 2012 after a redesign to improve national estimates. The NIS is one of a family of databases developed by the Healthcare Cost and Utilization Project (HCUP), an initiative sponsored by the Agency for Healthcare Research and Quality (AHRQ). The NIS was developed in 1988 as a nonmandatory database of hospital inpatient stays and represents approximately 20% of the discharges from US community hospitals covering 45 states, excluding rehabilitation and long-term acute care hospitals. The NIS sample records clinical and resource utilization data in a discharge abstract format, which includes primary and secondary diagnoses, procedures, patient demographic characteristics, hospital characteristics (e.g., ownership), expected payment source, total charges, discharge status, length of stay, and severity and comorbidity measures. Since the information included is limited to inpatient data, only morbidity and mortality during the hospitalization can be retrieved, however, may not be comparable to 30-day data presented on other databases (Murphy et al. 2013).

The NIS contains information on all patients regardless of payer, therefore including individuals covered by Medicare, Medicaid, private insurance, and the uninsured. Although the data entered only covers about 20% of the discharges in the United States, specific weights are included in the database to generate national estimates.

Researchers and policymakers use the NIS to identify, track, and analyze national trends in healthcare utilization, access, charges, quality, and outcomes. As of 2002, the NIS introduced elements for adjustment of the severity of illness and in 2005 implemented Diagnosis and Procedure Groups files with software tools to facilitate the use of ICD-9 diagnostic and procedure codes.

In 2012, the NIS was redesigned. Before 2012, the NIS was a sample of hospitals, retaining the corresponding discharges; after 2012, the NIS data corresponds to a sample of discharges from all the participating hospitals. Such modification renders more accurate estimates by reducing sampling error and narrowing the confidence intervals generated (https://www.hcup-us.ahrq.gov/nisoverview.jsp n.d.).

The NIS data is available for purchase to all participants, contingent upon a signed agreement to use the data for research purposes only and to make no attempt to identify the individuals in the database (http://www.hcup-us.ahrq.gov/nisoverview.jsp n.d.).

2.3.2 Clinical Databases

2.3.2.1 New York State Cardiac Registry

In 1988, the New York State Department of Health (NYS DOH) raised concern after identifying an up to fivefold disparity in mortality rates for CABG surgery and initiated a process to monitor the quality of cardiac surgery provided, considering the frequently large disparities in risk profiles among institutions. Parallel to these events, CMS publicly reported institutional mortality rates on an annual basis from 1986 to 1992. The risk-adjustment methodologies for these analyses were criticized due to the inaccuracies inherent to administrative data, prompting the NYS DOH to establish a mandatory patient-level clinical database for all cardiac surgery programs in New York State and develop well-structured risk models with reliable predictive strength. The first risk-adjusted institutional mortality rates were released to the public in 1990, and as a result of a subsequent lawsuit, the DOH was forced to release surgeon-specific mortality rates in 1992. Risk-adjusted mortality rates and outlier status of cardiac programs are published in an annual basis, and surgeon-specific results are reported on a rolling 3-year basis to accumulate enough data for meaningful statistical comparisons (Hannan et al. 2012).

A multiple logistic regression model was created to calculate the expected mortality as a function of patient-specific risk factors. The institutional and provider-specific risk-adjusted mortality rates are calculated by multiplying the statewide mortality rate by the ratio of the observed-to-expected mortality rates for a specific institution or provider. The expected mortality rate of the institution or provider under assessment is calculated by averaging the predicted mortality risk of all patients in the same group. Outliers in performance are identified outside the 95% confidence intervals of the statewide mortality rate. Individualized reports were initially sent to each cardiac surgery program, and by the year following the implementation of this initiative, a substantial improvement in outcomes was recorded. The NYS DOH has maintained the public reporting of cardiac surgery outcomes for cardiac surgery programs and individual cardiac surgeons since the development of this clinical registry. As of 1992, a coronary angioplasty reporting system was implemented, and annual reports have been released since 1997 (Hannan et al. 2012).

2.3.2.2 Northern New England Cardiovascular Disease Study Group

The Northern New England Cardiovascular Disease Study Group (NNECDSG) was founded in 1987 as a voluntary regional consortium to monitor and promote the quality improvement of cardiovascular care in Maine, New Hampshire, and Vermont. The NNECDSG maintains registries for all patients receiving CABG, percutaneous coronary interventions, and heart valve replacement surgery. Data is prospectively entered and risk-adjusted outcomes compared among institutions by using multivariable logistic regression models. Risk-adjusted comparisons identified differences in outcomes not entirely explained by variations in case mix but that may have resulted from differences in unmeasured quality of care variables among institutions. This registry has been used to explore quality improvement strategies by regular feedback of outcomes to the participating institutions, round-robin visits, and analysis of cause-specific mortality (O'Connor et al. 1991).

2.3.2.3 Veterans Administration Database

Starting in 1987, the Veterans Administration cardiac surgery programs were required to complete a datasheet including pre-, intra-, and postoperative data. Since then, the Veterans Administration Cardiac Database was established as a mandatory clinical registry with data entered by independent nursing personnel and submitted in a biannual basis. Risk adjustment for operative mortality and morbidity is conducted through multivariable logistic regression, and O/E ratios are reported to each participating institution to prompt program review and institute measures for quality improvement. This database has the restriction of including only veterans and, thus, is limited primarily to elderly men (Grover et al. 2001).

2.3.2.4 The Society of Thoracic Surgeons (STS) Adult Cardiac Surgery Database (ACSD)

Likewise to the NYS DOH, in 1987 the STS implemented a voluntary clinical database following the reporting of misleading raw mortality rates by the HCFA. The participation in the STS ACSD has progressively increased and covers over 90% of the cardiac surgery programs in the United States, representing the largest repository of clinical data in cardiac surgery. Designated data managers at an institutional level are responsible for the data entry, and intra- and inter-variable software-generated safe-checks are established to ensure consistency across data fields. Missing data has been reduced to a minimum with less than 1% in the majority of fields. The most commonly missing candidate predictor variables have been ejection fraction (5.5%), New York Heart Association (NYHA) class (4.7%), tricuspid insufficiency (3.9%), aortic insufficiency (3.7%), mitral insufficiency (3.1%), aortic stenosis (1.7%), and creatinine/dialysis (1.5%) (Shahian et al. 2009). The Duke Clinical Research Institute conducts a thorough data analysis and, through multivariable logistic regression, periodically creates risk models of operative mortality and standardized postoperative complications for CABG, mitral valve, and aortic valve surgery (Grover et al. 2001; Shahian et al. 2009; Caceres et al. 2010).

With the recent approval of transcatheter valve therapy (TVT) in the United States, in December 2012 the STS in conjunction with the American College of Cardiology (ACC) launched the STS/ACC TVT Registry, a new benchmarking tool to track real-world outcomes related to new and emerging TVT procedures. The TVT Registry serves as the main repository for clinical data related to TVT procedures and is positioned to capture outcome data for expanded indications, including additional devices and procedures that will likely emerge in the future. The registry is also structured to link clinical and administrative claims data to assess early and long-term outcomes. This registry forms the basis of a new platform suitable for post-approval studies in future generations of transcatheter valve devices (http://www.sts.org/news/sts-and-acc-launch-new-transcatheter-valve-therapy-registry n.d.).

2.4 Cardiac Surgery Risk Calculators

In an era of increasing emphasis on the quality of medical care, benchmarking of cardiac surgical outcomes is essential to allow reliable risk-adjusted comparisons. Cardiac surgery risk calculators represent the cornerstone in the prediction of surgical outcomes, allowing for the comparison of observed-to-expected rates and risk-adjusted event rates. Furthermore, risk calculators are useful tools for proper patient selection and informed patient consent. Multiple risk calculators have been developed, but two systems have been thoroughly validated and have become the major predictors of outcomes in cardiac surgery.

2.4.1 The STS Cardiac Surgery Risk Calculator

The STS database has served as the source of patient data to develop the STS cardiac surgery risk calculators. Although initially intended for CABG, iterations have been created for aortic and mitral valve surgery. At present, risk models have been established for CABG, aortic valve (AV) replacement, mitral valve (MV) replacement, MV repair, CABG/AV replacement, CABG/MV replacement, and CABG/MV repair. Risk models are developed through multivariable logistic regression, and predicted risks are calculated for specific outcome variables. Initial calculators focused on operative mortality, but in 2003 specific risk calculators were developed for nine endpoints: operative mortality, permanent stroke, renal failure, prolonged ventilation, deep sternal wound infection, major morbidity or mortality, prolonged postoperative length of stay (>14 days), and short postoperative length of stay (Shroyer et al. 2003). Subsequently, risk calculators for reoperation and prolonged ventilation have been incorporated (http://riskcalc.sts.org/stswebriskcalc/#/ n.d.). Definitions of each endpoint and predictor variables have been previously described by the STS (Shahian et al. 2009). The risk calculators for specific outcomes can be accessed at http://riskcalc.sts.org/stswebriskcalc/#/ (n.d.).

2.4.2 The European System for Cardiac Operative Risk Evaluation (EuroSCORE)

The EuroSCORE was developed in 1999, from nearly 20, 000 patients and 128 European centers, as a simplified tool to calculate the operative mortality risk in cardiac surgery. The initial version was structured as an additive score system, with values for each risk factor derived from a multivariable logistic regression model (Roques et al. 1999). The total score was calculated as the sum of the individual values of 17 participating variables and correlated to a corresponding predicted mortality risk. In 2003, a second iteration was developed, the logistic EuroSCORE, as a multivariable logistic regression formula; coefficients were determined for each participating variable, and the categorical or continuous values of each variable were entered in a logistic regression formula that calculated the predicted mortality risk as described under 2.2 (Michel et al. 2003). The additive system seemed to underestimate the outcomes in high-risk patients (EuroSCORE > 6), and the logistic EuroSCORE was developed to bridge this gap in the calculations. A third iteration was developed in 2011, the EuroSCORE II, a logistic regression formula similar to the logistic EuroSCORE, with several modifications to the participating variables (http://www.euroscore.org/calc.html n.d.).

Unlike the STS risk calculator, the EuroSCORE does not include calculations for morbidity endpoints and does not provide separate risk models for each type of cardiac surgical procedure; however, it adjusts for the number of surgical interventions, e.g., CABG with mitral valve surgery counts as two procedures and CABG with mitral and tricuspid valve surgery counts as three procedures. The EuroSCORE risk calculator can be accessed at http://www.euroscore.org/.

2.5 Limitations of Current Databases

Clinical databases have been successful in presenting early outcomes following cardiac surgery; however, midterm and long-term outcomes have been limited. Alternatively, administrative databases, although fraught with inferior data accuracy, have the potential to retrieve long-term endpoints through payer claims records. The difficulty to assign patient identifiers that could serve as relational links among databases has prevented the integration of early- and long-term outcome data. Likewise, the difficulty in merging clinical databases from different specialties has restricted the assessment of cardiac care outcomes to either surgical or medical modalities of treatment. In the last few years, several attempts have successfully linked the STS ACSD with the MedPAR data files and the ACC registries. As clinical and administrative databases evolve, relational links and the potential to study long-term outcomes will become more versatile; however, at the present, this process remains limited.

2.6 Summary

With the evolution of organized medicine, there has been a parallel expansion of a variety of multi-institutional registries, essential tools in the assessment of outcomes, and the implementation of quality improvement initiatives. The analysis of risk-adjusted results has been useful in identifying institutions with outlier results to facilitate the implementation of focused quality of care strategies. The data analysis of early outcomes in cardiac surgery has been satisfactory through clinical databases, but limitations still remain in the assessment of mid- and long-term outcomes. In the current landscape of scrutiny by consumers and third-party payer organizations, quality improvement remains at the forefront agenda in the healthcare systems; thus, proper risk adjustment through reliable regional and nationwide registries is essential for the accurate assessment of the quality of cardiac care.

References

https://plus.maths.org/content/florence-nightingale-compassionate-statistician.

http://riskcalc.sts.org/stswebriskcalc/#/.

https://www.cms.gov/research-statistics-data-and-systems/files-for-order/limiteddatasets/medpar-ldshospitalnational.html.

http://www.euroscore.org/calc.html.

https://www.hcup-us.ahrq.gov/nisoverview.jsp.

http://www.hcup-us.ahrq.gov/nisoverview.jsp.

https://www.oshpd.ca.gov/HID/Data_Request_Center/Types_of_Data.html.

https://www.resdac.org/cms-data/request/cms-data-request-center.

http://www.sts.org/news/sts-and-acc-launch-new-transcatheter-valve-therapy-registry.

http://www.sts.org/news/sts-national-database-establishes-important-link-cms-data.

Anderson RP. First publications from the society of thoracic surgeons national database. Ann Thorac Surg. 1994;57:6–7.

Austin PC. Propensity-score matching in the cardiovascular surgery literature from 2004 to 2006: a systematic review and suggestions for improvement. J Thorac Cardiovasc Surg. 2007;134:1128–35.

Austin PC. An introduction to propensity score methods for reducing the effects of confounding in observational studies. Multivar Behav Res. 2011;46:399–424.

Austin PC, Stuart EA. Moving towards best practice when using inverse probability of treatment weighting (IPTW) using the propensity score to estimate causal treatment effects in observational studies. Stat Med. 2015;34:3661–79.

Bewick V, Cheek L, Ball J. Statistics review 13: receiver operating characteristic curves. Crit Care. 2004;8:508–12.

Bewick V, Cheek L, Ball J. Statistics review 14: logistic regression. Crit Care. 2005;9:112–8.

Caceres M, Braud RL, Garrett HE Jr. A short history of the Society of Thoracic Surgeons national cardiac database: perceptions of a practicing surgeon. Ann Thorac Surg. 2010;89:332–9.

D'Agostino RB Jr. Propensity scores in cardiovascular research. Circulation. 2007;115:2340–3.

Deb S, Austin PC, Tu JV, Ko DT, Mazer CD, Kiss A, Fremes SE. A review of propensity-score methods and their use in cardiovascular research. Can J Cardiol. 2016;32:259–65.

Ellis H. Florence nightingale: creator of modern nursing and public health pioneer. J Perioper Pract. 2008;18:404–6.

Grover FL, Shroyer AL, Hammermeister K, Edwards FH, Ferguson TB Jr, Dziuban SW Jr, Cleveland JC Jr, Clark RE, McDonald G. A decade's experience with quality improvement in cardiac surgery using the veterans affairs and Society of Thoracic Surgeons national databases. Ann Surg. 2001;234:464–72.

Grunkemeier GL, Jin R. Receiver operating characteristic curve analysis of clinical risk models. Ann Thorac Surg. 2001;72:323–6.

Hannan EL, Cozzens K, King SB 3rd, Walford G, Shah NR. The New York state cardiac registries: history, contributions, limitations, and lessons for future efforts to assess and publicly report healthcare outcomes. J Am Coll Cardiol. 2012;59:2309–16.

Hosmer DW, Lemeshow S. Applied logistic regression. 2nd ed. New York: Wiley; 2000.
Michel P, Roques F, Nashef SA. EuroSCORE project group. Logistic or additive EuroSCORE for high-risk patients? Eur J Cardiothorac Surg. 2003;23:684–7.
Murphy M, Alavi K, Maykel J. Working with existing databases. Clin Colon Rectal Surg. 2013;26:5–11.
O'Connor GT, Plume SK, Olmstead EM, Coffin LH, Morton JR, Maloney CT, Nowicki ER, Tryzelaar JF, Hernandez F, Adrian L, et al. A regional prospective study of in-hospital mortality associated with coronary artery bypass grafting. The northern New England cardiovascular disease study group. JAMA. 1991;266:803–9.
Peduzzi P, Concato J, Kemper E, Holford TR, Feinstein AR. A simulation study of the number of events per variable in logistic regression analysis. J Clin Epidemiol. 1996;49:1373–9.
Roques F, Nashef SA, Michel P, Gauducheau E, de Vincentiis C, Baudet E, Cortina J, David M, Faichney A, Gabrielle F, Gams E, Harjula A, Jones MT, Pintor PP, Salamon R, Thulin L. Risk factors and outcome in European cardiac surgery: analysis of the EuroSCORE multinational database of 19030 patients. Eur J Cardiothorac Surg. 1999;15:816–22.
Shahian DM, O'Brien SM, Filardo G, Ferraris VA, Haan CK, Rich JB, Normand S-LT, DeLong ER, Shewan CM, Dokholyan RS, Peterson ED, Edwards FH, Anderson RP. The society of thoracic surgeons 2008 cardiac surgery risk models: part 1_coronary artery bypass grafting surgery. Ann Thorac Surg. 2009;88:2–22.
Shroyer LW, Coombs LP, Peterson ED, Eiken MC, Delong ER, Chen AY, Ferguson TB, Grover FL. The Society of Thoracic Surgeons: 30-day operative mortality and morbidity risk models. Ann Thor Surg. 2003;75:1856–64.
Weintraub WS, Grau-Sepulveda MV, Weiss JM, O'Brien SM, Peterson ED, Kolm P, Zhang Z, Klein LW, Shaw RE, McKay C, Ritzenthaler LL, Popma JJ, Messenger JC, Shahian DM, Grover FL, Mayer JE, Shewan CM, Garratt KN, Moussa ID, Dangas GD, Edwards FH. Comparative effectiveness of revascularization strategies. N Engl J Med. 2012;366:1467–76.
Weiss ES, Chang DD, Joyce DL, Nwakanma LU, Yuh DD. Optimal timing of coronary artery bypass after acute myocardial infarction: a review of California discharge data. J Thorac Cardiovasc Surg. 2008;135:503–11.
Welke KF, Peterson ED, Vaughan-Sarrazin MS, O'Brien SM, Rosenthal GE, Shook GJ, Dokholyan RS, Haan CK, Ferguson TB Jr. Comparison of cardiac surgery volumes and mortality rates between the Society of Thoracic Surgeons and Medicare databases from 1993 through 2001. Ann Thorac Surg. 2007;84:1538–46.
Zou KH, O'Malley AJ, Mauri L. Receiver-operating characteristic analysis for evaluating diagnostic tests and predictive models. Circulation. 2007;115:654–7.

Cardiac Physiology

3

Ali Dabbagh, Alireza Imani, and Samira Rajaei

Abstract

Cardiac physiology is one of the most interesting discussions both in basic science and clinic. Anatomy and physiology of the heart directly affect the clinical presentations of disease states. The heart is composed of pericardium (outmost layer), endocardium (innermost layer), and myocardium (middle layer), the last being more discussed here and consists of:

- Cardiac connective tissue cells
- Cardiomyocytes (which have contractile function)
- Cardiac electrical and conduction system cells (consisting of "impulse-generating cells" and "specialized conductive cells")

The main cardiac cells are cardiomyocytes with their unique structure having some shared features with both skeletal muscles and smooth muscles, though not completely similar with any of these two muscle types.

Cardiac cells have three different but "highly interrelated" physiologic features:

A. Dabbagh, M.D. (✉)
Cardiac Anesthesiology Department, Anesthesiology Research Center, Faculty of Medicine, Shahid Beheshti University of Medical Sciences, Tehran, Iran
e-mail: alidabbagh@sbmu.ac.ir

A. Imani, Ph.D.
Department of Physiology, School of Medicine, Tehran University of Medical Sciences, Tehran, Iran
e-mail: aimani@tums.ac.ir

S. Rajaei, M.D., Ph.D.
Department of Immunology, School of Medicine, Tehran University of Medical Sciences, Tehran, Iran
e-mail: samirarajaei@tums.ac.ir

A. Dabbagh et al. (eds.), *Postoperative Critical Care for Adult Cardiac Surgical Patients*, https://doi.org/10.1007/978-3-319-75747-6_3

- Action potential
- Excitation-contraction coupling (ECC)
- Contractile mechanisms

Each of the three is composed of numerous different physiologic chains to create together, and as a final outcome, a main goal: *cardiac contraction leading to cardiac output.*

There are a number of cardiac controllers which modulate cardiac function based on physiologic demands, which are discussed in this chapter.

And finally, a number of physiologic reflexes are involved in cardiac physiology discussed in the final part of the chapter.

Keywords
Cardiac physiology · Cardiac anatomy · Action potential · Excitation contraction coupling (ECC) · Chordae tendineae · Pericardium · Myocardium · Endocardium · Cardiomyocyte · Sarcolemma · T tubule · Sarcoplasmic reticulum · Spot desmosomes · Sheet desmosomes · Gap junction · His bundle · Coronary arteries · Ca^{2+} homeostasis · Ca^{2+}-induced Ca^{2+} release "CICR" · Actin · Myosin · Titin · Myosin binding protein C (MYBPC) · Tropomyosin · Troponin · Tropomodulin · Cardiac cycle · Cardiac work · Cardiac output · Ejection fraction · Frank-Starling relationship · Cardiac reflex · Bainbridge reflex · Baroreceptors reflex · Bezold-Jarisch reflex · Valsalva maneuver · Cushing reflex · Harvey cushing · Oculocardiac reflex · Chemoreceptor reflex

3.1 Introduction to Cardiac Physiology

3.1.1 The Physiologic Anatomy of the Heart

The normal adult heart is a physiologic muscular pump composed of two adjacent, parallel pumps (i.e., left and right); each of these separate pumps is composed of two chambers (i.e., atrium and ventricle); each atrium receives blood from drainage veins and conducts blood to the related ventricle; the ventricle would in turn pump the blood to the main artery connected to the related outflow tract, i.e., from the left ventricle outflow tract to the aorta and from the right ventricle outflow tract to the pulmonary artery. Afterward, the blood is sent forward, to the arterial tree in a propulsive manner. This cardiac contractile system is composed of two muscle masses named as "cardiac muscle syncytium": the atrial syncytium and the ventricular syncytium which are separated by a fine part of the cardiac conductive system (see following pages).

Grossly speaking, both the right atrium (RA) and left atrium (LA) have a delicate structure mainly composed of two muscle layers and are located above the related ventricle. On the other hand, the right ventricle (RV) and left ventricle (LV) are composed of three gross muscular layers, much thicker than atria. The two atria are separated anatomically by the interatrial septum, while the two ventricles are separated by the "thicker" interventricular septum. However, the two atria are connected as an electrical unit through the atrial electrical conduction system discussed later. The same is also correct for the ventricles, and they have a common electrical system with its divisions and branches spread throughout the ventricles.

The great veins are attached to the proximal chambers of the heart, i.e., atria; in other words, the superior and inferior venae cavae are attached to the right atrium and drain the deoxygenated blood from the upper and lower organs to the right heart, respectively. However, the right and left pulmonary veins bring oxygenated blood from the right and left lung to the left atrium. Afterward, the deoxygenated blood is sent from the right atrium through the right ventricle to the right ventricular outflow tract (RVOT) to enter the pulmonary artery; then, it goes to the lungs to be oxygenated. The oxygenated blood traverses the left atrium to the left ventricle and is pumped through the left ventricular outflow tract (LVOT) to the ascending aorta, aortic arch, and descending aorta to perfuse the whole body by oxygenated blood.

Each atrium is separated anatomically from its ventricle by an atrioventricular valve; on the right side, the tricuspid valve does this, and on the left side, the mitral valve separates the left atrium from the left ventricle; the tricuspid valve has three leaflets (or three cusps), while the mitral (bicuspid) valve has two leaflets (cusps). The leaflets of the atrioventricular valves are strengthened by the chordae tendineae, which are fibrous-connective bundles anchoring the ventricular wall to the inferior surface of the same side atrioventricular valve cusps; muscular extensions, named papillary muscles, are located between the ventricular wall and the chordae tendineae. The structure composed of chordae tendineae and papillary muscles prevents prolapsed of the atrioventricular valve from the ventricular cavity back to the atrial chamber during ventricular systole.

Also, each ventricle is separated from the related artery by a semilunar three-leaflet valve; the right ventricle is separated from the pulmonary artery by the pulmonary valve, while the aortic valve separates the left ventricle from the aorta (Fig. 3.1).

The heart is a muscular organ; its location is posterior to the sternal bone in the anterior mediastinum, a bit deviated to the left. Anatomically speaking, the heart is composed of three layers:

- "**Pericardium**": the outermost layer, covers the heart as a tissue sac and has itself three layers
  1. Fibrous pericardium (firm, outermost layer).
  2. Parietal pericardium (between fibrous pericardium and visceral pericardium).
  3. Visceral pericardium (innermost layer of pericardium) which is attached directly to the outer border of myocardial tissue; normally, a potential space exists between visceral and parietal pericardial layers which is filled with a few milliliters of serous tissue, functioning as a lubricant between the two layers, while there is continuous heart rhythm and myocardial contractions.

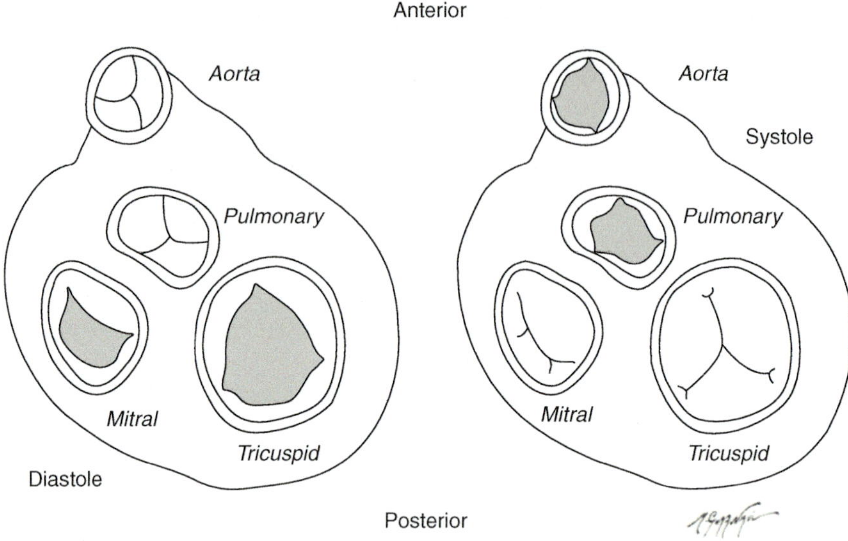

Fig. 3.1 The apex of the heart when viewed from above in systole and diastole; note the position of the valves and their relationships (Dabbagh 2014)

- "**Myocardium**": the middle layer, has the essential role of contraction and is composed mainly of
  1. Myocardial muscle tissue
  2. Coronary vascular system

Both of them are discussed in detail in the next paragraphs.

- "**Endocardium**": the innermost layer, covers the inner space of the cardiac chambers (Silver et al. 1971; Anderson et al. 2004; Anwar et al. 2007; Tops et al. 2007; Haddad et al. 2009; Silbiger and Bazaz 2009; Ho and McCarthy 2010; Rogers and Bolling 2010; Atkinson et al. 2011; Dell'Italia 2012; Silbiger 2012; Hong and Shaw 2017)

3.1.1.1 The Main Cell Types of the Myocardial Tissue

Here we discuss more about the myocardial muscle tissue and its ingredients. Based on a general classification, the cardiac muscle (myocardium) is mainly composed of three cell types:

- Cardiac *connective* tissue cells
- *Cardiomyocytes* (which have contractile function)
- Cardiac *conduction and electrical system cells* (which in turn consists of *impulse-generating* cells and specialized *conductive* cells)

3.1.1.2 Cardiac Connective Tissue Cells

The cardiomyocytes are arranged in a protective and supporting cellular bed known as *cardiac connective tissue cells*, which have the main following functions:

1. Supporting the cardiac muscle fibers as a physical protective structure
2. Transmission of the cardiomyocyte-produced mechanical force to cardiac chambers
3. Adding "tensile strength and stiffness" to the structure of the heart
4. Preventing excessive dilation and overexpansion of the heart
5. Keeping the heart within its original framework, returning the heart to its original shape after each contraction through the elastic fibers

The cardiac connective tissue would be modified according to the function of the related cardiac region; for example, *the amount of collagen in atria is different than in the ventricles* which shows the diversities and dissimilarities of anatomy that are the result of difference in function, both regarding "pressure and volume" of the physiologic work in different cardiac regions (Borg et al. 1982; Robinson et al. 1986, 1988; Rossi et al. 1998; Distefano and Sciacca 2012; Watson et al. 2012; Hong and Shaw 2017).

3.1.1.3 Cardiomyocyte (i.e., Cardiac Contractile Tissue Cell or Cardiac Muscle Cell)

The myocardium is composed of myocardial cells named as *heart muscle cell, cardiac myocytes*, or, briefly, *cardiomyocytes*. The following hierarchy could lead us to overall order seen in the fine and specialized structure of the myocardial histology.

- The cardiomyocytes are specialized muscle cells, ranging from 25 μm length in atria up to about 140 μm in ventricular cardiomyocytes and 25 μ width in ventricles.
- About half of a cardiomyocyte is composed of contractile parts (called myofibrils) arranged as contractile units called *sarcomere* (each cardiomyocyte contains a number of sarcomeres); sarcomere is the basic unit of contraction or better to say *contractile quantum of the heart.*
- The other half is composed of other cellular structures including nucleus, mitochondria (occupies about 30% of the heart volume), sarcoplasmic reticulum, and cytosol.
- These cells have contractile function similar to striated muscle cells; however, there is the main difference in their function: *their contraction is involuntary.*
- Each cardiomyocyte, instead of having many nuclei inside the cell (like the cellular structure seen in skeletal muscle cells), only has 1–2 nuclei.
- The internal structure of each cardiomyocyte is in turn composed of a wealth of cardiac myofibrils.
- In turn, each cardiac myofibril is composed of a vast number of sarcomeres; each sarcomere is located anatomically between two Z lines; thin filaments are attached perpendicularly to Z lines on each side, while thick filaments are arranged in between creating a parallel line-in-line fashion (Fig. 3.2).

Sarcolemma, T tubules, and sarcoplasmic reticulum: these cellular elements compose the other half of each cardiomyocyte. As a matter of fact, each cardiac cell

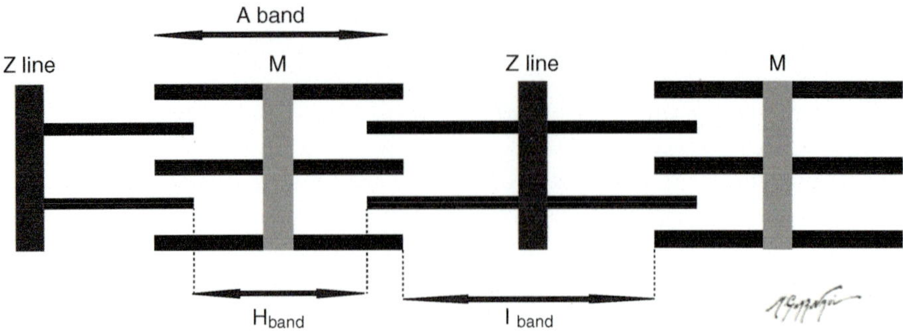

Fig. 3.2 Microscopic structure of a sarcomere (Dabbagh 2014)

is enveloped by a special membrane called *sarcolemma*, which not only covers the cardiomyocyte but also has a large network "invaginating" between the cells creating transverse tubules (*T tubules*); this feature of sarcolemma plays a central role in Ca^{2+} transfer in sarcoplasmic reticulum of the cardiomyocytes. In turn, Ca^{2+} has a pivotal role in all three main physiologic functions of the myocardium, including *excitation-contraction coupling* which in summary works as the "hinge" between the *electrical* and *mechanical* functions of the cardiomyocyte.

The *sarcoplasmic reticulum* (SR) is another cellular component of the cardiomyocyte with a specific dual mission for Ca^{2+} homeostasis: first, initial small Ca^{2+} during depolarization triggers Ca^{2+} release from SR, leading to contractility through junctional SR (JSR), and after that, Ca^{2+} is reabsorbed to the longitudinal SR (LSR) causing cardiac muscle relaxation.

Intercalated discs: *intercalated discs* are among the basic cellular structures found in cardiomyocytes; being **cardiac-specific structures**, intercalated discs function as the main communication port between adjacent cardiomyocytes; among the main roles of intercalated discs, these could be mentioned:

1. *Mechanical* connection between adjacent cardiomyocytes (include the fascia adherens and desmosomes)
2. *Electrochemical transport* between adjacent cardiomyocytes (i.e., rapid transduction and transmission of action potential)
3. *Synchronization* of cell contraction (Ehler 2016)

The above main roles of the intercalated discs are integral part of the myocardium working as a "physiologic" syncytium. Maybe another interesting feature of intercalated discs is that they are specific to cardiac muscle cells, while adult skeletal muscle cells are devoid of these specialized cellular structures. *Intercalated discs* perform their roles through three types of intercellular junctions:

1. Spot desmosomes
2. Sheet desmosomes
3. Gap junction

1. **Spot desmosomes** are intercellular connections which "anchor the intermediate-filament cytoskeleton" in the adjacent cells.
2. **Sheet desmosomes** are the place for contractile structures that connect two neighboring cells; it means that sheet desmosomes fasten and fix the contractile apparatus between the neighboring cells.
3. **Gap junctions** are specialized myocardial cell contacts which are primarily responsible for electrical and metabolic coupling of cells and signal transmission between adjacent cells causing rapid electrical wave progression in "cardiac syncytium" through a wide range of cellular and subcellular interactions which is beyond the scope of this chapter (Bennett et al. 2016; Vermij et al. 2017). Generally speaking, gap junctions have two main roles:
   - *Anchorage* which is an integral part of cardiac morphogenesis
   - *Communication* which is essential for cardiac conduction and cardiac action potential propagation

In general, intercalated discs could be an important potential source of cardiac diseases; i.e., some of the mutations in proteins of intercalated discs may lead to arrhythmic states like Brugada syndrome or arrhythmogenic cardiomyopathy (Kleber and Saffitz 2014; Calore et al. 2015; Tanaka et al. 2017; Vermij et al. 2017).

Gap junctions are composed of protein subunits including Connexins (mainly Connexin 43; while Connexin 40, Connexin 45, and Connexin 30.2 are also important); so, the cellular pathologies in gap junctions of cardiomyocytes (especially those related to Connexin 43) can have a major role in ischemia and some lethal arrhythmias. In human myocardium, Connexin 43 is the most common and important type of cardiac Connexins. Usually, the Purkinje cells have a high amount of gap junctions, while they do not have considerable amounts of contractile elements (Desplantez et al. 2007; Kurtenbach et al. 2014; Stroemlund et al. 2015; George and Poelzing 2016; Qiu et al. 2016; Krishnan et al. 2017).

Each cardiomyocyte is composed of a number of contractile units: let's say *contractile quantum* or the more familiar term *cardiac sarcomere*. Hence, sarcomere is the basic unit of contraction which we could consider it as the *contractile quantum* of the heart. Cardiac sarcomere has the main following characteristics:

- The primary function of cardiomyocyte (contractile function) is produced in each sarcomere.
- Each cardiomyocyte ranges from 25 to 140 μm in diameter, while each cardiac sarcomere is just about 1.6–2.2 μm in length.
- Nearly half of each cardiomyocyte is composed of contractile elements, arranged as contractile fibers, while the other half is composed of all other cellular structures like mitochondria, nucleus, cytosolic structures, and other intracellular organelles.
- Each sarcomere is defined as the contractile part of the myofibril located between two Z lines.

The contractile fibers in each sarcomere are classically divided as thick filaments and thin filaments; however, if the microscopic anatomy of sarcomere is viewed, each sarcomere is defined as the contractile part of the myofibril located between two Z lines and consists of the following parts:

- Z lines: when seen with a microscope present as thick lines; the margins of each sarcomere is defined by Z line in each side; Z stands for "Zuckung," a German name meaning "contraction" or "twitch"; so, each sarcomere is the region of myofilaments between two Z lines; the Z line is like an "anchor" to which the thin filaments are attached.
- Thin filaments: are attached perpendicularly to Z lines on each side; thin filaments are composed of two-stranded F actin, tropomyosin proteins, and troponin complex (troponin I, troponin T, and troponin C).
- Thick filaments: are in between them in a parallel fashion; these filaments are composed of myosin molecules and are located in the center of the sarcomere; the two ends of thick filaments are interspersed with thin filaments.
- "I" band: the light area of sarcomere on two sides of Z line contains thin filaments and is named "I" band; during myocardial contraction, "I" band shortens.
- "A" band: the central dark part of each sarcomere (between two I bands) contains thin and thick filaments and is called "A" band; each "A" band while located in center takes two "I" bands (each I band in one side of the single A band) plus two Z lines (each Z line attached to the other side of "I" band); this complex composes a sarcomere (as presented in figure).
- "H" band: is the central part of "A" band, composed mainly of thick filaments.

A full description of contractile proteins, thick filament, and thin filament is described in this chapter in later sections and also in Figs. 3.2, 3.3, 3.4, and 3.5.

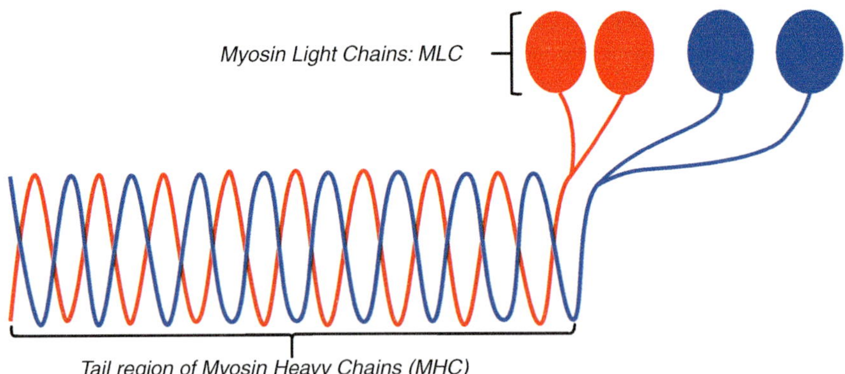

Fig. 3.3 Schematic presentation of a myosin molecule; modified from Dabbagh et al. (2017). Published with kind permission of © SpringerNature, 2017. All Rights Reserved

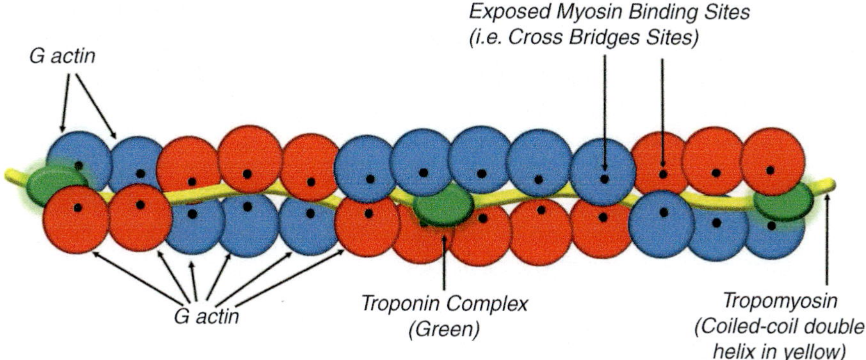

Fig. 3.4 Schematic presentation of a thin filament (also see Fig. 3.3a): each helix of F actin contains two strands of G actin each containing 13 G actin molecules (blue and red globes), myosin-binding sites which expose actin for crossbridging with myosin and located on each G actin (demonstrated as a black dot); troponin complex (green knobs) and tropomyosin double-strand coiled coils as yellow threads; modified from Dabbagh et al. (2017). Published with kind permission of © SpringerNature, 2017. All Rights Reserved

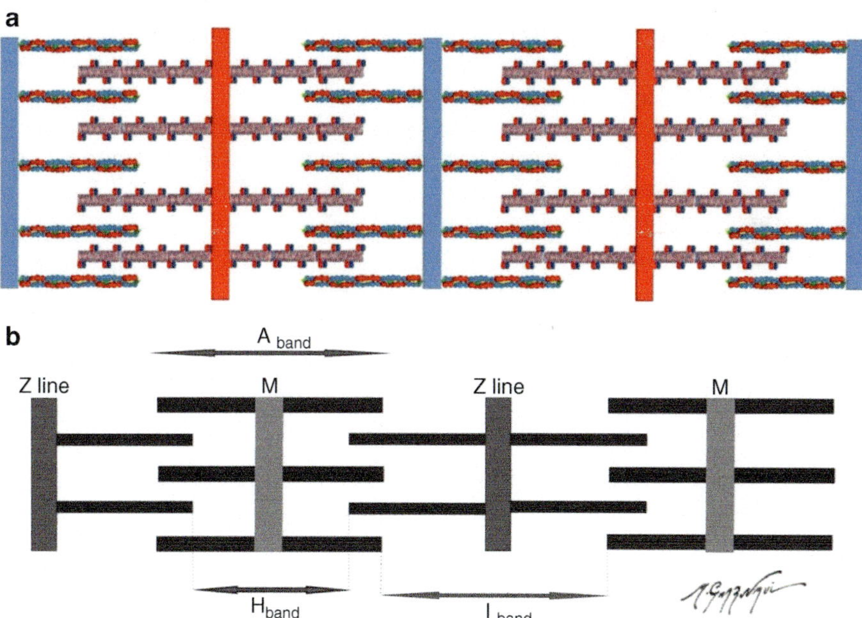

Fig. 3.5 (**a**) Schematic presentation of microscopic structure of a sarcomere from a wide view (also, see Fig. 9.7). (**b**) Schematic presentation of microscopic structure of a sarcomere (compare each part with its compared part in Section A); modified from Dabbagh (2014), Dabbagh et al. (2017). Published with kind permission of © SpringerNature, 2017. All Rights Reserved

Histological differences between cardiac muscle and skeletal muscle: one could find the following differences between cardiac muscle cell and striated muscle cell:

Cardiac muscle tissue is a complex of united and combined contractile cells, totally named as a syncytium; this syncytium is

- Composed of branched cells with the myofibers usually being fused at their ends.
- Cell length is definitely smaller than skeletal muscles; thin filaments in cardiac muscles do not have a constant length.
- Connections between adjacent cardiomyocytes are highly subdivided; creating a 3-D network which improves the function of the cardiac syncytium.
- A **relatively unique cardiac cellular structure** called intercalated discs has an integral role in creating this intercellular network, i.e., cardiac syncytium; one of the main ingredients of intercalated discs is gap junctions which are especial electrical link between cells and easily transmit electrical current between cells.
- Cardiomyocytes usually have one or two (rarely three to four) central nuclei.
- Enriched with *abundant mitochondria* which plays an essential role in *cellular energetics of cardiomyocytes*; the energy is delivered as ATP through oxidative phosphorylation for many processes including *excitation-contraction coupling*, the *contractile activity* of *sarcomere*, and the relationship between contractile filaments in systole and diastole.
- One of the most important functions of mitochondria is Ca^{2+} homeostasis (see below); this is why in cardiomyocytes, the mitochondria are located near the sarcoplasmic reticulum (SR)
- Both mitochondria and Ca^{2+} have a central role in cardiomyocyte necrosis; in such abnormal states, the role of mitochondria changes from an "ATP-producing engine" to "producers of excessive reactive oxygen species" which would release "pro-death proteins."
- The high rate of metabolism in these cells necessitates high vasculature in between all the cells having aerobic metabolism.
- The special Ca^{2+} metabolism of these cells is the main result for having fewer T tubules, while these T tubules are wider (cardiac T tubules are about five times more than skeletal muscles in diameter).
- Negligible Golgi vesicles are seen in cardiomyocytes; however, in skeletal muscles Golgi complex is not found.
- Studies in recent years have demonstrated unique proteins in cardiomyocytes which include a number of proteins constituting actin, myosin, and troponin filaments; also, natriuretic peptide A and natriuretic peptide B are specific to cardiomyocytes. Interestingly, some proteins are exclusively found in specific areas of the heart like atrial tissue, or some others are specific for intercalated discs and no other cardiac tissue (Abdelmeguid and Sorour 1992; Paniagua et al. 1996; Peters 1996; Lindskog et al. 2015; Pohjoismaki and Goffart 2017; Sun et al. 2017; Yester and Kuhn 2017).

Skeletal muscle cells have the following features due to their pattern of contraction, which is a pattern of neuromuscular junction unit:

- Longer, multinucleated and cylindrical shape.
- Usually not arranged as syncytium; instead, they are located side-by-side with no tight binding or gap junctions.
- Lower metabolism needs, necessitating medium vasculature, with lower amounts of mitochondria (about 2–3% of the cell).
- Both aerobic and anaerobic metabolism.
- Thick and thin filaments in skeletal muscles having a constant length.
- Heterochromatin, smooth sarcoplasm vesicles, and glycogen granules are seen more frequently in cardiac muscle cells (Severs 1985; Abdelmeguid and Sorour 1992; Peters 1996; Gordon et al. 2000; Kirchhoff et al. 2000; Lo 2000; Alberts et al. 2002; Burgoyne et al. 2008; Kobayashi et al. 2008; Meyer et al. 2010; Shaw and Rudy 2010; Workman et al. 2011; Anderson et al. 2012; Balse et al. 2012; Bingen et al. 2013; Delmar and Makita 2012; Eisner et al. 2012; Khan et al. 2012; Kubli and Gustafsson 2012; Miragoli et al. 2012; Orellana et al. 2012; Scriven and Moore 2012; Wang et al. 2012; Zhou and O'Rourke 2012; Barclay 2017; Bazgir et al. 2017; Bohnert et al. 2018).

3.1.1.4 Cardiac Conductive Tissue Cells

The synchronized *mechanical system* needs a delicate *electrochemical network*, known as *cardiac electrical network* or *cardiac electrical system* which is mainly composed of two cell types:

1. *Excitatory cells*: also known as "impulse-generating cells," mainly consist of the sinoatrial (SA) node
2. *Specialized conduction cells* known as *conductive cells* are composed of:
    - The *atrioventricular conduction* or internodal pathways
    - *AV node*
    - The *His bundle*
    - *Right and left branches* of the His bundle
    - The *Purkinje fiber cells* or the Purkinje fiber network distributed all over ventricles to conduct the electrical impulse all over the ventricles effectively and rapidly

This hierarchical pattern is schematically demonstrated in Fig. 3.6 and functions as the electrochemical backup for effective mechanical contraction of ventricles leading finally to an effective cardiac output (Desplantez et al. 2007; Dun and Boyden 2008; Anderson et al. 2009; Atkinson et al. 2011, 2013; Deng et al. 2012; Kennedy et al. 2016; Zack et al. 2016; Nakasuka et al. 2017).

3.1.2 Anatomy of the Coronary Arteries

The normal coronary arterial system has four main elements (Fig. 3.7); of course, a full description of abnormalities in coronary artery anatomy could be found elsewhere (Lluri and Aboulhosn 2014; Spicer et al. 2015; Villa et al. 2016; Yi et al. 2016; Foley et al. 2017; Hiltrop et al. 2017; Kokkinidis et al. 2017; Young et al. 2017):

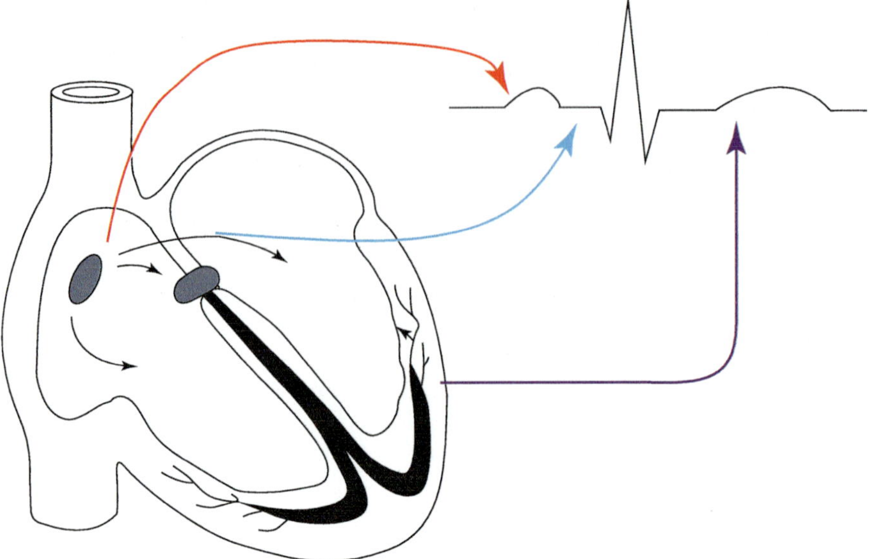

Fig. 3.6 Cardiac conductive system and its elements; in left, see the relationship of normal electrocardiography with the elements of the system. Modified from Dabbagh et al. (2017). Published with kind permission of © SpringerNature, 2017. All Rights Reserved

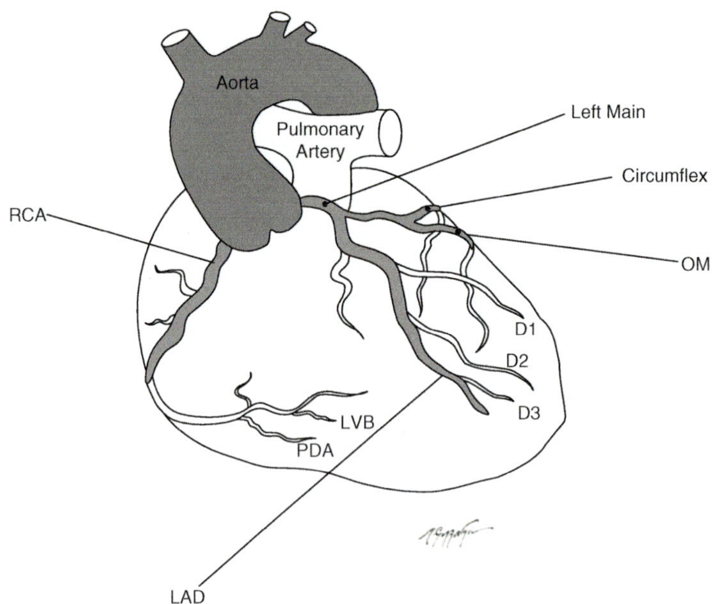

Fig. 3.7 Anatomy of normal epicardial coronary arteries (Dabbagh 2014)

- Left main coronary artery (LMCA)
- Left anterior descending coronary artery (LAD)
- Left circumflex coronary artery (LCX)
- Right coronary artery (RCA)

Left main coronary artery (LMCA): LMCA starts from the left coronary ostium in left Valsalva sinus and after passing a length (between 0–40 mm) is usually divided into two branches: LAD and LCX. At times, an extra branch is divided from the LMCA and passes parallel to the diagonal arterial system; this arterial branch is called the "ramus" branch.

Left anterior descending (LAD) artery: after LCX is separated from LMCA, the remainder of LMCA continues its path as left main coronary artery; LAD goes down the interventricular septum and reaches the apex

- The *diagonal branches* run as oblique derivations between LAD and LCX; the main role of diagonal branches is to perfuse the lateral wall of the left ventricle.
- Besides the diagonal branches, there are *septal branches* of LAD which perfuse the anterior two thirds (2/3) of the interventricular septum.

Left circumflex coronary artery (LCX): LMCA is divided into LAD and LCX often at a 90 degrees angle at the separation point; LCX has a number of ventricular branches which perfuse the lateral and posterior walls of the left ventricle (LV); these branches are called *obtuse marginal* or simply OM; in 40% of the patients, LCX perfuses the SA node; the other 60% are perfused by RCA.

Right coronary artery (RCA): originates from the right coronary ostium of the Valsalva sinus; so, its origin is from a different coronary ostium compared with the abovementioned coronary arteries; RCA then goes through the right atrioventricular groove (i.e., the groove located between the atria and ventricles toward right) to reach the posterior part of interventricular septum where it gives a branch called acute marginal artery; as mentioned, 60% are perfused by RCA. Finally, RCA is divided into two main branches:

- *Posterior descending artery* (PDA) to perfuse the posterior 1/3 of the interventricular septum and the inferior wall of LV and also the posteromedial papillary muscle; in the majority of the people (85%), PDA originates from RCA; these are called *right dominant*; however, in the other 15%, called *left dominant*, PDA originates from LCX.
- *Posterolateral branch* to perfuse the posterior part of LV wall.

3.2 Cellular Physiology

Among the main characteristic features of cardiomyocytes are their *very specialized* functional and histological features; these subspecialized anatomical and physiological features have key role in production, propagation, and transmission of "electrochemical and mechanical" functions of cardiomyocytes. Physiologically speaking, these electrochemical and mechanical functions are translated to three main domains:

1. Action potential
2. Excitation-contraction coupling (ECC)
3. Contractile mechanisms and their related processes

The following paragraph has been discussed above in detail; however, a briefing is brought here. The cardiac muscle is composed of two main syncytia: the atrial syncytium and the ventricular syncytium. In other words, in each syncytium, all the cells are interrelated with many widespread intercellular connections which are the result of cellular and histological arrangements of cardiomyocytes (discussed above). In some features, the cardiomyocytes resemble the skeletal muscles, being composed of actin and myosin filaments, contracting and relaxing in a well-cooperated and organized manner in order to produce the cardiac contractile force. The intercellular connections between cardiac muscles are mainly through the "intercalated discs" which are delicate pores located at the proximal and distal parts of each cardiomyocyte; these discs are able to transport great amounts of ions between the cardiomyocytes so transferring the ions from each cell to the next cell, which is mainly done through a special segment of intercalated discs called *gap junctions*. Hence, the term "syncytium" is not just an anatomical term but also a physiologic and electrochemical term; many proteins and other cellular elements are involved in the process. However, the two syncytia (atrial and ventricular) are separated not only physically by electrical insulator of fibrous skeleton but also electrochemically and physiologically by the AV node and AV bundle to act as independently functioning syncytium.

3.2.1 Action Potential

The normal cardiomyocytes have a specific pattern of fluctuating electrical potentials known as *action potentials*. As a matter of fact, the resting potential and the action potential of all cardiomyocytes are not the same; though, the mechanism of action potential production is similar. Action potential of cardiomyocytes, like many other cell types, is the result of ion chemical currents across the cellular membrane, with the final result presented as consecutive depolarization and repolarization which produces the cardiac electrical impulse. The impulse is generated and conducted over the cardiac "electrochemical" and "conduction" system (Shih 1994; Ravens and Cerbai 2008; Michael et al. 2009; Aronsen et al. 2013).

Normally, action potential of cardiomyocytes is composed of five phases which are produced due to the influx and efflux of ions, especially Na^+, Ca^{2+}, and K^+ ions, across the cell membrane.

The amplitude of normal action potential of cardiomyocytes is about 105 millivolts (mV) starting from a nadir of −80 to −90 mV reaching up to a peak of +15 to

+20 mV, then experiencing a plateau for about 0.2 ms, and finally turning down to the baseline which is the nadir of −80 to −90 mV (Morad and Tung 1982; Shih 1994; Lodish et al. 2000; Ravens and Cerbai 2008; Michael et al. 2009; Eisner et al. 2012; Aronsen et al. 2013).

The action potential in cardiomyocytes is much similar to the action potential of skeletal muscles; however, it has two main differentiating features:

- Although the fast Na^+ channels are present both in the skeletal muscle cells and cardiomyocytes, the slow (L)-type Ca^{2+} channels are present just in the cardiomyocytes and *not* in the skeletal muscle cells; however, in cardiomyocytes, after the start of action potential mainly by fast Na^+ channels, L-type Ca^{2+} channels open with a short time lag and then remain open for a few milliseconds to create the plateau of action potential. This property has two main effects; first to modulate heart rate in the physiologically defined range and second to augment cardiomyocyte contractions (Faber and Rudy 2000; Aronsen et al. 2013; Kusakari et al. 2017).

Besides Na^+ and Ca^{2+}, the third important ion in cardiomyocyte action potential is K^+. Just after cardiomyocyte depolarization, due to Ca^{2+} entry to the cell, there is abrupt and considerable decreases in K^+ outflux from the cell to the external milieu. This is also an important reason for delayed plateau of the action potential, mainly created by the slow (L)-type Ca^{2+} channels but also boosted by K^+ outflux. The permeability of the cardiomyocyte cell membrane to K^+ will return to normal after cessation of Ca^{2+} and Na^+ channels to normal potential (about 0.2–0.3 ms) which causes the return of K^+ outside the cell and ending action potential (Grunnet 2010; Humphries and Dart 2015; Zhao et al. 2017).

Based on the above transmembrane electrochemical currents, action potential has been arbitrarily divided into a number of phases. These phases of action potential in ventricular and atrial cardiomyocytes and also His bundle and Purkinje cells could be summarized as:

- Phase 0: early rapid upstroke of action potential caused by huge Na + influx through fast channels.
- Phase 1: short-term and incomplete repolarization due to K^+ outflux.
- Phase 2: slow (L)-type Ca^{2+} channels open, and there are Ca^{2+} influx and K^+ efflux; initiation of the contractions starts immediately afterward; this phase is also called plateau.
- Phase 3: large amounts of K^+ outflux which overcome the Ca^{2+} influx; again the action potential moves to negative levels to reach the resting potential; this phase, named resting potential phase, equals diastole.
- Phase 4: influx of very negligible amounts of K^+; however, the "3 Na^+–1 Ca^{2+} exchanger" also known as "NCX" has a very important role in relaxation phase, since it directly sends Ca^{2+} against its gradient into the exterior of myocardial cell and sends indirectly K^+ against its gradient to interior of myocardial cell; the failure of this exchanger or anti-port to function properly has been implicated as

one of the mechanisms involved in heart failure (Snyders 1999; Faber and Rudy 2000; Lodish et al. 2000; Rudy 2007; Ravens and Cerbai 2008; Grunnet 2010; Aronsen et al. 2013; Humphries and Dart 2015; Shattock et al. 2015; Limbu et al. 2016; Kusakari et al. 2017).

A brief and schematic presentation of these phases could be found in Table 3.1 and in Figs. 3.8, 3.9, and 3.10. The colors of phases between Table 3.1 and the figures are designed in concordance.

There are some differences between phases of action potential in "sinoatrial (SA) node and atrioventricular (AV) node cells" on one side with "ventricular and atrial cardiomyocytes and also His bundle and Purkinje cells" on the other side. The main result of these differences is creation of pacemaker cells versus other cell types of cardiomyocytes. These differences are mainly due to:

- Increased "Na^+ influx" during phase 4 of action potential
- Increased "Ca^{2+} influx" during phase 4 of action potential
- Decreased "K^+ influx" during phase 4 of action potential

A number of important events emerge due to these three differences, including:

- Resting potential of pacemaker cells is less negative than the other cardiac cells; it means that resting potential in majority of cardiac cells is −80 to −90 mV, while in

Table 3.1 Action potential in myocardial cells

Phase	Event in action potential	Ion current	Electrical status (mV)
Phase 0	Rapid upstroke: ***Depolarizaton***	Na^+ influx	Starts from -90 to -80 and goes up to about +10 to +15
Phase 1	Very short and initial ***repolarization*** which is "Incomplete repolarization"	K^+ outflux	Starts from +10 to + 15 and decreases to about +5
Phase 2	Initiation of contraction due to Ca^{2+} influx; this phase is also titled "***Plateau***" Usually determines the*action potential* ***duration*** and also, the a *refractory period*	Ca^{2+} influx due to opening of slow (L) type Ca^{2+} channels; also, K^+ outflux	Starts from + 5 and has a nearly steady level; maximum drop to 0
Phase 3	***Final Repolarization***	Huge K^+ outflux	Starts from about "0" Ends at -80 to -90
Phase 4	Resting potential *i.e.*no active potential)	K^+ influx and outflux	Stays at -80 to -90

Modified from Dabbagh et al. (2017). Published with kind permission of © SpringerNature, 2017. All Rights Reserved

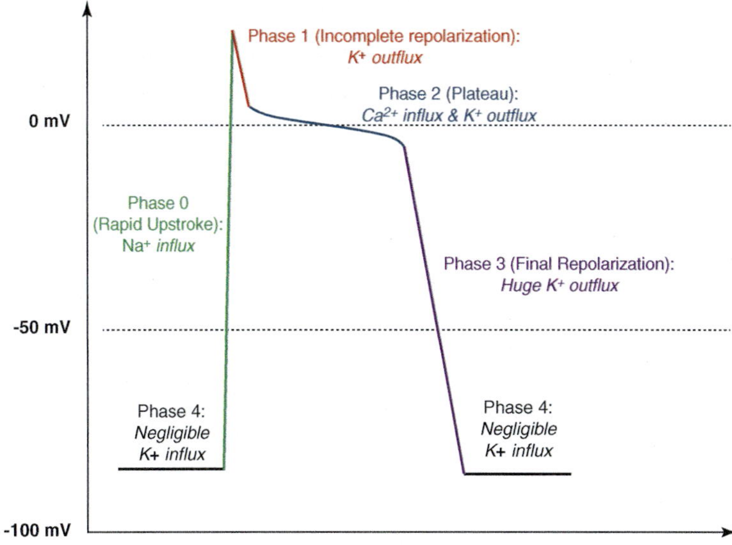

Fig. 3.8 Progress of action potential phases; modified from Dabbagh et al. (2017). Published with kind permission of © SpringerNature, 2017. All Rights Reserved (Marcotti et al. 2004; Parham et al. 2006; Wolf and Berul 2008; Amanfu and Saucerman 2011; Marionneau and Abriel 2015)

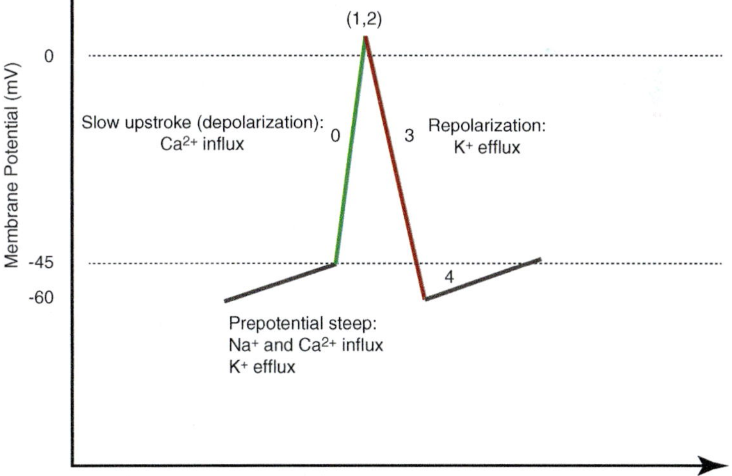

Fig. 3.9 Action potential (AP) in cardiac pacemaker cells; modified from Dabbagh et al. (2017). Published with kind permission of © SpringerNature, 2017. All Rights Reserved

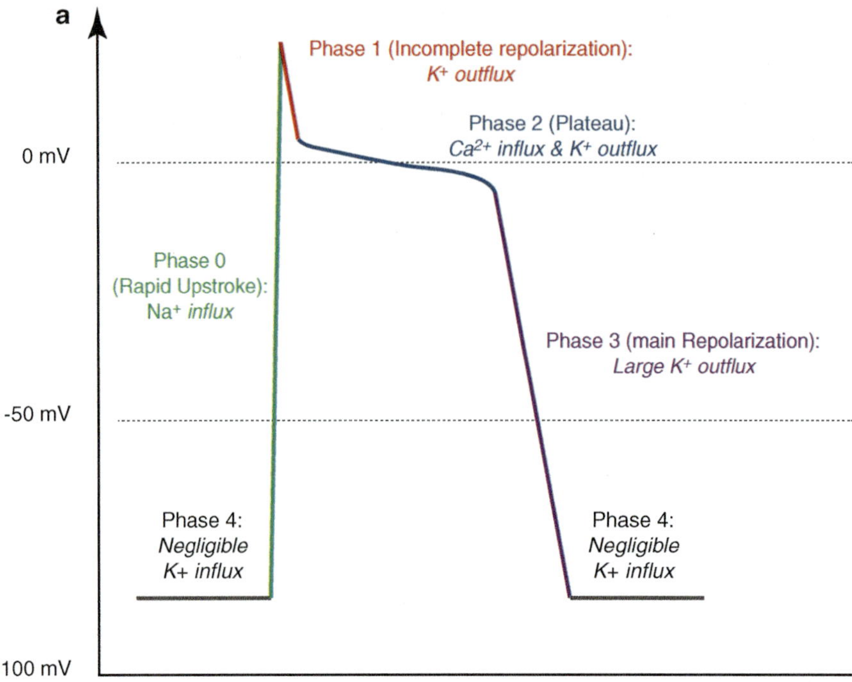

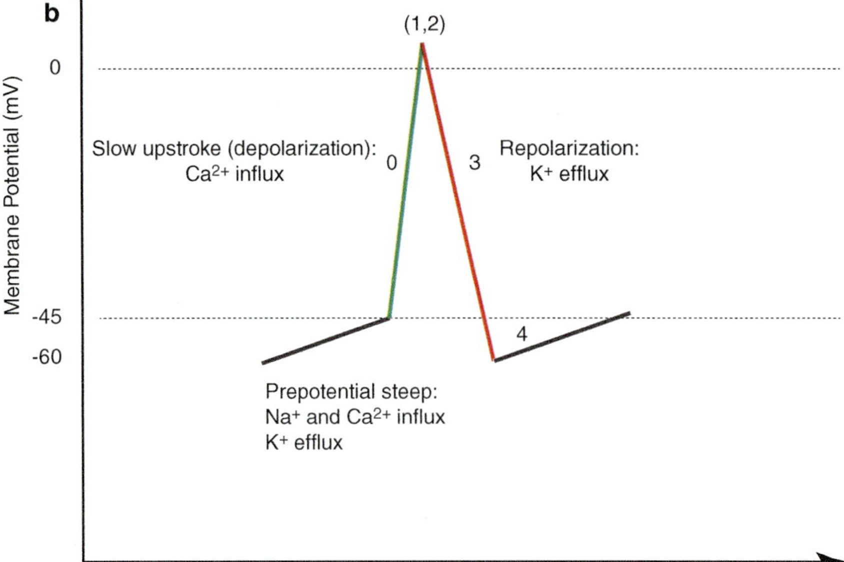

Fig. 3.10 The difference between action potential phases in normal (**a**) and pacemaker (**b**) cells; modified from Dabbagh et al. (2017). Published with kind permission of © SpringerNature, 2017. All Rights Reserved

pacemaker cells, it is just −50 to −60 mV; the main reason for this difference is that the flux of Na + and Ca2+ from outside to inside of *pacemaker cells* (i.e., Na + influx in pacemaker cells) continues during repolarization; so, changing the resting potential level from about −60 mV to upper levels in such a way that it reaches the needed voltage for threshold of depolarization (i.e., about −35 to −40 mV); this Na^+ current is called pacemaker "funny current of the heart" shortly named as I(f) of the heart; the funny current and Ca^{2+} influx are responsible for rhythmic, spontaneous pacemaker activity in pacemaker cells, especially SA node. Today, I(h) is used instead of I(f) which means hyperpolarization-dependent Na^+ current (Michael et al. 2009; Grunnet 2010; Kim et al. 2016).

- Phase 4 (diastole) of action potential is more abrupt and headed up, i.e., not as much flat as seen in the cardiac muscles' action potential, again due to the same Na^+ and Ca^{2+} currents in repolarization period (Grunnet 2010).
- Phase 1 of action potential is nearly eliminated.
- Phases 2 and 3 are nearly merged together.

Refractory period of cardiomyocytes: refractory period in cardiac action potential is the time period after termination of each action potential; during this time interval, no new impulse could be generated after any stimulus; the role of refractory period is to prevent premature contractions before the appropriate time for the start of the next cardiac contraction. Also, it has a protective role for the heart against "reentrant arrhythmias." However, *the time interval for refractory period* is not constant all over the cardiac cells, being shorter in the atrial cells (0.15 s) than the ventricular cells (0.3 s). Physiologically speaking, phase 2 (plateau) of action potential is the *main determinant factor* for duration of refractory period (Boyden et al. 1988; Szigligeti et al. 1996; Reuter et al. 2005; DiFrancesco 2006, 2010; Bucchi et al. 2007; DiFrancesco and Borer 2007; Zhang and Hancox 2009; Chen et al. 2010; Neco et al. 2010; Pott et al. 2011; Coronel et al. 2012; DiFrancesco and Noble 2012; Ednie and Bennett 2012; Shy et al. 2013; Strege et al. 2012; Torres-Jacome et al. 2013; Brunello et al. 2013; Goldhaber and Philipson 2013; Kim et al. 2013; Ottolia et al. 2013; Papaioannou et al. 2013; Sipido et al. 2013; Weisbrod et al. 2013; Yuniarti and Lim 2017).

3.2.2 Excitation-Contraction Coupling (ECC)

Excitation-contraction coupling (ECC): this term, used in 1952 for the first time, depicts a physiologic process which *transforms an electrochemical impulse to a mechanical contraction* which is seen in both skeletal and cardiac muscles. In other terms, it is the intermediary phase between action potential (electrochemical function of cardiomyocytes) and contraction (mechanical function) of the heart. Therefore, ECC could be imagined as a *joint* between the *electrochemical and mechanical limbs of cardiac function.*

ECC is one of the most important mechanisms in cardiac physiology, composed of three main delicate cellular and subcellular stages, each having their individual elements:

1. Functioning organelles of ECC including cell membrane L-type Ca^{2+} channels
2. Calcium ion (Ca^{2+}) and calcium release from intracellular calcium store (i.e., sarcoplasmic reticulum) which acts through ryanodine receptors (RyR2).
3. Controllers of ECC

A summary of these composing aspects and their related items are presented in the Tables 3.2 and 3.3 (Fabiato and Fabiato 1979; Fabiato 1985; Lodish et al. 2000;

Table 3.2 A summary of the composing elements of ECC

	The individual composing group of elements	The elements in each group
1	Functioning organelles of ECC	Cell membrane
		Thick and thin filaments
		T tubules
		Sarcoplasmic reticulum
2	Calcium ion (Ca^{2+})	Ca^{2+} influx to the cardiomyocytes (by L-type Ca^{2+} channels in *systole*)
		Ca^{2+} release inside the cell (by RyR in systole)
		Ca^{2+} efflux from the cardiomyocytes (by NCX in diastole)
		Ca^{2+} reuptake from the cell (by SERCA in diastole)
3	Controllers of ECC	Ryanodine receptor (RyR) family
		Dihydropyridine receptor (DHPR)
		Calmodulin

Abbott and Ritchie (1951), Sandow (1952), Hamilton et al. (2000), Periasamy and Huke (2001), Tang et al. (2002), Scoote et al. (2003), Yang et al. (2003), Bickler and Fahlman (2004), Scoote and Williams (2004), Reuter et al. (2005), Vangheluwe et al. (2006), Periasamy et al. (2008), Currie (2009), Kerckhoffs et al. (2009), Koivumaki et al. (2009), Neco et al. (2010), Williams et al. (2010), Malik and Morgan (2011), McDonald (2011), Prosser et al. (2011), Rybakova et al. (2011), Tavi and Westerblad (2011), Eisner et al. (2012), Ibrahim et al. (2012), Jafri (2012), Lu et al. (2012), Nakada et al. (2012), Scriven and Moore (2012), ter Keurs (2012), Goldhaber and Philipson (2013), Shy et al. (2013), Sipido et al. (2013), and Solaro et al. (2013), and Dabbagh (2014)

Table 3.3 A summary of ECC process

	Event	Protein or channel in charge	The main phenomenon	Result
1	Initial Ca^{2+} influx (Ca^{2+} entry to the cell)	$\boldsymbol{I}_{CaL}$ DHPR	DHPR channel opens	Triggers CICR (opening of RyR-2)
2	Ca^{2+} release (CICR) due to opening of RyR-2	RyR-2	Channel opens and huge Ca^{2+} is released from SR	Starts myocardial contraction
3	Ca^{2+} recycling, from cytosol back to SR, i.e., Ca^{2+} reuptake and Ca^{2+} efflux	SERCA2a (mainly) and NCX	Recollection of Ca^{2+} from cytosol	Starts myocardial relaxation
4	Modulation of SERCA2a	PLB	Stopping Ca^{2+} reuptake by SERCA2a	Stops myocardial relaxation; the next contraction could now start

Modified from Dabbagh et al. (2017). Published with kind permission of © SpringerNature, 2017. All Rights Reserved

Dulhunty 2006; Berisha and Nikolaev 2017; Hong and Shaw 2017; Tuomainen and Tavi 2017; Zhou and Hong 2017).

3.2.2.1 Which Parts of Cardiomyocyte Are the Functioning Organelles of ECC?

1. *Cell membrane* (which is responsible for electrical function, i.e., action potential; discussed before)
2. *Thick and thin filaments* (which are responsible for mechanical function, i.e., contractile function; discussed later in this chapter)
3. *Mitochondria* (ECC needs a great amount of energy; mitochondria are responsible for supporting ECC regarding its energy needs in the form of ATP, through oxidative phosphorylation; discussed before)
4. *Sarcoplasmic reticulum:* SR (which is the intracellular calcium store; discussed here)
5. *Transverse tubules* of cardiomyocytes (known as T tubules; discussed here)

As mentioned by Dulhunty, there is a "macromolecular protein complex or calcium release unit handling ECC" composed of a series of "cellular structures starting from extracellular space and involving the cellular surface membrane, transverse tubules, the cytoplasm, the sarcoplasmic reticulum membrane and reaching inside the lumen of the sarcoplasmic reticulum". This macromolecular protein complex plays an integrated role in production of ECC (Dulhunty 2006; Park et al. 2014; Arias-Calderon et al. 2016; London 2017).

Sarcoplasmic reticulum: SR is divided into longitudinal SR (LSR) and junctional SR (JSR). LSR releases Ca^{2+} reserves into the cell as fast as possible in just a few milliseconds, which would activate cardiomyocyte contractile structures. Junctional SR contains huge "Ca^{2+} releasing channels" acting through "ryanodine receptors." These receptors form a protein network which would enhance the release of Ca^{2+} in response to the primary Ca^{2+} influx. The role of "ryanodine receptors" is more recognized when considering the following fact:

For *cardiac cell* contraction, nearly 75% of cytoplasmic Ca^{2+} is released from SR.

T tubules: T tubules are invaginations of the cardiomyocyte cell membrane into the interior space of the cardiac muscle cells and transmit the action potential of the cell membrane to the internal parts of the cardiomyocyte. The role of T tubules is conducting the depolarization phase of action potential, as rapidly as possible, from the cell membrane to the interior of the cell; for this purpose, action potential is transmitted through the T tubules to the "longitudinal sarcoplasmic reticulum."

During some cardiac diseases like heart failure or ventricular hypertrophy, the "loss of integrity in transverse tubules" is one of the main etiologies for impaired availability of Ca^{2+} for sarcomere contractile functions; leading to impaired Ca^{2+} movements and its availability for contraction of the sarcomere myofilaments.

T tubules of cardiomyocytes have some *unique features*:

1. Ca^{2+} is the main mediator playing the most important role in cardiomyocyte action potential, ECC, and also muscle contraction. Although the start of action potential in *cardiac muscles* is similar to skeletal muscle, its continuation is dependent on the role of Ca^{2+} (see subtitle of *action potential*). As mentioned above, the role of Ca^{2+} is also important in the release of intracellular Ca^{2+} reservoirs: "the CICR phenomenon"; CICR is one of the mechanisms explaining why structural disintegration and disturbance of T tubules are an early happening in heart failure.
2. Although cardiac cell action potential is the main trigger for Ca^{2+} release, the first Ca^{2+} release is from the large Ca^{2+} reservoirs of T tubules and T tubules would trigger the release of more Ca^{2+} from SR. As mentioned before, the influx of Ca^{2+} from ECF to interior of cardiac cells through slow (L)-type calcium channels located on the T tubule strengthens the depolarization of *cardiac muscle* cells and causes the plateau phase of depolarization; this feature is special to depolarization of cardiac cells, while in skeletal muscle depolarization, the influx of Ca^{2+} to skeletal cells, through T tubule's slow (L)-type calcium channels, *does not* have any significant role.
3. T tubules are invagination of the cell membrane to the cells; it means that T tubules are in fact part of the extracellular fluid (ECF); so, they have continuous exchange of Ca^{2+} with ECF. Any decrease in Ca^{2+} concentration of the blood results in decreased Ca^{2+} concentration of ECF, which in turn would reduce Ca^{2+} concentration in the intracellular milieu; this is why any decrease in plasma levels of Ca^{2+} is associated with decreased cardiac contractility.

3.2.2.2 Ca^{2+} Homeostasis

Ca^{2+} homeostasis in cardiomyocytes is so important, and any perturbation in its equilibrium state would result in cardiac disturbances. Intracellular Ca^{2+} is considered as a second messenger in cardiac sarcomeres, while its concentration and trends of change exert important effects on "mitochondrial energetic," "cell death or apoptosis," and "the intracellular buffering capacity for controlling stress."

To have this equilibrium in a continuous manner for a lifelong time, a delicate balance between Ca^{2+} influx and Ca^{2+} efflux in cardiomyocytes is a prerequisite: the Ca^{2+} balance has a central role in each cardiac cycle, composed of a systole (contraction) and a diastole (relaxation); although there are a number of states in which influx would exceed efflux or vice versa, a number of subcellular mechanisms work together to modify these fluxes and reach the final equilibrium in such a way to increase the efficacy of myocardial contractions as a result of control in Ca^{2+}homeostasis.

Ca^{2+} surge and Ca^{2+} reuptake are both located inside the cardiomyocytes, and also, both are among the main features of systole and diastole, respectively. This dual phase is seen in all aspects of Ca^{2+} homeostasis, including cardiac contraction, Ca^{2+} flow direction, Ca^{2+} concentration inside each cell, and Ca^{2+} release and reuptake in all potential intracellular elements including mitochondria.

However, this "*dual-phase pattern of* Ca^{2+}" is controlled mainly by four mechanisms:

1. Ca^{2+} influx to the cardiomyocytes (mainly by L-type channels in *systole*: contraction phase)
2. Ca^{2+} release inside the cell (by ryanodine receptor (RyR) in *systole*: contraction phase)
3. Ca^{2+} efflux from the cardiomyocytes (mainly by $3Na^+–1Ca^{2+}$ exchanger (NCX) in *diastole*: relaxation phase)
4. Ca^{2+} reuptake from the cell (by sarcoendoplasmic reticulum Ca^{2+} transport ATPase (SERCA) in *diastole*: relaxation phase)

One of the main etiologic mechanisms for heart failure is "reduced and sluggish Ca^{2+} release and/or slow removal of Ca^{2+}." In these patients, reduced and delayed function of L-type Ca^{2+} channel, slow release of Ca^{2+} from SR, and "delayed activation" of Na^+–Ca^{2+} exchanger (NCX) are among the most important mechanisms involved in the pathogenesis of the disease state (Hohendanner et al. 2014; Zhao et al. 2017).

3.2.2.3 What Are the Controllers of ECC?

The exact mechanisms of ECC are delicately controlled and regulated *mainly* by these proteins:

1. Ryanodine receptor (RyR) family (a class of intracellular Ca^{2+} receptors)
2. Dihydropyridine receptor (DHPR)
3. Calmodulin

Let's once more stress on the fact that Ca^{2+} cycling is the ultimate goal of ECC and the main mechanism responsible for its course, including commencement, continuation, and termination of ECC.

Ca^{2+} would enter the cardiomyocyte cytosol through L-type Ca^{2+} channels (also known as dihydropyridine (DHP)) in cytosol. This primary Ca^{2+} influx would trigger Ca^{2+} release from subsarcolemma SR (i.e., the specific part of the SR which is under the sarcolemma).

> Ca^{2+} cycling is the ultimate goal of ECC and the main managing mechanism.

The functional steps in ECC are as follows (Fabiato and Fabiato 1977, 1978; Fabiato 1983; Swaminathan et al. 2012; Van Petegem 2012; Mattiazzi et al. 2015; Dickson et al. 2016):

1. ECC is started by Ca^{2+} entry into cells through L-type Ca^{2+} channels (i.e., DHP).
2. This initial small amounts of Ca^{2+} trigger type 2 ryanodine receptor (i.e., RyR2)
3. RyR2 is located on the JSR, and when triggered, RyR2 causes huge amounts of Ca^{2+} to be released from SR (the release of large Ca^{2+} amounts after the initial small Ca^{2+} influx is called Ca^{2+}-induced Ca^{2+} release (CICR), a phenomenon first explained by Alexandre Fabiato).

4. In turn, the necessary Ca^{2+} for contraction is released from SR reservoirs.
5. Immediately afterward, interaction of Ca^{2+} with contractile proteins of sarcomere occurs.
6. The above interaction between Ca^{2+} and contractile proteins produces mechanical force of contraction.
7. The Ca^{2+} surge would be resolved by later Ca^{2+}reuptake.
8. Ca^{2+} reuptake is primarily done through a recycling mechanism in SR (SR acts as a very huge intracellular Ca^{2+} reservoir) which happens after occurrence of the contraction.
9. The rest of Ca^{2+} is effluxed outside the cell by a exchanger and anti-port called Na^{+}/Ca^{2+} exchanger (NCX).
10. Ca^{2+} reuptake by SR ends contraction and starts relaxation; Ca^{2+} reuptake is a primary function of a specific protein called sarcoendoplasmic reticulum Ca^{2+} transport ATPase (SERCA) which is an ATP-dependent Ca^{2+} pump in SR; SERCA is also the main protein component of SR.
11. The second main protein of SR is phospholamban which inhibits the function of SERCA; in other words "phospholamban is a major regulator of SERCA pump."
12. SERCA activates Ca^{2+} reuptake and initiates myocardial relaxation, while phospholamban ends the Ca^{2+} reuptake through inhibition of SERCA and, hence, ends the relaxation phase.

Besides SERCA, calmodulin, and phospholamban, there are a number of other main proteins involved in Ca^{2+} reserve and adjustment called calsequestrin, calreticulin, and calmodulin.

Calsequestrin is a Ca^{2+} storing reservoir inside the sarcoplasmic reticulum containing large amounts of calcium which keeps calcium inside SR against its gradient; the release of calcium form calsequestrin is among the main triggering factors for contraction.

Calmodulin (CaM) is an abbreviation for **cal**cium-**modul**ated prote**in**; a small-sized protein with the following characteristics:

- Each molecule of calmodulin binds to $4Ca^{2+}$ ions.
- Calmodulin controls and modulates (i.e., excites or inhibits) two main Ca^{2+} ports which have essential role in ECC,
- Calmodulin controls both slow (L)-type Ca^{2+} channel (located in transverse tubules of the sarcolemma) and also RyR located at JSR,
- So, calmodulin is a multifunctional protein which does its functions through signal transduction and plays the role of the "boss" who controls all the Ca^{2+} bottlenecks in cardiomyocyte.

3.2.3 Contractile Mechanisms and Their Related Processes

The contractile function of the heart is a unique function produced in each of the cardiomyocytes. As mentioned in the previous parts of this chapter (under the title *Cardiac contractile tissue cells*), the cardiac muscle is composed of two muscle masses: "atrial syncytium" and "ventricular syncytium." We can assume each of the two syncytia as a separate "military band" with all the cardiomyocytes working and acting in a cooperated, regulated, and arranged manner, the same as each soldier acts in a military group during a "military march." So, the physical outcome of cardiomyocyte function is force generation, and its physiological outcome is cardiac contraction which in turn would produce cardiac output. However, cardiac output (i.e., physiological role of the heart) is set in a widespread spectrum, in such a way that the body demands are met well in severe exercise as well as deep sleep. Such an adaptive and cooperative capacity for fulfilling demands in a wide range of body physiologic needs is directly dependent on the contractile properties of sarcomere. Part of these mechanisms is discussed here; but, the full nature of these mechanisms, in health or in disease, is far beyond the scope of this book.

As described in the previous pages (under the title *Cardiac contractile tissue cells*), each cardiomyocyte is composed of a number of contractile units or let's say *contractile quantum* which is called *cardiac sarcomere*. So, the main function of cardiomyocyte is produced in sarcomere. As mentioned, each sarcomere is margined by a line named "Z" line; so, each sarcomere is the region of myofilaments between two Z lines. Thin and thick filaments are the main contractile elements of sarcomere.

It would be worth to know that genetic disturbances (including mutations) are an important source for creating pathologies in sarcomere myofilaments; these pathologies would be the origin for a number of cardiac diseases (named sarcomere diseases with genetic origin); among them, a number of hypertrophic or dilated cardiomyopathies, rhythm disorders, and sudden cardiac death could be mentioned.

However, when considering the cellular mechanisms of contraction, the story is much more complicated, containing the following steps:

- Contraction of the cardiomyocyte is composed of a repeated and continuous contraction-relaxation process, being the main function of the sarcomeres.
- We should know that the engine of this contractile process is started with an *ignition switch*, Ca^{2+}, which is the initiator of the contractile process.
- Cardiomyocyte action potential releases Ca^{2+} indirectly from sarcoplasmic reticulum (SR) and directly from DHPR of T tubules.
- At the next step, Ca^{2+} starts the contraction-relaxation process; known as "cross-bridge cycling."
- The contraction-relaxation process is done through the contractile proteins, located in thick and thin filaments discussed in previous sections of this chapter.
- Ca^{2+} concentration which is necessary for activation of concentration in cardiomyocytes is always lower than the "saturation" level: it has been demonstrated that *decreased myofilament response* to effects of Ca^{2+} in the contractile system is one of the main mechanisms for heart failure.

The very unique contractile proteins of sarcomere could be classified as "functional classification" and "structural classification."

1. **Functional classification of sarcomere proteins** divides the sarcomere contractile proteins functionally as two protein classes:
   (a) *Contractile proteins*: the contractile proteins and their supporting structures are mainly composed of actin, myosin, and titin; cardiac contraction is the final outcome of interactions between myofilaments, presented at cellular level as *crossbridges* of myosin head with active site of actin,
   (b) *Regulatory proteins*: contraction of all muscles including cardiac sarcomeres is a very delicate and ordered phenomenon needing precise regulatory and control systems; in sarcomeres, this regulatory function is a duty by the *regulatory proteins* which work "shoulder to shoulder" of contractile proteins to control their crossbridge-induced contractions; the main regulatory proteins are "troponin," "tropomyosin," "tropomodulin," and "myosin-binding protein C"; when sarcomere is in relaxation phase, these proteins attach to actin and myosin to prevent contraction. However, when action potential goes to the activation phase, Ca^{2+} is attached to troponin in order to activate interactions between myosin head and actin; contraction starts immediately afterward.
2. **Structural classification of sarcomere proteins** divides the sarcomere contractile proteins in one of the two following classes:
   - Thick filament
   - Thin filament

These two filaments are formed as inter-digit strands going "in between" each other and coming out in a sliding manner; this sliding back-and-forth movement of thin and thick filaments forms the cardiac "systole" and "diastole," respectively.

Thick Filament

The contractile proteins are the "workforce" of the myocardium; the more the *crossbridges* of actin and myosin, the more the contractile force of the sarcomere. Crossbridges are the result of interactions between myosin head and actin after trigger of Ca^{2+}.

Myosin is the largest and heaviest protein of sarcomere among the others which are in form of rods; being about 15 nm in diameter, it composes thick filament of myofibrils and interacts with actin during contractions as crossbridges; myosin rods are made of myosin molecules in the following features and characteristics:

- One myosin heavy chain (MHC) plus two myosin light chains (MLC) are composed together as a single strand.
- Two single strands twist round each other to produce one molecule of myosin.
- Each myosin molecule has two functional domains, a head (composed of four MLCs and the lever like end of two MHCs) coming out of the main molecule.
- Myosin heads are the *main location* for interactions with actin and create hinge-shaped features, coming out of the bouquet like "lever arm" and are inhibited by

TnI; after interaction with Ca^{2+}, they attach to actin in order to produce crossbridges.
- Three hundred molecules of myosin are attached together in a parallel fashion to form the myosin rod, in which its microscopic figure is similar to a number of parallel golf clubs forming a bouquet, twisting together in an orderly fashion forming the *body of myosin rod*; while their heads are exposed out of the bouquet, the bodies are attached together.

Crossbridges between actin and myosin (the principal mechanism of muscle contraction) are formed repetitively and released after a very short period of time; great amounts of ATP molecules are used for production of actin-myosin interactions and crossbridges leading to muscle contractions. These interactions cause a rotation in myosin along actin filament; the main interaction site is the head and hinge region of myosin.

Myosin-binding protein C (MYBPC) is another important and determining protein of sarcomere, being among the regulator proteins; a number of life-threatening arrhythmias and some types of hypertrophic cardiomyopathies are the results of genetic impairments in this protein; new treatments of heart failure are in development regarding the role of this protein.

Titin is the third most common filament in sarcomere (after actin and myosin), being the main factor for passive features of the myocardium in lower ventricular volumes; this is why the main role of titin is muscular assembly of the heart and its elasticity features. Regarding the molecular structure, titin is a giant filamentous protein, extending as long as "half sarcomere from Z line to M line"; this giant structure of titin provides a continuous link between the Z line and the M line inside each sarcomere; so, titin functions as an extensible filamentous protein to preserve the structural integrity of sarcomere and also to function in sarcomere to reach its normal length after systolic contraction and returning to normal length in diastole. This is why titin has a central role in patients with ischemic or diastolic heart failure.

As it is demonstrated in Figs. 3.5 and 3.11, the force created by titin helps keep the thick filament in its central position in sarcomere, maintaining the balance inside the sarcomere between sarcomere structures during systole and diastole.

Titin could be divided into two main parts: the *extensible part* which is located in the "I band" area of sarcomere and the *non-extensible part* located in the "A band" area of sarcomere. Also, the extensible parts of titin are mainly composed of two segments, both taking part in passive force development of sarcomere during stretch:

- Immunoglobulin-like segment
- PEVK segment in which four amino acids are abundant: proline (P), glutamate (E), valine (V), and lysine (K)

Finally, if we want to describe titin in just a two-word phrase, we could name titin as *molecular spring* of the sarcomere which creates elastic properties for the sarcomere.

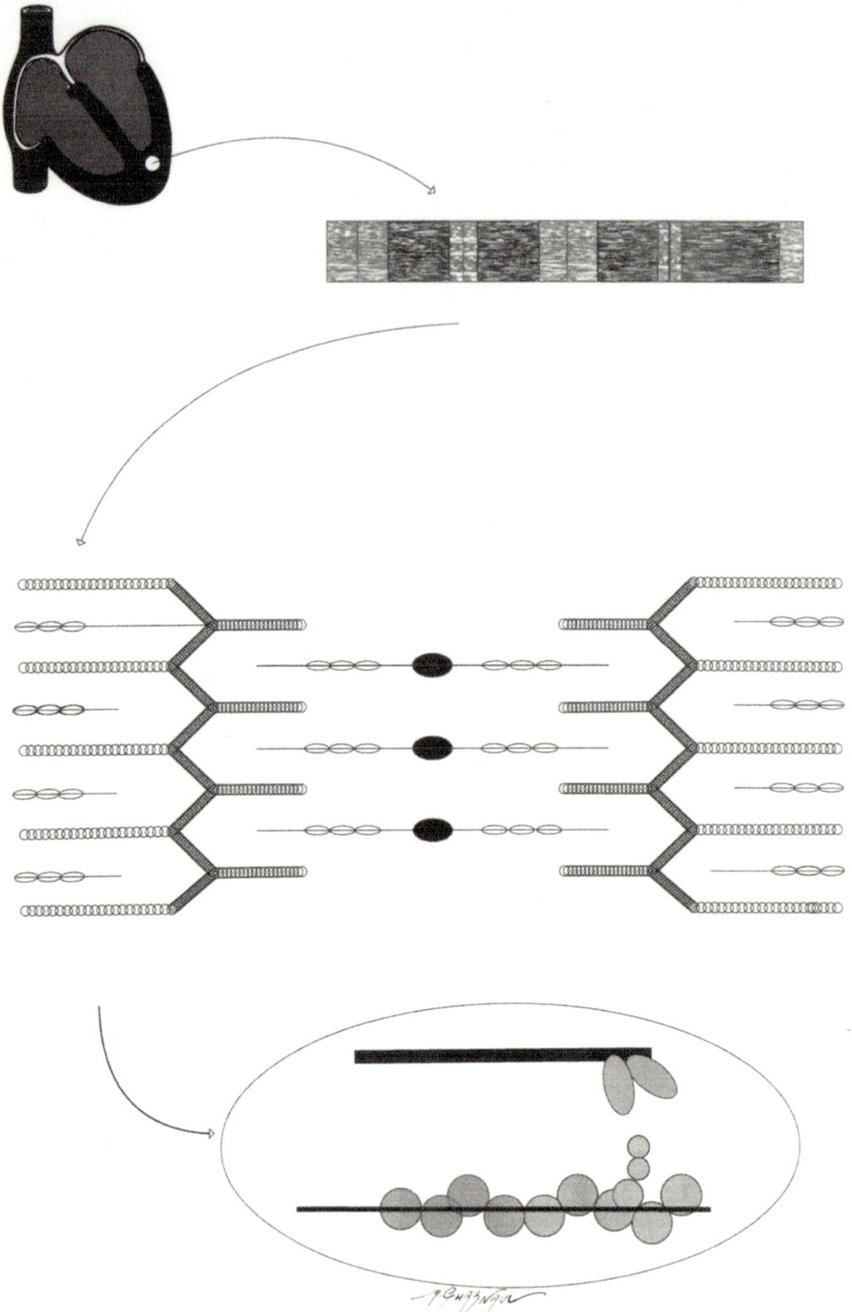

Fig. 3.11 Detailed sarcomere anatomy in different aspects; also, see Figs. 3.2, 3.3, 3.4, and 3.5 (Dabbagh 2014)

Thin filament is composed of the following ingredients discussed here; if we consider an "imaginary unit" for thin filament, this unit consists of:

- Two F actin strands
- Two tropomyosin strands (i.e., two TM)
- Three troponin complex (i.e., three Tn)

These "imaginary units" are attached together in a row, from head to tail, to compose the thin filament in such a way that:

- F actin (the actin strand) makes the foundation of the filament.
- The two tropomyosin strands lie in the two grooves of the filament as long as the entire thin filament.
- Troponin complexes are attached to actin filament at defined intervals.

Actin: actin is one of the main contractile proteins and also a main protein of the thin filament; actin filaments are double-stranded filaments composed of actin molecules, arranged in a special configuration; actin is a 43 kd, 7 nm globular protein *G actin*; 13 G actin monomers are polymerized to form the two-stranded filament *F actin* which is a 360 degrees twisted filament as the contractile element. F actin in cardiomyocytes is mainly "alpha actin" isomer. Pathogenic mutations in actin-related genes are responsible for some cardiac diseases like idiopathic dilated cardiomyopathy.

Tropomyosin (TM) is a part of the thin filament, being an inhibitory protein; this protein is formed as α-coiled coil dimmers attached head to tail; in other words, each TM molecule is attached to another TM molecule; then, these two twist round each other to create the first coil, and afterward, the first coil twists once more round itself to produce the coiled coil; this final configuration is repeatedly formed in thin filament and is located inside the groove of F actin between two adjacent lines of actin monomers in such a way that each TM is in attachment with seven actin monomers; however, this line of repeated TM molecules are attached together from the head of one molecule to the tail of the next and so on. This special configuration of TM has a very determining role in coordination and cooperation of the functions of thin filament.

Troponin is part of the thin filament; each troponin complex is attached to one actin monomer after each seven repeated monomers; troponin is in fact a complex of three proteins totally named as troponin complex (Tn):

- Troponin C (TnC) is the Ca^{2+} receptor protein in the contraction-relaxation process; four Ca^{2+} could attach to each TnC molecule.
- Troponin I (TnI) binds to actin to inhibit actin-myosin interaction.
- Troponin T (TnT) is responsible for attachment of troponin to TM; it binds to TM on one side and on the other side binds to TnC and TnI.

Tropomodulin is a regulatory filament located at the end of actin to prevent excessive elongation of the filament.

Now, let's once go back to Ca^{2+} which is the *ignition switch* of the contraction-relaxation process. When Ca^{2+} binds to TnC, there is a structural change in TnI which would move away from F actin, in such a way to expose the special site on actin for attachment of myosin head; after Ca^{2+} removal from TnC, TnI resumes its primary structural form to inhibit the actin-myosin attachment. TnI-actin interaction has an inhibitory nature; hence, the release of TnI from actin causes detachment of actin from one myosin head and its attachment to another myosin head; the detachment-attachment of actin-myosin head is an ATP-consuming process.

TnC and TnI form the head of Tn, while TnT forms the tail of Tn. These three subunits of troponin have determining roles in contraction-relaxation phases of cardiomyocytes. There are a series of *pathogenic mutations* in amino acid sequence of TnI, resulting in impaired function of TnI as an inhibitory protein in cardiomyocyte contractile system, leading to some type of "diastolic dysfunction" or "hypertrophic/restrictive cardiomyopathies"; also, TnI has the diagnostic role in myocardial infarction.

The specific site for Ca^{2+} in TnC is the unique location and the sole place which has a direct and central role in contraction process of cardiomyocytes through Ca^{2+}, performing its function through the following mechanism:

- When Ca^{2+} is attached to TnC, it would induce a "structural change" in troponin.
- This configuration change will result in dissociation of tropomyosin from actin.
- Then, when actin is released, "myosin attachment site" on actin filament is freed.
- Myosin attachment site could start anew the "crossbridge formation."
- "Inappropriate phosphorylation of sarcomere contractile proteins" especially *troponin* and *myosin* should be mentioned among the important etiologies for heart failure (like ventricular hypertrophy, diabetic cardiomyopathy, or heart failure).

The following factors are the main determinants of force generation in cardiac sarcomere:

- Ca^{2+} activation level (i.e., level of sensitivity of sarcomere proteins to Ca^{2+}).
- Sarcomere length (i.e., the Frank-Starling relationship).
- Myofilament phosphorylation and other changes in sarcomere proteins (this is why in some cardiac pathologies phosphorylation of cardiac contractile proteins has a central role in progress of the disease).

On the other hand, the two latter factors could affect the sensitivity of contractile filaments to Ca^{2+} (Fig. 3.11 and Table 3.4).

Table 3.4 A summary of the main sarcomere proteins

	Thick filament	Thin filament
Contractile proteins	Myosin Titin	Actin
Regulatory proteins	Myosin-binding protein C	Tropomyosin Troponin Tropomodulin

McLachlan and Stewart (1975), Hill et al. (1980), White et al. (1987), Pan et al. (1989), Schoenberg (1993), Thierfelder et al. (1994), Farah and Reinach (1995), Marston et al. (1998), Redwood et al. (1999), Wick (1999), Gordon et al. (2000), Linke (2000a, b), Morimoto and Goto (2000), Craig and Lehman (2001), Agarkova et al. (2003), Marston and Redwood (2003), Agarkova and Perriard (2005), Granzier et al. (2005), Bragadeesh et al. (2007), LeWinter et al. (2007), Vahebi et al. (2007), Hitchcock-DeGregori (2008), Kobayashi et al. (2008), Ohtsuki and Morimoto (2008), Rice et al. (2008), Teerlink (2009), Campbell (2010), Offer and Ranatunga (2010), Gautel (2011), Kruger and Linke (2011), Malik et al. (2011), Malik and Morgan (2011), McDonald (2011), Posch et al. (2011), Tardiff (2011), Balse et al. (2012), Eisner et al. (2012), Herzog et al. (2012), Kajioka et al. (2012), Knoll (2012), Kuster et al. (2012), ter Keurs (2012), and Dabbagh (2014)

3.3 Cardiac Cycle and Cardiac Work

3.3.1 Normal Cardiac Cycle

The final goal of all cardiac treatments (medical, surgical, or interventional) is to change the situation from a diseased pathologic heart toward a normal physiologic heart, which would pump the blood appropriately. In other words, our interventions need to go, as much as possible, toward a normal physiologic heart which could pump the blood appropriately with appropriate force and in appropriate time manner. In other words, we need to go, as much as possible, toward a normal cardiac physiology or, more specifically, a normal *cardiac cycle*, filling normally in diastole (with appropriate time schedule and normal pressure, without overpressurizing the pulmonary vasculature) and then ejecting enough blood in systole. The above process could be translated into a four-phase repetitive cycle, as follows:

Phase 1—**diastolic filling** during which the atrioventricular valves (i.e., mitral and tricuspid) open, while aortic and pulmonary valves are closed. In this phase, the ventricular cavity is filled with blood based on three factors:

- Pressure gradient between atria and ventricles
- Ventricular diastolic compliance
- Atrial contraction (atrial kick)

Phase 2—**isovolumic systole** during which the ventricular cavity pressure raises without any volume change. The atrioventricular valves are closed in early stages of this phase. However, in a fraction of time, the intracavity pressure increases to a critical level which is more than aortic and pulmonary valves, going to the next phase.

Phase 3—**systolic ejection** in which the blood is pushed with a high pressure to the aorta or pulmonary bed, i.e., blood ejection, to perfuse each of the two vascular beds. The size of the ventricles decreases as the blood ejects and their blood content exits as fast as possible.

Phase 4—**isovolumic relaxation** in which both ventricles are relaxed, starting to increase their size. The aortic and pulmonary valves are closed due to decreased intraventricular pressure, while mitral and tricuspid valves begin to open at the end of this phase. Again, the cardiac cycle goes to phase 1 to start a new cycle (Tanaka et al. 1993; Gibson and Francis 2003; Chatterjee 2012).

3.3.2 Cardiac Work

Cardiac work: cardiac work implies the product of myocardial performance and is the algebraic sum of two different items; first, the *external work* which is equivalent to the total myocardial energy used for ejecting the blood out of the ventricles to the systemic and pulmonary vascular bed. The second parameter is the *internal work* which is the total energy needed by myocardial tissue to maintain cell energetic, myocardial integrity, and homeostasis of cardiomyocytes. For calculating the external work, we use the product of "*stroke work* multiplied by *ventricular cavity pressure*." Also, the external work is equal to "end diastolic volume (preload)" multiplied by "mean arterial pressure (afterload)." However, we usually calculate the external work by calculating the area under curve of pressure-volume loop of the left ventricle (i.e., LV pressure-volume AUC). The main myocardial need for energy reserve and its oxygen consumption is used for external work; however, myocardial ischemia would jeopardize mainly the external work. There are a number of clinical indices for assessment of cardiac work. Since we could not measure the cellular energetic easily in clinical practice, we use a number of indices which are discussed here. These are stroke volume, cardiac output, and ejection fraction.

Stroke volume: each "stroke volume" is the amount of the blood ejected from the heart in each ventricular beat. Stroke volume (SV) is the result of "end diastolic volume (EDV) minus end systolic volume (ESV)" or, simply, "SV = EDV - ESV." According to this equation, both EDV and ESV could affect SV. However, which factors could affect EDV and ESV?

- EDV depends directly at two factors:
  1. **Venous return** is the returned blood to the ventricles from veins, i.e., from inferior and superior vena cava (IVC and SVC) to RV and from pulmonary veins to LV.
  2. Diastolic time of ventricular filling or simply **filling time** which is the time in diastole that the blood accumulates in ventricles; the longer the filling time, the more would be SV.
- ESV depends on three factors:
  1. **Preload** is the amount of ventricular stretching; the more stretch in the ventricle, the more contractile force; this is discussed more in the section of "Frank-Starling relationship"; the relationship between preload and ESV is a converse relationship.

2. **Contractility** is the contractile force of the myocardium; this factor has a converse relationship with ESV; i.e., the more contractility, the less volume would remain in the ventricle; however, there are a multitude of factors affecting contractility which are discussed later.
3. **Afterload** is the resistance against the pumping action of ventricles; there is a direct relationship between ESV and afterload; for LV, afterload is mainly the systemic vascular resistance (SVR) which is about 90% of LV afterload; however, pulmonary vascular resistance (PVR) produces about 50% of RV afterload, and the RV wall stress is responsible for the other half of RV afterload.

Cardiac output abbreviated as CO is the amount of blood which is pumped out of the heart during a 1 min interval; so, CO is the product of SV multiplied by heart rate; so, "cardiac output (mL/min) = stroke volume (mL/beat) × heart rate (beat/min)" or simply CO = HR × SV.

Ejection fraction: another important variable is ejection fraction or more commonly known as "EF". EF is calculated based on this equation: EF=SV/EDV. (In this formula, EDV stands for end diastolic volume.) Usually EF is expressed in percentage. Normal EF is usually between 55 and 70%, though more than 50% is considered normal for EF and consider patients having EF > 50% as good LV performance. EF is directly a very determining index of cardiac function and global clinical outcome. Patients with EF < 30% are often considered as very high-risk cases impressing the global outcome.

Among the above three main factors (i.e., SV, ESV, and EDV), the cardiac work is much related to EDV and less to the other two factors; this is due to the length-tension concept of sarcomere which affects the cardiac contractility, cardiac work, and cardiac output more than the others. To understand this latter fact, we have to discuss Frank-Starling relationship in the next paragraph (Germano et al. 1995; Ababneh et al. 2000; Rozanski et al. 2000; Sharir et al. 2006; Lomsky et al. 2008; Mahadevan et al. 2008).

3.3.3 Frank-Starling Relationship

Otto Frank in 1895 and Ernest Starling, two decades later, demonstrated in animal models that the heart has a very important basic and intrinsic characteristic: "length-dependent activation" or the "Frank-Starling relationship."

The Frank-Starling relationship tells us that in the physiologic range, the more blood accumulated in each of the ventricles in diastole, the more pump output would be pushed out in systole. This interesting feature is seen even when the heart is removed out from the body to work in a lab environment. So, the Frank-Starling relationship tells us that the heart has a wide range of capacity for adaptation against preload, afterload, and their related imposed work; this fundamental concept of cardiac physiology explains the ability of the heart to change its contractile response under different physiologic and pathologic states, in such a way to save the cardiac output as much appropriate as possible to physiologic body demands. This adaptation capacity is both due to the cellular structure of the heart (especially the sarcomere structure) and also the effects of neurohormonal effectors and the cardiac reflexes. So, considering these length-force changes, we reach to a final conclusion which is the general concept that Frank-Starling relationship: within a defined length of sarcomere, there is a clear and direct "optimal interaction length" for sarcomere; however, in human sarcomere, this "optimal length" between actin and myosin is when the sarcomere length equals 2.2 μ. The cellular basis for Frank-Starling relationship is in general known as "length-dependent activation," which is a mechanism seen in every other sarcomere in all of the cardiomyocytes. In physiologic measurements of the Frank-Starling relationship, any sudden increase in diastolic length of a contractile segment of cardiomyocyte (i.e., sarcomere) would result in a sudden increase of its systolic force reaching a plateau after a short time. Before this plateau, the more length of sarcomere, the more force produced by myocardium; however, after reaching this plateau, the sarcomere could not produce more contraction since the actin and myosin heads start going far from each other and the sarcomere length goes far from its optimal length. Meanwhile, any sudden decrease in diastolic length of the contractile elements would result in decreased systolic force, again reaching a plateau phase after a short time. Though Frank-Starling relationship has been discovered for more than 100 years, its underlying mechanism(s) are not fully clear yet. In other words, its cellular and subcellular mechanisms are not limited to one single mechanism. Instead, Frank-Starling relationship is "the end product of a complex system of interacting elements"; however, there are many different molecular mechanisms cooperating together in each of the cardiac sarcomeres "to produce strain-dependent activation." Here, two main classes for its mechanisms have been introduced:

- First, "increased diastolic tension" results in "increased number of cross-bridges" which in turn will improve the "myofilaments overlap" status, favoring more effective contractions. In other words, the interdigitations of actin and myosin in diastole will become more effective in producing systolic contractions. Though this is the main mechanism, another proposed mechanism seems important.
- Second, improved efficacy of sarcomere contractile function to produce increased contractile force in response to Ca^{2+} concentration is seen when the length of the sarcomere is increased. In other words, according to this mechanism, Frank-Starling relationship is due to improved response of myofilaments to Ca^{2+} when the length of the sarcomere is increased. The interested reader could find more extended explanations in other sources, being beyond the scope of this chapter (Markwalder and Starling 1914; Patterson et al. 1914; Fuchs and Smith 2001; Solaro 2007; Bollensdorff et al. 2011; Campbell 2011; Ribaric and Kordas 2012; Cingolani et al. 2013; Goldhaber and Philipson 2013; Chaui-Berlinck and Monteiro 2017; Sequeira and van der Velden 2017).

3.4 Cardiac Reflexes

3.4.1 Bainbridge Reflex

Bainbridge reflex was described first in 1915 by Francis Bainbridge (English physiologist, 1874–1921). He discovered and demonstrated that "saline or blood infusion into the jugular vein of the anesthetized dog" would result in reflex tachycardia. This reflex is also called the "atrial reflex" and involves increased heart rate in response to dilation of "the main systemic veins, left and right atrium." In response to dilation of the right atrium, stretch receptors located in the right atrium (i.e., venoatrial stretch receptors) are activated and send their impulse through the vagus nerve (tenth cranial nerve) to CNS; this is why the reflex is blocked if the patient is premedicated with atropine. Also, in animal studies, this reflex is blocked by "bilateral vagotomy or combined cholinergic and beta-adrenergic blockades." After being processed in the CNS, the response to the afferent impulse would result in increased sympathetic tone, which in turn would cause increased contractility and tachycardia which finally helps emptying of the heart. Simply saying, the "Bainbridge reflex" causes "hypervolemia-induced tachycardia." The efferent limb of the reflex is mediated through the sympathetic pathways. In cardiovascular physiologic pathways, the Bainbridge reflex plays an important role and has control over heart rate and other hemodynamic variables; also, the effects of the Bainbridge reflex are in contrary to the effects of the "carotid baroreceptor reflex." This reflex is sensed in the atria through the atrial type B mechanoreceptors; these receptors are located at the junction of venae cavae and the right atria and the junction of pulmonary veins and left atria, which in turn would trigger the neural pathway of the reflex (Vatner and Zimpfer 1981; Boettcher et al. 1982; Hakumaki 1987; Hajdu et al. 1991; Barbieri et al. 2002; Crystal and Salem 2012; Kuhtz-Buschbeck et al. 2017).

3.4.2 Baroreceptors Reflex (or Carotid Sinus Reflex)

This reflex results in regulation of blood pressure, especially if it is highly elevated or severely depressed; however, the reflex is usually elicited in systolic blood pressures over 150–170 mmHg; the other part of the reflex is not often seen when the systolic blood pressure is below 50–60 mmHg. However, in patients with underlying hypertension or atherosclerosis or in the elderly, the reflex thresholds might be altered, and at times, the reflex would not be seen partially or totally. The main receptors of this reflex are located in the walls of carotid arteries and aortic arch, and its sequence is as follows:

- The circumferential and longitudinal stretch receptors are located in carotid sinus and aortic arch; increased blood pressure triggers these receptors leading to impulse firing.

- The transport of impulse from carotid sinus is through the ninth cranial nerve and from the aortic arch through the tenth cranial nerve.
- The impulses from these two locations are sent to the nucleus solitaries in the medullary cardio-regulatory and vasomotor centers.
- The nucleus solitaries, however, have two different parts: the first part is lateral and rostral, known as the "pressor center," and the second part is located at the central and caudal part which is known as the "depressor" center; in these two parts, the limbic and hypothalamic inputs are integrated to create the final response as either of the two following responses:
- Decreased *sympathetic* tone (mainly through inhibition of sympathetic chain and sympathetic nerves) leading to hypotension and bradycardia and also decreased vascular tone, leading to blood vessel dilation (i.e., systemic vasodilation).
- Increased *parasympathetic* tone (mainly through vagus nerve) leading to decreased heart rate and decreased myocardial contractility.
- These interactions would bring the blood pressure to normal, hence relieving the pressure over the baroreceptors.
- If the initial event is decreased blood pressure, the decreased tone on the baroreceptors would initiate the opposite response (Vasquez et al. 1997; Pilowsky and Goodchild 2002; Campagna and Carter 2003; Kashihara 2009; de Leeuw et al. 2017; Kuhtz-Buschbeck et al. 2017).

3.4.3 Bezold-Jarisch Reflex

This reflex, known as a "cardioinhibitory" reflex, was described first by *von Bezold* and *Hirt* in 1867; it was more studied and completed in the late 1930s by *Adolf Jarisch* and *Richter*. Describing the reflex in brief, it is a triad of "bradycardia, hypotension, and peripheral vasodilation" usually accompanied with hypopnea or apnea. Also, coronary artery vasodilation has been mentioned among the items of the reflex. This reflex seems to have some cardioprotective effects; for example, it is seen during some myocardial stress states including during acute phase of myocardial ischemia, infarction, or reperfusion syndrome, especially when involving posterior or inferior myocardial walls.

The main physiologic phenomenon underlying the reflex is *parasympathetic* overactivity; however, some degrees of *sympathetic* inhibition have an etiologic role in the reflex. The sequence of the reflex in brief is as follows:

- The reflex is initiated after mechanical stimuli (like volume overload or pressure) or chemical stimuli (like metabolites of myocardial ischemia or chemicals like veratrum alkaloids) which trigger the specific receptors of the reflex in the heart.
- The sensors of the reflex are located in a number of locations over the cardiac walls including the left ventricle wall, the atrial walls, atrial-caval junctions, and other cardiac chambers.
- The majority of the afferent fibers are nonmyelinated C fibers (75% of the afferent pathways located over all the cardiac chambers) and myelinated fibers (25%

of the afferent pathways located in the atrial walls and the atrial-caval junctions).

- The afferent fibers inhibit the medullary vasomotor center which would have two effects: directly leads to bradycardia and also suppresses the sympathetic output.
- Decreased sympathetic output leads to decreased peripheral vascular tone leading to peripheral vasodilation, presented as systemic hypotension (Robertson et al. 1985; Hakumaki 1987; Meyrelles et al. 1997; Campagna and Carter 2003; Kashihara et al. 2004; Salo et al. 2007; Kashihara 2009; Kuhtz-Buschbeck et al. 2017; Raut et al. 2017).

3.4.4 Valsalva Maneuver

The "Valsalva maneuver" first described by Valsalva in 1704 is the name for a cardiac reflex starting with a forced expiration against a "closed glottis"; this act results in sudden increase of intrathoracic pressure resulting in increased central venous pressure (CVP); the increased CVP) would cause decreased venous return which leads to decreased "cardiac output" and decreased blood pressure. The decreased blood pressure would be sensed by baroreceptors located in the arterial system and would stimulate the sympathetic pathways leading to tachycardia. After glottis opening, venous return would be resumed leading to increased contractility, and finally, the blood pressure returns to normal which this time would inhibit the baroreceptors leading to "normalized" heart rate; all these changes are as a matter of fact "a sequence of rapid changes in preload and afterload stress" imposed to the heart; this maneuver has a number of clinical therapeutic and diagnostic implications (Sharpey-Schafer 1955; Porth et al. 1984; Smith 2012; Wang et al. 2013; Goldstein and Cheshire 2017).

3.4.5 Cushing Reflex

The Cushing reflex was introduced in 1901–1902 by Harvey Cushing (1869–1939) and is presented clinically as a triad of:

- Bradycardia
- Hypertension: presented as increased systolic blood pressure and wide pulse pressure
- Respiratory depression: presented as respiratory irregularity leading to bradypnea and apnea

This reflex is due to increased ICP (often an abrupt increase of ICP), and many times this clinical presentation is associated with cerebral herniation and death; in other words, the Cushing reflex is associated with the cerebral perfusion status; increased cerebrospinal fluid (CSF) production or its decreased reabsorption or, in another way, a mass effect in the CNS would lead to increased intracranial pressure which causes cerebral ischemia; however, cerebral ischemia would trigger sympathetic activity in an attempt to compensate for reduced cerebral perfusion leading to increased heart rate, blood pressure, and myocardial contractility; the increased blood pressure would be sensed by the baroreceptors in the aortic arch and carotid sinus, which leads to reflex bradycardia, well known in Cushing reflex; finally, the triad usually seen after elicitation of Cushing reflex is "increased systolic and pulse pressure with bradycardia and respiratory irregularity" all due to increased intracranial pressure (Grady and Blaumanis 1988; Dickinson 1990; Ayling 2002; Fodstad et al. 2006; Molnar et al. 2008; Wan et al. 2008; Robbins et al. 2016).

3.4.6 Oculocardiac Reflex

This reflex is elicited due to traction on the extraocular muscles (especially rectus medialis) or pain in the eyeball. The pathway of this reflex is as follows:

- The afferent limb of the reflex passes through the ophthalmic division of the fifth cranial nerve (trigeminal nerve); the other branches of the trigeminal nerve (maxillary and mandibular branches) might also be involved.
- The impulses go to CNS, i.e., trigeminal sensory nucleus.
- The efferent limb of the reflex is the tenth cranial nerve (vagus nerve) which causes sinus bradycardia as the final clinical presentation of the reflex; at times, junctional rhythms, asystole or other types of arrhythmias, atrioventricular blocks, or hypotension may occur.

The frequency of occurrence of the reflex is diminished with aging and also could be somewhat prevented by anticholinergic pretreatment, like atropine (Lang et al. 1991; Smith 1994; Gao et al. 1997; Seshubabu 1998; Kim et al. 2000, 2012; Paton et al. 2005; Chung et al. 2008; Yi and Jee 2008; Arasho et al. 2009; Simon 2010; Tsai and Heitz 2012; Karaman et al. 2016; Nicholson et al. 2017).

3.4.7 Chemoreceptor Reflex

This reflex is another important one among the cardiac reflexes.

- Chemoreceptors are located in carotid body and aortic arch.
- Acidosis, hypercarbia (increased CO_2 pressure in the blood), or a drop in blood oxygen pressure triggers the chemoreceptors.
- Afferent nerves are the ninth (glossopharyngeal) and tenth (vagus) cranial nerves.
- These nerves send the impulses to the medulla.
- The response would be increased sympathetic tone to compensate for hypoxia and hypercarbia.

- However, if hypoxia and hypercarbia do not resolve, the response would be as parasympathetic stimulation to decrease heart rate and oxygen demands (Schultz and Sun 2000; Schultz and Li 2007; Ding et al. 2011; Schultz 2011; Campanucci et al. 2012; Schultz et al. 2012; Schultz and Marcus 2012; Dampney 2016).

References

Ababneh AA, Sciacca RR, Kim B, Bergmann SR. Normal limits for left ventricular ejection fraction and volumes estimated with gated myocardial perfusion imaging in patients with normal exercise test results: influence of tracer, gender, and acquisition camera. J Nucl Cardiol. 2000;7:661–8.

Abbott BC, Ritchie JM. Early tension relaxation during a muscle twitch. J Physiol. 1951;113:330–5.

Abdelmeguid NE, Sorour JM. A comparative ultrastructural study of the cardiac and skeletal striated muscles of the skink. Funct Dev Morphol. 1992;2:147–50.

Agarkova I, Ehler E, Lange S, Schoenauer R, Perriard JC. M-band: a safeguard for sarcomere stability? J Muscle Res Cell Motil. 2003;24:191–203.

Agarkova I, Perriard JC. The M-band: an elastic web that crosslinks thick filaments in the center of the sarcomere. Trends Cell Biol. 2005;15:477–85.

Alberts B, Johnson A, Lewis J, et al., editors. Molecular biology of the cell. 4th ed. New York: Garland Science; 2002.

Amanfu RK, Saucerman JJ. Cardiac models in drug discovery and development: a review. Crit Rev Biomed Eng. 2011;39:379–95.

Anderson EJ, Katunga LA, Willis MS. Mitochondria as a source and target of lipid peroxidation products in healthy and diseased heart. Clin Exp Pharmacol Physiol. 2012;39:179–93.

Anderson RH, Razavi R, Taylor AM. Cardiac anatomy revisited. J Anat. 2004;205:159–77.

Anderson RH, Yanni J, Boyett MR, Chandler NJ, Dobrzynski H. The anatomy of the cardiac conduction system. Clin Anat. 2009;22:99–113.

Anwar AM, Geleijnse ML, Soliman OI, McGhie JS, Frowijn R, Nemes A, van den Bosch AE, Galema TW, Ten Cate FJ. Assessment of normal tricuspid valve anatomy in adults by real-time three-dimensional echocardiography. Int J Card Imaging. 2007;23:717–24.

Arasho B, Sandu N, Spiriev T, Prabhakar H, Schaller B. Management of the trigeminocardiac reflex: facts and own experience. Neurol India. 2009;57:375–80.

Arias-Calderon M, Almarza G, Diaz-Vegas A, Contreras-Ferrat A, Valladares D, Casas M, Toledo H, Jaimovich E, Buvinic S. Characterization of a multiprotein complex involved in excitation-transcription coupling of skeletal muscle. Skelet Muscle. 2016;6:15.

Aronsen JM, Swift F, Sejersted OM. Cardiac sodium transport and excitation-contraction coupling. J Mol Cell Cardiol. 2013;61:11–9.

Atkinson A, Inada S, Li J, Tellez JO, Yanni J, Sleiman R, Allah EA, Anderson RH, Zhang H, Boyett MR, Dobrzynski H. Anatomical and molecular mapping of the left and right ventricular his-Purkinje conduction networks. J Mol Cell Cardiol. 2011;51:689–701.

Atkinson AJ, Logantha SJ, Hao G, Yanni J, Fedorenko O, Sinha A, Gilbert SH, Benson AP, Buckley DL, Anderson RH, Boyett MR, Dobrzynski H. Functional, anatomical, and molecular investigation of the cardiac conduction system and arrhythmogenic atrioventricular ring tissue in the rat heart. J Am Heart Assoc. 2013;2:e000246.

Ayling J. Managing head injuries. Emerg Med Serv. 2002;31:42.

Balse E, Steele DF, Abriel H, Coulombe A, Fedida D, Hatem SN. Dynamic of ion channel expression at the plasma membrane of cardiomyocytes. Physiol Rev. 2012;92:1317–58.

Barbieri R, Triedman JK, Saul JP. Heart rate control and mechanical cardiopulmonary coupling to assess central volume: a systems analysis. Am J Phys Regul Integr Comp Phys. 2002;283:R1210–20.

Barclay CJ. Energy demand and supply in human skeletal muscle. J Muscle Res Cell Motil. 2017;38(2):143–55.
Bazgir B, Fathi R, Rezazadeh Valojerdi M, Mozdziak P, Asgari A. Satellite cells contribution to exercise mediated muscle hypertrophy and repair. Cell J. 2017;18:473–84.
Bennett BC, Purdy MD, Baker KA, Acharya C, McIntire WE, Stevens RC, Zhang Q, Harris AL, Abagyan R, Yeager M. An electrostatic mechanism for Ca(2+)-mediated regulation of gap junction channels. Nat Commun. 2016;7:8770.
Berisha F, Nikolaev VO. Cyclic nucleotide imaging and cardiovascular disease. Pharmacol Ther. 2017;175:107–15.
Bickler PE, Fahlman CS. Moderate increases in intracellular calcium activate neuroprotective signals in hippocampal neurons. Neuroscience. 2004;127:673–83.
Bingen BO, Askar SF, Schalij MJ, Kazbanov IV, Ypey DL, Panfilov AV, Pijnappels DA. Prolongation of minimal action potential duration in sustained fibrillation decreases complexity by transient destabilization. Cardiovasc Res. 2013;97(1):161–70.
Boettcher DH, Zimpfer M, Vatner SF. Phylogenesis of the Bainbridge reflex. Am J Phys. 1982;242:R244–6.
Bohnert KR, McMillan JD, Kumar A. Emerging roles of ER stress and unfolded protein response pathways in skeletal muscle health and disease. J Cell Physiol. 2018;233(1):67–78.
Bollensdorff C, Lookin O, Kohl P. Assessment of contractility in intact ventricular cardiomyocytes using the dimensionless 'Frank-Starling Gain' index. Pflugers Arch. 2011;462:39–48.
Borg TK, Sullivan T, Ivy J. Functional arrangement of connective tissue in striated muscle with emphasis on cardiac muscle. Scan Electron Microsc. 1982:1775–84.
Boyden PA, Gardner PI, Wit AL. Action potentials of cardiac muscle in healing infarcts: response to norepinephrine and caffeine. J Mol Cell Cardiol. 1988;20:525–37.
Bragadeesh TK, Mathur G, Clark AL, Cleland JG. Novel cardiac myosin activators for acute heart failure. Expert Opin Investig Drugs. 2007;16:1541–8.
Brunello L, Slabaugh JL, Radwanski PB, Ho HT, Belevych AE, Lou Q, Chen H, Napolitano C, Lodola F, Priori SG, Fedorov VV, Volpe P, Fill M, Janssen PM, Gyorke S. Decreased RyR2 refractoriness determines myocardial synchronization of aberrant Ca2+ release in a genetic model of arrhythmia. Proc Natl Acad Sci U S A. 2013;110:10312–7.
Bucchi A, Barbuti A, Baruscotti M, DiFrancesco D. Heart rate reduction via selective 'funny' channel blockers. Curr Opin Pharmacol. 2007;7:208–13.
Burgoyne T, Muhamad F, Luther PK. Visualization of cardiac muscle thin filaments and measurement of their lengths by electron tomography. Cardiovasc Res. 2008;77:707–12.
Calore M, Lorenzon A, De Bortoli M, Poloni G, Rampazzo A. Arrhythmogenic cardiomyopathy: a disease of intercalated discs. Cell Tissue Res. 2015;360:491–500.
Campagna JA, Carter C. Clinical relevance of the Bezold-Jarisch reflex. Anesthesiology. 2003;98:1250–60.
Campanucci VA, Dookhoo L, Vollmer C, Nurse CA. Modulation of the carotid body sensory discharge by NO: an up-dated hypothesis. Respir Physiol Neurobiol. 2012;184:149–57.
Campbell KS. Short-range mechanical properties of skeletal and cardiac muscles. Adv Exp Med Biol. 2010;682:223–46.
Campbell KS. Impact of myocyte strain on cardiac myofilament activation. Pflugers Arch. 2011;462:3–14.
Chatterjee K. Pathophysiology of systolic and diastolic heart failure. Med Clin North Am. 2012;96:891–9.
Chaui-Berlinck JG, Monteiro LHA. Frank-Starling mechanism and short-term adjustment of cardiac flow. J Exp Biol. 2017;220(Pt 23):4391–8.
Chen PS, Joung B, Shinohara T, Das M, Chen Z, Lin SF. The initiation of the heart beat. Circ J. 2010;74:221–5.
Chung CJ, Lee JM, Choi SR, Lee SC, Lee JH. Effect of remifentanil on oculocardiac reflex in paediatric strabismus surgery. Acta Anaesthesiol Scand. 2008;52:1273–7.
Cingolani HE, Perez NG, Cingolani OH, Ennis IL. The Anrep effect: 100 years later. Am J Phys Heart Circ Phys. 2013;304:H175–82.

Coronel R, Janse MJ, Opthof T, Wilde AA, Taggart P. Postrepolarization refractoriness in acute ischemia and after antiarrhythmic drug administration: action potential duration is not always an index of the refractory period. Heart Rhythm. 2012;9:977–82.
Craig R, Lehman W. Crossbridge and tropomyosin positions observed in native, interacting thick and thin filaments. J Mol Biol. 2001;311:1027–36.
Crystal GJ, Salem MR. The Bainbridge and the "reverse" Bainbridge reflexes: history, physiology, and clinical relevance. Anesth Analg. 2012;114:520–32.
Currie S. Cardiac ryanodine receptor phosphorylation by CaM kinase II: keeping the balance right. Front Biosci. 2009;14:5134–56.
Dabbagh A. Cardiac physiology. In: Dabbagh A, Esmailian F, Aranki S, editors. Postoperative critical care for cardiac surgical patients. 1st ed. New York: Springer; 2014. p. 1–39.
Dabbagh A, Imani A, Rajaei S. Pediatric cardiovascular physiology. In: Dabbagh A, Conte AH, Lubin L, editors. Congenital heart disease in pediatric and adult patients: anesthetic and perioperative management. 1st ed. New York: Springer; 2017. p. 65–116.
Dampney RA. Central neural control of the cardiovascular system: current perspectives. Adv Physiol Educ. 2016;40:283–96.
de Leeuw PW, Bisognano JD, Bakris GL, Nadim MK, Haller H, Kroon AA. Sustained reduction of blood pressure with baroreceptor activation therapy: results of the 6-year open follow-up. Hypertension. 2017;69:836–43.
Dell'Italia LJ. Anatomy and physiology of the right ventricle. Cardiol Clin. 2012;30:167–87.
Delmar M, Makita N. Cardiac connexins, mutations and arrhythmias. Curr Opin Cardiol. 2012;27:236–41.
Deng D, Jiao P, Ye X, Xia L. An image-based model of the whole human heart with detailed anatomical structure and fiber orientation. Comput Math Methods Med. 2012;2012:891070.
Desplantez T, Dupont E, Severs NJ, Weingart R. Gap junction channels and cardiac impulse propagation. J Membr Biol. 2007;218:13–28.
Dickinson CJ. Reappraisal of the Cushing reflex: the most powerful neural blood pressure stabilizing system. Clin Sci (Lond). 1990;79:543–50.
Dickson EJ, Jensen JB, Hille B. Regulation of calcium and phosphoinositides at endoplasmic reticulum-membrane junctions. Biochem Soc Trans. 2016;44:467–73.
DiFrancesco D. Funny channels in the control of cardiac rhythm and mode of action of selective blockers. Pharmacol Res. 2006;53:399–406.
DiFrancesco D. The role of the funny current in pacemaker activity. Circ Res. 2010;106:434–46.
DiFrancesco D, Borer JS. The funny current: cellular basis for the control of heart rate. Drugs. 2007;67(Suppl 2):15–24.
DiFrancesco D, Noble D. The funny current has a major pacemaking role in the sinus node. Heart Rhythm. 2012;9:299–301.
Ding Y, Li YL, Schultz HD. Role of blood flow in carotid body chemoreflex function in heart failure. J Physiol. 2011;589:245–58.
Distefano G, Sciacca P. Molecular pathogenesis of myocardial remodeling and new potential therapeutic targets in chronic heart failure. Ital J Pediatr. 2012;38:41.
Dulhunty AF. Excitation-contraction coupling from the 1950s into the new millennium. Clin Exp Pharmacol Physiol. 2006;33:763–72.
Dun W, Boyden PA. The Purkinje cell; 2008 style. J Mol Cell Cardiol. 2008;45:617–24.
Ednie AR, Bennett ES. Modulation of voltage-gated ion channels by sialylation. Compr Physiol. 2012;2:1269–301.
Ehler E. Cardiac cytoarchitecture - why the "hardware" is important for heart function! Biochim Biophys Acta. 2016;1863:1857–63.
Eisner D, Bode E, Venetucci L, Trafford A. Calcium flux balance in the heart. J Mol Cell Cardiol. 2012;58:110–7.
Faber GM, Rudy Y. Action potential and contractility changes in [Na(+)](i) overloaded cardiac myocytes: a simulation study. Biophys J. 2000;78:2392–404.
Fabiato A. Calcium-induced release of calcium from the cardiac sarcoplasmic reticulum. Am J Phys. 1983;245:C1–14.

Fabiato A. Time and calcium dependence of activation and inactivation of calcium-induced release of calcium from the sarcoplasmic reticulum of a skinned canine cardiac Purkinje cell. J Gen Physiol. 1985;85:247–89.
Fabiato A, Fabiato F. Calcium release from the sarcoplasmic reticulum. Circ Res. 1977;40: 119–29.
Fabiato A, Fabiato F. Calcium-induced release of calcium from the sarcoplasmic reticulum of skinned cells from adult human, dog, cat, rabbit, rat, and frog hearts and from fetal and new-born rat ventricles. Ann N Y Acad Sci. 1978;307:491–522.
Fabiato A, Fabiato F. Calcium and cardiac excitation-contraction coupling. Annu Rev Physiol. 1979;41:473–84.
Farah CS, Reinach FC. The troponin complex and regulation of muscle contraction. FASEB J. 1995;9:755–67.
Fodstad H, Kelly PJ, Buchfelder M. History of the cushing reflex. Neurosurgery. 2006;59:1132–7; discussion 1137
Foley JR, Plein S, Greenwood JP. Assessment of stable coronary artery disease by cardiovascular magnetic resonance imaging: current and emerging techniques. World J Cardiol. 2017;9:92–108.
Fuchs F, Smith SH. Calcium, cross-bridges, and the frank-Starling relationship. News Physiol Sci. 2001;16:5–10.
Gao L, Wang Q, Xu H, Tao Z, Wu F. The oculocardiac reflex in cataract surgery in the elderly. Br J Ophthalmol. 1997;81:614.
Gautel M. Cytoskeletal protein kinases: titin and its relations in mechanosensing. Pflugers Arch. 2011;462:119–34.
George SA, Poelzing S. Cardiac conduction in isolated hearts of genetically modified mice—Connexin43 and salts. Prog Biophys Mol Biol. 2016;120:189–98.
Germano G, Kiat H, Kavanagh PB, Moriel M, Mazzanti M, Su HT, Van Train KF, Berman DS. Automatic quantification of ejection fraction from gated myocardial perfusion SPECT. J Nucl Med. 1995;36:2138–47.
Gibson DG, Francis DP. Clinical assessment of left ventricular diastolic function. Heart. 2003;89:231–8.
Goldhaber JI, Philipson KD. Cardiac sodium-calcium exchange and efficient excitation-contraction coupling: implications for heart disease. Adv Exp Med Biol. 2013;961:355–64.
Goldstein DS, Cheshire WP Jr. Beat-to-beat blood pressure and heart rate responses to the Valsalva maneuver. Clin Auton Res. 2017;27(6):361–7.
Gordon AM, Homsher E, Regnier M. Regulation of contraction in striated muscle. Physiol Rev. 2000;80:853–924.
Grady PA, Blaumanis OR. Physiologic parameters of the Cushing reflex. Surg Neurol. 1988;29:454–61.
Granzier H, Wu Y, Siegfried L, LeWinter M. Titin: physiological function and role in cardiomyopathy and failure. Heart Fail Rev. 2005;10:211–23.
Grunnet M. Repolarization of the cardiac action potential. Does an increase in repolarization capacity constitute a new anti-arrhythmic principle? Acta Physiol. 2010;198(Suppl 676):1–48.
Haddad F, Couture P, Tousignant C, Denault AY. The right ventricle in cardiac surgery, a perioperative perspective: I. Anatomy, physiology, and assessment. Anesth Analg. 2009;108:407–21.
Hajdu MA, Cornish KG, Tan W, Panzenbeck MJ, Zucker IH. The interaction of the Bainbridge and Bezold-Jarisch reflexes in the conscious dog. Basic Res Cardiol. 1991;86:175–85.
Hakumaki MO. Seventy years of the Bainbridge reflex. Acta Physiol Scand. 1987;130:177–85.
Hamilton SL, Serysheva I, Strasburg GM. Calmodulin and excitation-contraction coupling. News Physiol Sci. 2000;15:281–4.
Herzog JA, Leonard TR, Jinha A, Herzog W. Are titin properties reflected in single myofibrils? J Biomech. 2012;45:1893–9.
Hill TL, Eisenberg E, Greene L. Theoretical model for the cooperative equilibrium binding of myosin subfragment 1 to the actin-troponin-tropomyosin complex. Proc Natl Acad Sci U S A. 1980;77:3186–90.

Hiltrop N, Bennett J, Desmet W. Circumflex coronary artery injury after mitral valve surgery: a report of four cases and comprehensive review of the literature. Catheter Cardiovasc Interv. 2017;89:78–92.

Hitchcock-DeGregori SE. Tropomyosin: function follows structure. Adv Exp Med Biol. 2008;644:60–72.

Ho SY, McCarthy KP. Anatomy of the left atrium for interventional electrophysiologists. PACE. 2010;33:620–7.

Hohendanner F, McCulloch AD, Blatter LA, Michailova AP. Calcium and IP3 dynamics in cardiac myocytes: experimental and computational perspectives and approaches. Front Pharmacol. 2014;5:35.

Hong T, Shaw RM. Cardiac T-tubule microanatomy and function. Physiol Rev. 2017;97:227–52.

Humphries ES, Dart C. Neuronal and cardiovascular potassium channels as therapeutic drug targets: promise and pitfalls. J Biomol Screen. 2015;20:1055–73.

Ibrahim M, Siedlecka U, Buyandelger B, Harada M, Rao C, Moshkov A, Bhargava A, Schneider M, Yacoub MH, Gorelik J, Knoll R, Terracciano CM. A critical role for Telethonin in regulating t-tubule structure and function in the mammalian heart. Hum Mol Genet. 2012;22(2):372–83.

Jafri MS. Models of excitation-contraction coupling in cardiac ventricular myocytes. Methods Mol Biol. 2012;910:309–35.

Kajioka S, Takahashi-Yanaga F, Shahab N, Onimaru M, Matsuda M, Takahashi R, Asano H, Morita H, Morimoto S, Yonemitsu Y, Hayashi M, Seki N, Sasaguri T, Hirata M, Nakayama S, Naito S. Endogenous cardiac troponin T modulates Ca(2+)-mediated smooth muscle contraction. Sci Rep. 2012;2:979.

Karaman T, Demir S, Dogru S, Sahin A, Tapar H, Karaman S, Kaya Z, Suren M, Arici S. The effect of anesthesia depth on the oculocardiac reflex in strabismus surgery. J Clin Monit Comput. 2016;30:889–93.

Kashihara K. Roles of arterial baroreceptor reflex during bezold-jarisch reflex. Curr Cardiol Rev. 2009;5:263–7.

Kashihara K, Kawada T, Li M, Sugimachi M, Sunagawa K. Bezold-Jarisch reflex blunts arterial baroreflex via the shift of neural arc toward lower sympathetic nerve activity. Jpn J Physiol. 2004;54:395–404.

Kennedy A, Finlay DD, Guldenring D, Bond R, Moran K, McLaughlin J. The cardiac conduction system: generation and conduction of the cardiac impulse. Crit Care Nurs Clin North Am. 2016;28:269–79.

Kerckhoffs RC, Campbell SG, Flaim SN, Howard EJ, Sierra-Aguado J, Mulligan LJ, McCulloch AD. Multi-scale modeling of excitation-contraction coupling in the normal and failing heart. Conf Proc IEEE Eng Med Biol Soc. 2009;2009:4281–2.

Khan MU, Cheema Y, Shahbaz AU, Ahokas RA, Sun Y, Gerling IC, Bhattacharya SK, Weber KT. Mitochondria play a central role in nonischemic cardiomyocyte necrosis: common to acute and chronic stressor states. Pflugers Arch. 2012;464:123–31.

Kim B, Takeuchi A, Koga O, Hikida M, Matsuoka S. Mitochondria Na(+)-Ca (2+) exchange in cardiomyocytes and lymphocytes. Adv Exp Med Biol. 2013;961:193–201.

Kim BB, Qaqish C, Frangos J, Caccamese JF Jr. Oculocardiac reflex induced by an orbital floor fracture: report of a case and review of the literature. J Oral Maxillofac Surg. 2012;70:2614–9.

Kim HS, Kim SD, Kim CS, Yum MK. Prediction of the oculocardiac reflex from pre-operative linear and nonlinear heart rate dynamics in children. Anaesthesia. 2000;55:847–52.

Kim Y, Boucher M, Argaez C. Ifunny channel inhibitors: an emerging option for heart failure. Ottawa, ON: CADTH Issues in Emerging Health Technologies; 2016. Canadian Agency for Drugs and Technologies in Health Copyright (c) CADTH 2017. You are permitted to reproduce this document for non-commercial purposes, provided it is not modified when reproduced and appropriate credit is given to CADTH.

Kirchhoff S, Kim JS, Hagendorff A, Thonnissen E, Kruger O, Lamers WH, Willecke K. Abnormal cardiac conduction and morphogenesis in connexin 40 and connexin 43 double-deficient mice. Circ Res. 2000;87:399–405.

Kleber AG, Saffitz JE. Role of the intercalated disc in cardiac propagation and arrhythmogenesis. Front Physiol. 2014;5:404.
Knoll R. Myosin binding protein C: implications for signal-transduction. J Muscle Res Cell Motil. 2012;33:31–42.
Kobayashi T, Jin L, de Tombe PP. Cardiac thin filament regulation. Pflugers Arch. 2008;457:37–46.
Koivumaki JT, Korhonen T, Takalo J, Weckstrom M, Tavi P. Regulation of excitation-contraction coupling in mouse cardiac myocytes: integrative analysis with mathematical modelling. BMC Physiol. 2009;9:16.
Kokkinidis DG, Waldo SW, Armstrong EJ. Treatment of coronary artery in-stent restenosis. Expert Rev Cardiovasc Ther. 2017;15:191–202.
Krishnan S, Fiori MC, Cuello LG, Altenberg GA. A cell-based assay to assess Hemichannel function. Yale J Biol Med. 2017;90:87–95.
Kruger M, Linke WA. The giant protein titin: a regulatory node that integrates myocyte signaling pathways. J Biol Chem. 2011;286:9905–12.
Kubli DA, Gustafsson AB. Mitochondria and mitophagy: the yin and yang of cell death control. Circ Res. 2012;111:1208–21.
Kuhtz-Buschbeck JP, Schaefer J, Wilder N. Mechanosensitivity: from Aristotle's sense of touch to cardiac mechano-electric coupling. Prog Biophys Mol Biol. 2017;130(Pt B):126–31.
Kurtenbach S, Kurtenbach S, Zoidl G. Gap junction modulation and its implications for heart function. Front Physiol. 2014;5:82.
Kusakari Y, Urashima T, Shimura D, Amemiya E, Miyasaka G, Yokota S, Fujimoto Y, Akaike T, Inoue T, Minamisawa S. Impairment of excitation-contraction coupling in right ventricular hypertrophied muscle with fibrosis induced by pulmonary artery banding. PLoS One. 2017;12:e0169564.
Kuster DW, Bawazeer AC, Zaremba R, Goebel M, Boontje NM, van der Velden J. Cardiac myosin binding protein C phosphorylation in cardiac disease. J Muscle Res Cell Motil. 2012;33:43–52.
Lang S, Lanigan DT, van der Wal M. Trigeminocardiac reflexes: maxillary and mandibular variants of the oculocardiac reflex. Can J Anaesth. 1991;38:757–60.
LeWinter MM, Wu Y, Labeit S, Granzier H. Cardiac titin: structure, functions and role in disease. Clin Chim Acta. 2007;375:1–9.
Limbu B, Shah K, Weinberg SH, Deo M. Role of cytosolic calcium diffusion in murine cardiac purkinje cells. Clin Med Insights Cardiol. 2016;10:17–26.
Lindskog C, Linne J, Fagerberg L, Hallstrom BM, Sundberg CJ, Lindholm M, Huss M, Kampf C, Choi H, Liem DA, Ping P, Varemo L, Mardinoglu A, Nielsen J, Larsson E, Ponten F, Uhlen M. The human cardiac and skeletal muscle proteomes defined by transcriptomics and antibody-based profiling. BMC Genomics. 2015;16:475.
Linke WA. Stretching molecular springs: elasticity of titin filaments in vertebrate striated muscle. Histol Histopathol. 2000a;15:799–811.
Linke WA. Titin elasticity in the context of the sarcomere: force and extensibility measurements on single myofibrils. Adv Exp Med Biol. 2000b;481:179–202; discussion 203-176.
Lluri G, Aboulhosn J. Coronary arterial development: a review of normal and congenitally anomalous patterns. Clin Cardiol. 2014;37:126–30.
Lo CW. Role of gap junctions in cardiac conduction and development: insights from the connexin knockout mice. Circ Res. 2000;87:346–8.
Lodish H, Berk A, Zipursky SL, et al. Section 21.2: the action potential and conduction of electric impulses. In: Molecular cell biology. 4th ed. New York: W. H. Freeman; 2000.
Lomsky M, Johansson L, Gjertsson P, Bjork J, Edenbrandt L. Normal limits for left ventricular ejection fraction and volumes determined by gated single photon emission computed tomography—a comparison between two quantification methods. Clin Physiol Funct Imaging. 2008;28:169–73.
London B. Defining the complexity of the junctional membrane complex. Circ Res. 2017;120: 11–2.
Lu X, Ginsburg KS, Kettlewell S, Bossuyt J, Smith GL, Bers DM. Measuring local gradients of intra-mitochondrial [Ca] in cardiac myocytes during SR Ca release. Circ Res. 2012;112(3): 424–31.

Mahadevan G, Davis RC, Frenneaux MP, Hobbs FD, Lip GY, Sanderson JE, Davies MK. Left ventricular ejection fraction: are the revised cut-off points for defining systolic dysfunction sufficiently evidence based? Heart. 2008;94:426–8.

Malik FI, Hartman JJ, Elias KA, Morgan BP, Rodriguez H, Brejc K, Anderson RL, Sueoka SH, Lee KH, Finer JT, Sakowicz R, Baliga R, Cox DR, Garard M, Godinez G, Kawas R, Kraynack E, Lenzi D, Lu PP, Muci A, Niu C, Qian X, Pierce DW, Pokrovskii M, Suehiro I, Sylvester S, Tochimoto T, Valdez C, Wang W, Katori T, Kass DA, Shen YT, Vatner SF, Morgans DJ. Cardiac myosin activation: a potential therapeutic approach for systolic heart failure. Science. 2011;331:1439–43.

Malik FI, Morgan BP. Cardiac myosin activation part 1: from concept to clinic. J Mol Cell Cardiol. 2011;51:454–61.

Marcotti W, Johnson SL, Kros CJ. A transiently expressed SK current sustains and modulates action potential activity in immature mouse inner hair cells. J Physiol. 2004;560:691–708.

Marionneau C, Abriel H. Regulation of the cardiac Na channel Na1.5 by post-translational modifications. J Mol Cell Cardiol. 2015;82:36–47.

Markwalder J, Starling EH. On the constancy of the systolic output under varying conditions. J Physiol. 1914;48:348–56.

Marston S, Burton D, Copeland O, Fraser I, Gao Y, Hodgkinson J, Huber P, Levine B, el-Mezgueldi M, Notarianni G. Structural interactions between actin, tropomyosin, caldesmon and calcium binding protein and the regulation of smooth muscle thin filaments. Acta Physiol Scand. 1998;164:401–14.

Marston SB, Redwood CS. Modulation of thin filament activation by breakdown or isoform switching of thin filament proteins: physiological and pathological implications. Circ Res. 2003;93:1170–8.

Mattiazzi A, Bassani RA, Escobar AL, Palomeque J, Valverde CA, Vila Petroff M, Bers DM. Chasing cardiac physiology and pathology down the CaMKII cascade. Am J Phys Heart Circ Phys. 2015;308:H1177–91.

McDonald KS. The interdependence of Ca2+ activation, sarcomere length, and power output in the heart. Pflugers Arch. 2011;462:61–7.

McLachlan AD, Stewart M. Tropomyosin coiled-coil interactions: evidence for an unstaggered structure. J Mol Biol. 1975;98:293–304.

Meyer T, Stuerz K, Guenther E, Edamura M, Kraushaar U. Cardiac slices as a predictive tool for arrhythmogenic potential of drugs and chemicals. Expert Opin Drug Metab Toxicol. 2010;6:1461–75.

Meyrelles SS, Bernardes CF, Modolo RP, Mill JG, Vasquez EC. Bezold-Jarisch reflex in myocardial infarcted rats. J Auton Nerv Syst. 1997;63:144–52.

Michael G, Xiao L, Qi XY, Dobrev D, Nattel S. Remodelling of cardiac repolarization: how homeostatic responses can lead to arrhythmogenesis. Cardiovasc Res. 2009;81:491–9.

Miragoli M, Novak P, Ruenraroengsak P, Shevchuk AI, Korchev YE, Lab MJ, Tetley TD, Gorelik J. Functional interaction between charged nanoparticles and cardiac tissue: a new paradigm for cardiac arrhythmia? Nanomedicine (London). 2012;8(5):725–37.

Molnar C, Nemes C, Szabo S, Fulesdi B. Harvey cushing, a pioneer of neuroanesthesia. J Anesth. 2008;22:483–6.

Morad M, Tung L. Ionic events responsible for the cardiac resting and action potential. Am J Cardiol. 1982;49:584–94.

Morimoto S, Goto T. Role of troponin I isoform switching in determining the pH sensitivity of Ca(2+) regulation in developing rabbit cardiac muscle. Biochem Biophys Res Commun. 2000;267:912–7.

Nakada T, Flucher BE, Kashihara T, Sheng X, Shibazaki T, Horiuchi-Hirose M, Gomi S, Hirose M, Yamada M. The proximal C-terminus of alpha1C subunits is necessary for junctional membrane targeting of cardiac L-type calcium channels. Biochem J. 2012;448:221–31.

Nakasuka K, Miyamoto K, Noda T, Kamakura T, Wada M, Nakajima I, Ishibashi K, Inoue Y, Okamura H, Nagase S, Aiba T, Kamakura S, Shimizu W, Noguchi T, Anzai T, Yasuda S, Ohte N, Kusano K. "Window Sliding" analysis combined with high-density and rapid electroanatomical mapping: its efficacy and the outcome of catheter ablation of atrial tachycardia. Heart Vessel. 2017;32(8):984–96.

Neco P, Rose B, Huynh N, Zhang R, Bridge JH, Philipson KD, Goldhaber JI. Sodium-calcium exchange is essential for effective triggering of calcium release in mouse heart. Biophys J. 2010;99:755–64.

Nicholson D, Kossler A, Topping K, Stary CM. Exaggerated oculocardiac reflex elicited by local anesthetic injection of an empty orbit: a case report. A&A Pract. 2017;9(12):337–8.

Offer G, Ranatunga KW. Crossbridge and filament compliance in muscle: implications for tension generation and lever arm swing. J Muscle Res Cell Motil. 2010;31:245–65.

Ohtsuki I, Morimoto S. Troponin: regulatory function and disorders. Biochem Biophys Res Commun. 2008;369:62–73.

Orellana JA, Sanchez HA, Schalper KA, Figueroa V, Saez JC. Regulation of intercellular calcium signaling through calcium interactions with connexin-based channels. Adv Exp Med Biol. 2012;740:777–94.

Ottolia M, Torres N, Bridge JH, Philipson KD, Goldhaber JI. Na/Ca exchange and contraction of the heart. J Mol Cell Cardiol. 2013;61:28–33.

Pan BS, Gordon AM, Luo ZX. Removal of tropomyosin overlap modifies cooperative binding of myosin S-1 to reconstituted thin filaments of rabbit striated muscle. J Biol Chem. 1989;264:8495–8.

Paniagua R, Royuela M, Garcia-Anchuelo RM, Fraile B. Ultrastructure of invertebrate muscle cell types. Histol Histopathol. 1996;11:181–201.

Papaioannou VE, Verkerk AO, Amin AS, de Bakker JM. Intracardiac origin of heart rate variability, pacemaker funny current and their possible association with critical illness. Curr Cardiol Rev. 2013;9:82–96.

Parham WA, Mehdirad AA, Biermann KM, Fredman CS. Hyperkalemia revisited. Tex Heart Inst J. 2006;33:40–7.

Park KH, Weisleder N, Zhou J, Gumpper K, Zhou X, Duann P, Ma J, Lin PH. Assessment of calcium sparks in intact skeletal muscle fibers. J Vis Exp. 2014;84:e50898.

Paton JF, Boscan P, Pickering AE, Nalivaiko E. The yin and yang of cardiac autonomic control: vago-sympathetic interactions revisited. Brain Res Brain Res Rev. 2005;49:555–65.

Patterson SW, Piper H, Starling EH. The regulation of the heart beat. J Physiol. 1914;48:465–513.

Periasamy M, Bhupathy P, Babu GJ. Regulation of sarcoplasmic reticulum Ca2+ ATPase pump expression and its relevance to cardiac muscle physiology and pathology. Cardiovasc Res. 2008;77:265–73.

Periasamy M, Huke S. SERCA pump level is a critical determinant of Ca(2+)homeostasis and cardiac contractility. J Mol Cell Cardiol. 2001;33:1053–63.

Peters NS. New insights into myocardial arrhythmogenesis: distribution of gap-junctional coupling in normal, ischaemic and hypertrophied human hearts. Clin Sci (Lond). 1996;90:447–52.

Pilowsky PM, Goodchild AK. Baroreceptor reflex pathways and neurotransmitters: 10 years on. J Hypertens. 2002;20:1675–88.

Pohjoismaki JL, Goffart S. The role of mitochondria in cardiac development and protection. Free Radic Biol Med. 2017;106:345–54.

Porth CJ, Bamrah VS, Tristani FE, Smith JJ. The Valsalva maneuver: mechanisms and clinical implications. Heart Lung. 1984;13:507–18.

Posch MG, Waldmuller S, Muller M, Scheffold T, Fournier D, Andrade-Navarro MA, De Geeter B, Guillaumont S, Dauphin C, Yousseff D, Schmitt KR, Perrot A, Berger F, Hetzer R, Bouvagnet P, Ozcelik C. Cardiac alpha-myosin (MYH6) is the predominant sarcomeric disease gene for familial atrial septal defects. PLoS One. 2011;6:e28872.

Pott C, Eckardt L, Goldhaber JI. Triple threat: the Na+/Ca2+ exchanger in the pathophysiology of cardiac arrhythmia, ischemia and heart failure. Curr Drug Targets. 2011;12:737–47.

Prosser BL, Hernandez-Ochoa EO, Schneider MF. S100A1 and calmodulin regulation of ryanodine receptor in striated muscle. Cell Calcium. 2011;50:323–31.

Qiu J, Zhou S, Liu Q. Phosphorylated AMP-activated protein kinase slows down the atrial fibrillation progression by activating Connexin43. Int J Cardiol. 2016;208:56–7.

Raut MS, Maheshwari A, Dubey S. Sudden hemodynamic instability during off-pump coronary artery bypass grafting surgery: role of Bezold-Jarisch reflex. J Cardiothorac Vasc Anesth. 2017;31(6):2139–40.
Ravens U, Cerbai E. Role of potassium currents in cardiac arrhythmias. Europace. 2008;10:1133–7.
Redwood CS, Moolman-Smook JC, Watkins H. Properties of mutant contractile proteins that cause hypertrophic cardiomyopathy. Cardiovasc Res. 1999;44:20–36.
Reuter H, Pott C, Goldhaber JI, Henderson SA, Philipson KD, Schwinger RH. Na(+)–Ca^{2+} exchange in the regulation of cardiac excitation-contraction coupling. Cardiovasc Res. 2005;67:198–207.
Ribaric S, Kordas M. Simulation of the frank-Starling law of the heart. Comput Math Methods Med. 2012;2012:267834.
Rice JJ, Wang F, Bers DM, de Tombe PP. Approximate model of cooperative activation and crossbridge cycling in cardiac muscle using ordinary differential equations. Biophys J. 2008;95:2368–90.
Robbins MS, Robertson CE, Kaplan E, Ailani J, Lt C, Kuruvilla D, Blumenfeld A, Berliner R, Rosen NL, Duarte R, Vidwan J, Halker RB, Gill N, Ashkenazi A. The sphenopalatine ganglion: anatomy, pathophysiology, and therapeutic targeting in headache. Headache. 2016;56: 240–58.
Robertson D, Hollister AS, Forman MB, Robertson RM. Reflexes unique to myocardial ischemia and infarction. J Am Coll Cardiol. 1985;5:99B–104B.
Robinson TF, Cohen-Gould L, Factor SM, Eghbali M, Blumenfeld OO. Structure and function of connective tissue in cardiac muscle: collagen types I and III in endomysial struts and pericellular fibers. Scanning Microsc. 1988;2:1005–15.
Robinson TF, Factor SM, Sonnenblick EH. The heart as a suction pump. Sci Am. 1986;254:84–91.
Rogers JH, Bolling SF. Valve repair for functional tricuspid valve regurgitation: anatomical and surgical considerations. Semin Thorac Cardiovasc Surg. 2010;22:84–9.
Rossi MA, Abreu MA, Santoro LB. Images in cardiovascular medicine. Connective tissue skeleton of the human heart: a demonstration by cell-maceration scanning electron microscope method. Circulation. 1998;97:934–5.
Rozanski A, Nichols K, Yao SS, Malholtra S, Cohen R, DePuey EG. Development and application of normal limits for left ventricular ejection fraction and volume measurements from 99mTc-sestamibi myocardial perfusion gates SPECT. J Nucl Med. 2000;41:1445–50.
Rudy Y. Modelling the molecular basis of cardiac repolarization. Europace. 2007;9(Suppl 6):vi17–9.
Rybakova IN, Greaser ML, Moss RL. Myosin binding protein C interaction with actin: characterization and mapping of the binding site. J Biol Chem. 2011;286:2008–16.
Salo LM, Woods RL, Anderson CR, McAllen RM. Nonuniformity in the von Bezold-Jarisch reflex. Am J Phys Regul Integr Comp Phys. 2007;293:R714–20.
Sandow A. Excitation-contraction coupling in muscular response. Yale J Biol Med. 1952;25:176–201.
Schoenberg M. Equilibrium muscle crossbridge behavior: the interaction of myosin crossbridges with actin. Adv Biophys. 1993;29:55–73.
Schultz HD. Angiotensin and carotid body chemoreception in heart failure. Curr Opin Pharmacol. 2011;11:144–9.
Schultz HD, Del Rio R, Ding Y, Marcus NJ. Role of neurotransmitter gases in the control of the carotid body in heart failure. Respir Physiol Neurobiol. 2012;184:197–203.
Schultz HD, Li YL. Carotid body function in heart failure. Respir Physiol Neurobiol. 2007;157:171–85.
Schultz HD, Marcus NJ. Heart failure and carotid body chemoreception. Adv Exp Med Biol. 2012;758:387–95.
Schultz HD, Sun SY. Chemoreflex function in heart failure. Heart Fail Rev. 2000;5:45–56.
Scoote M, Poole-Wilson PA, Williams AJ. The therapeutic potential of new insights into myocardial excitation-contraction coupling. Heart. 2003;89:371–6.
Scoote M, Williams AJ. Myocardial calcium signalling and arrhythmia pathogenesis. Biochem Biophys Res Commun. 2004;322:1286–309.

Scriven DR, Moore ED. Ca(2+) channel and Na(+)/Ca(2+) exchange localization in cardiac myocytes. J Mol Cell Cardiol. 2012;58:22–31.
Sequeira V, van der Velden J. The frank-Starling law: a jigsaw of titin proportions. Biophys Rev. 2017;9:259–67.
Seshubabu G. The oculocardiac reflex in cataract surgery in the elderly. Br J Ophthalmol. 1998;82:589.
Severs NJ. Intercellular junctions and the cardiac intercalated disk. Adv Myocardiol. 1985;5:223–42.
Sharir T, Kang X, Germano G, Bax JJ, Shaw LJ, Gransar H, Cohen I, Hayes SW, Friedman JD, Berman DS. Prognostic value of poststress left ventricular volume and ejection fraction by gated myocardial perfusion SPECT in women and men: gender-related differences in normal limits and outcomes. J Nucl Cardiol. 2006;13:495–506.
Sharpey-Schafer EP. Effects of Valsalva's manoeuvre on the normal and failing circulation. Br Med J. 1955;1:693–5.
Shattock MJ, Ottolia M, Bers DM, Blaustein MP, Boguslavskyi A, Bossuyt J, Bridge JH, Chen-Izu Y, Clancy CE, Edwards A, Goldhaber J, Kaplan J, Lingrel JB, Pavlovic D, Philipson K, Sipido KR, Xie ZJ. Na^+/Ca^{2+} exchange and Na^+/K^+-ATPase in the heart. J Physiol. 2015;593:1361–82.
Shaw RM, Rudy Y. Cardiac muscle is not a uniform syncytium. Biophys J. 2010;98:3102–3; discussion 3104–3105.
Shih HT. Anatomy of the action potential in the heart. Tex Heart Inst J. 1994;21:30–41.
Shy D, Gillet L, Abriel H. Cardiac sodium channel Na(V)1.5 distribution in myocytes via interacting proteins: the multiple pool model. Biochim Biophys Acta. 2013;1833(4):886–94.
Silbiger JJ. Anatomy, mechanics, and pathophysiology of the mitral annulus. Am Heart J. 2012;164:163–76.
Silbiger JJ, Bazaz R. Contemporary insights into the functional anatomy of the mitral valve. Am Heart J. 2009;158:887–95.
Silver MD, Lam JH, Ranganathan N, Wigle ED. Morphology of the human tricuspid valve. Circulation. 1971;43:333–48.
Simon JW. Complications of strabismus surgery. Curr Opin Ophthalmol. 2010;21:361–6.
Sipido KR, Acsai K, Antoons G, Bito V, Macquaide N. T-tubule remodelling and ryanodine receptor organization modulate sodium-calcium exchange. Adv Exp Med Biol. 2013;961:375–83.
Smith G. Management of supraventricular tachycardia using the Valsalva manoeuvre: a historical review and summary of published evidence. Eur J Emerg Med. 2012;19:346–52.
Smith RB. Death and the oculocardiac reflex. Can J Anaesth. 1994;41:760.
Snyders DJ. Structure and function of cardiac potassium channels. Cardiovasc Res. 1999;42:377–90.
Solaro RJ. Mechanisms of the frank-Starling law of the heart: the beat goes on. Biophys J. 2007;93:4095–6.
Solaro RJ, Henze M, Kobayashi T. Integration of troponin I phosphorylation with cardiac regulatory networks. Circ Res. 2013;112:355–66.
Spicer DE, Henderson DJ, Chaudhry B, Mohun TJ, Anderson RH. The anatomy and development of normal and abnormal coronary arteries. Cardiol Young. 2015;25:1493–503.
Strege P, Beyder A, Bernard C, Crespo-Diaz R, Behfar A, Terzic A, Ackerman M, Farrugia G. Ranolazine inhibits shear sensitivity of endogenous Na (+) current and spontaneous action potentials in HL-1 cells. Channels. 2012;6(6):457–62.
Stroemlund LW, Jensen CF, Qvortrup K, Delmar M, Nielsen MS. Gap junctions—guards of excitability. Biochem Soc Trans. 2015;43:508–12.
Sun T, Dong YH, Du W, Shi CY, Wang K, Tariq MA, Wang JX, Li PF. The role of MicroRNAs in myocardial infarction: from molecular mechanism to clinical application. Int J Mol Sci. 2017;18(4):E745.
Swaminathan PD, Purohit A, Hund TJ, Anderson ME. Calmodulin-dependent protein kinase II: linking heart failure and arrhythmias. Circ Res. 2012;110:1661–77.
Szigligeti P, Pankucsi C, Banyasz T, Varro A, Nanasi PP. Action potential duration and force-frequency relationship in isolated rabbit, guinea pig and rat cardiac muscle. J Comp Physiol B. 1996;166:150–5.

Tanaka H, Matsuyama TA, Takamatsu T. Towards an integrated understanding of cardiac arrhythmogenesis–growing roles of experimental pathology. Pathol Int. 2017;67:8–16.
Tanaka Y, Nakamura K, Kuroiwa N, Odachi M, Mawatari K, Onimaru M, Sanada J, Arima T. Isovolumetric relaxation flow in patients with ischemic heart disease. J Am Coll Cardiol. 1993;21:1357–64.
Tang W, Sencer S, Hamilton SL. Calmodulin modulation of proteins involved in excitation-contraction coupling. Front Biosci. 2002;7:d1583–9.
Tardiff JC. Thin filament mutations: developing an integrative approach to a complex disorder. Circ Res. 2011;108:765–82.
Tavi P, Westerblad H. The role of in vivo Ca(2)(+) signals acting on Ca(2)(+)-calmodulin-dependent proteins for skeletal muscle plasticity. J Physiol. 2011;589:5021–31.
Teerlink JR. A novel approach to improve cardiac performance: cardiac myosin activators. Heart Fail Rev. 2009;14:289–98.
ter Keurs HE. The interaction of Ca^{2+} with sarcomeric proteins: role in function and dysfunction of the heart. Am J Phys Heart Circ Phys. 2012;302:H38–50.
Thierfelder L, Watkins H, MacRae C, Lamas R, McKenna W, Vosberg HP, Seidman JG, Seidman CE. Alpha-tropomyosin and cardiac troponin T mutations cause familial hypertrophic cardiomyopathy: a disease of the sarcomere. Cell. 1994;77:701–12.
Tops LF, van der Wall EE, Schalij MJ, Bax JJ. Multi-modality imaging to assess left atrial size, anatomy and function. Heart. 2007;93:1461–70.
Torres-Jacome J, Gallego M, Rodriguez-Robledo JM, Sanchez-Chapula JA, Casis O. Improvement of the metabolic status recovers cardiac potassium channel synthesis in experimental diabetes. Acta Physiol. 2013;207(3):447–59.
Tsai JC, Heitz JW. Oculocardiac reflex elicited during debridement of an empty orbit. J Clin Anesth. 2012;24:426–7.
Tuomainen T, Tavi P. The role of cardiac energy metabolism in cardiac hypertrophy and failure. Exp Cell Res. 2017;360(1):12–8.
Vahebi S, Ota A, Li M, Warren CM, de Tombe PP, Wang Y, Solaro RJ. p38-MAPK induced dephosphorylation of alpha-tropomyosin is associated with depression of myocardial sarcomeric tension and ATPase activity. Circ Res. 2007;100:408–15.
Van Petegem F. Ryanodine receptors: structure and function. J Biol Chem. 2012;287:31624–32.
Vangheluwe P, Sipido KR, Raeymaekers L, Wuytack F. New perspectives on the role of SERCA2's Ca^{2+} affinity in cardiac function. Biochim Biophys Acta. 2006;1763:1216–28.
Vasquez EC, Meyrelles SS, Mauad H, Cabral AM. Neural reflex regulation of arterial pressure in pathophysiological conditions: interplay among the baroreflex, the cardiopulmonary reflexes and the chemoreflex. Braz J Med Biol Res. 1997;30:521–32.
Vatner SF, Zimpfer M. Bainbridge reflex in conscious, unrestrained, and tranquilized baboons. Am J Phys. 1981;240:H164–7.
Vermij SH, Abriel H, van Veen TA. Refining the molecular organization of the cardiac intercalated disc. Cardiovasc Res. 2017;113(3):259–75.
Villa AD, Sammut E, Nair A, Rajani R, Bonamini R, Chiribiri A. Coronary artery anomalies overview: the normal and the abnormal. World J Radiol. 2016;8:537–55.
Wan WH, Ang BT, Wang E. The cushing response: a case for a review of its role as a physiological reflex. J Clin Neurosci. 2008;15:223–8.
Wang Q, Lin JL, Wu KH, Wang DZ, Reiter RS, Sinn HW, Lin CI, Lin CJ. Xin proteins and intercalated disc maturation, signaling and diseases. Front Biosci. 2012;17:2566–93.
Wang Z, Yuan LJ, Cao TS, Yang Y, Duan YY, Xing CY. Simultaneous beat-by-beat investigation of the effects of the Valsalva maneuver on left and right ventricular filling and the possible mechanism. PLoS One. 2013;8:e53917.
Watson CJ, Phelan D, Xu M, Collier P, Neary R, Smolenski A, Ledwidge M, McDonald K, Baugh J. Mechanical stretch up-regulates the B-type natriuretic peptide system in human cardiac fibroblasts: a possible defense against transforming growth factor-beta mediated fibrosis. Fibrogenesis Tissue Repair. 2012;5:9.

Weisbrod D, Peretz A, Ziskind A, Menaker N, Oz S, Barad L, Eliyahu S, Itskovitz-Eldor J, Dascal N, Khananshvili D, Binah O, Attali B. SK4 Ca^{2+} activated K^+ channel is a critical player in cardiac pacemaker derived from human embryonic stem cells. Proc Natl Acad Sci U S A. 2013;110:E1685–94.
White SP, Cohen C, Phillips GN Jr. Structure of co-crystals of tropomyosin and troponin. Nature. 1987;325:826–8.
Wick M. Filament assembly properties of the sarcomeric myosin heavy chain. Poult Sci. 1999;78:735–42.
Williams GS, Smith GD, Sobie EA, Jafri MS. Models of cardiac excitation-contraction coupling in ventricular myocytes. Math Biosci. 2010;226:1–15.
Wolf CM, Berul CI. Molecular mechanisms of inherited arrhythmias. Curr Genomics. 2008;9:160–8.
Workman AJ, Smith GL, Rankin AC. Mechanisms of termination and prevention of atrial fibrillation by drug therapy. Pharmacol Ther. 2011;131:221–41.
Yang D, Song LS, Zhu WZ, Chakir K, Wang W, Wu C, Wang Y, Xiao RP, Chen SR, Cheng H. Calmodulin regulation of excitation-contraction coupling in cardiac myocytes. Circ Res. 2003;92:659–67.
Yester JW, Kuhn B. Mechanisms of cardiomyocyte proliferation and differentiation in development and regeneration. Curr Cardiol Rep. 2017;19:13.
Yi C, Jee D. Influence of the anaesthetic depth on the inhibition of the oculocardiac reflex during sevoflurane anaesthesia for paediatric strabismus surgery. Br J Anaesth. 2008;101:234–8.
Yi Y, Jin ZY, Wang YN. Advances in myocardial CT perfusion imaging technology. Am J Transl Res. 2016;8:4523–31.
Young ML, McLeary M, Chan KC. Acquired and congenital coronary artery abnormalities. Cardiol Young. 2017;27:S31–s35.
Yuniarti AR, Lim KM. The effect of electrical conductivity of myocardium on cardiac pumping efficacy: a computational study. Biomed Eng Online. 2017;16:11.
Zack F, Rodewald AK, Blaas V, Buttner A. Histologic spectrum of the cardiac conducting tissue in non-natural deaths under 30 years of age: an analysis of 43 cases with special implications for sudden cardiac death. Int J Legal Med. 2016;130:173–8.
Zhang YH, Hancox JC. Regulation of cardiac Na^+–Ca^{2+} exchanger activity by protein kinase phosphorylation—still a paradox? Cell Calcium. 2009;45:1–10.
Zhao CY, Greenstein JL, Winslow RL. Mechanisms of the cyclic nucleotide cross-talk signaling network in cardiac L-type calcium channel regulation. J Mol Cell Cardiol. 2017;106:29–44.
Zhou K, Hong T. Cardiac BIN1 (cBIN1) is a regulator of cardiac contractile function and an emerging biomarker of heart muscle health. Sci China Life Sci. 2017;60:257–63.
Zhou L, O'Rourke B. Cardiac mitochondrial network excitability: insights from computational analysis. Am J Phys Heart Circ Phys. 2012;302:H2178–89.

Cardiovascular Pharmacology in Adult Patients Undergoing Cardiac Surgery

4

Ali Dabbagh, Ardeshir Tajbakhsh, Zahra Talebi, and Samira Rajaei

Abstract

The word "drug" originated from a French word "drogue," which also came from "droge-vate" from Middle Dutch meaning "dry barrels" (*Harper, Douglas. "drug". Online Etymology Dictionary*). This concept is referring to the preservation of pharmaceutical plants in barrels. As Claude Bernard quoted in 1865, "*everything is poisonous, nothing is poisonous, and it is all a matter of dose*" (Bernard, Claude. An introduction to the study of experimental study; 1865). Therefore in this chapter, we are reviewing some clinical pharmacological titles including inotropes, vasoactive agents, diuretics, antihypertensive agents, antiarrhythmic agents, anesthetic drugs, agents affecting autonomic nervous systems, anticoagulation and thrombolysis drugs, blood products, and antibiotics.

In this chapter, we emphasize on main clinical consideration and dosage in addition to indications and contraindications, in other words when will the drug

A. Dabbagh, M.D. (✉)
Faculty of Medicine, Cardiac Anesthesiology Department, Anesthesiology Research Center, Shahid Beheshti University of Medical Sciences, Tehran, Iran

Cardiac Anesthesiology Fellowship Program, Shahid Beheshti University of Medical Sciences, Tehran, Iran
e-mail: alidabbagh@sbmu.ac.ir

A. Tajbakhsh, M.D.
Anesthesiology Department, Anesthesiology Research Center, Faculty of Medicine, Shahid Beheshti University of Medical Sciences, Tehran, Iran

Z. Talebi, Pharm D
Anesthesiology Research Center, Shahid Beheshti University of Medical Sciences, Tehran, Iran

S. Rajaei, M.D., Ph.D.
Department of Immunology, School of Medicine, Tehran University of Medical Sciences, Tehran, Iran
e-mail: samirarajaei@tums.ac.ir

A. Dabbagh et al. (eds.), *Postoperative Critical Care for Adult Cardiac Surgical Patients*, https://doi.org/10.1007/978-3-319-75747-6_4

be poisonous as quoted above. The aim of this chapter is to have a practical, clinical, and logical approach in pharmaceutical management of patients with heart disease.

Keywords
Heart disease · Cardiology · Cardiac medications · Adult cardiac surgery Pharmacology · Vasoactive agents · Inotropes · Phenylephrine hydrochloride Vasopressin · Epinephrine · Dopamine hydrochloride · Norepinephrine bitartrate Levophed · Milrinone lactate · Dobutamine phosphate · Levosimendan · Glyceryl trinitrate · Nitroglycerin · Hydralazine · Prostaglandin E1 · Alprostadil · Sodium pentacyanonitrosylferrate · Sodium nitroprusside · Phentolamine mesylate Phentolamine · Regitine · Angiotensin-converting enzyme (ACE) inhibitors Angiotensin II receptor blockers (ARBs) · Calcium channel blockers (CCBs) Diuretics · Pulmonary hypertension · Nitric oxide · Phosphodiesterase 5 (PDE 5) inhibitors · Endothelin receptor blockers · Anti-arrhythmic agents · Analgesic agents · Sedative drugs · Intravenous anesthetic agents · Ramsay sedation scale (Ramsay) · Sedation-agitation scale (SAS) · Richmond agitation-sedation scale (RASS) · Volatile anesthetics · Neuromuscular blocking agents · Stress ulcer Anticoagulants (oral and parenteral forms) · Antiplatelet agents · Thrombolytic agents · Novel oral anticoagulants · Antifibrinolytic agents · Antibiotic prophylaxis

4.1 Vasoactive Agents

In order to define these agents, a classification could be made by dividing them into two different subclasses:

- Vasoactive agents (either vasopressors or vasodilators)
- Inotropes (positive or negative inotropes)

It should be kept in mind that this classification could not precisely divide these drugs. There may be some overlaps between these subclasses. Also, most of currently available agents share some aspect of each of these classification (Holmes 2005; Bangash et al. 2012; Bracht et al. 2012; Noori and Seri 2012; Jentzer et al. 2015).

Therefore another classification with a wider domain could classify these agents into four different categories mentioned below:

1. Pure vasopressors, i.e., *pure vasoconstrictors* (phenylephrine and vasopressin).
2. Inoconstrictors *which have both vasoconstrictor and inotropic activity* (mainly epinephrine, dopamine, and norepinephrine).
3. Inodilators *which have both vasodilator and inotropic activity* (mainly milrinone, dobutamine, and levosimendan).

Table 4.1 Receptor types targeted by current vasoactive pharmaceuticals

Specific adrenoceptor	The main target organ(s)	Clinical response
α1 (including α_{1A}, α_{1B}, α_{1D})	Arteries, arterioles, veins; however, α effects predominate over β in splanchnic circulation	Arterial constriction
α2 (including α_{2A}, α_{2B}, α_{2C})	Gastrointestinal (GI) tract Cutaneous circulation	Decreased GI tone Decreased motility Decreased amount of GI secretions
β1	Heart (β 1 ≫ β 2 in coronary circulation)	Increased heart rate Augmented myocardial contractility
β2	The vessels of the skeletal muscles	Dilation of the vessels
	Coronary arterial bed	Dilation of the vessels
	Smooth muscles in the tracheobronchial tree	Relaxation of the smooth muscles
β3	Adipose tissue	Enhancement of lipolysis in adipose tissue, thermogenesis in skeletal muscle

Modified from Dabbagh A., et al. "Cardiovascular Pharmacology in Pediatric Patients with Congenital Heart Disease"; in "Congenital Heart Disease in Pediatric and Adult Patients; Anesthetic and Perioperative Management". Dabbagh A., Hernandez Conte A., Lubin L. Springer 2017, pp. 117–195. Published with kind permission of © SpringerNature, 2017. All Rights Reserved. Dabbagh et al. (2017a)

Table 4.2 Myocardial receptors characterized by their properties

Receptor type	Chronotropy	Inotropy	Lusitropy	Bathmotropy	Dromotropy
β_1	+	+	+	+	+
M_2	–	–	–	–	–

Modified from Dabbagh A., et al. "Cardiovascular Pharmacology in Pediatric Patients with Congenital Heart Disease"; in "Congenital Heart Disease in Pediatric and Adult Patients; Anesthetic and Perioperative Management". Dabbagh A., Hernandez Conte A., Lubin L. Springer 2017, pp. 117–195. Published with kind permission of © SpringerNature, 2017. All Rights Reserved. Dabbagh et al. (2017a)
– = decrease, + = increase

4. Pure vasodilators which affect the arterial system (arterial dilators) and/or the venous system (venodilators); these agents have no inotropic activity (include mainly nitroglycerin, hydralazine, alprostadil, sodium nitroprusside, phentolamine mesylate).

Considering autonomic receptors and their functions in specific organs could help understanding the agent's mechanism of action. Therefore following Tables 4.1 and 4.2 describe a summary of common receptors involved when using these agents (Kee 2003; Trappe et al. 2003; Bangash et al. 2012).

4.1.1 Pure Vasopressors, i.e., Pure Vasoconstrictors

4.1.1.1 Phenylephrine

Drug name: Phenylephrine hydrochloride

Class: Alpha adrenergic agonists

CAS number: 61-76-7

Mechanism of action: Phenylephrine is used in clinical content as a direct peripheral α-1 adrenergic stimulant which causes peripheral vasoconstriction. This sympathomimetic amine used to treat systemic hypotension as bolus or infusion regiment. This effect could cause reflex bradycardia and hence decreasing cardiac output; therefore heart rate monitoring should be used wherever phenylephrine is being administered. Phenylephrine has many indications including (Chierchia et al. 1984; Cannesson et al. 2012; Ryu et al. 2012; Panchal et al. 2015; Chan et al. 2017; Li et al. 2017a):

- The most important indication is increasing blood pressure in adults with clinically important hypotension resulting primarily from vasodilation, in such settings as septic shock or anesthesia.
- Peri-intubation hypotension preventing post-reperfusion syndrome during adult liver transplantation.
- Prolongation of the effects of local anesthetics.
- Prevention and treatment of nasal congestion.
- Hemorrhoids.

Dosing

Bolus intravenous administration is 50–250 μg; however, the most frequently reported initial bolus dose is 50 or 100 μg.

Continuous intravenous infusion is 0.5 μg/kg/min to 1.4 μg/kg/min, titrated to blood pressure goal which should be administrated through a central venous catheter if possible.

Common Adverse Effect of Phenylephrine

- Exacerbation of angina, heart failure, and pulmonary arterial hypertension
- Vasoconstriction of peripheral vascular beds which can decrease the blood flow in vital organs including the skin, renal, heart, and mesenteric vessels
- Nausea and vomiting
- Headache
- Nervousness

Cautions: This drug has sulfite in its formulation; hence hypersensitivity reactions could occur in susceptible patients. Also, extravasation of this drug into the skin and subcutaneous tissue could cause necrosis of tissue.

4.1.1.2 Vasopressin

Name of drug: Vasopressin

Class: Pituitary

CAS number: 11000-17-2

Vasopressin is exogenous form of antidiuretic hormone that is secreted from the pituitary gland. This agent mainly acts on renal parenchyma and blood vessels. Vasopressin reduces urine output and augments water reabsorption. Also this agent could increase blood pressure by inducing vasoconstriction. Vasopressin, acting thorough V1 and V2 receptors, is often used in management of refractory vasodilatory shock. Low dose of this drug could be prescribed in management of septic patients irresponsible to other agents.

Mechanism of Action and Indications for Drug Use: V1 receptors located in the peripheral vessels induce intense vasoconstriction, and V2 receptors in collecting tubules of renal parenchyma could reabsorb water and decrease urine output. This mechanism of action which is indifferent from adrenergic pathway is especially important when adrenergic receptors are downregulated or in the setting of metabolic acidosis in which catecholamines could not yield their function. On the other hand, the antidiuretic effect of this agent, opposed to catecholamines, could help in maintaining the perfusion of end organs.

Vasopressin Indications

- Diabetes insipidus
- Polyuria
- CPR
- Abdominal radiographic procedures
- Diagnostic procedures
- Gastrointestinal hemorrhage
- Vasodilatory shock
- Hypotension due to angiotensin-converting enzyme inhibitors
- Hemodynamic rescue in catecholamine-resistant vasoplegic shock after resection of a pheochromocytoma

Vasopressin is indicated for management of low systemic vascular resistant caused by excessive adrenergic blockade in which case direct adrenergic agonist could not be useful. Due to various scenarios in which this agent could be prescribed, different doses and regiment are introduced. In CPR when dealing with asystole, pulseless ventricular fibrillation or tachycardia, 40 units intravenously once followed by 20 cm^3 normal saline could improve outcome. In diabetes insipidus five to ten units intramuscularly or subcutaneously two to four times/day could be beneficial. The usual dose of vasopressin administrated is 0.2–2 mili-units/kg/min infusion, which can be titrated to achieve desired effect; however, the dose should be weaned and discontinued as soon as possible. 4–8 mili-units/kg/min doses have been reported in some clinical trials to treat vasodilatory shock. There are rare reports of adverse effects following low doses of vasopressin; hence with administering higher doses, these adverse effects increase in severity and frequency.

When prescribing vasopressin, cardiovascular side effects should always be kept in mind, including cardiac arrest, decreased cardiac output, increased systemic vascular resistance, bradycardia, and myocardial ischemia. These cardiovascular complications have been estimated to be 25%. Skin necrosis was also reported when these agents extravasated. Hyponatremia is reported in prolonged usage; therefore serum sodium level should be measured daily when administering this agent. Terlipressin is analogue of vasopressin that acts mostly by V1 receptors and has longer half-life. This agent could be used in norepinephrine-resistant shocks with doses from 7 μg/kg twice a day to 2 μg/kg every 4 h. The logical use of vasopressin and terlipressin would be their role as a rescue therapy and the last resort therapy in refractory shock states unresponsive to norepinephrine and epinephrine (O'Brien et al. 2002; Holmes et al. 2003, 2004; Motta et al. 2005; Choong and Kissoon 2008; Leone and Martin 2008; Meyer et al. 2008; Mossad et al. 2008; Singh et al. 2009; Stahl et al. 2010; Meyer et al. 2011; Russell 2011; Biban and Gaffuri 2013; Bihari et al. 2014; Sharawy 2014; Brissaud et al. 2016; Gordon and Gordon 2016; Desborough et al. 2017; Li et al. 2017b; Mirhosseini et al. 2017).

4.1.2 Inoconstrictors

When prescribing catecholamines, we should always think of factors affecting patient's response to the specific agent we are using. The underlying disease and the ongoing treatment are two of the most important factors which should always be evaluated (Bangash et al. 2012; Bracht et al. 2012).

4.1.2.1 Epinephrine

Name of drug: Epinephrine, adrenalin

CAS number: 51-43-4

Drug group: α and β adrenergic receptor agonist

Mechanism of effect: All adrenergic receptors are activated by epinephrine. This agent imitates sympathetic stimulation except the effects on facial arteries and sweating. Epinephrine is the most potent adrenergic agonist which has positive inotropic and chronotropic effects and enhanced conduction in the heart (β1), smooth muscle relaxation in the vasculature and bronchial tree (β2), and vasoconstriction (α1).

Low doses of this agent (<0.1–0.2 μg/kg/min) mainly activate the β adrenoceptors with inotropic effects. Higher doses result in vasoconstrictor effect which takes the lead. Other effects of this agent include bronchial dilation, mydriasis, glycogenolysis, tachyarrhythmia, myocardial ischemia, pulmonary hypertension, hyperglycemia, and lactic acidosis. Epinephrine also reduces splanchnic and hepatic perfusion and increases metabolic workload of the liver. So this hypermetabolism that impairs oxygen exchange, glycolysis, and suppression of insulin cause lactic acidosis.

Indications of epinephrine

Indication	Specific effects of the indication
Cardiopulmonary resuscitation and rhythm disturbances	Epinephrine could increase diastolic perfusion pressure, and as a result, coronary perfusion pressure and cerebral perfusion pressure would be maintained. These effects are through activation of α1 adrenergic receptors. On the other hand, effects of this agent on β adrenergic receptors would increase cardiac work and therefore reduce subendocardial perfusion; therefore the use of epinephrine in cardiogenic shock should be with caution. Finally epinephrine is the drug of choice in cardiopulmonary resuscitation
Anaphylaxis and anaphylactoid reactions	Epinephrine is the drug of choice in case of severe anaphylaxis and emergencies. In these cases either subcutaneous injection or intravascular injection would be life-saving
Bronchospasm	In case of dealing with severe asthma or acute bronchospasm, epinephrine would be a choice of therapy with especial attention to its cardiovascular effects
Gastrointestinal and renal bleeding	Epinephrine could be used in treatment of bleeding by selective intra-arterial administration in the setting of angiography
As adjunct to local anesthetics	Could increase half-life of local anesthetics by reducing its distribution
Other uses	Treatment of severe hypoglycemia, premature labor, radiation nephritis, control of local skin or mucosal bleeding, as adjuvant to radiocontrast dyes

Routes of administration: The following routes could be used for administration of epinephrine:

- Intravenous
- Intramuscular
- Subcutaneous
- Infusion through intravenous line or central line
- Intra-arterial (very rarely, e.g., in radiographic assessments)
- Through endotracheal tube in cardiopulmonary bypass
- Intraosseous
- Inhalational through pulmonary devices like metered dose inhalers or nebulizers (usually used for children above 4 years)
- Local administration in control for mucosal or skin bleeding

Epinephrine dose

Specific dose of Epinephrine	Specific effects of the dose
Very-low-dose epinephrine	0.01–0.05 μg/kg/min; this dose would mostly activate β adrenoceptors and therefore does not significantly change cardiovascular responses
Low-dose epinephrine infusion	0.05 μg/kg/min to 0.1 μg/kg/min. Low-dose epinephrine activates adrenergic receptors as follows: (β2 > β1 > α1). These changes results in reducing SVR and blood pressure and simultaneously increasing myocardial contractility. Some studies propose that before any inotropic effect occurs, heart rate should raise first
Moderate-dose epinephrine infusion	0.1 μg/kg/min to 0.5 μg/kg/min; the prominent effect is mediated through α1 adrenergic activation

Specific dose of Epinephrine	Specific effects of the dose
High-dose epinephrine infusion	0.5 μg/kg/min to 1 μg/kg/min. This dose would affect mostly α1 > β1, β2 so SVR, cardiac index, and diastolic blood pressure would increase. Also these vasoconstrictions would lead to increased plasma glucose and lactate
Very-high-dose epinephrine infusion	More than 1.5 μg/kg/min; this dose would result in significant increase in SVR; therefore by increasing afterload, a significant reduction in cardiac index in both sides would be expected. These changes lead to increase in oxygen demand and imbalance of supply and demand
During cardiac arrest	1 mg of epinephrine is suggested as the usual dose in CPR every 3–5 min. This dose predominately activates α adrenergic receptors which results in vasoconstriction in root of aorta to increase diastolic pressure to improve coronary perfusion pressure. This dose of epinephrine could be administered through intravenous and intraosseous
The endotracheal dose during cardiac arrest	Ten times higher and should be diluted and followed by five manual ventilation maneuvers to assist its absorption in emergency situations
Cautions	Inadvertent injection of epinephrine could result in life-threatening event. Some of its complications would be very high blood pressure, chest pain and myocardial ischemia, rupture of aneurysms, or aortic injuries. In susceptible patients with arrhythmia, this agent could potentiate volatile-induced dysrhythmias

Clutter et al. (1980), Kee (2003), Trappe et al. (2003), Cooper (2008), Kleinman et al. (2010), Watt et al. (2011), Bangash et al. (2012), Bracht et al. (2012), Noori and Seri (2012), Atkins et al. (2015), de Caen et al. (2015), Jentzer et al. (2015), Maconochie et al. (2015), Maslov et al. (2015), Simons and Sampson (2015), Lucas et al. (2016), Cruickshank (2017), Minton and Sidebotham (2017), Shao and Li (2017), Yildirim et al. (2017), and Zhang et al. (2017a)

4.1.2.2 Dopamine

Name of drug: Dopamine hydrochloride

CAS Number: 62-31-7

Drug group: Selective agonist of β-1 adrenergic receptors

Mechanism of effect: Dopamine is synthesized by DOPA decarboxylase from DOPA (L-3, 4-**d**ihydr**o**xy**p**henyl**a**lanine) which is converted from L-tyrosine and L-phenylalanine. Dopamine could be transformed to norepinephrine by dopamine β-hydroxylase. This agent has different roles in human body including neurotransmitter and catecholamine which has chronotropic and inotropic effect on the heart. Dopamine can directly activate β adrenoreceptors and also can release norepinephrine from its reservoir.

Clinical effects of dopamine: Dopamine could be classified as an inoconstrictor with weaker effect compared to epinephrine or norepinephrine. Dopamine's effect on alpha and beta adrenergic receptors is related directly to the dose of dopamine administered, and also it has interindividual variability (Table 4.3):

Table 4.3 Dopamine doses and their effects

Dose of dopamine	Type of affected receptor(s)					
	α1 adrenoceptor	α2 adrenoceptor	β1 adrenoceptor	β2 adrenoceptor	Dopamine 1 receptor (D1)	Dopamine 2 receptor (D2)
0.5–2 μg/kg/min	0	0	+	0	+++	+++
2–10 μg/kg/min	+	+	+++	+++	++++	++++
10–20 μg/kg/min	+++	+	+++	+	++++	++++

Modified from Dabbagh A., et al. "Cardiovascular Pharmacology in Pediatric Patients with Congenital Heart Disease"; in "Congenital Heart Disease in Pediatric and Adult Patients; Anesthetic and Perioperative Management". Dabbagh A., Hernandez Conte A., Lubin L. Springer 2017, pp. 117–195. Published with kind permission of © SpringerNature, 2017. All Rights Reserved

+ = increase; – = decrease; 0 = no change

Specific dose of dopamine		Specific effects of the dose
Low-dose dopamine	0.5–2 μg/kg/min	Induces vasodilatory effects by dopamine receptors especially on mesenteric, renal, cerebral, and coronary vessels. Renal artery vasodilation results in increased renal blood flow and increased glomerular filtration rate. Low-dose dopamine was considered "renal dose of dopamine," but there is no conclusive evidence about its beneficial use in acute renal failure. As mentioned above, vasodilatory effect of dopamine would not affect peripheral vascular bed, because this effect would be neutralized by alpha activity of this agent
Medium-dose dopamine	2–10 μg/kg/min	This dose has inotropic effects through β-1 adrenoceptors and chronotropic effects by stimulation of sinoatrial node. This increase in myocardial contractility results in elevating oxygen consumption of myocardium and also increase in systolic blood pressure. On the other hand, diastolic blood pressure is not much affected. Therefore perfusion pressure of end organs will be increased due to increased cardiac output and relatively constant peripheral vascular resistance
High-dose dopamine	10–20 μg/kg/min	Causes vasoconstriction through α adrenoceptor stimulation. The first effect site would be muscular arterial tone afterward and with higher doses renal and mesenteric vessels would be affected. So very high doses of dopamine would decrease peripheral perfusion and may lead to ischemia of end organs

Time of effect: 5 min after initiating dopamine infusion, dopamine reaches its biophase and therefore started to act. Also its plasma half-life is about 2 min. So 10 min after cessation of infusion, its effect would fade away. It should be kept in mind that in patient with chronic use of monoamine oxidase inhibitors (MAOI), dopamine's effect would last longer; therefore, careful titration is mandatory.

Indications

1. Shock: In order to increase cardiac index and/or systemic vascular resistance, this agent would be helpful.
2. Cardiopulmonary resuscitation: Dopamine is indicated in return of spontaneous circulation (ROSC) cases in which increased cardiac output is desired.
3. Heart failure: In refractory cases and short-term usage, dopamine is indicated in these patients.
4. Acute renal failure: Currently no evidence supports dopamine administration for prophylaxis or treatment of acute renal failure. Hence historically low-dose dopamine was considered to be effective due to its vasodilatory effect on renal vascular bed.
5. Hepatorenal syndrome: Although dopamine is a part of treatment in these patients, no beneficial effect is documented in long-term use.

Dopamine dose and administration: Bolus doses of dopamine should be avoided; therefore this agent is usually administered by intravenous catheter or in some rare emergency situations through intraosseous path. It is preferential to administer dopamine through central venous catheter or large peripheral catheters (antecubital is preferred). Infusion through small veins, i.e., dorsal veins of the hand and ankle, could cause extravasation, so it should be avoided. This agent can be diluted by DW 5%, and concentration from 400 to 3200 μg/mL is used in clinical practice. Higher concentrations are being used in patients with fluid restriction.

Warnings and Contraindications

- As mentioned above MAOIs will increase dopamine's half-life; therefore if there is a history of using MAOIs (2–3 weeks), dopamine dose should be reduced.
- Pheochromocytoma and uncorrected tachyarrhythmia or VF are contraindications for dopamine administration.
- Hypersensitivity to this agent in patients with history of allergic reactions to sulfite is reported in some formulations.
- Administration of dopamine with IV fluids could result in overhydration. Therefore careful volume titration is mandatory.
- *Common adverse effects* include tachycardia, palpitation, nausea, vomiting, dyspnea, hypotension, angina, vasoconstriction, and headaches.

General precautions: During administration of dopamine, it is advised to use ECG, BP, and urine output monitoring in order to diagnose and treat complications (e.g., hypovolemia, hypoxia, hypercapnia, hypotension, hypertension, and arrhythmia) in time. Dilution of this agent with dextrose should be accounted in diabetic patients. On the other hand, with abrupt cessation of this, recurrence of hypotension could occur; therefore, gradual and careful titration plus expanding blood volume is advised.

Dopaminergic activity and its effect on the immunologic and neurohormonal systems: Dopamine decreases secretion of prolactin, thyroid hormone, and growth hormone and also increases glucocorticoid hormones. These changes would be significant in chronically and critically ill patient under prolonged use of this agent. However, dopamine interactions with immunologic system are diverse and dose dependent, acting through different receptors including D1–5 and also α and β adrenergic receptors. Below, the list of currently known immunomodulatory roles of dopamine could be found:

Specific effect on immune system	Effect of dopamine
Synthesis of adhesion molecules and cytokines	Decreased by dopamine
Chemotaxis of neutrophils	Decreased by dopamine
Proliferation of T-cell lymphocytes mediated	Impaired by dopamine through D1–5 receptors
Natural killer cell's activity	Facilitation mediated by D1 receptors (D1/D5)
Natural killer cell's activity	Suppression mediated by D2 receptors (D2/D3/D4)
Dendritic cells (DCs): links between innate and adaptive immune system	DCs produce and store dopamine and therefore stimulate D1 and D2 receptors through autocrine manner
Differentiation of CD 4(+) T cells to T helper 1 or T helper 2	Enhanced by dopamine
Regulatory T cells synthetize dopamine	Dopamine in turn suppresses T cells

Elenkov et al. (2000), Kee (2003), Trappe et al. (2003), Beck et al. (2004), Cooper (2008), Bangash et al. (2012), Bracht et al. (2012), Prado et al. (2013), Zhao et al. (2013), Pacheco et al. (2014), Eftekhar-Vaghefi et al. (2015), Franz et al. (2015), Herrera et al. (2015), Jentzer et al. (2015), Scanzano and Cosentino (2015), CID=681 (2016), Levite (2016), Rizza et al. (2016), Motyl et al. (2017), Pinoli et al. (2017), and Zhang et al. (2017b)

4.1.2.3 Norepinephrine

Name of drug: Norepinephrine bitartrate (Levophed)

Class: Alpha and beta adrenergic agonists

CAS number: 69815-49-2

Norepinephrine is released mostly by postganglionic adrenergic nerve endings and differs from epinephrine by a lack of methyl group. This agent activates α-1 and β-1 adrenoreceptors in the vessels and heart, respectively.

Norepinephrine is a potent α-1 agonist which is responsible for vasoconstriction more than β adrenoreceptors; therefore its main clinical effect would be increase in SVR and blood pressure. On the other hand, the cardiac output is often decreased or unchanged due to baroreceptor reflex through vagal activation. Also norepinephrine causes hyperglycemia in prolonged infusions more than other inotropic agents (Table 4.4).

Indications	Norepinephrine is indicated in circumstances which other vasopressor agents fail, and a potent vasoconstrictor is required, for instance, in vasoplegia syndrome. Other indications are listed below: • Shock: after adequate volume resuscitation, this agent would be prescribed for vasoconstriction and increasing SVR • Anaphylactic shock: in anaphylaxis resistant to epinephrine, 0.05–0.1 μg/kg/min IV infusion of norepinephrine is indicated to maintain SVR • Hypotension during anesthesia: an alternative to phenylephrine or ephedrine is norepinephrine, although its use is not common • CPR: severe hypotension due to low peripheral vascular resistance could be treated with this agent in ACLS • Pericardial tamponade to temporarily increase cardiac filling pressure • Myocardial infraction: to treat the hypotension in selected cases • Adjunct to local anesthetics: an alternative to epinephrine that increases half-life of local anesthetics hence not commonly used

Dose and administration	Norepinephrine dose varies from 0.02 to 0.2 μg/kg/min Route of administration: norepinephrine is administered through central venous catheter or in emergency situations from antecubital vein or femoral vein. Extravasation results in severe necrosis, and the treatment would be infiltration of phentolamine to the affected area. This agent should not be used in the same catheter with alkaline solution which deactivates the drug. It is preferred to change the administration site periodically in order to limit the complications. The lowest effective dose with the shortest duration of infusion is recommended
Warnings and contraindications	• As epinephrine its use in conjunction to local anesthetics in extremities (e.g., fingers, ears, or genitalia) is contraindicated • Every patient treated with norepinephrine should be monitored for ECG, blood pressure, hypovolemia, hypoxia, acidosis, and site of injection (in order to rule out extravasation). Patients with occlusive vascular diseases, arteriosclerosis, diabetes mellitus, hypertension, or hyperthyroidism are at risk of complications and need more careful attention
General precautions	The main precautions in using norepinephrine would be as follows: • Prolonged administration: causes decrease in cardiac output, edema, focal myocarditis, subpericardial hemorrhage, necrosis of end organs, i.e., intestine, hepatic, and renal • Arrhythmias: susceptible patients would be the ones with acute MI, hypoxia, and hypercapnia • Common adverse effects: respiratory difficulty, headaches, dizziness, and tremor • Cardiovascular and renal effects: severe vasoconstriction in end organs would limit their blood flow. Also increased cardiac work (due to decreased preload and increased afterload) would result in imbalance of oxygen supply and demand

De Backer et al. (2010), Mossad et al. (2011), Bangash et al. (2012), Vasu et al. (2012), Mehta et al. (2013), Rizza et al. (2016), Rossano et al. (2016), and Hamzaoui et al. (2017)

4.1.3 Inodilators (Mainly Milrinone, Dobutamine, and Levosimendan)

The main inodilators are milrinone, dobutamine, and levosimendan. Table 4.5 summarizes their characteristics.

4.1.3.1 Milrinone

Name of drug: Milrinone lactate

CAS number: 78415-72-2

Drug group: Cardiotonic drug, phosphodiesterase III inhibitor

Mechanism of effect: Milrinone acts through inhibition of phosphodiesterase (PDE) III in cardiomyocytes and vascular smooth muscle cells. This enzyme degrades cAMP, so by inhibiting its action, intracellular cAMP levels are elevated, and this in turn activates protein kinase A (PKA). PKA will activate contractile elements of cardiomyocytes. This results in increased contractility, arterial dilation,

Table 4.4 A summary of the main vasopressor agents

Drug	Dose	Receptors	Inotropy	HR[a]	SVR	PVR	Renal vascular resistance	Half-life	Adverse effects
Epinephrine (CAS number: 51-43-4)	Cardiac arrest: Children: IV bolus: 0.01 mg/kg every 3–5 min Low cardiac output: Continuous IV infusion: 0.01–1 μg/kg/min	Lower doses: $\beta_1, \beta_2 > \alpha_1$ Higher doses: $\alpha_1 > \beta_1, \beta_2$	+ +	+ +	0,- +	0,– +	– +	<2 min	Tachyarrhythmias If extravasation occurs, skin necrosis is possible
Norepinephrine (CAS number: 51-41-2)	Continuous IV infusion: 0.05–0.3 μg/kg/min (maximum dose, 2 μg/kg/min)	$\alpha_1 > \beta_1, \beta_2$	+	+	+	+	–	<2 min	Hypertension Bradycardia Myocardial ischemia If extravasation occurs, skin necrosis is possible
Dopamine (CAS number: 51-61-6)	Continuous IV infusion: 2–5 μg/kg/min 5–10 μg/kg/min 10–20 μg/kg/min	DA_1, DA_2 $\beta_1, \beta_2 > \alpha_1$ $\alpha_1 > \beta_1, \beta_2$	0 + +	0 + +	0 0,- +	0 0 +	– 0 +	2 min	Hypertension, tachyarrhythmias
Dobutamine (CAS number: 34368-04-2)	Continuous IV infusion: 2–20 μg/kg/min	$\beta_1 > \alpha_1, \beta_2$	+	+	–	–	0	2 min	Tachyarrhythmias
Isoproterenol (CAS number: 7683-59-2)	Continuous IV infusion: 0.01–0.2 μg/kg/min	β_1, β_2	+	+	–	–	–	8–50 min	Tachyarrhythmias

(continued)

Table 4.4 (continued)

Drug	Dose	Receptors	Inotropy	HR[a]	SVR	PVR	Renal vascular resistance	Half-life	Adverse effects
Calcium chloride (CAS number: 7440-70-2)	5–10 mg/kg IV bolus; 10 mg/kg/h infusion 20 mg/kg intracardiac (in ventricular cavity)	Contractile proteins	+	0,–	+	0,+	0	N/A	Hypertension
Milrinone (CAS number: 78415-72-2)	Continuous IV infusion: 0.25–0.75 μg/kg/min	Phosphodiesterase III, inhibitor/↑ cAMP	+	+	–	–	–	2.3 hours	Hypotension, ventricular arrhythmias, headache
Nesiritide (CAS number: 124584-08-3)	Continuous IV infusion: 0.01 μg/kg/min; if necessary, titrate by 0.005 μg/kg/min every 3 h to maximum of 0.03 μg/kg/min[b]	B-natriuretic peptide	0	0	–	–	+	60 min	Hypotension, increased levels of serum creatinine
Levosimendan (CAS number: 141505-33-1)	6–12 μg/kg load; 0.05–0.1 μg/kg/min	Troponin C, increasing Ca^{2+}sensitivity; ATP-sensitive K^+ channels for vasodilation	+	0	–	–	–	1 h	Hypotension, tachyarrhythmias, nausea, headache
Digoxin (CAS number: 20830-75-5)	Oral: 5–15 μg/kg/day divided every 12 h IV: 4–12 μg/kg/day divided every 12 h	Inhibition of the Na^+/K^+ ATPase in myocardium	+	–	–	–	–	36–48 hours with normal renal function; however, in patients with underlying, half life is considerably longer	Nausea and vomiting Dizziness, headache, dysrhythmia

Phenylephrine (CAS number: 59-42-7)	Bolus intravenous dose: 5–20 µg/kg which could be repeated each 10–20 min Intravenous infusion dose: 0.1–0.5 µg/kg/min Increase/decrease rate of infusion by minimum of 10 µg/min at intervals no longer than Q 15 min Titration parameter: MAP; SBP adjusted for age	Selective α1 agonist	0/+	0/– May decrease heart rate if blood pressure goes very high	+++	0/+	++	5 min		Bradycardia, arrhythmia, myocardial ischemia If extravasation occurs, skin necrosis is possible
Vasopressin (CAS number: 11000-17-2)	0.04 units/min	Agonist of vasopressin 1 (V1) receptors	0	0	+	0		**10–30 min**		Hypertension Bradycardia Arrhythmia Vasoconstriction Distal limb ischemia If extravasation occurs, skin necrosis is possible

Modified from Dabbagh A., et al. "Cardiovascular Pharmacology in Pediatric Patients with Congenital Heart Disease"; in "Congenital Heart Disease in Pediatric and Adult Patients; Anesthetic and Perioperative Management". Dabbagh A., Hernandez Conte A., Lubin L. Springer 2017, pp. 117–195. Published with kind permission of © SpringerNature, 2017. All Rights Reserved (Dabbagh et al. 2017a)

+ = increase; – = decrease; 0 = no change

[a] *v* vasopressin, *HR* heart rate, *SVR* systemic vascular resistance, *PVR* pulmonary vascular resistance, *DA* dopamine, *cAMP* cyclic adenosine monophosphate, *cGMP* cyclic guanosine monophosphate

[b] Recommended dose in *Moss and Adams' Heart disease in Infants, Children, and Adolescent* 2013: 1 µg/kg load; 0.1–0.2 µg/kg/min

Table 4.5 A summary and comparison between the main inodilators

Drug	Dose	HR	MAP	PCWP	CO	SVR	Adverse effects
Milrinone (CAS number: 78415-72-2)	0.25–0.75 μg/kg/min Increase/decrease by minimum of 0.125 μg/kg/min at intervals no longer than Q 6 h *Parameters for titration of drug*: blood pressure, CO, CI	0/+	0/–	–	+	–	Arrhythmia, thrombocytopenia, myocardial ischemia, hypotension/vasodilation *No increase* in myocardial oxygen demand
Dobutamine (CAS number: 34368-04-2)	2.5–20 μg/kg/min Increase/decrease by 1 μg/kg/min at intervals no longer than Q 30 min *Parameters for titration of drug*: blood pressure, CO, CI	0/+	0	–	+	–	Arrhythmia, may potentiate hypokalemia, increases myocardial oxygen demand, and so, may lead to myocardial ischemia, hypotension/vasodilation
Levosimendan (CAS number: 141505-33-1)	Loading dose: 6–12 μg/kg over 10 min then intravenous infusion of 0.05–0.2 μg/kg/min	0/+	0/–	–	+		Headache and/or hypotension may be induced due to vasodilatory effects of drug *No* risk of arrhythmia *No* renal or hepatic dose adjustment needed *No increase* in myocardial oxygen demand

Modified from Dabbagh A., et al. "Cardiovascular Pharmacology in Pediatric Patients with Congenital Heart Disease"; in "Congenital Heart Disease in Pediatric and Adult Patients; Anesthetic and Perioperative Management". Dabbagh A., Hernandez Conte A., Lubin L. Springer 2017, pp. 117–195. Published with kind permission of © SpringerNature, 2017. All Rights Reserved (Dabbagh et al. 2017a)

+ = increase; – = decrease; 0 = no change

and weak effect on chronotropism; therefore this agent is often called inodilator. As mentioned above, milrinone acts through different pathway in comparison to catecholamines. This agent does not have any effect on adrenergic receptors nor Na/K ATPase activity. The positive inotropic effect of this agent is caused by augmentation of myocardial contractility and improved Frank-Starling curve in heart failure. Also milrinone favors diastolic relaxation. These effects are present in plasma level of 100–300 ng/mL.

Indications	• Low cardiac output state (LCOS) • Acute treatment of heart failure or cardiogenic shock • Pulmonary hypertension
Dosage	**Loading dose**: 25–75 μg/kg (as a bolus dose during CPB); if the patient is not under cardiopulmonary bypass, this dose should be administered intravenously in 10–60 min, with precise control of blood pressure **Maintenance dose**: 0.25–0.75 μg/kg/min as intravenous continuous infusion, the treatment can begin with the infusion, recognizing that therapeutic plasma levels will not be achieved for the next several hours **Note**: milrinone is metabolized in the kidney; therefore in patients with kidney diseases, there should be dose adjustments in order to reach the therapeutic dose of 100–300 ng/mL
Routes of administration	**Intravenous** either central or peripheral vein; ports of cardiopulmonary bypass circuit could be considered in this category **Intraosseous** (e.g., during cardiopulmonary resuscitation) **Inhalational route**, in case of pulmonary hypertension, could minimize systemic effect of this agent **Oral route** which may increase morbidity **Note**: milrinone may be diluted before administration by half saline, normal saline, or normal saline with 5% dextrose; also, IV administration of milrinone should not be continued for more than 48 h due to accumulation of intracellular cAMP which may cause arrhythmias
Adverse effects and pharmaceutical precautions	**Hypersensitivity** to the drug or its formulation **Cardiac collapse and severe hypotension**: may occur in a number of patients, including but not limited to patients with obstructive valve lesions (e.g., pulmonary valve stenosis, aortic valve stenosis, or hypertrophic subaortic stenosis) receiving milrinone **Increased atrioventricular (AV) node transmission** which would be significant in patients with atrial flutter or fibrillation; in these patients it is recommended to administer cardiac glycosides before starting milrinone **Electrolyte imbalance**: when milrinone is added to diuretics, it leads to increased renal perfusion and electrolyte imbalance

Fleming et al. (2008), Begum et al. (2011), Knight and Yan (2012), Majure et al. (2013), Brunner et al. (2014), Ogawa et al. (2014), Ventetuolo and Klinger (2014), Bianchi et al. (2015), Ferrer-Barba et al. (2016), Gist et al. (2016), Chong et al. (2018), Duman et al. (2017), Gavra et al. (2017), Kelly et al. (2017), Lomis et al. (2017), Nanayakkara et al. (2017), Touchan and Guglin (2017), and Tremblay et al. (2017)

4.1.3.2 Dobutamine

Name of drug: Dobutamine phosphate

CAS number: 34368-04-2

Mechanism of action: Dobutamine, a synthetic analogue of dopamine, has positive inotropic effect through adrenergic receptors. Dobutamine in contrast to dopamine does not have any effect on DA receptors; therefore its main target is β1 receptors; also dobutamine has effects on β2 and α1 receptors. By activating β2 adrenergic receptors, systemic vascular resistance would be reduced. Dobutamine would increase patient's heart rate, but the rate of this effect is not as much as dopamine. Therefore in patients with ventricular dysfunction, dobutamine would be a better choice than dopamine.

Indications	• Cardiogenic shock • Acute heart failure • Low cardiac output sate • Myocarditis • MI • Heart failure • After cardiac surgery
Dosage	• **Maintenance dose**: 2–20 μg/kg/min • **High doses** (more than 20 μg/kg/min): results in tachycardia and ventricular ectopy therefore could cause myocardial ischemia and should be avoided • **Note**: due to vasodilatory effect of dobutamine, in hypotensive patients this agent could be co-administered with norepinephrine or dopamine
Side effects	• Tachycardia • Hypotension • Ectopic heartbeats • Phlebitis
Contraindications	• Cardiac dysrhythmia • Obstructive heart lesions • Correction of hypovolemia is mandatory before administration of dobutamine • Dobutamine has more effect on SVR and heart rate than phosphodiesterase inhibitors but less than isoproterenol

Kee (2003), Holmes (2005), Noori and Seri (2012), Jentzer et al. (2015), Parthenakis et al. (2016), Rossano et al. (2016), Shang et al. (2017), Stratton et al. (2017), and Touchan and Guglin (2017)

4.1.3.3 Levosimendan

Name of drug: Levosimendan

CAS number: 141505-33-1

New class of drugs named calcium sensitizers are introduced into practice. The most common drug in this category is levosimendan mainly used for acute decompensated heart failure and low cardiac output state. This agent by stabilizing calcium binding to cardiac troponin C (TnC) will increase myocyte calcium sensitivity. Also by opening ATP-sensitive potassium channels in vessels, this agent has vasodilatory effects. Therefore this agent does not increase myocardial oxygen demand and has cardioprotective effects.

Levosimendan does not need any adjustment neither renal nor hepatic. There have not been any evidences for dysrhythmia while administering, but its main complications would be hypotension and headache.

The loading dose is 6–12 μg/kg over 10 min followed by an infusion of 0.1–0.2 μg/kg/min. Its effects would be observed after 5 min and will be peaked in 10–30 min with the duration of 1–2 h.

There are many evidences about decreasing mortality with levosimendan administration. Also this agent would ameliorate post-cardiac arrest myocardial dysfunction (Mebazaa et al. 2007; Landoni et al. 2012; Lechner et al. 2012; Papp et al. 2012; Nieminen et al. 2013; Li and Hwang 2015; Silvetti et al. 2015; Ferrer-Barba et al. 2016; Fuchs et al. 2016; Kushwah et al. 2016; Rizza et al. 2016; Hummel et al. 2017a, 2017b; Shang et al. 2017; Yandrapalli et al. 2017).

4.1.4 Pure Vasodilators

4.1.4.1 Nitroglycerin

Name of drug: Glyceryl trinitrate

CAS number: 55-63-0

Nitroglycerin is a nitric oxide (NO) donor which preferentially acts on venous system. This venodilation decreases preload and myocardial wall stress that results in decreased cardiac work. This agent also dilates coronary circulation.

Dosage: Nitroglycerine infused at 0.5–2 μg/kg/min leads to venodilation with higher doses 2–5 μg/kg/min; nitroglycerine improves cardiac index and decreases pulmonary and systematic blood pressure (Hari and Sinha 2011).

Indications: Nitroglycerine is the first choice in treatment of hypertension in patients with ischemic heart. Also it is used for the control of heart failure in setting of acute myocardial infarction. This agent also had been used for induction of controlled hypotension in perioperative patients.

Contraindications: Pericardial tamponade, restrictive cardiomyopathy or constrictive pericarditis, elevated intracranial pressure, and concomitant use of phosphodiesterase inhibitors.

4.1.4.2 Hydralazine

Name of drug: Hydralazine

CAS number: 86-54-4

Hydralazine is a pure vasodilator by directly relaxing vascular smooth muscle. Its vasodilatory effect is more pronounced in arterioles which results in decreasing peripheral vascular resistance. Hydralazine's effect is more on diastolic blood pressure than systolic. This agent also increases heart rate and stroke volume and cardiac output. Also this agent elevates renal and cerebral blood flow.

Its oral dose is 0.75 mg/kg daily and can be increased up to 7.5 mg/kg (till 200 mg daily). Parenteral formulation is also available with bolus dose of 0.2–0.6 mg/kg, repeated every 4 h, which is used in severe hypertension. The elimination half-life would be increased in uremic patients; therefore careful titration should be made in aforementioned patients.

Hydralazine is contraindicated in coronary artery disease and mitral valvular rheumatic heart disease. Its side effects are headache, dizziness, pyridoxine insufficiency, peripheral neuritis, drug-induced systemic lupus erythematous, and blood dyscrasias. Due to these side effects, CNS findings and cell blood count should be monitored during treatment (Hari and Sinha 2011; Watt et al. 2011; Ostrye et al. 2014; Flynn et al. 2016).

4.1.4.3 Alprostadil

Name of drug: Prostaglandin E1

CAS number: 745-65-3

Alprostadil (prostaglandin E1): There are a number of pharmacologic effects attributed to this drug including stimulation of smooth muscle contraction in the intestine and uterus accompanied with vasodilation, platelet aggregation inhibition, and a number of other effects. Doses of 1–10 μg/kg could induce vasodilation and then reduce blood pressure, augment cardiac output, and increase heart rate.

There is limited use of this drug in adult cardiovascular diseases, except for a number of effects including its use in the treatment of acidosis in patients with restricted systemic blood flow. Increased blood pressure and decreased "pulmonary artery/aortic pressure" ratio are also among its effects (Carroll et al. 2006; Cuthbert 2011; Strobel and Lu le 2015; Lakshminrusimha et al. 2016).

4.1.4.4 Sodium Nitroprusside

Name of drug: Sodium pentacyanonitrosylferrate

CAS number: 13755-38-9

Mechanism of action	• Sodium nitroprusside (SNP) is a vasodilator which acts through the release of nitric oxide (NO) • This increase in local NO would result in increase in tissue levels of cGMP in arterial and venous system • The final effect would be relaxation of smooth muscles in the vessel's wall
Clinical effects	• SNP would improve cardiac function by decreasing afterload • On the other hand in hypovolemia, this agent could result in severe hypotension. Therefore careful selection of patients in order to minimize complication is mandatory for sodium nitroprusside • In obstructive disease such as aortic stenosis or hypertrophic obstructive cardiomyopathy, this decrease in afterload would be disastrous • Plasma half-life of sodium nitroprusside is 3–4 min; therefore its action is seen within second and lasts for 1–2 min
Side effects	• SNP would also react with oxyhemoglobin in large dose or long-term infusions. This reaction produces methemoglobin and cyanide anions • If cyanide accumulates in tissue, it would bind to cytochrome oxidase that impairs oxidative phosphorylation • This side effect would be minimized by reducing total dose and avoiding long infusions • The diagnosis suspected in patients receiving high dose of SNP and who present with signs of impaired oxygen delivery despite adequate circulation

Dose and administration route	• The initial dose of SNP is recommended to be 0.3 μg/kg/min IBW which is administered by continuous IV infusion • The maintenance dose should be titrated upward to a maximum of 10 μg/kg/min IBW • The best predictor of toxicity is mean dose that is in relation with cyanide levels • The risk of cyanide toxicity increases when total dose greater than 500 μg/kg is administered faster than 2 μg/kg/min of IBW • Another route of administration is inhalational form. This form reduce systemic side effects and is specially indicated in patients with pulmonary hypertension

Friederich and Butterworth (1995), Varon and Marik (2003), Moffett and Price (2008), Thomas et al. (2009), Hottinger et al. (2014), Ehlert et al. (2016), Moffett et al. (2016), Nazir et al. (2016), and Roeleveld and Zwijsen (2017)

4.1.4.5 Phentolamine (Regitine)

Name of drug: Phentolamine mesylate

CAS number: 50-60-2

Phentolamine is a short-duration agent which acts through blocking alpha adrenergic receptors. It causes vasodilation, and to a lesser degree, this agent has positive inotropic and chronotropic effect. High doses of this drug cause tachycardia and arrhythmia by blocking α_2 adrenergic receptors.

As described above, vasodilation causes decrease in afterload and therefore increases cardiac output. On the other hand, this agent would decrease pulmonary vascular resistance and could be beneficial in patients suffering from pulmonary hypertension. It may cause tachycardia, arrhythmia, and hypotension. Its pharmacological characteristics could be found in Table 4.6 (Allen et al. 2013).

4.1.5 Antihypertensive Agents

Blood pressure is the force exerted by blood against the walls of vessels. The degree of that depends on the work being done by the heart and the resistance of the vessels. Hypertension is a long-term medical condition in which blood pressure is elevated persistently. This phenomenon may lead to end organ damage including the heart, kidney, retina, or brain. Currently a vast variety of antihypertensive agents are being used (Flynn 2011; Chu et al. 2014; Dhull et al. 2016).

The current antihypertensive agents could be categorized mainly as follows:

Angiotensin-converting enzyme (ACE) inhibitors: Captopril, enalapril, lisinopril, and ramipril are common drugs in this subclass. Dose, half-life, and side effects are summarized in Table 4.7 (Chaturvedi et al. 2014a, b; Dhull et al. 2016).

Angiotensin II receptor antagonists (ARBs): The prototype drugs in this subclass are losartan and valsartan; however, other members of the group include candesartan, eprosartan, irbesartan, olmesartan, and telmisartan. Table 4.8 is a summary of main ARBs (Chaturvedi et al. 2014a, b; Dhull et al. 2016).

Table 4.6 A summary of vasoactive drugs including *vasodilator* and *vasoconstrictor* drugs used in congenital heart diseases

Drug	Dose	Receptors	Indication	Half-life (duration)	Adverse effects/notes
Vasopressin (11000-17-2)	0.01–0.05 units/kg/h	V_1, V_2	Refractory hypotension after conventional drugs have failed, heart failure, vasodilatory shock, e.g., septic shock	10–30 min	Splanchnic ischemia due to its vasoconstrictor action
Phenylephrine (59-42-7)	0.02–0.3 μg/kg/min	α_1	Hypotension during anesthesia	5 min	Nausea, vomiting, headache, nervousness
Nitroglycerin (55-63-0)	0.2–10 μg/kg/min	Vascular myocyte/ guanylyl cyclase, cGMP ↑	Post-cardiac surgery for valvular regurgitation; cardiac surgeries where coronaries are involved, e.g., arterial switch operation, Ross operation, and repair for anomalous left coronary artery from pulmonary artery; and systemic hypertension	1–4 min	Hypotension, tachycardia, methemoglobinemia leading to cyanosis, acidosis, convulsions, and coma
Nitroprusside (13755-38-9)	0.2–5 μg/kg/min	Vascular myocyte/ guanylyl cyclase, cGMP ↑	Systemic hypertension, e.g., after repair of coarctation of aorta, malignant hypertension of renal vascular origin; acute, severe valvular regurgitation, low cardiac output state following cardiac surgery, especially after valvular surgery, acute heart failure	2 min	Excessive hypotension, cyanide toxicity

Inhaled nitric oxide (10102-43-9)	10–40 ppm	Vascular myocyte/cGMP ↑	Pulmonary hypertension of the newborn	2–6 s	Nitric oxide should not be used for long term, as it results in methemoglobinemia
Prostaglandin E1 (745-65-3)	0.01–0.4 μg/kg/min	Vascular myocyte/cAMP ↑	In newborns who have congenital heart defects (e.g., pulmonary stenosis, tricuspid atresia) and who depend on patent ductus for survival	0.5–10 min	Hypotension, cardiac arrest, edema
Fenoldopam (67227-57-0)	0.025–0.3 μg/kg/min Initial dose, titrate To maximum dose 0.8 μg/kg/min	DA-1, α2	Severe hypertension	3–5 min	Hypotension, tachycardia
Nicardipine (55985-32-5)	1–3 μg/kg/min IV infusion, maximum 15 mg/h	Calcium channel antagonist	Severe hypertension	14.4 h	Headache, hypotension, nausea/vomiting, tachycardia
Phentolamine mesylate (50-60-2)	1 mg, 0.1 mg/kg, or 3 mg/m^2	α adrenergic blocking agent, an imidazoline	Hypertension crisis, hypertension in pheochromocytoma, extravasation of catecholamines pulmonary artery hypertension	15–30 min	Abdominal pain, nausea, vomiting, diarrhea, exacerbation of peptic ulcer, orthostatic hypotension

Modified from Dabbagh A., et al. "Cardiovascular Pharmacology in Pediatric Patients with Congenital Heart Disease"; in "Congenital Heart Disease in Pediatric and Adult Patients; Anesthetic and Perioperative Management". Dabbagh A., Hernandez Conte A., Lubin L. Springer 2017, pp. 117–195. Published with kind permission of © SpringerNature, 2017. All Rights Reserved (Dabbagh et al. 2017a)

Table 4.7 The main ACE inhibitors

Drug	Dose	Half-life	Adverse effects
Captopril (CAS number: 62571-86-2)	Oral: 25 mg orally 2–3 times a day 1 h before meals	1–2.3 h	Cough Headache Rash
Enalapril (CAS number: 75847-73-3)	Initial dose (oral tablets or solution): 5 mg orally once a day Maintenance dose (oral tablets or solution): 10–40 mg orally/day Maximum dose: 40 mg orally daily	10–12 h	Dizziness Hypotension Hyperkalemia Angioedema
Lisinopril (CAS number: 83915-83-7)	Initial dose: 5–10 mg orally once a day Maintenance dose: 20–40 mg orally once a day Maximum dose: 80 mg orally once a day	11–13 h	

Modified from Dabbagh A., et al. "Cardiovascular Pharmacology in Pediatric Patients with Congenital Heart Disease"; in "Congenital Heart Disease in Pediatric and Adult Patients; Anesthetic and Perioperative Management". Dabbagh A., Hernandez Conte A., Lubin L. Springer 2017, pp. 117–195. Published with kind permission of © SpringerNature, 2017. All Rights Reserved (Dabbagh et al. 2017a)

Table 4.8 The main ARBs

Drug	Dose	Half-life	Adverse effects
Losartan (CAS number: 114798-26-4)	Initial dose: 50 mg orally once a day Maximum dose: 100 mg orally once a day	1.5–2 h Active metabolite: 6–9 h	Headache Dizziness Hypoglycemia Hypotension Hyperkalemia Diarrhea
Valsartan (CAS number: 137862-53-4)	Initial dose: 80–160 mg orally once a day Maintenance dose: 80–320 mg orally once a day	4–5 h	

Modified from Dabbagh A., et al. "Cardiovascular Pharmacology in Pediatric Patients with Congenital Heart Disease"; in "Congenital Heart Disease in Pediatric and Adult Patients; Anesthetic and Perioperative Management". Dabbagh A., Hernandez Conte A., Lubin L. Springer 2017, pp. 117–195. Published with kind permission of © SpringerNature, 2017. All Rights Reserved (Dabbagh et al. 2017a)

Calcium channel blockers (CCBs): There are two types of calcium channel blockers: dihydropyridines and non-dihydropyridines. Their main drugs are summarized in Table 4.9 (Chaturvedi et al. 2014a, b; Dhull et al. 2016; Smith et al. 2016; Green et al. 2017; Latorre et al. 2017; Tran et al. 2017).

Diuretics: Tables 4.10, 4.11, and 4.12 are summaries of diuretic agents which could be classified in four groups listed below (Bayat et al. 2015; Dhull et al. 2016; McCammond et al. 2016; Al-Naher et al. 2017; Jiang et al. 2017; Ng and Yap 2018):

Table 4.9 The main calcium channel blockers

Drug	Dose	Half-life	Adverse effects
Amlodipine (CAS number: 88150-42-9)	Initial dose: 5 mg orally once a day Maintenance dose: 5–10 mg orally once a day Maximum dose: 10 mg/day	30–50 h	Fatigue Somnolence Nausea Flushing Edema Dizziness Palpitations Abdominal pain
Nifedipine (CAS number: 21829-25-4)	– Initial dose: 30–60 mg orally once a day – Maintenance dose: 30–90 mg orally once a day – Maximum dose: up to 120 mg/day	2–7 h	
Isradipine (CAS number: 75695-93-1)	Immediate-release capsules: 2.5 mg orally twice a day Controlled-release tablets: 5 mg orally once a day	Biphasic, initial half-life 1.5–2 h, terminal elimination half-life approximately 8 h	

Modified from Dabbagh A., et al. "Cardiovascular Pharmacology in Pediatric Patients with Congenital Heart Disease"; in "Congenital Heart Disease in Pediatric and Adult Patients; Anesthetic and Perioperative Management". Dabbagh A., Hernandez Conte A., Lubin L. Springer 2017, pp. 117–195. Published with kind permission of © SpringerNature, 2017. All Rights Reserved (Dabbagh et al. 2017a)

Table 4.10 The main loop diuretics

IV: intravenous			
Drug	Dose	Half-life	Adverse effects
Furosemide (CAS number: 54-31-9)	Oral: 80 mg/day IV, intramuscular: 0.5–2 mg/kg/dose every 6–24 h Continuous IV infusion: 0.1–0.4 mg/kg/h	0.5–2 h; 9 h in end-stage renal disease	Hypokalemia Metabolic alkalosis Hypomagnesemia Hyperuricemia Hyponatremia
Ethacrynic acid (CAS number: 58-54-8)	50–200 mg orally/day	2–4 h	

Modified from Dabbagh A., et al. "Cardiovascular Pharmacology in Pediatric Patients with Congenital Heart Disease"; in "Congenital Heart Disease in Pediatric and Adult Patients; Anesthetic and Perioperative Management". Dabbagh A., Hernandez Conte A., Lubin L. Springer 2017, pp. 117–195. Published with kind permission of © SpringerNature, 2017. All Rights Reserved (Dabbagh et al. 2017a)

Table 4.11 Spironolactone: the main mineralocorticoid (aldosterone) receptor antagonist

Drug	Dose	Half-life	Adverse effects
Spironolactone (CAS number: 52-01-7)	Oral: 50–100 mg orally/day in single or divided doses	1.4 h; active metabolites: 12–20 h	Hyperkalemia Gynecomastia diarrhea Vomiting Nausea Dizziness

Table 4.12 Thiazide and thiazide-like diuretics

Drug	Dose	Half-life	Adverse effects
Chlorothiazide (CAS number: 58-94-6)	Oral or IV: 500–1000 mg once or twice a day	45–120 min	Hypokalemia Hypomagnesemia Hyperuricemia Hyponatremia
Hydrochlorothiazide (CAS number: 58-93-5)	Oral: initial dose, 25 mg orally once daily Maintenance dose: may increase to 50 mg orally daily	6–15 h	
Metolazone (Zaroxolyn) (CAS number: 17560-51-9)	Oral: initial dose, 2.5 mg orally once a day or	6–20 h	

Modified from Dabbagh A., et al. "Cardiovascular Pharmacology in Pediatric Patients with Congenital Heart Disease"; in "Congenital Heart Disease in Pediatric and Adult Patients; Anesthetic and Perioperative Management". Dabbagh A., Hernandez Conte A., Lubin L. Springer 2017, pp. 117–195. Published with kind permission of © SpringerNature, 2017. All Rights Reserved (Dabbagh et al. 2017a)

Specific type of diuretic agents	Members of this diuretic type
Loop diuretics	Bumetanide Ethacrynic acid Furosemide Torsemide
Potassium-sparing diuretics (mineralocorticoid "aldosterone" receptor antagonists)	Spironolactone Amiloride Triamterene
Thiazide diuretics	Epitizide Hydrochlorothiazide Chlorothiazide Bendroflumethiazide
Thiazide-like diuretics	Indapamide Chlorthalidone Metolazone

Adrenergic receptor antagonists (alpha- and/or beta-blockers): Some of these agents are discussed under the anti-arrhythmic categories; however, others are discussed in the Table 4.13.

Vasodilators: These subclass include nitroglycerine, nitroprusside, hydralazine, and minoxidil; most of them are discussed in previous chapter of pure vasodilators, and others are presented in Table 4.14 (Hari and Sinha 2011; Ostrye et al. 2014; Dhull et al. 2016; Flynn et al. 2016).

Table 4.13 A number of adrenoceptor blocking agents

Drug	Dose	Half-life	Adverse effects
β-blockers			
Metoprolol (CAS number: 37350-58-6)	Oral: initial dose, 100 mg orally/day in single or divided doses Maintenance dose: 100–450 mg orally/day	3–4 h (7–9 h in poor CYP2D6 metabolizers)	Bradyarrhythmias Hypotension Headache Dizziness Fatigue
Esmolol (CAS number: 103598-03-4)	IV: administer 500 μg/kg IV as a bolus dose over 1 min followed by a maintenance infusion of 50 μg/kg/min IV for 4 min	4–7 min	
Propranolol (CAS number: 525-66-6)	Oral dose: 40 mg orally 2 times a day Maintenance dose: 120–240 mg orally daily	3–6 h	
Mixed alpha + beta blocker			
Carvedilol (CAS number: 72956-09-3)	Initial dose: 6.25 mg orally twice a day Maximum dose: 50 mg orally twice a day	7–10 h	Blurred vision Cold sweats Confusion Shortness of breath Swelling of face, Tightness in chest Wheezing
Labetalol (CAS number: 36894-69-6)	IV: – Initial dose: 20 mg by slow IV injection over a 2-min period – Additional injections of 40–80 mg can be given at 10 min intervals until a desired supine blood pressure is achieved or a total of 300 mg has been used	5.5 h after IV administration	
Peripheral alpha-blockers			
Prazosin (CAS number: 19216-56-9)	Initial dose: 1 mg orally 2 or 3 times a day Maintenance dose: 1–20 mg orally/day in divided doses	2–4 h	Dizziness, headache, drowsiness, weakness, palpitation, nausea
Terazosin (CAS number: 63590-64-7)	Initial dose: 1 mg orally once a day at bedtime Maintenance dose: 1–5 mg orally once a day Maximum dose: 20 mg/day	Approximately 12 h	
Alpha-2 adrenergic agonists			
Clonidine (CAS number: 4205-90-7)	– Initial dose: 0.1 mg orally 2 times a day – Maintenance dose: 0.2–0.6 mg orally/day in divided doses – Maximum dose: 2.4 mg orally/day in divided doses	6–20 h	Dry mouth Constipation Dizziness Drowsiness Sedation Major depression (for methyldopa)
Methyldopa (CAS number: 555-30-6)	Initial dose: 250 mg orally 2–3 times a day or 250–500 mg IV over 30–60 min every 6 h, up to a maximum of 3 g/day Maintenance dose: 500 mg to 2 g orally divided in 2–4 doses, up to a maximum of 3 g/day	2–8 h after single oral dose or 4–12 h multiple oral doses	

Modified from Dabbagh A., et al. "Cardiovascular Pharmacology in Pediatric Patients with Congenital Heart Disease"; in "Congenital Heart Disease in Pediatric and Adult Patients; Anesthetic and Perioperative Management". Dabbagh A., Hernandez Conte A., Lubin L. Springer 2017, pp. 117–195. Published with kind permission of © SpringerNature, 2017. All Rights Reserved (Dabbagh et al. 2017a)

Driscoll et al. (2015), Xue et al. (2015), Klugman et al. (2016), McCammond et al. (2016), Rossano et al. (2016), and Zou et al. (2016)

Table 4.14 Common vasodilators

Drug	Dose	Half-life	Adverse effects
Hydralazine (CAS number: 86-54-4)	Initial dose: 10 mg orally 4 times a day for the first 2–4 days, increase to 25 mg orally 4 times a day for the balance of the first week Week 2 and subsequent weeks: 50 mg orally 4 times a day Maintenance dose: adjust dosage to the lowest effective levels	2–4 h	Headache Retention of salt and water Reflex tachycardia Palpitation
Minoxidil (CAS number: 38304-91-5)	Initial dose: 5 mg orally once a day Maintenance dose: 10–40 mg/day Maximum dose: 100 mg/day	4 h	Hypertrichosis Retention of salt and water Nausea Pericardial effusion

Modified from Dabbagh A., et al. "Cardiovascular Pharmacology in Pediatric Patients with Congenital Heart Disease"; in "Congenital Heart Disease in Pediatric and Adult Patients; Anesthetic and Perioperative Management". Dabbagh A., Hernandez Conte A., Lubin L. Springer 2017, pp. 117–195. Published with kind permission of © SpringerNature, 2017. All Rights Reserved (Dabbagh et al. 2017a)

4.2 Drugs Used in Pulmonary Hypertension

Pulmonary hypertension affects the arteries of the lungs and right cardiac chambers. Pulmonary hypertension and right heart failure reduce left ventricular filling pressure, decreased cardiac output which results in systemic hypotension. Table 4.14 summarizes drugs used in this disease.

Since 1987 when NO was recognized as endothelial-derived vasodilator, its use in clinical scenarios has been extended. This agent is constructed from oxygen and L-arginine by nitric oxide synthases, and most of its action is through soluble guanylate cyclase (sGC) that catalyzes cyclic guanosine monophosphate (cGMP) as second messenger. Inhaled NO (iNO) is a selective pulmonary vasodilator which is administered through the lungs.

Phosphodiesterase inhibitors like milrinone inhibit breakdown of cyclic adenosine monophosphate and therefore increase its intracellular concentration. These agents also could be used in pulmonary hypertension patients.

Other agents which are efficient in these patients include prostacyclin analogues (epoprostenol, iloprost, treprostinil), phosphodiesterase 5 inhibitors (sildenafil and tadalafil), phosphodiesterase 3 inhibitors (mainly milrinone), endothelin receptor antagonists (bosentan, ambrisentan, and macitentan), and soluble guanylate cyclase stimulator (riociguat) (Poor and Ventetuolo 2012; Ventetuolo and Klinger 2014; Vorhies and Ivy 2014; Abman et al. 2015; Jentzer and Mathier 2016; Hansmann et al. 2016; Jortveit et al. 2016; Kim et al. 2016; Kozlik-Feldmann et al. 2016; Lakshminrusimha et al. 2016; Latus et al. 2016; Smith et al. 2016; Chong et al. 2018; Gavra et al. 2017; Green et al. 2017; Kelly et al. 2017).

4.2.1 Nitric Oxide

As described above, NO is an important cellular signaling molecule. This agent is a potent vasodilator and its half-life is about few seconds in the blood. Nitroglycerine and amyl nitrite were found to be precursors to NO. This lipophilic molecule is synthesized from transformation of L-arginine by nitric oxide synthase (NOS). NO is administered through inhalation (iNO), and therefore its first line of action is in smooth muscle cells of pulmonary vessels that leads to accumulation of cGMP and hence dilate pulmonary circulation system.

iNO is rapidly reached to its biophase through alveolar-capillary membranes and metabolized by circulatory erythrocytes. Therefore there are least possible systemic side effects (Kim et al. 2016; Moffett et al. 2016).

Dose: This agent is administered by nasal cannula, face mask, or endotracheal tube. The initial dose is 2–5 ppm and the maximum dose is 40 ppm. Higher doses would cause systemic side effects without increasing drug's effect. It is administered by specific instruments which have high costs. The most important side effects are methemoglobinemia and direct lung injury. Routine monitoring of methemoglobin is recommended in every patients receiving iNO. Also rebound pulmonary hypertension is reported by abrupt cessation of iNO (Atz and Wessel 1997; Mossad 2001; Gao and Raj 2010; Pritts and Pearl 2010; Abman et al. 2015; Latus et al. 2015; Hansmann et al. 2016; Kim et al. 2016; Moffett et al. 2016; Garcia-Rivas et al. 2017; Giesinger et al. 2017; Klinger and Kadowitz 2017; Lai et al. 2017; McMahon and Bryan 2017).

4.2.2 Phosphodiesterase 5 (PDE 5) Inhibitors

Sildenafil, tadalafil, and vardenafil are among the agents in this group. Among them, sildenafil and tadalafil are more commonly used for pulmonary hypertension.

Sildenafil: Phosphodiesterase 5 (PDE 5) breaks down cGMP, so sildenafil, as inhibitor of this enzyme, leads to accumulation of cGMP and vasodilation. There are both intravenous and oral formulations of sildenafil. Therefore unlike NO, systemic effects commonly occur. This could be hazardous in critically ill patients due to life-threatening systemic hypotension. The recommended initial oral dose is 5 mg every 8 h which could be increased with the maximum dose of 20 mg every 8 h. This titration should be based on clinical effect of this agent. Intravenous dose is 2.5–10 mg three times a day. Other information of sildenafil could be found in Table 4.15 (Shah and Ohlsson 2011; Beghetti et al. 2014; Vorhies and Ivy 2014; Wang et al. 2014; Dodgen and Hill 2015; Perez and Laughon 2015; Lakshminrusimha et al. 2016; Gamidov et al. 2017; Kniotek and Boguska 2017; Unegbu et al. 2017).

Table 4.15 Pharmacological agents used in the management of pulmonary hypertension

Drug	Recommended dose	Adverse effects	Clinical considerations
Inhaled nitric oxide (iNO): mechanism of action is increasing cGMP, pulmonary vasodilation			
iNO (CAS number: 10102-43-9)	2–5 ppm to a maximum of 40 ppm	Lung injury Methemoglobinemia Rebound pulmonary hypertension	Should not be over administered to prevent side effects Its cost may suggest to consider the drug as the last choice
Prostacyclin/prostacyclin analogues: their mechanism of action is pulmonary and systemic vasodilation through increasing cAMP; also, antiplatelet aggregation			
Epoprostenol (CAS number: 35121-78-9)	– Initial dose: 2 ng/kg/min via continuous IV infusion and titrate up in increments of 2 ng/kg/min every 15 min or longer until a tolerance limit is established or further increases in infusion rate not clinically warranted	Flushing, headache, nausea, diarrhea, jaw discomfort, hypotension, thrombocytopenia	Potential risk of hypotension and bleeding in patients receiving anticoagulants, platelet inhibitors, or other vasodilators
Iloprost (CAS number: 73873-87-7)	– Initial dose: 2.5 μg inhaled orally once; if tolerated, increase to 5 μg – Maintenance dose: 2.5 or 5 μg inhaled orally 6–9 times/day – Maximum dose: 45 μg/day (5 μg/dose 9 times/day)	Cough, wheeze, headache, flushing, jaw pain, hypotension (at higher doses)	Potential risk of exacerbation of reactive airway disease
Treprostinil (IV/subcutaneous) (CAS number: 81846-19-7)	– Initial dose: 1.25 ng/kg/min – Maintenance dose: increase infusion rate by 1.25 ng/kg/min/week for the first 4 weeks	Flushing, headache, nausea, diarrhea, musculoskeletal discomfort, rash, hypotension, thrombocytopenia, and pain at subcutaneous infusion site	Similar to epoprostenol
Treprostinil (inhaled)	– Initial dose: 3 breaths (18 μg) per treatment session 4 times a day – Maintenance dose: increase by an additional 3 breaths at about 1–2 week intervals – Maximum dose: 9 breaths (54 μg) per treatment session 4 times a day	Cough, headache, nausea, dizziness, flushing, and throat irritation	Reactive airway symptoms and hypotension may occur at high doses

Table 4.15 (continued)

Drug	Recommended dose	Adverse effects	Clinical considerations
Treprostinil (oral)	– Initial dose: 0.25 mg orally every 12 h or 0.125 mg every 8 h – Maintenance dose: titrate to the highest tolerated dose in increments of 0.25 or 0.5 mg twice a day or 0.125	Headache, nausea, jaw pain, extremity pain, hypokalemia, abdominal discomfort, and flushing	If "twice daily" dosing is not tolerated, consider "three times daily" dosing
PDE-5 inhibitors: inhibit phosphodiesterase-5, leading to pulmonary vasodilation and inhibition of vascular remodeling			
Sildenafil (CAS number: 171599-83-0)	– Initial dose: 5 or 20 mg orally three times a day, 4–6 h apart – Maximum dose: 20 mg orally three times a day	Headache, flushing, rhinitis, dizziness, hypotension, peripheral edema, dyspepsia, diarrhea, myalgia, and back pain	Co-administration of nitrates is contraindicated Sensorineural hearing loss and ischemic optic neuropathy have been reported
Tadalafil (CAS number: 171596-29-5)	– Oral dose: 40 mg orally once a day	Similar to sildenafil No significant effect on vision	Similar to sildenafil
Antagonists of endothelin receptor: counteract with the effects of both endothelin receptors (ET_A and ET_B), vasodilation of the pulmonary vascular system, and remodeling inhibition			
Ambrisentan (CAS number: 177036-94-1)	– Initial dose: 5 mg orally once a day	Peripheral edema, nasal congestion, headache, flushing, anemia, nausea, and decreased sperm count	Baseline liver enzymes and hemoglobin are needed Monitor based on clinical parameters
Bosentan (CAS number: 147536-97-8)	– Initial dose: 62.5 mg orally twice a day for 4 weeks – Maintenance dose: following initial dose, increase to 125 mg orally twice a day	Abdominal pain, vomiting, extremity pain, fatigue, flushing, headache, edema, nasal congestion, anemia, and decreased sperm count Potential risk of dose dependent increases in amino-transaminase levels	Liver enzymes and hemoglobin levels should be monitored and, in patients with moderate or severe degrees of hepatic impairment, should be used cautiously Also, concomitant use of CYP3A4 inducers and inhibitors should be considered as important caution

(continued)

Table 4.15 (continued)

Drug	Recommended dose	Adverse effects	Clinical considerations
Macitentan (CAS number: 441798-33-0)	10 mg orally once a day	Nasal congestion, headache, flushing, anemia, and decreased sperm count	The incidence of serum aminotransferase elevation is low Obtain baseline liver enzymes and hemoglobin and monitor as clinically indicated teratogenicity REMS*
sGC stimulator: its action mechanism is stimulation of soluble guanylate cyclase leading to pulmonary vasodilation associated with inhibition of vascular remodeling			
Riociguat (CAS number: 625115-55-1)	– Initial dose: 1 mg orally 3 times a day – Maximum dose: 2.5 mg orally 3 times a day	Headache, dizziness, dyspepsia, nausea, diarrhea, hypotension, vomiting, anemia, gastroesophageal reflux, and constipation	Co-administration of nitrates and/or PDE-5 inhibitors is contraindicated Teratogenicity is a potential risk

Modified from Dabbagh A., et al. "Cardiovascular Pharmacology in Pediatric Patients with Congenital Heart Disease"; in "Congenital Heart Disease in Pediatric and Adult Patients; Anesthetic and Perioperative Management". Dabbagh A., Hernandez Conte A., Lubin L. Springer 2017, pp. 117–195. Published with kind permission of © SpringerNature, 2017. All Rights Reserved (Dabbagh et al. 2017a)

4.2.3 Endothelin Receptor Blockers (ET Blockers)

Endothelin receptor located on endothelium and vascular smooth muscles is responsible for vasoconstriction. Endothelin receptor blockers oppose this reaction and therefore are used in pulmonary hypertensive patients. Bosentan, a prototype of nonselective ET blockers, inhibits both ET_A and ET_B receptor activities with a higher affinity for the A subtype. This agent improves symptoms, exercise tolerance, and hemodynamics by decreasing pulmonary vascular resistance in these patients.

ET-1 antagonist and bosentan could elevate hepatic enzyme, so monitoring of hepatic function is mandatory. Almost 10% of patients on treatment with bosentan had abnormal liver function tests. The common dosing for is as follows:

- Initial dose: 62.5 mg orally twice a day for 4 weeks.
- Maintenance dose: Following initial dose, increase to 125 mg orally twice a day.
- Doses above 125 mg twice a day did not appear to confer additional benefit sufficient enough to offset increased risk of hepatotoxicity.

Other side effects are headaches, edema, hypotension, palpitation, anemia, and dyspepsia (Allen et al. 2013; Liu et al. 2013; Abman et al. 2015; Latus et al. 2015; Hansmann et al. 2016; Kim et al. 2016; Moffett et al. 2016; Arora et al. 2017).

4.2.4 Milrinone

Milrinone is discussed in detail throughout the previous paragraphs under "inodilators."

4.3 Anti-arrhythmic Agents

As the medications for treatment of arrhythmia increased, the need for classification became important. The most widely used classification in this era is Vaughan Williams. The basic of this classification is grouping of agents according to the physiology of myocardial cells, discussed in Chap. 3. The mechanism of each class of anti-arrhythmic could be schematized by Fig. 4.1. Also Tables 4.16 and 4.17

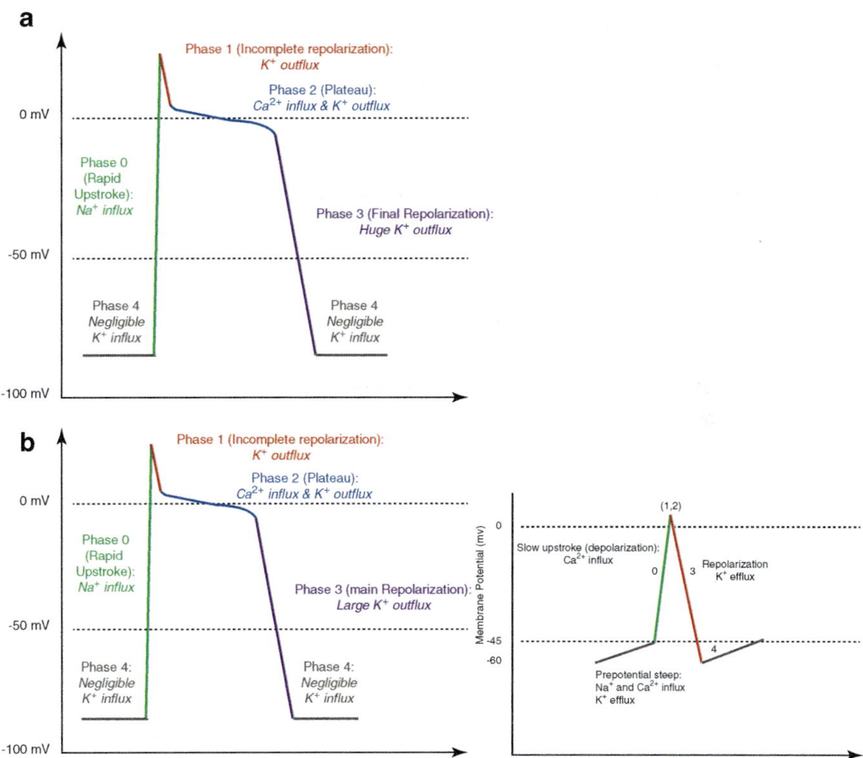

Fig. 4.1 (**a**) Progress of action potential phases in normal myocardial cells; (**b**) Comparison of action potential phases between normal myocardial cells and pacemaker cells. Modified from Dabbagh A., et al. "Pediatric Cardiovascular Physiology"; in "Congenital Heart Disease in Pediatric and Adult Patients; Anesthetic and Perioperative Management". Dabbagh A., Hernandez Conte A., Lubin L. Springer 2017, pp. 65–116. Published with kind permission of © SpringerNature, 2017. All Rights Reserved (Dabbagh 2014, Dabbagh et al. 2017a, b)

Table 4.16 Vaughan Williams classification of anti-arrhythmic agents (Vaughan Williams 1989, 1992; Zipes et al. 2006; Moffett et al. 2016; Yerokun et al. 2016; Dabbagh et al. 2017a, b)

Class of drugs	Drugs (alphabetic order)	Mechanism of action
Class I a	Disopyramide, procainamide, quinidine	*Fast Na channel blockers*: depress phase 0, prolonging repolarization
Class I b	Lidocaine, mexiletine, phenytoin, tocainide	*Fast Na channel blockers*: selectively depress phase 0 in abnormal/ischemic tissue, shorten repolarization
Class I c	Flecainide, moricizine, propafenone	*Fast Na channel blockers*: markedly depress phase 0, with minimal effect on repolarization
Class II	Atenolol, bisoprolol, carvedilol, esmolol, metoprolol, propranolol, timolol	*Beta-blockers*: decreases slope of phase 4
Class III	Amiodarone, dofetilide, ibutilide, sotalol	Potassium (K) channel blockers which prolong the cardiac action potential: mainly prolong phase 3
Class IV	Diltiazem, verapamil	Slow calcium (Ca) channel blockers: prolong phase 2
Class V	Adenosine, digoxin, magnesium sulfate	Variable mechanism

summarize their characteristics (Marcotti et al. 2004; Parham et al. 2006; Wolf and Berul 2008; Amanfu and Saucerman 2011; Marionneau and Abriel 2015; Moffett et al. 2016; Bond et al. 2017; Cata et al. 2017; Khan et al. 2017).

4.4 Analgesic Agents, Sedative Drugs, and Intravenous Anesthetic Agents

One of the most needs of patients in perioperative period is analgesia. This could be due to residual pain from surgical site, new manipulations, changing the surgical dressings, or frequent tracheal suctioning. Therefore one of the skills every physician should encounter is dealing with analgesics and sedatives (Lucas et al. 2016).

In order to manage these conditions, we should have the ability to assess pain and anxiety. Numerous scales are introduced in order to define conditions. Some of them are listed below and are discussed in another chapter of the book "Postoperative Central Nervous System Monitoring in Adult Cardiac Surgery" in detail:

- Ramsay sedation scale (Ramsay)
- Sedation-agitation scale (SAS)
- Richmond agitation-sedation scale (RASS)

Sedation and analgesia is a great challenge in patients with cardiac diseases due to low cardiorespiratory reserve; therefore monitoring and vigilance are the keys for a successful management. Overtreatment could cause cardiopulmonary insufficiency and cardiac arrest; on the other hand, under treatment would increase cardiopulmonary demand and may lead to cardiac arrest. Appropriate choice of analgesic

Table 4.17 Individual anti-arrhythmic agents

Medication	Dosing	Indication	Adverse events	Specific clinical considerations
Class I a				
Procainamide (CAS number: 51-06-9)	IV: Loading dose: 15–18 mg/kg IM: 50 mg/kg	Atrial tachycardia, JET, VT	Hypotension and pro-arrhythmia	Procainamide and NAPA concentrations are used as serum markers of therapy
Disopyramide (CAS number: 3737-09-5)	Oral: 400–800 mg/day	Ventricular arrhythmias	Anticholinergic effects	May be ineffective in patients with hypokalemia and toxic effects may be enhanced in patients with hyperkalemia
Quinidine (CAS number: 56-54-2)	Tablet (sulfate):100–600 mg/dose orally every 4–6 h IV: 800 mg	SVT, VT, atrial tachycardia ventricular premature complexes	Hypotension (particularly with IV formulation)	There are two forms of drug available (sulfate and gluconate) IV route is not routinely recommended because of hypotension
Class I b				
Lidocaine (CAS number: 137-58-6)	Initial dose: 50–100 mg IV bolus Following bolus administration: 1–4 mg/min continuous	PVCs, VT, VF	Hypotension and numbness	
Mexiletine (CAS number: 31828-71-4)	400 mg loading dose (in rapid control) followed by 200 mg in 8 h	Ventricular arrhythmias	Development or exacerbation of arrhythmias and hypotension	Limit use to those with life-threatening arrhythmias, lack of evidence for improved survival for class I anti-arrhythmic agents
Phenytoin (CAS number: 57-41-0)	Oral 100 mg 2–4 times daily IV 100 mg by direct IV injection at 5-min intervals until a total of 1 g is given	VT, PAT	Hypotension, severe cardiotoxic reactions (e.g., decreased cardiac output, atrial or ventricular conduction depression, ventricular depression)	IV use contraindicated in patients with sinus bradycardia, SA block, second- or third-degree AV block, or Adams-Stokes syndrome

(continued)

Table 4.17 (continued)

Medication	Dosing	Indication	Adverse events	Specific clinical considerations
Tocainide: no longer sold in US				
Class I c				
Flecainide (CAS number: 54143-55-4)	Initial dose: 50 mg orally every 12 h Maintenance dose: may be increased in increments of 50 mg bid every 4 days	SVT	Potential for pro-arrhythmia in patients with congenital heart disease	Caution use in patients with congenital heart disease; milk feeds may decrease absorption; level monitoring may assist in guiding therapy
Moricizine: withdrawn from the market				
Propafenone (CAS number: 54063-53-5)	Immediate release: 150 mg orally every 8 h	Paroxysmal atrial fibrillation/flutter and paroxysmal supraventricular tachyarrhythmias, VT, atrial fibrillation	Bradycardia and pro-arrhythmia	
Class II (beta-blockers)				
Atenolol (CAS number: 29122-68-7)	Oral: initial dose, 50 mg orally once a day	SVT, VT	Bradycardia, hypotension, and hypoglycemia	
Bisoprolol: no indication in arrhythmia				
Carvedilol: no indication in arrhythmia				
Esmolol (CAS number: 103598-03-4)	IV: bolus, 500 μg/kg IV over 1 min IV: continuous infusion, 25–200 μg/kg/min IV	Sinus tachycardia; atrial and ventricular tachyarrhythmias	Bradycardia, hypotension, and hypoglycemia	
Metoprolol (CAS number: 37350-58-6)	Oral: children 1–17 year, 1–2 mg/kg/day given twice daily (max, 6 mg/kg/day or 200 mg/day)	SVT, VT	Bradycardia, hypotension, and hypoglycemia	
Propranolol (CAS number: 525-66-6)	Oral: 100 mg orally/day in single or divided doses)	SVT, VT	Bradycardia, hypotension, and hypoglycemia	

Timolol: no indication in arrhythmia				
Class III				
Amiodarone (CAS number: 1951-25-3)	– Loading infusions: 150 mg over the first 10 min (15 mg/min), followed by 360 mg over the next 6 h (1 mg/min) – Maintenance infusion: 540 mg over the remaining 18 h (0.5 mg/min	Atrial tachycardia, flutter, and fibrillation, JET, VT, and VF	Bradycardia, hypotension, torsade de pointes, hepatotoxicity, thyroid dysfunction, skin color alteration, corneal deposits, and pulmonary fibrosis	Patients may require 1–2 weeks of loading dose (higher doses) at the beginning of therapy due to the long half-life of amiodarone Extensive laboratory monitoring at baseline required due to high incidence of adverse events
Dofetilide (CAS number: 115256-11-6)	Initially, 500 μg twice daily; modify dosage according to Clcr and QTc interval	SVT	Arrhythmias (torsade de pointes)	Arrhythmogenic, contraindicated in congenital or acquired long QT syndromes; baseline QT or QTc interval > 440 ms (500 ms in patients with ventricular conduction abnormalities) Severe renal impairment (calculated Clcr <20 mL/min)
Ibutilide (CAS number: 122647-32-9)	*Atrial flutter and/or fibrillation* IV **Adults** weighing ≥60 kg: initially, 1 or 2 mg Adults weighing <60 kg: initially, 0.01 mg/kg (10 μg/kg). Repeat after 10 min if needed, *Atrial flutter and/or fibrillation following coronary bypass graft or valvular surgery* IV Adults weighing ≥60 kg: 1 or 2 infusions of 0.5 mg each (given 10 min apart) Adults weighing <60 kg: 1 or 2 infusions of 0.005 mg/kg (5 μg/kg) each (given 10 min apart)	SVT, atrial flutter and/or fibrillation following coronary bypass graft or valvular surgery	Arrhythmia, CHF, renal failure	Atrial arrhythmias of not so recent onset are less likely to respond to the drug. Efficacy not determined in atrial arrhythmias of >90 days' duration (AHFS 2016)

(continued)

Table 4.17 (continued)

Medication	Dosing	Indication	Adverse events	Specific clinical considerations
Sotalol (CAS number: 3930-20-9)	Oral: 80 mg orally 2 times a day IV: 75 mg IV infused over 5 h once or twice daily	Atrial arrhythmia, VT	Bradycardia, hypotension, hypoglycemia, and torsade de pointes	Dosing for infants <2 years is controversial; ECG monitoring for QT prolongation necessary; women at greater risk for TdP than men
Class IV				
Diltiazem (CAS number: 42399-41-7)	IV Initially, 15–20 mg (or 0.25 mg/kg) by direct IV injection over 2 min. 20–25 mg (or 0.35 mg/kg) can be administrated 15 min after the initial if needed Maintenance infusion: 5–15 mg/h; titrate dose to heart rate	SVT	Hypotension, renal or hepatic injury, slowing cardiac conduction, possible transient VPB on conversion of PSVT to sinus rhythm	IV diltiazem contraindicated • In patients with VT. • Patients with atrial flutter or fibrillation with an accessory pathway if concurrent or recent (e.g., within a few hours) administration of IV β adrenergic blockers
Verapamil (CAS number: 52-53-9)	IV: initial dose, 5–10 mg Oral: 240–320 mg/day orally in 3 or 4 divided doses	SVT	Hypotension and bradycardia	IV use is not recommended in patients who are <1 year old because of the risk of cardiovascular collapse
Class V				
Adenosine (CAS number: 58-61-7)	IV: first dose 6 mg bolus from peripheral and second dose 12 mg	SVT	Gasping, chest pain, flushing, and wide complex tachycardia	Rapid flush required immediately after adenosine infusion; should be given at a site closest to the heart Life support equipment should be nearby when administering adenosine

Digoxin (CAS number: 20830-75-5)	IV: initial 8–12 μg/kg Maintenance: 2.4–3.6 μg/kg once a day	Atrial fibrillation and flutter, sinus tachycardia, paroxysmal supraventricular tachycardias	Bradycardia, nausea/vomiting, and visual disturbances	Adverse events from digoxin toxicity may occur in patients with kidney dysfunction, electrolyte disturbances, or drug interactions
Magnesium sulfate (CAS number: 7487-88-9)	3–4 g (30–40 mL of a 10% solution) IV over 30 s	VT (torsade de pointes) Prevention of JET	Hypotension Muscle weakness, sedation	May cause hypotension on infusion; rate of infusion should be dictated by patient condition

Modified from Dabbagh A., et al. "Cardiovascular Pharmacology in Pediatric Patients with Congenital Heart Disease"; in "Congenital Heart Disease in Pediatric and Adult Patients; Anesthetic and Perioperative Management". Dabbagh A., Hernandez Conte A., Lubin L. Springer 2017, pp. 117–195. Published with kind permission of © SpringerNature, 2017. All Rights Reserved (Dabbagh et al. 2017a, b; Moffett et al. 2016)

IV intravenous, *SVT* supraventricular tachycardia, *AV* atrioventricular, *JET* junctional ectopic tachycardia, *VT* ventricular tachycardia, *VF* ventricular fibrillation, *PVC* premature ventricular contraction or sedative could be helpful to keep away these circumstances. Neuromuscular blocking drugs are also helpful in some cases, and careful use of them is advised in mechanically ventilated patients with hemodynamic instability or CNS insult. Volatile anesthetics have a crucial role in operative theatre, but their use in postoperative period is not usual. Tables 4.18, 4.19, 4.20, and 4.21 summarize agents listed above (Friesen and Williams 2008; Verghese and Hannallah 2010; Galante 2011; Twite and Friesen 2014; Lucas et al. 2016; Maldifassi et al. 2016; Bourenne et al. 2017; Feng et al. 2017; Herzog-Niescery et al. 2017; Romantsik et al. 2017).

Table 4.18 Analgesic agents (opioids and non-opioids)

Medication	Dosing	Indication	Adverse events and specific clinical considerations
Fentanyl (opioid) (CAS number: 437-38-7)	Bolus: 1–2 μg/kg Infusion: 1–10 μg/kg/h **Transdermal** fentanyl patches are available	Analgesia	Chest wall rigidity with rapid bolus or high doses; rapid tolerance with infusion, respiratory depression, depressed consciousness, hypotension, nausea/vomiting, decreased GI motility/ileus, urinary retention Preferred for a rapid onset of analgesia in acutely distressed patients Individualize dose for each patient More rapid onset of action and a shorter half-life than morphine Renal failure does not appear to largely affect pharmacokinetics Onset: 30 s Duration: 30–45 min
Remifentanil (opioid) (CAS number: 132875-61-7)	Bolus:1–3 μg/kg/dose Infusion (preferred): 0.4–1 μg/kg/min	Analgesia	Half-life: 10–15 min, has been associated with bradycardia and hypotension particularly during rapid infusion Has no liver or renal elimination
Morphine (opioid) (CAS number: 57-27-2)	Bolus: 0.05–0.1 mg/kg Infusion: 0.025–0.1 mg/kg/h Single dose: 0.1 mg/kg	Analgesia	Peak: 20 min Respiratory depression, depressed consciousness, hallucinations, hypotension, nausea/vomiting, decreased GI motility/ileus, urinary retention, histamine release: flushing, tachycardia, pruritus may occur Withdrawal symptoms when moderate to high-doses are used for up to or more than 1 week

Table 4.18 (continued)

Medication	Dosing	Indication	Adverse events and specific clinical considerations
Methadone (opioid) (CAS number: 76-99-3)	0.1–0.2 mg/kg q 8-12 h	Analgesia; opioid tolerance	Use for opioid wean protocol
Hydromorphone (CAS number: 466-99-9)	**Oral**: 0.03–0.08 mg/kg/dose q 4 h **Single IV** dose: 0.01–0.02 mg/kg q 4 h **Continuous IV** infusions: 1 μg/kg/h Titration based on pain scale	Analgesia	Respiratory depression, depressed consciousness, hallucinations, hypotension, nausea/vomiting, decreased GI motility/ileus, urinary retention Individualize dose for each patient More rapid onset of action and a shorter half-life than morphine Withdrawal symptoms when moderate to high-doses are used for up to or more than 1 week
Acetaminophen (non-opioid: inhibits prostaglandin synthesis) (CAS number: 103-90-2)	10–15 mg/kg q 6 h	Non-opioid analgesia	Do not use when there is significant hepatic disease
Ketorolac (non-opioid: nonsteroidal anti-inflammatory agent (cyclooxygenase-1 and 2 inhibitor) (CAS number: 74103-06-3)	0.5 mg/kg q 6 h; max 30 mg; do not administer for more than 48–72 h	Non-opioid analgesia	Injection site pain, abdominal pain, constipation, diarrhea, flatulence, indigestion, nausea/vomiting, headache Inhibition of platelet function: may cause bleeding Use with caution in patients with preexisting renal insufficiency Use lowest effective dose for the shortest period of time

Modified from Dabbagh A., et al. "Cardiovascular Pharmacology in Pediatric Patients with Congenital Heart Disease"; in "Congenital Heart Disease in Pediatric and Adult Patients; Anesthetic and Perioperative Management". Dabbagh A., Hernandez Conte A., Lubin L. Springer 2017, pp. 117–195. Published with kind permission of © SpringerNature, 2017. All Rights Reserved (Dabbagh et al. 2017a)

4.5 Stress Ulcer Prevention and Treatment

Stress ulcers are acute ulceration due to inflammatory response to physical or thermal trauma, shock, sepsis, and emotional and some other stress factors. They are usually located at the proximal portion of the stomach and restricted to mucosa. This phenomenon initiated with disturbed microcirculation and focal ischemia. So, the main pathogenic factor is temporary decrease in gastric blood flow which can be complicated by bleeding, endotoxemia, and sepsis.

Table 4.19 Sedative drugs and intravenous anesthetics

Medication	Dosing	Indication	Mechanism of action	Clinical considerations
Propofol (CAS number: 2078-54-80)	Bolus: 1–3 mg/kg Infusion: 100–200 μg/kg/min	Procedural sedation	Modulation of $GABA_A$ receptor complex	>4 h (risk of propofol infusion syndrome)
Midazolam (CAS number: 59467-70-8)	Infusion: 0.025–0.1 mg/kg/h Average: 0.05–0.1 mg/kg/h	Amnesia, sedation, anxiolysis	Modulation of $GABA_A$ receptor complex	Rapid tolerance with infusion Onset: 1–5 min Duration: 20–30 min
Lorazepam (CAS number: 846-49-1)	Bolus: 0.025–0.1 mg/kg q 4 h Infusion:0.025 mg/kg/h	Amnesia, sedation, anxiolysis	Modulation of $GABA_A$ receptor complex	Risk of tolerance with infusion Onset: 1–5 min Duration: 20–30 min
Dexmedetomidine (CAS number: 113775-47-6)	0.3–0.7 μg/kg/h	Sedation; some analgesia	Synthetic central α2 agonist (purely α2)	For short-term ICU sedation; bradycardia and heart block half-life: 6–12 min
Clonidine (CAS number: 4205-90-7)	Infusion: 0.25–1 μg/kg/h	Analgesia, sedation	α1 and α2 adrenoreceptor agonist	May lead to hypotension
Etomidate (CAS number: 33125-97-2)	0.2–0.4 mg/kg	Sedation	Modulation of $GABA_A$ receptor complex	Onset: 1 min Duration:3–5 min
Ketamine (CAS number: 6740-88-1)	Bolus: 1.5–2 mg/kg May administer incremental doses of 0.5–1 mg/kg every 5–15 min as needed	Analgesia, sedation	NMDA receptor antagonist	Hallucinations, dysphoria Excessive salivation, tachycardia onset, 3–5 min, and duration, 20–30 min

Modified from Dabbagh A., et al. "Cardiovascular Pharmacology in Pediatric Patients with Congenital Heart Disease"; in "Congenital Heart Disease in Pediatric and Adult Patients; Anesthetic and Perioperative Management". Dabbagh A., Hernandez Conte A., Lubin L. Springer 2017, pp. 117–195. Published with kind permission of © SpringerNature, 2017. All Rights Reserved (Dabbagh et al. 2017a)

Table 4.20 Volatile anesthetics

Drug	MAC Value %	Comments
Isoflurane	1.15	Cardiac depression Irritant of respiratory tract, which may lead to laryngospasm
Sevoflurane	2.1	Shortened recovery time and more rapid recovery of perception, which might produce a state of restlessness Decreases the chance of postoperative nausea and vomiting
Desflurane	6–7.25	Not suitable for mask induction anesthesia because of its pungent smell, respiratory tract irritation, apnea, and laryngospasm
Xenon	71	When a mixture of 30 volume% oxygen and 70 volume% xenon is used, the analgesic effect is excellent Extremely costly Increases pulmonary artery pressure
Nitrous oxide	105, so could never be a sole anesthetic agent	Not widely used in cardiac surgery and *should not be used* on newborns and children with pulmonary infections In combination with other agents, reduces the need for volatile anesthetics
Enflurane	1.6	Possible epileptic effects and the possibility of raising hepatic enzymes
Halothane	0.75	Increased sensitivity of myocardium to circulating catecholamines Rise in hepatic enzymes May lead to intraoperative arrhythmia

Modified from Dabbagh A., et al. "Cardiovascular Pharmacology in Pediatric Patients with Congenital Heart Disease"; in "Congenital Heart Disease in Pediatric and Adult Patients; Anesthetic and Perioperative Management". Dabbagh A., Hernandez Conte A., Lubin L. Springer 2017, pp. 117–195. Published with kind permission of © SpringerNature, 2017. All Rights Reserved (Dabbagh et al. 2017a)
MAC Minimum Alveolar Concentration

Postoperative period in patients undergoing cardiac surgery would be a stressful tread and hence makes the patient susceptible for stress ulceration. Stress ulcer prophylaxis is achieved with either sucralfate, histamine type 2 blockers, or proton-pump inhibitors. The only agent that has prophylactic effect and does not raise gastric pH is sucralfate. This is important because alkalization of gastric content results in colonization and therefore could be a risk factor for aspiration pneumonia. Table 4.22 summarizes the drugs used for prophylaxis of this complication (Griffin 1998; Langford and Mehta 2006; Reveiz et al. 2010; Giglia et al. 2016).

Table 4.21 Neuromuscular blocking agents (depolarizing, non-depolarizing)

	Succinylcholine	Pancuronium	Vecuronium	Cisatracurium	Atracurium	Rocuronium
Initial dose	1–2 mg/kg	0.06–0.15 mg/kg	0.08–0.1 mg/kg	0.1–0.15 mg/kg	0.4–0.5 mg/kg (0.3–0.4 mg/kg for 1 month to 2 years of age)	0.6–1.2 mg/kg
Onset of effect	< 1 min	2–5 min	1–3 min	1–3 min	1–3 min	<1 min
Duration	10 min	90–100 min	35–45 min	45–60 min	25–35 min	26–40 min
Continuous infusion dose	N/A	1–2 μg/kg/min	0.8–1.2 μg/kg/min	1–10 μg/kg/min	2–12 μg/kg/min	10–12 μg/kg/min
Recovery	10–20 min	120–180 min	45–60 min	90 min	40–60 min	30–60 min
Renal failure	No change	Increased effect	Increased effect	No change	No change	
Hepatic failure	Increased effect (decrease dose)	Mild increased effect	Variable	Minimal to no change	Minimal to no change	30% increased effect
Active metabolites	Yes	Yes	Yes	No	No	Yes
Adverse effects	Apnea bradyarrhythmia Cardiac arrest Cardiac dysrhythmia Hyperkalemia Hypersensitivity reaction Malignant hyperthermia Prolonged neuromuscular block Respiratory depression Rhabdomyolysis tachyarrhythmia	Apnea Bronchospasm Hypertension Prolonged neuromuscular block Respiratory failure Tachyarrhythmia	Anaphylaxis Apnea Bronchospasm Hypotension Muscle weakness Prolonged neuromuscular block Tachyarrhythmia	Bradyarrhythmia Bronchospasm Hypotension	Anaphylaxis Bradyarrhythmia Bronchospasm Edema Erythema Hives Hypersensitivity reaction Hypotension at larger than recommended doses Laryngeal spasm Muscle weakness Paralysis Tachyarrhythmia, at higher doses	Hypotension Hypertension Tachycardia Pruritus Nausea Wheezing Allergic reactions

Modified from Dabbagh A., et al. "Cardiovascular Pharmacology in Pediatric Patients with Congenital Heart Disease"; in "Congenital Heart Disease in Pediatric and Adult Patients; Anesthetic and Perioperative Management". Dabbagh A., Hernandez Conte A., Lubin L. Springer 2017, pp. 117–195. Published with kind permission of © SpringerNature, 2017. All Rights Reserved (Dabbagh et al. 2017a)

Table 4.22 Stress ulcer prevention and treatment drugs

Agent	Dosing	Adverse effects/comments
H2 blockers		
Ranitidine (CAS number: 66357-35-5)	Off-label: 150 mg PO or NG q12hr 50 mg (2 mL) IM or intermittent IV bolus or infusion q6-8 h	Headache, dizziness, mental status changes, thrombocytopenia Dose adjustment needed for renal dysfunction Potential increased risk of nosocomial pneumonia
Famotidine (CAS number: 76824-35-6)	Oral, IV, or nasogastric (NG) tube: 20 mg twice daily	
Proton-pump inhibitors (PPI)		
Omeprazole (CAS number: 73590-58-6)	40 mg orally	Respiratory effects No adjustment needed for renal or liver dysfunction Potential increased risk of nosocomial pneumonia Potential increased risk of *Clostridium difficile* infection Many drug interactions IV administration ONLY for patients who cannot tolerate PO/NG administration
Esomeprazole (CAS number: 217087-09-7)	20 or 40 mg orally once daily for up to 8 weeks	
Lansoprazole (CAS number: 103577-45-3)	30 mg PO Q24 Hours	
Sucralfate		
Sucralfate (CAS number: 54182-58-0)	1 g four times/day orally	Lower rate of clinically important GI bleeding than antacids Associated with fewer nosocomial pneumonia s than PPI and H2 blockers

Modified from Dabbagh A., et al. "Cardiovascular Pharmacology in Pediatric Patients with Congenital Heart Disease"; in "Congenital Heart Disease in Pediatric and Adult Patients; Anesthetic and Perioperative Management". Dabbagh A., Hernandez Conte A., Lubin L. Springer 2017, pp. 117–195. Published with kind permission of © SpringerNature, 2017. All Rights Reserved (Dabbagh et al. 2017a)

4.6 Anticoagulation and Thrombolysis Drugs

Four main classes could be described in order to have better understanding on these agents (Ageno et al. 2012; Moffett et al. 2016):

- Anticoagulants (oral and parenteral forms)
- Antiplatelet agents
- Thrombolytic agents
- Novel oral anticoagulants

4.6.1 Oral Anticoagulants

Warfarin, dabigatran, rivaroxaban, and apixaban are the main drugs in this category. The most commonly used drug is warfarin which inhibits vitamin K epoxide reductase. These agents are used mostly in prophylaxis and treatment of venous thrombosis, pulmonary emboli, systemic embolic complications (e.g., stroke) associated with atrial fibrillation, prophylaxis and treatment of thromboembolic complications associated with cardiac valve replacement, and reduction in the risk of death, recurrent MI, and thromboembolic events (e.g., stroke, systemic embolization) after MI. Other agents (including dabigatran, rivaroxaban, and apixaban) may be used in adults with congenital heart problems. Their mechanism of action, half-life, and other characteristics are described in Tables 4.23 and 4.24.

4.6.2 Antiplatelet Agents

Antiplatelet agents are used extensively in adult patients, especially in patients with acute coronary syndrome, cerebral vascular events, and thromboembolic events. Also, after CABG, there is a common practice of using dual antiplatelet therapy (DAPT) to improve clinical outcome, though a number of studies have questioned DAPT practice. However, commonness of DAPT mandates more vigilance on these drug effects and their interactions. The antiplatelet agents decrease platelet aggregation especially in arterial circulation unlike anticoagulants which effect mostly in venous circulation.

Based on their mechanism of action, these agents could be classified as follows:

- *Salicylic acid family* including aspirin and triflusal.
- **Aspirin** is an irreversible cyclooxygenase inhibitor (inhibition of COX-1 and COX-2 activity).
- **Triflusal** (Disgren®) is a salicylate, which blocks cyclooxygenase and phosphodiesterase and also preserves vascular prostacyclin.
- *Adenosine diphosphate (ADP) receptor inhibitors* that block P2Y12 component of ADP receptor on platelet surface (including **clopidogrel** "Plavix®," prasugrel "Effient®," **ticagrelor** "Brilinta®," and **ticlopidine** "Ticlid®").
- *Phosphodiesterase inhibitors* which increase plasma level of cellular cAMP and block platelet aggregation in response to ADP like **cilostazol** (Pletal®) which is a selective **phosphodiesterase 3** inhibitor or **dipyridamole** "Persantine®" which is both a **phosphodiesterase 5** inhibitor and an adenosine deaminase inhibitor (Gresele et al. 2011).
- *Glycoprotein IIB/IIIA inhibitors* including **abciximab** "ReoPro®," **eptifibatide** "Integrilin®," and **tirofiban** "Aggrastat®." These agents are only available in intravenous formulations.
- *Protease-activated receptor-1 (PAR-1) antagonists*, mainly **vorapaxar** "Zontivity®," block thrombin-responsive receptors in platelets and prevent thrombin generation (Capodanno et al. 2012; Wang 2015).
- *Thromboxane inhibitors* including thromboxane synthase inhibitors and thromboxane receptor antagonists like **terutroban.**

Pharmacological properties are presented in Table 4.25 (Dixon et al. 2009; Capodanno et al. 2012; Mauri et al. 2014; Bomb et al. 2015; Giglia et al. 2016; Yerokun et al. 2016; Degrauwe et al. 2017; Gaudino et al. 2017; Janssen et al. 2017; Salem et al. 2017).

Table 4.23 Oral anticoagulant dosing, monitoring, and preoperative discontinuation

Anticoagulant	Half-life ($t_{1/2}$)/dose	Monitoring	Discontinue prior to surgery (days)/reversal agent	Mechanism of action
Warfarin (Coumadin®) http://packageinserts.bms.com/pi/pi_coumadin.pdf. *Accessed April 9, 2016*	• 20–60 h • Individualized dosing • Initial bolus dosing of 0.2 mg/kg (maximum initial dose 10 mg) with adjustments on subsequent days based on daily INR • Alternative regime without bolus: age 2–12 years old, 0.09 mg/kg/day; age more than 12 years old, 0.08 mg/kg/day	• PT/INR	• Minimum of 5 days without reversal agents • Reversal agents – **Vitamin K** 10 mg PO/IVPB for emergent *normalization* of PT/INR; IVPB initial effect at 2 h and full correction within 24 h 5 mg PO and 1 mg IVPB produce similar effects on INR at 24 h 0.5-1 mg orally for reducing PT/INR into *therapeutic range* (for <2.5 mg use IV form administered orally) Ineffective in hepatic disease due to inability to produce factors *Oral* route not effective in biliary disease SQ not recommended due to unpredictable absorption and reversal characteristics – **Prothrombin complex concentrate** (PCC, factor IX complex, Profilnine®) 25–50 units/kg with vitamin K to prevent rebound increase in INR – **Recombinant-activated factor VII** For intracranial hemorrhage, doses vary; 20-40 μg/kg have been used; available as 1-, 2-, 5- and 8-mg vial sizes; use lowest dose rounded to nearest vial size and repeat if needed due to risk of arterial and venous thrombotic and thromboembolic events	Inhibits vitamin K epoxide reductase; in this way, warfarin prevents vitamin K1 regeneration after γ-carboxylation **Both ADULT and PEDIATRIC LABELING are available**

(continued)

Table 4.23 (continued)

Anticoagulant	Half-life ($t_{1/2}$)/dose	Monitoring	Discontinue prior to surgery (days)/reversal agent	Mechanism of action
Dabigatran (Pradaxa®) https://www.pradaxa.com/ *Accessed April 9, 2016*	• 12–17 h in healthy subjects • CrCl >30 mL/min: 150 mg BID • CrCl 30–50 mL/min + dronedarone or ketoconazole: 75 mg BID • CrCl 15–30 mL/min: 75 • Mg BID	No readily available method • Activated partial thromboplastin time (aPTT) demonstrates presence but not degree of anticoagulation • Prothrombin time (PT) insensitive • Thrombin time (TT)-normal value rules out presence of dabigatran • Ecarin clotting time (ECT)—linear dose relationship; not routinely available	• CrCl ≥50 mL/min: 1–2 days • CrCl 30–50 mL/min: 2–4 days • CrCl <30 mL/min: ≥5 days • Dialysis may remove up to 62% within 2 h • pINN: idarucizumab (dabigatran antidote) has been approved in 2015 by the FDA • Glund et al. (2015) and Pollack et al. (2015)	Dabigatran is among direct thrombin inhibitors (DTIs) **ONLY ADULT LABELING is available; PEDIATRIC LABELING not available yet**
Rivaroxaban (Xarelto®) http://www.xareltohcp.com/ *Accessed April 9, 2016*	• 5–9 h in healthy subjects • Atrial fibrillation • VTE prophylaxis • VTE treatment	No readily available method • Prolongs aPTT, PT/INR • No direct effect on platelet aggregation	• At least 1 day (24 h) • No reversal agent available and unlikely to be dialyzable due to high protein binding	Direct factor Xa inhibitor (orally active) **ONLY ADULT LABELING is available; PEDIATRIC LABELING not available yet**

Apixaban (Eliquis®) http://packageinserts.bms.com/pi/pi_eliquis.pdf *Accessed April 9, 2016*	• ~12 h following repeated dosing • Atrial fibrillation	No readily available method • Prolongs aPTT, PT/INR • No direct effect on platelet aggregation	• 24–48 h prior to surgery depending on risk, location, and ability to control bleeding • No reversal agent and unlikely to be dialyzable due to high protein binding • Activated charcoal may be useful in overdose situations	Direct factor Xa inhibitor **PEDIATRIC LABELING not available yet**

Modified from Dabbagh A., et al. "Cardiovascular Pharmacology in Pediatric Patients with Congenital Heart Disease"; in "Congenital Heart Disease in Pediatric and Adult Patients; Anesthetic and Perioperative Management". Dabbagh A., Hernandez Conte A., Lubin L. Springer 2017, pp. 117–195. Published with kind permission of © SpringerNature, 2017. All Rights Reserved (Dabbagh et al. 2017a)

CrCl clearance of creatinine, *VTE* venous

Table 4.24 Parenteral anticoagulant dosing and monitoring *in adults*

Anticoagulant	Half-life ($t_{1/2}$)/dose	Monitoring	Discontinue prior to surgery (hours)/ reversal agent
Unfractionated heparin (UFH)	• 60–90 min • VTE: 80 units/kg bolus, then 18 units/kg/h • ACS: 60 units/kg bolus, then 12 units/kg/h • Prophylaxis: 5000 units SQ BID or TID	aPTT Anti-Xa activity level (UFH levels) Activated clotting time (ACT; intraoperatively)	• 4–6 h • Protamine 1 mg/100 units of heparin (max 50 mg at a rate not to exceed 5 min) – Dose adjust based on time since heparin held: >60 min: 0.5 mg/100 units; >2 h 0.25 mg/100 units
Low-molecular-weight heparin Dalteparin (Fragmin®) *www.pfizer.com/files/products/uspi_fragmin.pdf Accessed 18 July* Enoxaparin (Lovenox®) *http://products.sanofi.us/lovenox/lovenox.html#section-14.1 Accessed 18 July*	• 4.5–7 h • **VTE treatment:** **Dalteparin**: 200 units/kg SQ daily **Enoxaparin**: 1 mg/kg SQ BID or 1.5 mg/kg SQ daily • **VTE prophylaxis** **Dalteparin** 5000 units SQ daily **Enoxaparin** 30 mg SQ BID or 40 mg SQ daily • **ACS** **Dalteparin**120 units/kg SQ every 12 h **Enoxaparin** 1 mg/kg SQ every 12 h	• Anti-Xa activity level (LMWH level) • Dalteparin treatment doses should not be used in patients with CrCl ≤30 mL/min • Enoxaparin 1 mg/kg SQ daily may be considered in patients with chronic stable kidney disease and CrCl ≤30 mL/min who are not dialysis dependent; anti-Xa and serum creatinine monitoring is highly recommended	• 24 h • Protamine – <8 h after last dose: 1 mg/1 mg enoxaparin or per 100 units of dalteparin – 8–12 h after last dose or if repeat is necessary: 0.5 mg/1 mg enoxaparin or per 100 units of dalteparin – >12 h after last dose: administration of protamine may not be necessary • The anti-factor Xa activity is never completely reversed (typically 60% is reversed)

Direct thrombin inhibitors Argatroban® *http://us.gsk.com/products/assets/us_argatroban.pdf* *Accessed 31 July 2012* Bivalirudin (Angiomax®) *www.angiomax.com/Downloads/Angiomax_PI_2010_PN1601-12.pdf.* *Accessed 18 July 2012*	• **Argatroban**50 min **Treatment of HIT**: 2 μg/kg/min initial dose; adjust for hepatic insufficiency and critically ill patients with multi-system organ failure • **Bivalirudin**25 min **CPB dosing in setting of HIT**: **On pump**:1 mg/kg bolus, 50 mg for pump then 2.5 mg/kg/h; goal ACT >2.5x baseline **Off pump:** 0.75 mg/kg bolus, 1.75 mg/kg/h: Goal ACT >300 s	• aPTT	• 2 h • No reversal agent – Case reports suggest that recombinant factor VIIa 90 μg/kg × 1 may reverse the anticoagulant effect (Schulman and Bijsterveld)
Factor Xa inhibitor Fondaparinux (Arixtra®) *http://us.gsk.com/products/assets/us_arixtra.pdf* *Accessed 31 July 2012*	• 17–21 h • VTE **Prophylaxis**: 2.5 mg SQ daily **Treatment:** <50 kg: 5 mg SQ daily 50–100 kg: 7.5 mg SQ daily >100 kg: 10 mg SQ daily	• Not routinely available. International standards for anti-Xa activity for UFH/LMWH do not apply	• 48 h • No reversal agent – Case reports suggest that recombinant factor VIIa 90 μg/kg × 1 reverse the anticoagulant effect (Schulman and Bijsterveld)

Modified from Dabbagh A., et al. "Cardiovascular Pharmacology in Pediatric Patients with Congenital Heart Disease"; in "Congenital Heart Disease in Pediatric and Adult Patients; Anesthetic and Perioperative Management". Dabbagh A., Hernandez Conte A., Lubin L. Springer 2017, pp. 117–195. Published with kind permission of © SpringerNature, 2017. All Rights Reserved (Dabbagh et al. 2017a)

Table 4.25 Oral and intravenous antiplatelet agents

Antiplatelet agent	Mechanism of action	Dose	Duration of effect	Half-life	Discontinue prior to surgery/monitor/reversal
Oral antiplatelet agents					
Aspirin	Cyclooxygenase inhibitor Inhibiting formation of thromboxane (TXA2) Inhibiting platelet activation and aggregation	75 mg to 325 mg orally once a day	7 days (since the affected platelets should be replaced)	5–20 min	3–5 days is needed before surgery to discontinue the drug No routine monitor For reversal, platelets (4–20 units/kg) may be given
Clopidogrel (Plavix®) http://www.plavix.com/Index.aspx *Accessed April 9, 2016*	Irreversibly blocks P2Y12 ADP receptor on platelet surface	75 mg orally once a day	7 days (since the affected platelets should be replaced)	The t½ of the drug is around 6 h; however, t½ of the active metabolite is about 30 min	5–7 days No routine monitor No reversal agent available, platelets 4–20 units/kg
Prasugrel (Effient®) http://www.effient.com/Pages/index.aspx *Accessed April 9, 2016*	Irreversibly blocks P2Y12 ADP receptor on platelet surface	Initial dose: 60 mg orally once Maintenance dose: 10 mg orally once a day	7 days (since the affected platelets should be replaced)	The active metabolite has an elimination half-life of about 7 h	7 days
Ticagrelor (Brilinta®) http://www.brilinta.com/ *Accessed April 9, 2016*	Reversibly blocks P2Y12 ADP receptor on platelet surface		48 h	6–13 h including active metabolite	3–5 days

Intravenous antiplatelet agents					
Abciximab (Reopro®) http://www.reopro.com/Pages/index.aspx *Accessed August 8, 2012*	Irreversible inhibitor of glycoprotein IIb/IIIa	IV: 0.25 mg/kg bolus followed by an 18–24 h infusion of 10 μg/min	24 h	Plasma: 30 min; dissociation half-life from GP IIb/IIIa receptors: up to 4 h (Schror 2003)	24 h
Eptifibatide (Integrilin®) http://www.integrilin.com/integrilin/index.html *Accessed August 8, 2012*	Reversible glycoprotein IIb/IIIa inhibitor	Initial: 180 μg/kg intravenous bolus Maintenance: 2 μg/kg/min continuous infusion	4 h	Plasma elimination half-life is approximately 2.5 h	4 h
Tirofiban (Aggrastat®) http://www.aggrastat.com/ *Accessed August 8, 2012*	Reversible glycoprotein IIb/IIIa inhibitor	Initial dose: 25 μg/kg IV within 5 min Maintenance dose: 0.15 μg/kg/min IV infusion for up to 18 h	4 h	2 h	4 h
Dipyridamole; both IV and oral (Persantine®)	Inhibition of the activity of adenosine deaminase and phosphodiesterase activity leading to blockade of platelet aggregation in response to ADP	75–100 mg orally 3–4 times a day	40 min	10–12 h	No routine monitoring No reversal agent available, platelets 10–20 units/kg

Modified from Dabbagh A., et al. "Cardiovascular Pharmacology in Pediatric Patients with Congenital Heart Disease"; in "Congenital Heart Disease in Pediatric and Adult Patients; Anesthetic and Perioperative Management". Dabbagh A., Hernandez Conte A., Lubin L. Springer 2017, pp. 117–195. Published with kind permission of © SpringerNature, 2017. All Rights Reserved (Dabbagh et al. 2017a)

4.6.3 Thrombolytic Agents

Thrombolytic agents are serine proteases which convert plasminogen to plasmin in order to lyses clots. Streptokinase and urokinase are historically first agents of this class. Another agent is tissue plasminogen activator (tPA) which is a natural agent.

Alteplase, reteplase, and tenecteplase are fibrin-specific agents. On the other hand, streptokinase is classified as a non-fibrin-specific agent. Streptokinase is indicated in acute myocardial infarction, pulmonary emboli, deep vein thrombosis, and occluded arteriovenous cannula. Table 4.26 described pharmacologic properties of this class of drugs.

4.6.4 Antifibrinolytic Agents

Tranexamic acid and ε-aminocaproic acid (EACA) are two members of this group. Both of them have been recommended to use in order to decrease intraoperative and postoperative bleeding. These lysine-like drugs interfere with formation of plasmin from plasminogen. They block binding sites of the plasminogen activators and decrease plasmin production rate. Evidences recommended their use in cardiac surgery and orthopedic surgery in which tourniquet is being used, and they are strategies in order to reduce blood transfusion. Table 4.27 presented details of these agents (Eaton 2008; Schouten et al. 2009; Faraoni and Goobie 2014).

Table 4.26 Thrombolytic agents

Thrombolytic Agent	Mechanism of action	Half-life	Dose	Discontinue prior to surgery/ monitor/reversal
Alteplase (TPA) Reteplase Tenecteplase Urokinase Streptokinase	Biosynthetic forms of the enzyme *human tissue-type plasminogen activator* (tPA)	5–10 min	**Urokinase** loading: 4400 units/kg, maintenance: 4400 units/kg/h for 6-12 h **Streptokinase** loading: 2000 units/kg maintenance: 2000 units/kg/h for 6–12 h **tPA** 0.1–0.6 mg/kg/h for 6 h	Monitor: fibrinogen, TCT, PT, aPTT No reversal agent available

Modified from Dabbagh A., et al. "Cardiovascular Pharmacology in Pediatric Patients with Congenital Heart Disease"; in "Congenital Heart Disease in Pediatric and Adult Patients; Anesthetic and Perioperative Management". Dabbagh A., Hernandez Conte A., Lubin L. Springer 2017, pp. 117–195. Published with kind permission of © SpringerNature, 2017. All Rights Reserved (Dabbagh et al. 2017a)

Table 4.27 Dosing antifibrinolytic agents

Agent	Dose regimen
Epsilon-aminocaproic acid (Amicar®) (CAS number: 60-32-2)	IV: 4–5 g IV infusion during the first hour of treatment, followed by a continuous infusion of 1 g/h
Tranexamic acid (Cyclokapron®) (CAS number: 1197-18-8)	5.4 mg/kg loading dose followed by 5 mg/kg/h with an additional 20 mg/L bypass pump prime

Modified from Dabbagh A., et al. "Cardiovascular Pharmacology in Pediatric Patients with Congenital Heart Disease"; in "Congenital Heart Disease in Pediatric and Adult Patients; Anesthetic and Perioperative Management". Dabbagh A., Hernandez Conte A., Lubin L. Springer 2017, pp. 117–195. Published with kind permission of © SpringerNature, 2017. All Rights Reserved (Dabbagh et al. 2017a)

4.7 Antibiotic Prophylaxis in Perioperative Period

Cardiothoracic surgeries are classified as clean surgeries; therefore the risk of infection is very low in these patients. On the other hand, infection in these patients could be life-threatening. Organ infections or deep surgical infections (e.g., mediastinitis, endocarditis, or osteomyelitis) are rare but could lead to catastrophic events. The aim of antibiotic prophylaxis is prevention of surgical site infection with cost-effective, safe, and appropriate spectrum antimicrobial agents. The selection of antibiotics might be according to Surgical Care Improvement Project (SCIP) guidelines. It is recommended to use cephalosporin as the primary prophylactic antibiotic for cardiac surgery and should be administered within 1 h before incision so the plasma and tissue level reached their suitable level. In patients who are allergic to penicillin, vancomycin within 2 h of incision could be used.

Although risk factors of superficial and deep surgical infections are different from each other, a comprehensive list of risk factors are listed below (Mehta et al. 2000; Allpress et al. 2004; Nateghian et al. 2004; Lepelletier et al. 2005; Iarussi et al. 2008; Costello et al. 2010; Bucher et al. 2011; Vijarnsorn et al. 2012):

- Higher classes of ASA (American Society of Anesthesiologist score)
- Younger patients
- Prolonged preoperative stay
- Prolonged ICU stay (>3 days)
- Prolonged inotropic support in ICU
- Prolonged mechanical ventilation (>2 days)
- Longer surgical procedures
- More units of postoperative blood transfusions
- Prolonged intubation
- Extubation failure (especially when repeated failure occurs)
- Prolonged hospital length of stay (>14 days)
- Prolonged postoperative hospital stay
- Reopen procedures

- Increased leukocyte band cell counts during preoperative period and on first postoperative day
- Elevated serum lactate levels in the first postoperative day

Common antibiotics used in these settings and their clinical pharmacologic properties are described in detail in Tables 4.28 and 4.29.

Table 4.28 Antibiotic prophylaxis for cardiac surgeries

Procedure	Common pathogens	Recommended antibiotic prophylaxis	Postoperative duration of antibiotic treatment
Congenital cardiac procedures	• *Staph epidermidis* • *Staph aureus* • *Coagulase-negative Staphylococcus* • *Escherichia coli* • *Pseudomonas Aeruginosa* • *Haemophilus influenzae non-type b*	**Cefazolin** OR **Vancomycin** for known MRSA or high risk for MRSA, or major reaction to beta-lactams	Discontinue within 48–72 h of surgical end time
Ventricular assist devices (VADs)	*Staph epidermidis* *Staph aureus* *Streptococcus* *Corynebacterium* Enteric-Gram-negative bacilli *Candida*	Vancomycin 15 mg/kg IV within 60 min prior to surgical incision and q12h × 48 h Piperacillin-tazobactam 3.375 g IV within 60 min prior to surgical incision and q6h × 48 h Fluconazole 400 mg IV within 60 min prior to surgical incision and q24h × 48 h Mupirocin (Bactroban®) 2% nasal ointment applied to nares the night before and morning of surgery (if nasal culture is positive for *S. aureus*)	Gram-negative coverage tailored to patient flora and/or institutional susceptibility × 48 h Mupirocin (Bactroban®) 2% nasal ointment to nares BID for 5 days (if nasal culture is positive for *S. aureus*)

Modified from Dabbagh A., et al. "Cardiovascular Pharmacology in Pediatric Patients with Congenital Heart Disease"; in "Congenital Heart Disease in Pediatric and Adult Patients; Anesthetic and Perioperative Management". Dabbagh A., Hernandez Conte A., Lubin L. Springer 2017, pp. 117–195. Published with kind permission of © SpringerNature, 2017. All Rights Reserved (Dabbagh et al. 2017a)

Staph epidermidis, Staph aureus, Streptococcus, Corynebacterium, enteric Gram-negative bacilli

Table 4.29 Commonly used antibiotics for prophylaxis in cardiac surgical patients

Antibiotic agent	Intraoperative re-dosing with normal renal function	Timing of the first dose	Time for effect	Re-dosing time (min)
Cefazolin (CAS number: 25953-19-9)	25 mg/kg q 6–8 h (max 1000 mg; if greater than 80 kg, use 2000 mg)	Begin 60 min or less before incision	30	Every 6–8 h
Cefotaxime (CAS number: 63527-52-6)	20–30 mg/kg	Begin 60 min or less before incision	30	Every 6 h
Cefuroxime (CAS number: 55268-75-2)	50 mg/kg	Within 1 h prior to incision	15–60	Every 4 h
Clindamycin (CAS number: 18323-44-9)	5–10 mg/kg up to 900 mg	Begin 60 min or less before incision	30	Every 6–8 h
Vancomycin (CAS number: 1404-90-6)	10 mg/kg (up to 1000 mg if >50 kg)	Begin 60–120 min before incision	60	Every 6 h

Modified from Dabbagh A., et al. "Cardiovascular Pharmacology in Pediatric Patients with Congenital Heart Disease"; in "Congenital Heart Disease in Pediatric and Adult Patients; Anesthetic and Perioperative Management". Dabbagh A., Hernandez Conte A., Lubin L. Springer 2017, pp. 117–195. Published with kind permission of © SpringerNature, 2017. All Rights Reserved (Dabbagh et al. 2017a)

References

Abman SH, Hansmann G, Archer SL, Ivy DD, Adatia I, Chung WK, Hanna BD, Rosenzweig EB, Raj JU, Cornfield D, Stenmark KR, Steinhorn R, Thebaud B, Fineman JR, Kuehne T, Feinstein JA, Friedberg MK, Earing M, Barst RJ, Keller RL, Kinsella JP, Mullen M, Deterding R, Kulik T, Mallory G, Humpl T, Wessel DL. Pediatric pulmonary hypertension: guidelines from the american heart association and american thoracic society. Circulation. 2015;132:2037–99.

Ageno W, Gallus AS, Wittkowsky A, Crowther M, Hylek EM, Palareti G. Oral anticoagulant therapy: antithrombotic therapy and prevention of thrombosis, 9th ed: American College of Chest Physicians Evidence-Based Clinical Practice Guidelines. Chest. 2012;141:e44S–88S.

Al-Naher A, Wright D, Devonald MAJ, Pirmohamed M. Renal function monitoring in heart failure—what is the optimal frequency? A narrative review. Br J Clin Pharmacol. 2017;84(1):5–17.

Allen HD, Driscoll DJ, Shaddy RE, Feltes TF. Moss & Adams' heart disease in infants, children, and adolescents: including the fetus and young adult. Philadelphia, PA: Lippincott Williams & Wilkins; 2013.

Allpress AL, Rosenthal GL, Goodrich KM, Lupinetti FM, Zerr DM. Risk factors for surgical site infections after pediatric cardiovascular surgery. Pediatr Infect Dis J. 2004;23:231–4.

Amanfu RK, Saucerman JJ. Cardiac models in drug discovery and development: a review. Crit Rev Biomed Eng. 2011;39:379–95.

Arora TK, Arora AK, Sachdeva MK, Rajput SK, Sharma AK. Pulmonary hypertension: molecular aspects of current therapeutic intervention and future direction. J Cell Physiol. 2017. https://doi.org/10.1002/jcp.26191.

Atkins DL, Berger S, Duff JP, Gonzales JC, Hunt EA, Joyner BL, Meaney PA, Niles DE, Samson RA, Schexnayder SM. Part 11: pediatric basic life support and cardiopulmonary resuscitation quality: 2015 American Heart Association guidelines update for cardiopulmonary resuscitation and emergency cardiovascular care. Circulation. 2015;132:S519–25.

Atz AM, Wessel DL. Inhaled nitric oxide in the neonate with cardiac disease. Semin Perinatol. 1997;21:441–55.

Bangash MN, Kong ML, Pearse RM. Use of inotropes and vasopressor agents in critically ill patients. Br J Pharmacol. 2012;165:2015–33.

Bayat F, Faritous Z, Aghdaei N, Dabbagh A. A study of the efficacy of furosemide as a prophylaxis of acute renal failure in coronary artery bypass grafting patients: a clinical trial. ARYA Atheroscler. 2015;11:173–8.

Beck G, Brinkkoetter P, Hanusch C, Schulte J, van Ackern K, van der Woude FJ, Yard BA. Clinical review: immunomodulatory effects of dopamine in general inflammation. Crit Care. 2004;8:485–91.

Beghetti M, Wacker Bou Puigdefabregas J, Merali S. Sildenafil for the treatment of pulmonary hypertension in children. Expert Rev Cardiovasc Ther. 2014;12:1157–84.

Begum N, Shen W, Manganiello V. Role of PDE3A in regulation of cell cycle progression in mouse vascular smooth muscle cells and oocytes: implications in cardiovascular diseases and infertility. Curr Opin Pharmacol. 2011;11:725–9.

Bianchi MO, Cheung PY, Phillipos E, Aranha-Netto A, Joynt C. The effect of milrinone on splanchnic and cerebral perfusion in infants with congenital heart disease prior to surgery: an observational study. Shock. 2015;44:115–20.

Biban P, Gaffuri M. Vasopressin and terlipressin in neonates and children with refractory septic shock. Curr Drug Metab. 2013;14:186–92.

Bihari D, Prakash S, Bersten A. Low-dose vasopressin in addition to noradrenaline may lead to faster resolution of organ failure in patients with severe sepsis/septic shock. Anaesth Intensive Care. 2014;42:671–4.

Bomb R, Oliphant CS, Khouzam RN. Dual antiplatelet therapy after coronary artery bypass grafting in the setting of acute coronary syndrome. Am J Cardiol. 2015;116:148–54.

Bond R, Olshansky B, Kirchhof P. Recent advances in rhythm control for atrial fibrillation. F1000Res. 2017;6:1796.

Bourenne J, Hraiech S, Roch A, Gainnier M, Papazian L, Forel JM. Sedation and neuromuscular blocking agents in acute respiratory distress syndrome. Ann Transl Med. 2017;5:291.

Bracht H, Calzia E, Georgieff M, Singer J, Radermacher P, Russell JA. Inotropes and vasopressors: more than haemodynamics! Br J Pharmacol. 2012;165:2009–11.

Brissaud O, Botte A, Cambonie G, Dauger S, de Saint Blanquat L, Durand P, Gournay V, Guillet E, Laux D, Leclerc F, Mauriat P, Boulain T, Kuteifan K. Experts' recommendations for the management of cardiogenic shock in children. Ann Intensive Care. 2016;6:14.

Brunner N, de Jesus Perez VA, Richter A, Haddad F, Denault A, Rojas V, Yuan K, Orcholski M, Liao X. Perioperative pharmacological management of pulmonary hypertensive crisis during congenital heart surgery. Pulm Circ. 2014;4:10–24.

Bucher BT, Warner BW, Dillon PA. Antibiotic prophylaxis and the prevention of surgical site infection. Curr Opin Pediatr. 2011;23:334–8.

Cannesson M, Jian Z, Chen G, Vu TQ, Hatib F. Effects of phenylephrine on cardiac output and venous return depend on the position of the heart on the Frank-Starling relationship. J Appl Physiol. 2012;113:281–9.

Capodanno D, Bhatt DL, Goto S, O'Donoghue ML, Moliterno DJ, Tamburino C, Angiolillo DJ. Safety and efficacy of protease-activated receptor-1 antagonists in patients with coronary artery disease: a meta-analysis of randomized clinical trials. J Thromb Haemost. 2012;10:2006–15.

Carroll SJ, Ferris A, Chen J, Liberman L. Efficacy of prostaglandin E1 in relieving obstruction in coarctation of a persistent fifth aortic arch without opening the ductus arteriosus. Pediatr Cardiol. 2006;27:766–8.

Cata JP, Ramirez MF, Velasquez JF, Di AI, Popat KU, Gottumukkala V, Black DM, Lewis VO, Vauthey JN. Lidocaine stimulates the function of natural killer cells in different experimental settings. Anticancer Res. 2017;37:4727–32.
Chan MJ, Chung T, Glassford NJ, Bellomo R. Near-infrared spectroscopy in adult cardiac surgery patients: a systematic review and meta-analysis. J Cardiothorac Vasc Anesth. 2017;31:1155–65.
Chaturvedi S, Lipszyc DH, Licht C, Craig JC, Parekh R. Pharmacological interventions for hypertension in children. Cochrane Database Syst Rev. 2014a;2:Cd008117.
Chaturvedi S, Lipszyc DH, Licht C, Craig JC, Parekh R. Pharmacological interventions for hypertension in children. Cochrane Database Syst Rev. 2014b;9:498–580.
Chierchia S, Davies G, Berkenboom G, Crea F, Crean P, Maseri A. Alpha-adrenergic receptors and coronary spasm: an elusive link. Circulation. 1984;69:8–14.
Chong LYZ, Satya K, Kim B, Berkowitz R. Milrinone dosing and a culture of caution in clinical practice. Cardiol Rev. 2018;26(1):35–42.
Choong K, Kissoon N. Vasopressin in pediatric shock and cardiac arrest. Pediatr Crit Care Med. 2008;9:372–9.
Chu PY, Campbell MJ, Miller SG, Hill KD. Anti-hypertensive drugs in children and adolescents. World J Cardiol. 2014;6:234–44.
CID=681 NCfBIPCD. 2016. Dopamine.
Clutter WE, Bier DM, Shah SD, Cryer PE. Epinephrine plasma metabolic clearance rates and physiologic thresholds for metabolic and hemodynamic actions in man. J Clin Invest. 1980;66:94–101.
Cooper BE. Review and update on inotropes and vasopressors. AACN Adv Crit Care. 2008;19:5–13; quiz 14–15.
Costello JM, Graham DA, Morrow DF, Morrow J, Potter-Bynoe G, Sandora TJ, Pigula FA, Laussen PC. Risk factors for surgical site infection after cardiac surgery in children. Ann Thorac Surg. 2010;89:1833–41; discussion 1841–1832.
Cruickshank JM. The role of beta-blockers in the treatment of hypertension. Adv Exp Med Biol. 2017;956:149–66.
Cuthbert AW. Lubiprostone targets prostanoid EP(4) receptors in ovine airways. Br J Pharmacol. 2011;162:508–20.
Dabbagh A. Cardiac physiology. In: Dabbagh A, Esmailian F, Aranki S, editors. Postoperative critical care for cardiac surgical patients. 1st ed. Berlin: Springer; 2014. p. 1–39.
Dabbagh A, Talebi Z, Rajaei S. Cardiovascular pharmacology i heart disease. In: Dabbagh A, Conte AH, Lubin L, editors. Congenital heart disease in pediatric and adult patients: anesthetic and perioperative management. 1st ed. Berlin: Springer; 2017a. p. 117–95.
Dabbagh A, Imani A, Rajaei S. Pediatric cardiovascular physiology. In: Dabbagh A, Conte AH, Lubin L, editors. Congenital heart disease in pediatric and adult patients: anesthetic and perioperative management. 1st ed. Berlin: Springer; 2017b. p. 65–116.
De Backer D, Biston P, Devriendt J, Madl C, Chochrad D, Aldecoa C, Brasseur A, Defrance P, Gottignies P, Vincent JL. Comparison of dopamine and norepinephrine in the treatment of shock. N Engl J Med. 2010;362:779–89.
de Caen AR, Berg MD, Chameides L, Gooden CK, Hickey RW, Scott HF, Sutton RM, Tijssen JA, Topjian A, van der Jagt EW, Schexnayder SM, Samson RA. Part 12: pediatric advanced life support: 2015 American Heart Association guidelines update for cardiopulmonary resuscitation and emergency cardiovascular care. Circulation. 2015;132:S526–42.
Degrauwe S, Pilgrim T, Aminian A, Noble S, Meier P, Iglesias JF. Dual antiplatelet therapy for secondary prevention of coronary artery disease. Open Heart. 2017;4:e000651.
Desborough MJ, Oakland K, Brierley C, Bennett S, Doree C, Trivella M, Hopewell S, Stanworth SJ, Estcourt LJ. Desmopressin use for minimising perioperative blood transfusion. Cochrane Database Syst Rev. 2017;7:Cd001884.
Dhull RS, Baracco R, Jain A, Mattoo TK. Pharmacologic treatment of pediatric hypertension. Curr Hypertens Rep. 2016;18:32.
Dixon BS, Beck GJ, Vazquez MA, Greenberg A, Delmez JA, Allon M, Dember LM, Himmelfarb J, Gassman JJ, Greene T, Radeva MK, Davidson IJ, Ikizler TA, Braden GL, Fenves AZ, Kaufman

JS, Cotton JR Jr, Martin KJ, McNeil JW, Rahman A, Lawson JH, Whiting JF, Hu B, Meyers CM, Kusek JW, Feldman HI. Effect of dipyridamole plus aspirin on hemodialysis graft patency. N Engl J Med. 2009;360:2191–201.

Dodgen AL, Hill KD. Safety and tolerability considerations in the use of sildenafil for children with pulmonary arterial hypertension. Drug Healthc Patient Saf. 2015;7:175–83.

Driscoll A, Currey J, Tonkin A, Krum H. Nurse-led titration of angiotensin converting enzyme inhibitors, beta-adrenergic blocking agents, and angiotensin receptor blockers for people with heart failure with reduced ejection fraction. Cochrane Database Syst Rev. 2015;12:Cd009889.

Duman E, Karakoc F, Pinar HU, Dogan R, Firat A, Yildirim E. Higher dose intra-arterial milrinone and intra-arterial combined milrinone-nimodipine infusion as a rescue therapy for refractory cerebral vasospasm. Interv Neuroradiol. 2017;23(6):636–43.

Eaton MP. Antifibrinolytic therapy in surgery for congenital heart disease. Anesth Analg. 2008;106:1087–100.

Eftekhar-Vaghefi S, Esmaeili-Mahani S, Elyasi L, Abbasnejad M. Involvement of mu opioid receptor signaling in the protective effect of opioid against 6-hydroxydopamine-induced SH-SY5Y human neuroblastoma cells apoptosis. Basic Clin Neurosci. 2015;6:171–8.

Ehlert A, Manthei G, Hesselmann V, Mathias K, Bein B, Pluta R. A case of hyperacute onset of vasospasm after aneurysmal subarachnoid hemorrhage and refractory vasospasm treated with intravenous and intraventricular nitric oxide: a mini review. World Neurosurg. 2016;91:673.e611–8.e611.

Elenkov IJ, Wilder RL, Chrousos GP, Vizi ES. The sympathetic nerve—an integrative interface between two supersystems: the brain and the immune system. Pharmacol Rev. 2000;52:595–638.

Faraoni D, Goobie SM. The efficacy of antifibrinolytic drugs in children undergoing noncardiac surgery: a systematic review of the literature. Anesth Analg. 2014;118:628–36.

Feng AY, Kaye AD, Kaye RJ, Belani K, Urman RD. Novel propofol derivatives and implications for anesthesia practice. J Anaesthesiol Clin Pharmacol. 2017;33:9–15.

Ferrer-Barba A, Gonzalez-Rivera I, Bautista-Hernandez V. Inodilators in the management of low cardiac output syndrome after pediatric cardiac surgery. Curr Vasc Pharmacol. 2016;14:48–57.

Fleming GA, Murray KT, Yu C, Byrne JG, Greelish JP, Petracek MR, Hoff SJ, Ball SK, Brown NJ, Pretorius M. Milrinone use is associated with postoperative atrial fibrillation after cardiac surgery. Circulation. 2008;118:1619–25.

Flynn JT. Management of hypertension in the young: role of antihypertensive medications. J Cardiovasc Pharmacol. 2011;58:111–20.

Flynn JT, Bradford MC, Harvey EM. Intravenous hydralazine in hospitalized children and adolescents with hypertension. J Pediatr. 2016;168:88–92.

Franz D, Contreras F, Gonzalez H, Prado C, Elgueta D, Figueroa C, Pacheco R. Dopamine receptors D3 and D5 regulate CD4(+)T-cell activation and differentiation by modulating ERK activation and cAMP production. J Neuroimmunol. 2015;284:18–29.

Friederich JA, Butterworth JF. Sodium nitroprusside: twenty years and counting. Anesth Analg. 1995;81:152–62.

Friesen RH, Williams GD. Anesthetic management of children with pulmonary arterial hypertension. Paediatr Anaesth. 2008;18:208–16.

Fuchs C, Ertmer C, Rehberg S. Effects of vasodilators on haemodynamic coherence. Best Pract Res Clin Anaesthesiol. 2016;30:479–89.

Galante D. Intraoperative management of pulmonary arterial hypertension in infants and children—corrected and republished article. Curr Opin Anaesthesiol. 2011;24:468–71.

Gamidov SI, Ovchinnikov RI, Popova AY, Izhbaev SK. Phosphodiesterase type 5 inhibitors in the treatment of erectile dysfunction: past, present and future. Urologiia. 2017;1:103–7.

Gao Y, Raj JU. Regulation of the pulmonary circulation in the fetus and newborn. Physiol Rev. 2010;90:1291–335.

Garcia-Rivas G, Jerjes-Sanchez C, Rodriguez D, Garcia-Pelaez J, Trevino V. A systematic review of genetic mutations in pulmonary arterial hypertension. BMC Med Genet. 2017;18:82.

Gaudino M, Antoniades C, Benedetto U, Deb S, Di Franco A, Di Giammarco G, Fremes S, Glineur D, Grau J, He GW, Marinelli D, Ohmes LB, Patrono C, Puskas J, Tranbaugh R, Girardi LN,

Taggart DP. Mechanisms, consequences, and prevention of coronary graft failure. Circulation. 2017;136:1749–64.

Gavra P, Laflamme M, Denault AY, Theoret Y, Perrault LP, Varin F. Use of nebulized milrinone in cardiac surgery; comparison of vibrating mesh and simple jet nebulizers. Pulm Pharmacol Ther. 2017;46:20–9.

Giesinger RE, More K, Odame J, Jain A, Jankov RP, McNamara PJ. Controversies in the identification and management of acute pulmonary hypertension in preterm neonates. Pediatr Res. 2017;82(6):901–14.

Giglia TM, Witmer C, Procaccini DE, Byrnes JW. Pediatric cardiac intensive care society 2014 consensus statement: pharmacotherapies in cardiac critical care anticoagulation and thrombolysis. Pediatr Crit Care Med. 2016;17:S77–88.

Gist KM, Goldstein SL, Joy MS, Vinks AA. Milrinone dosing issues in critically ill children with kidney injury: a review. J Cardiovasc Pharmacol. 2016;67:175–81.

Glund S, Moschetti V, Norris S, Stangier J, Schmohl M, van Ryn J, Lang B, Ramael S, Reilly P. A randomised study in healthy volunteers to investigate the safety, tolerability and pharmacokinetics of idarucizumab, a specific antidote to dabigatran. Thromb Haemost. 2015;113: 943–51.

Gordon NK, Gordon R. The organelle of differentiation in embryos: the cell state splitter. Theor Biol Med Model. 2016;13:35.

Green JB, Hart B, Cornett EM, Kaye AD, Salehi A, Fox CJ. Pulmonary vasodilators and anesthesia considerations. Anesthesiol Clin. 2017;35:221–32.

Gresele P, Momi S, Falcinelli E. Anti-platelet therapy: phosphodiesterase inhibitors. Br J Clin Pharmacol. 2011;72:634–46.

Griffin MR. Epidemiology of nonsteroidal anti-inflammatory drug-associated gastrointestinal injury. Am J Med. 1998;104:23S–9S; discussion 41S–42S.

Hamzaoui O, Scheeren TWL, Teboul JL. Norepinephrine in septic shock: when and how much? Curr Opin Crit Care. 2017;23:342–7.

Hansmann G, Apitz C, Abdul-Khaliq H, Alastalo TP, Beerbaum P, Bonnet D, Dubowy KO, Gorenflo M, Hager A, Hilgendorff A, Kaestner M, Koestenberger M, Koskenvuo JW, Kozlik-Feldmann R, Kuehne T, Lammers AE, Latus H, Michel-Behnke I, Miera O, Moledina S, Muthurangu V, Pattathu J, Schranz D, Warnecke G, Zartner P. Executive summary. Expert consensus statement on the diagnosis and treatment of paediatric pulmonary hypertension. The European Paediatric pulmonary vascular disease network, endorsed by ISHLT and DGPK. Heart. 2016;102(Suppl 2):ii86–ii100.

Hari P, Sinha A. Hypertensive emergencies in children. Indian J Pediatr. 2011;78:569–75.

Herrera AJ, Espinosa-Oliva AM, Carrillo-Jimenez A, Oliva-Martin MJ, Garcia-Revilla J, Garcia-Quintanilla A, de Pablos RM, Venero JL. Relevance of chronic stress and the two faces of microglia in Parkinson's disease. Front Cell Neurosci. 2015;9:312.

Herzog-Niescery J, Seipp HM, Weber TP, Bellgardt M. Inhaled anesthetic agent sedation in the ICU and trace gas concentrations: a review. J Clin Monit Comput. 2017. https://doi.org/10.1007/s10877-017-0055-6.

Holmes CL. Vasoactive drugs in the intensive care unit. Curr Opin Crit Care. 2005;11:413–7.

Holmes CL, Landry DW, Granton JT. Science review: vasopressin and the cardiovascular system part 1—receptor physiology. Crit Care. 2003;7:427–34.

Holmes CL, Landry DW, Granton JT. Science review: vasopressin and the cardiovascular system part 2—clinical physiology. Crit Care. 2004;8:15–23.

Hottinger DG, Beebe DS, Kozhimannil T, Prielipp RC, Belani KG. Sodium nitroprusside in 2014: a clinical concepts review. J Anaesthesiol Clin Pharmacol. 2014;30:462–71.

Hummel J, Rucker G, Stiller B. Prophylactic levosimendan for the prevention of low cardiac output syndrome and mortality in paediatric patients undergoing surgery for congenital heart disease. Cochrane Database Syst Rev. 2017a;8:Cd011312.

Hummel J, Rucker G, Stiller B. Prophylactic levosimendan for the prevention of low cardiac output syndrome and mortality in paediatric patients undergoing surgery for congenital heart disease. Cochrane Database Syst Rev. 2017b;3:Cd011312.

Iarussi T, Marolla A, Pardolesi A, Patea RL, Camplese P, Sacco R. Sternectomy and sternum reconstruction for infection after cardiac surgery. Ann Thorac Surg. 2008;86:1680–1.

Janssen PWA, Claassens DMF, Willemsen LM, Bergmeijer TO, Klein P, Ten Berg JM. Perioperative management of antiplatelet treatment in patients undergoing isolated coronary artery bypass grafting in Dutch cardiothoracic centres. Neth Hear J. 2017;25(9):482–9.

Jentzer JC, Coons JC, Link CB, Schmidhofer M. Pharmacotherapy update on the use of vasopressors and inotropes in the intensive care unit. J Cardiovasc Pharmacol Ther. 2015;20:249–60.

Jentzer JC, Mathier MA. Pulmonary hypertension in the intensive care unit. J Intensive Care Med. 2016;31(6):369–85.

Jiang M, Karasawa T, Steyger PS. Aminoglycoside-induced cochleotoxicity: a review. Front Cell Neurosci. 2017;11:308.

Jortveit J, Leirgul E, Eskedal L, Greve G, Fomina T, Dohlen G, Tell GS, Birkeland S, Oyen N, Holmstrom H. Mortality and complications in 3495 children with isolated ventricular septal defects. Arch Dis Child. 2016;101(9):808–13.

Kee VR. Hemodynamic pharmacology of intravenous vasopressors. Crit Care Nurse. 2003;23:79–82.

Kelly LE, Ohlsson A, Shah PS. Sildenafil for pulmonary hypertension in neonates. Cochrane Database Syst Rev. 2017;8:Cd005494.

Khan SU, Winnicka L, Saleem MA, Rahman H, Rehman N. Amiodarone, lidocaine, magnesium or placebo in shock refractory ventricular arrhythmia: a Bayesian network meta-analysis. Heart Lung. 2017;46:417–24.

Kim JS, McSweeney J, Lee J, Ivy D. Pediatric cardiac intensive care society 2014 consensus statement: pharmacotherapies in cardiac critical care pulmonary hypertension. Pediatr Crit Care Med. 2016;17:S89–s100.

Kleinman ME, Chameides L, Schexnayder SM, Samson RA, Hazinski MF, Atkins DL, Berg MD, de Caen AR, Fink EL, Freid EB, Hickey RW, Marino BS, Nadkarni VM, Proctor LT, Qureshi FA, Sartorelli K, Topjian A, van der Jagt EW, Zaritsky AL. Part 14: pediatric advanced life support: 2010 American Heart Association guidelines for cardiopulmonary resuscitation and emergency cardiovascular care. Circulation. 2010;122:S876–908.

Klinger JR, Kadowitz PJ. The nitric oxide pathway in pulmonary vascular disease. Am J Cardiol. 2017;120:S71–s79.

Klugman D, Goswami ES, Berger JT. Pediatric cardiac intensive care society 2014 consensus statement: pharmacotherapies in cardiac critical care antihypertensives. Pediatr Crit Care Med. 2016;17:S101–8.

Knight WE, Yan C. Cardiac cyclic nucleotide phosphodiesterases: function, regulation, and therapeutic prospects. Horm Metab Res. 2012;44:766–75.

Kniotek M, Boguska A. Sildenafil can affect innate and adaptive immune system in both experimental animals and patients. J Immunol Res. 2017;2017:4541958.

Kozlik-Feldmann R, Hansmann G, Bonnet D, Schranz D, Apitz C, Michel-Behnke I. Pulmonary hypertension in children with congenital heart disease (PAH-CHD, PPHVD-CHD). Expert consensus statement on the diagnosis and treatment of paediatric pulmonary hypertension. The European Paediatric Pulmonary Vascular Disease Network, endorsed by ISHLT and DGPK. Heart. 2016;102(Suppl 2):ii42–8.

Kushwah S, Kumar A, Sahana KS. Levosimendan. A promising future drug for refractory cardiac failure in children? Indian Heart J. 2016;68(Suppl 1):S57–60.

Lai MY, Chu SM, Lakshminrusimha S, Lin HC. Beyond the inhaled nitric oxide in persistent pulmonary hypertension of the newborn. Pediatr Neonatol. 2017. https://doi.org/10.1016/j.pedneo.2016.09.011.

Lakshminrusimha S, Mathew B, Leach CL. Pharmacologic strategies in neonatal pulmonary hypertension other than nitric oxide. Semin Perinatol. 2016;40:160–73.

Landoni G, Biondi-Zoccai G, Greco M, Greco T, Bignami E, Morelli A, Guarracino F, Zangrillo A. Effects of levosimendan on mortality and hospitalization. A meta-analysis of randomized controlled studies. Crit Care Med. 2012;40:634–46.

Langford RM, Mehta V. Selective cyclooxygenase inhibition: its role in pain and anaesthesia. Biomed Pharmacother. 2006;60:323–8.

Latorre R, Castillo K, Carrasquel-Ursulaez W, Sepulveda RV, Gonzalez-Nilo F, Gonzalez C, Alvarez O. Molecular determinants of BK channel functional diversity and functioning. Physiol Rev. 2017;97:39–87.

Latus H, Delhaas T, Schranz D, Apitz C. Treatment of pulmonary arterial hypertension in children. Nat Rev Cardiol. 2015;12:244–54.

Latus H, Kuehne T, Beerbaum P, Apitz C, Hansmann G, Muthurangu V, Moledina S. Cardiac MR and CT imaging in children with suspected or confirmed pulmonary hypertension/pulmonary hypertensive vascular disease. Expert consensus statement on the diagnosis and treatment of paediatric pulmonary hypertension. The European Paediatric Pulmonary Vascular Disease Network, endorsed by ISHLT and DGPK. Heart. 2016;102(Suppl 2):ii30–5.

Lechner E, Hofer A, Leitner-Peneder G, Freynschlag R, Mair R, Weinzettel R, Rehak P, Gombotz H. Levosimendan versus milrinone in neonates and infants after corrective open-heart surgery: a pilot study. Pediatr Crit Care Med. 2012;13:542–8.

Leone M, Martin C. Role of terlipressin in the treatment of infants and neonates with catecholamine-resistant septic shock. Best Pract Res Clin Anaesthesiol. 2008;22:323–33.

Lepelletier D, Perron S, Bizouarn P, Caillon J, Drugeon H, Michaud JL, Duveau D. Surgical-site infection after cardiac surgery: incidence, microbiology, and risk factors. Infect Control Hosp Epidemiol. 2005;26:466–72.

Levite M. Dopamine and T cells: dopamine receptors and potent effects on T cells, dopamine production in T cells, and abnormalities in the dopaminergic system in T cells in autoimmune, neurological and psychiatric diseases. Acta Physiol (Oxford). 2016;216:42–89.

Li H, Kim HW, Shin SE, Seo MS, An JR, Ha KS, Han ET, Hong SH, Firth AL, Choi IW, Han IY, Lee DS, Yim MJ, Park WS. The vasorelaxant effect of mitiglinide via activation of voltage-dependent K+ channels and SERCA pump in aortic smooth muscle. Life Sci. 2017a;188:1–9.

Li J, Tang B, Zhang W, Wang C, Yang S, Zhang B, Gao X. Relationship and mechanism of Kv2.1 expression to ADH secretion in rats with heart failure. Am J Transl Res. 2017b;9:3687–95.

Li MX, Hwang PM. Structure and function of cardiac troponin C (TNNC1): implications for heart failure, cardiomyopathies, and troponin modulating drugs. Gene. 2015;571:153–66.

Liu C, Chen J, Gao Y, Deng B, Liu K. Endothelin receptor antagonists for pulmonary arterial hypertension. Cochrane Database Syst Rev. 2013;2:Cd004434.

Lomis N, Gaudreault F, Malhotra M, Westfall S, Shum-Tim D, Prakash S. A novel milrinone nanoformulation for use in cardiovascular diseases: preparation and in vitro characterization. Mol Pharm. 2017;

Lucas SS, Nasr VG, Ng AJ, Joe C, Bond M, DiNardo JA. Pediatric cardiac intensive care society 2014 consensus statement: pharmacotherapies in cardiac critical care: sedation, analgesia and muscle relaxant. Pediatr Crit Care Med. 2016;17:S3–s15.

Maconochie IK, de Caen AR, Aickin R, Atkins DL, Biarent D, Guerguerian AM, Kleinman ME, Kloeck DA, Meaney PA, Nadkarni VM, Ng KC, Nuthall G, Reis AG, Shimizu N, Tibballs J, Pintos RV. Part 6: pediatric basic life support and pediatric advanced life support: 2015 international consensus on cardiopulmonary resuscitation and emergency cardiovascular care science with treatment recommendations. Resuscitation. 2015;95:e147–68.

Majure DT, Greco T, Greco M, Ponschab M, Biondi-Zoccai G, Zangrillo A, Landoni G. Meta-analysis of randomized trials of effect of milrinone on mortality in cardiac surgery: an update. J Cardiothorac Vasc Anesth. 2013;27:220–9.

Maldifassi MC, Baur R, Sigel E. Functional sites involved in modulation of the GABA receptor channel by the intravenous anesthetics propofol, etomidate and pentobarbital. Neuropharmacology. 2016;105:207–14.

Marcotti W, Johnson SL, Kros CJ. A transiently expressed SK current sustains and modulates action potential activity in immature mouse inner hair cells. J Physiol. 2004;560:691–708.

Marionneau C, Abriel H. Regulation of the cardiac Na channel Na1.5 by post-translational modifications. J Mol Cell Cardiol. 2015;82:36–47.

Maslov MY, Wei AE, Pezone MJ, Edelman ER, Lovich MA. Vascular dilation, tachycardia, and increased inotropy occur sequentially with increasing epinephrine dose rate, plasma and myocardial concentrations, and cAMP. Heart Lung Circ. 2015;24:912–8.

Mauri L, Kereiakes DJ, Yeh RW, Driscoll-Shempp P, Cutlip DE, Steg PG, Normand SL, Braunwald E, Wiviott SD, Cohen DJ, Holmes DR Jr, Krucoff MW, Hermiller J, Dauerman HL, Simon DI, Kandzari DE, Garratt KN, Lee DP, Pow TK, Ver Lee P, Rinaldi MJ, Massaro JM. Twelve or 30 months of dual antiplatelet therapy after drug-eluting stents. N Engl J Med. 2014;371:2155–66.

McCammond AN, Axelrod DM, Bailly DK, Ramsey EZ, Costello JM. Pediatric cardiac intensive care society 2014 consensus statement: pharmacotherapies in cardiac critical care fluid management. Pediatr Crit Care Med. 2016;17:S35–48.

McMahon TJ, Bryan NS. Biomarkers in pulmonary vascular disease: gauging response to therapy. Am J Cardiol. 2017;120:S89–s95.

Mebazaa A, Nieminen MS, Packer M, Cohen-Solal A, Kleber FX, Pocock SJ, Thakkar R, Padley RJ, Poder P, Kivikko M. Levosimendan vs dobutamine for patients with acute decompensated heart failure: the SURVIVE randomized trial. JAMA. 2007;297:1883–91.

Mehta PA, Cunningham CK, Colella CB, Alferis G, Weiner LB. Risk factors for sternal wound and other infections in pediatric cardiac surgery patients. Pediatr Infect Dis J. 2000;19:1000–4.

Mehta S, Granton J, Gordon AC, Cook DJ, Lapinsky S, Newton G, Bandayrel K, Little A, Siau C, Ayers D, Singer J, Lee TC, Walley KR, Storms M, Cooper DJ, Holmes CL, Hebert P, Presneill J, Russell JA. Cardiac ischemia in patients with septic shock randomized to vasopressin or norepinephrine. Crit Care. 2013;17:R117.

Meyer S, Gortner L, McGuire W, Baghai A, Gottschling S. Vasopressin in catecholamine-refractory shock in children. Anaesthesia. 2008;63:228–34.

Meyer S, McGuire W, Gottschling S, Mohammed Shamdeen G, Gortner L. The role of vasopressin and terlipressin in catecholamine-resistant shock and cardio-circulatory arrest in children: review of the literature. Wien Med Wochenschr. 2011;161:192–203.

Minton J, Sidebotham DA. Hyperlactatemia and cardiac surgery. J Extra Corpor Technol. 2017;49:7–15.

Mirhosseini SM, Sanjari Moghaddam A, Tahmaseb Pour P, Dabbagh A. Refractory vasoplegic syndrome in an adult patient with infective endocarditis: a case report and literature review. J Tehran Heart Cent. 2017;12:27–31.

Moffett BS, Price JF. Evaluation of sodium nitroprusside toxicity in pediatric cardiac surgical patients. Ann Pharmacother. 2008;42:1600–4.

Moffett BS, Salvin JW, Kim JJ. Pediatric cardiac intensive care society 2014 consensus statement: pharmacotherapies in cardiac critical care antiarrhythmics. Pediatr Crit Care Med. 2016;17:S49–58.

Mossad E, Motta P, Sehmbey K, Toscana D. The hemodynamic effects of phenoxybenzamine in neonates, infants, and children. J Clin Anesth. 2008;20:94–8.

Mossad EB. Pro: intraoperative use of nitric oxide for treatment of pulmonary hypertension in patients with congenital heart disease is effective. J Cardiothorac Vasc Anesth. 2001;15:259–62.

Mossad EB, Motta P, Rossano J, Hale B, Morales DL. Perioperative management of pediatric patients on mechanical cardiac support. Paediatr Anaesth. 2011;21:585–93.

Motta P, Mossad E, Toscana D, Zestos M, Mee R. Comparison of phenoxybenzamine to sodium nitroprusside in infants undergoing surgery. J Cardiothorac Vasc Anesth. 2005;19:54–9.

Motyl KJ, Beauchemin M, Barlow D, Le PT, Nagano K, Treyball A, Contractor A, Baron R, Rosen CJ, Houseknecht KL. A novel role for dopamine signaling in the pathogenesis of bone loss from the atypical antipsychotic drug risperidone in female mice. Bone. 2017;103:168–76.

Nanayakkara S, Bergin P, Mak V, Crannitch K, Kaye DM. Extended release oral milrinone as an adjunct to heart failure therapy. Intern Med J. 2017;47:973–4.

Nateghian A, Taylor G, Robinson JL. Risk factors for surgical site infections following open-heart surgery in a Canadian pediatric population. Am J Infect Control. 2004;32:397–401.

Nazir SA, Khan JN, Mahmoud IZ, Greenwood JP, Blackman DJ, Kunadian V, Been M, Abrams KR, Wilcox R, Adgey AAJ, McCann GP, Gershlick AH. Efficacy and Mechanism Evaluation. In: The REFLO-STEMI (REperfusion Facilitated by LOcal adjunctive therapy in ST-Elevation

Myocardial Infarction) trial: a randomised controlled trial comparing intracoronary administration of adenosine or sodium nitroprusside with control for attenuation of microvascular obstruction during primary percutaneous coronary intervention. Southampton (UK): NIHR Journals Library Copyright (c) Queen's Printer and Controller of HMSO 2016. This work was produced by Nazir et al. under the terms of a commissioning contract issued by the Secretary of State for Health. This issue may be freely reproduced for the purposes of private research and study and extracts (or indeed, the full report) may be included in professional journals provided that suitable acknowledgement is made and the reproduction is not associated with any form of advertising. Applications for commercial reproduction should be addressed to: NIHR Journals Library, National Institute for Health Research, Evaluation, Trials and Studies Coordinating Centre, Alpha House, University of Southampton Science Park, Southampton SO16 7NS, UK; 2016.

Ng KT, Yap JLL. Continuous infusion vs. intermittent bolus injection of furosemide in acute decompensated heart failure: systematic review and meta-analysis of randomised controlled trials. Anaesthesia. 2018;73(2):238–47.

Nieminen MS, Fruhwald S, Heunks LM, Suominen PK, Gordon AC, Kivikko M, Pollesello P. Levosimendan: current data, clinical use and future development. Heart Lung Vess. 2013;5:227–45.

Noori S, Seri I. Neonatal blood pressure support: the use of inotropes, lusitropes, and other vasopressor agents. Clin Perinatol. 2012;39:221–38.

O'Brien A, Clapp L, Singer M. Terlipressin for norepinephrine-resistant septic shock. Lancet. 2002;359:1209–10.

Ogawa R, Stachnik JM, Echizen H. Clinical pharmacokinetics of drugs in patients with heart failure: an update (part 2, drugs administered orally). Clin Pharmacokinet. 2014;53:1083–114.

Ostrye J, Hailpern SM, Jones J, Egan B, Chessman K, Shatat IF. The efficacy and safety of intravenous hydralazine for the treatment of hypertension in the hospitalized child. Pediatr Nephrol. 2014;29:1403–9.

Pacheco R, Contreras F, Zouali M. The dopaminergic system in autoimmune diseases. Front Immunol. 2014;5:117.

Panchal AR, Satyanarayan A, Bahadir JD, Hays D, Mosier J. Efficacy of bolus-dose phenylephrine for peri-intubation hypotension. J Emerg Med. 2015;49:488–94.

Papp Z, Edes I, Fruhwald S, De Hert SG, Salmenpera M, Leppikangas H, Mebazaa A, Landoni G, Grossini E, Caimmi P, Morelli A, Guarracino F, Schwinger RH, Meyer S, Algotsson L, Wikstrom BG, Jorgensen K, Filippatos G, Parissis JT, Gonzalez MJ, Parkhomenko A, Yilmaz MB, Kivikko M, Pollesello P, Follath F. Levosimendan: molecular mechanisms and clinical implications: consensus of experts on the mechanisms of action of levosimendan. Int J Cardiol. 2012;159:82–7.

Parham WA, Mehdirad AA, Biermann KM, Fredman CS. Hyperkalemia revisited. Tex Heart Inst J. 2006;33:40–7.

Parthenakis F, Maragkoudakis S, Marketou M, Patrianakos A, Zacharis E, Vardas P. Myocardial inotropic reserve: an old twist that constitutes a reliable index in the modern era of heart failure. Am J Cardiovasc Drugs. 2016;57:311–4.

Perez KM, Laughon M. Sildenafil in term and premature infants: a systematic review. Clin Ther. 2015;37:2598.e2591–607.e2591.

Pinoli M, Marino F, Cosentino M. Dopaminergic regulation of innate immunity: a review. J NeuroImmune Pharmacol. 2017;12(4):602–23.

Pollack CV Jr, Reilly PA, Eikelboom J, Glund S, Verhamme P, Bernstein RA, Dubiel R, Huisman MV, Hylek EM, Kamphuisen PW, Kreuzer J, Levy JH, Sellke FW, Stangier J, Steiner T, Wang B, Kam CW, Weitz JI. Idarucizumab for dabigatran reversal. N Engl J Med. 2015;373:511–20.

Poor HD, Ventetuolo CE. Pulmonary hypertension in the intensive care unit. Prog Cardiovasc Dis. 2012;55:187–98.

Prado C, Bernales S, Pacheco R. Modulation of T-cell mediated immunity by dopamine receptor d5. Endocr Metab Immune Disord Drug Targets. 2013;13:184–94.

Pritts CD, Pearl RG. Anesthesia for patients with pulmonary hypertension. Curr Opin Anaesthesiol. 2010;23:411–6.

Reveiz L, Guerrero-Lozano R, Camacho A, Yara L, Mosquera PA. Stress ulcer, gastritis, and gastrointestinal bleeding prophylaxis in critically ill pediatric patients: a systematic review. Pediatr Crit Care Med. 2010;11:124–32.

Rizza A, Bignami E, Belletti A, Polito A, Ricci Z, Isgro G, Locatelli A, Cogo P. Vasoactive drugs and hemodynamic monitoring in pediatric cardiac intensive care: an italian survey. World J Pediatr Congenit Heart Surg. 2016;7:25–31.

Roeleveld PP, Zwijsen EG. Treatment strategies for paradoxical hypertension following surgical correction of coarctation of the aorta in children. World J Pediatr Congenit Heart Surg. 2017;8:321–31.

Romantsik O, Calevo MG, Norman E, Bruschettini M. Clonidine for sedation and analgesia for neonates receiving mechanical ventilation. Cochrane Database Syst Rev. 2017;5:Cd012468.

Rossano JW, Cabrera AG, Jefferies JL, Naim MP, Humlicek T. Pediatric cardiac intensive care society 2014 consensus statement: pharmacotherapies in cardiac critical care chronic heart failure. Pediatr Crit Care Med. 2016;17:S20–34.

Russell JA. Bench-to-bedside review: vasopressin in the management of septic shock. Crit Care. 2011;15:226.

Ryu HG, Jung CW, Lee HC, Cho YJ. Epinephrine and phenylephrine pretreatments for preventing postreperfusion syndrome during adult liver transplantation. Liver Transpl. 2012;18:1430–9.

Salem S, Askandar S, Khouzam RN. Aspirin monotherapy vs. dual antiplatelet therapy in diabetic patients following coronary artery bypass graft (CABG): where do we stand? Ann Transl Med. 2017;5:213.

Scanzano A, Cosentino M. Adrenergic regulation of innate immunity: a review. Front Pharmacol. 2015;6:171.

Schouten ES, van de Pol AC, Schouten AN, Turner NM, Jansen NJ, Bollen CW. The effect of aprotinin, tranexamic acid, and aminocaproic acid on blood loss and use of blood products in major pediatric surgery: a meta-analysis. Pediatr Crit Care Med. 2009;10:182–90.

Shah PS, Ohlsson A. Sildenafil for pulmonary hypertension in neonates. Cochrane Database Syst Rev. 2011;8:Cd005494.

Shang G, Yang X, Song D, Ti Y, Shang Y, Wang Z, Tang M, Zhang Y, Zhang W, Zhong M. Effects of levosimendan on patients with heart failure complicating acute coronary syndrome: a meta-analysis of randomized controlled trials. Am J Cardiovasc Drugs. 2017;17(6):453–63.

Shao H, Li CS. Epinephrine in out-of-hospital cardiac arrest: helpful or harmful? Chin Med J. 2017;130:2112–6.

Sharawy N. Vasoplegia in septic shock: do we really fight the right enemy? J Crit Care. 2014;29:83–7.

Silvetti S, Silvani P, Azzolini ML, Dossi R, Landoni G, Zangrillo A. A systematic review on levosimendan in paediatric patients. Curr Vasc Pharmacol. 2015;13:128–33.

Simons FE, Sampson HA. Anaphylaxis: unique aspects of clinical diagnosis and management in infants (birth to age 2 years). J Allergy Clin Immunol. 2015;135:1125–31.

Singh VK, Sharma R, Agrawal A, Varma A. Vasopressin in the pediatric cardiac intensive care unit: myth or reality. Ann Pediatr Cardiol. 2009;2:65–73.

Smith KA, Ayon RJ, Tang H, Makino A, Yuan JX. Calcium-sensing receptor regulates cytosolic [Ca 2+] and plays a major role in the development of pulmonary hypertension. Front Physiol. 2016;7:517.

Stahl W, Bracht H, Radermacher P, Thomas J. Year in review 2009: critical care—shock. Crit Care. 2010;14:239.

Stratton L, Berlin DA, Arbo JE. Vasopressors and inotropes in sepsis. Emerg Med Clin North Am. 2017;35:75–91.

Strobel AM, Lu le N. The critically ill infant with congenital heart disease. Emerg Med Clin North Am. 2015;33:501–18.

Thomas C, Svehla L, Moffett BS. Sodium-nitroprusside-induced cyanide toxicity in pediatric patients. Expert Opin Drug Saf. 2009;8:599–602.
Touchan J, Guglin M. Temporary mechanical circulatory support for cardiogenic shock. Curr Treat Options Cardiovasc Med. 2017;19:77.
Tran KC, Leung AA, Tang KL, Quan H, Khan NA. Efficacy of calcium channel blockers on major cardiovascular outcomes for the treatment of hypertension in asian populations: a meta-analysis. Can J Cardiol. 2017;33:635–43.
Trappe HJ, Brandts B, Weismueller P. Arrhythmias in the intensive care patient. Curr Opin Crit Care. 2003;9:345–55.
Tremblay JA, Beaubien-Souligny W, Elmi-Sarabi M, Desjardins G, Denault AY. Point-of-care ultrasonography to assess portal vein pulsatility and the effect of inhaled milrinone and epoprostenol in severe right ventricular failure: a report of 2 cases. A A Case Rep. 2017;9:219–23.
Twite MD, Friesen RH. The anesthetic management of children with pulmonary hypertension in the cardiac catheterization laboratory. Anesthesiol Clin. 2014;32:157–73.
Unegbu C, Noje C, Coulson JD, Segal JB, Romer L. Pulmonary hypertension therapy and a systematic review of efficacy and safety of PDE-5 inhibitors. Pediatrics. 2017;139(3):e20161450.
Varon J, Marik PE. Clinical review: the management of hypertensive crises. Crit Care. 2003;7:374–84.
Vasu TS, Cavallazzi R, Hirani A, Kaplan G, Leiby B, Marik PE. Norepinephrine or dopamine for septic shock: systematic review of randomized clinical trials. J Intensive Care Med. 2012;27:172–8.
Vaughan Williams EM. Relevance of cellular to clinical electrophysiology in interpreting antiarrhythmic drug action. Am J Cardiol. 1989;64:5j–9j.
Vaughan Williams EM. The relevance of cellular to clinical electrophysiology in classifying antiarrhythmic actions. J Cardiovasc Pharmacol. 1992;20(Suppl 2):S1–7.
Ventetuolo CE, Klinger JR. Management of acute right ventricular failure in the intensive care unit. Ann Am Thorac Soc. 2014;11:811–22.
Verghese ST, Hannallah RS. Acute pain management in children. J Pain Res. 2010;3:105–23.
Vijarnsorn C, Winijkul G, Laohaprasitiporn D, Chungsomprasong P, Chanthong P, Durongpisitkul K, Soonswang J, Nana A, Subtaweesin T, Sriyoschati S, Pooliam J. Postoperative fever and major infections after pediatric cardiac surgery. J Med Assoc Thail. 2012;95:761–70.
Vorhies EE, Ivy DD. Drug treatment of pulmonary hypertension in children. Paediatr Drugs. 2014;16:43–65.
Wang A. Review of vorapaxar for the prevention of atherothrombotic events. Expert Opin Pharmacother. 2015;16:2509–22.
Wang RC, Jiang FM, Zheng QL, Li CT, Peng XY, He CY, Luo J, Liang ZA. Efficacy and safety of sildenafil treatment in pulmonary arterial hypertension: a systematic review. Respir Med. 2014;108:531–7.
Watt K, Li JS, Benjamin DK Jr, Cohen-Wolkowiez M. Pediatric cardiovascular drug dosing in critically ill children and extracorporeal membrane oxygenation. J Cardiovasc Pharmacol. 2011;58:126–32.
Wolf CM, Berul CI. Molecular mechanisms of inherited arrhythmias. Curr Genomics. 2008;9:160–8.
Xue H, Lu Z, Tang WL, Pang LW, Wang GM, Wong GW, Wright JM. First-line drugs inhibiting the renin angiotensin system versus other first-line antihypertensive drug classes for hypertension. Cochrane Database Syst Rev. 2015;1:Cd008170.
Yandrapalli S, Tariq S, Aronow WS. Advances in chemical pharmacotherapy for managing acute decompensated heart failure. Am J Cardiovasc Drugs. 2017;18:471–85.
Yerokun BA, Williams JB, Gaca J, Smith PK, Roe MT. Indications, algorithms, and outcomes for coronary artery bypass surgery in patients with acute coronary syndromes. Coron Artery Dis. 2016;27:319–26.
Yildirim A, Lubbers HT, Yildirim A. Drug-induced anaphylaxis. Adrenalin as emergency drug in anaphylaxis. Swiss Dent J. 2017;127:242–3.

Zhang Q, Liu B, Zhao L, Qi Z, Shao H, An L, Li C. Efficacy of vasopressin-epinephrine compared to epinephrine alone for out of hospital cardiac arrest patients: a systematic review and meta-analysis. Am J Emerg Med. 2017a;35:1555–60.

Zhang X, Liu Q, Liao Q, Zhao Y. Potential roles of peripheral dopamine in tumor immunity. J Cancer. 2017b;8:2966–73.

Zhao W, Huang Y, Liu Z, Cao BB, Peng YP, Qiu YH. Dopamine receptors modulate cytotoxicity of natural killer cells via cAMP-PKA-CREB signaling pathway. PLoS One. 2013;8:e65860.

Zipes DP, Camm AJ, Borggrefe M, Buxton AE, Chaitman B, Fromer M, Gregoratos G, Klein G, Moss AJ, Myerburg RJ, Priori SG, Quinones MA, Roden DM, Silka MJ, Tracy C, Smith SC Jr, Jacobs AK, Adams CD, Antman EM, Anderson JL, Hunt SA, Halperin JL, Nishimura R, Ornato JP, Page RL, Riegel B, Priori SG, Blanc JJ, Budaj A, Camm AJ, Dean V, Deckers JW, Despres C, Dickstein K, Lekakis J, McGregor K, Metra M, Morais J, Osterspey A, Tamargo JL, Zamorano JL. ACC/AHA/ESC 2006 guidelines for management of patients with ventricular arrhythmias and the prevention of sudden cardiac death: a report of the American College of Cardiology/American Heart Association Task Force and the European Society of Cardiology Committee for Practice Guidelines (Writing Committee to Develop Guidelines for Management of Patients With Ventricular Arrhythmias and the Prevention of Sudden Cardiac Death). J Am Coll Cardiol. 2006;48:e247–346.

Zou Z, Yuan HB, Yang B, Xu F, Chen XY, Liu GJ, Shi XY. Perioperative angiotensin-converting enzyme inhibitors or angiotensin II type 1 receptor blockers for preventing mortality and morbidity in adults. Cochrane Database Syst Rev. 2016;1:Cd009210.

Cardiovascular Monitoring in Postoperative Care of Adult Cardiac Surgical Patients

5

Ali Dabbagh

Abstract

One of the fundamental functions in each intensive care unit is monitoring, while we can consider respiratory monitoring, cardiovascular monitoring, and cerebral monitoring as the main three monitoring functions of ICU. Though, in the current world of increasing health technology, the sophisticated bedside examinations of the clinicians could not be replaced by any of these technologic improvements. On the other hand, continuous hemodynamic assessments after cardiac operations are the cornerstone of postoperative cardiac surgeries. The main cardiovascular monitoring methods involve—but are not confined to—the following pages, though more detailed explanations could be found in details in related texts. Noninvasive and invasive blood pressure, central venous and pulmonary artery pressure, cardiac output monitoring modalities, and the normal range for measured hemodynamic variables are among the main topics that the reader could be familiar with after reading this chapter.

Keywords

Noninvasive · Blood pressure · Monitoring · Automated blood pressure measurement · Riva-Rocci · Korotkoff · Mean arterial pressure · Compartment syndrome Invasive blood pressure monitoring · Radial artery · Complications · Femoral artery · Axillary artery · Brachial artery · Dorsalis pedis artery · Posterior tibialis Superficial temporal artery · Zeroing · Calibration · Central venous pressure Central venous pressure curves · Sedillot's triangle · Ultrasound-guided CVC insertion · Complications of central venous catheter · Pulmonary artery pressure monitoring · Pulmonary artery catheter · Swan-Ganz · Complications of pulmonary artery

A. Dabbagh, M.D.
Faculty of Medicine, Cardiac Anesthesiology Department, Anesthesiology Research Center, Shahid Beheshti University of Medical Sciences, Tehran, Iran

Cardiac Anesthesiology Fellowship Program, Shahid Beheshti University of Medical Sciences, Tehran, Iran
e-mail: alidabbagh@sbmu.ac.ir

A. Dabbagh et al. (eds.), *Postoperative Critical Care for Adult Cardiac Surgical Patients*, https://doi.org/10.1007/978-3-319-75747-6_5

catheter · Cardiac output monitoring · Fick principle · Transpulmonary lithium indicator dilution · Partial carbon dioxide (CO_2) rebreathing · Esophageal Doppler · Pulse contour analysis · Bioimpedance and bioreactance · Ultrasonic cardiac output monitor · Other noninvasive systems · Transpulmonary lithium indicator dilution · Partial carbon dioxide (CO_2) rebreathing · FloTrac/Vigileo LiDCO® system · PiCCO® system · PRAM · Bioimpedance and Bioreactance® USCOM · ClearSight system · Normal values for hemodynamic parameters

5.1 Noninvasive Blood Pressure Monitoring

In 1896, Scipione Riva-Rocci, using a cuff over the upper arm, described the completed method in measuring systolic blood pressure for the first time; afterward, in 1905, Nicolai Sergeivich Korotkoff a Russian surgeon described the method of measuring blood pressure by auscultation now well known as the Korotkoff sounds, from I to V, although Korotkoff himself could recognize four stages which were "first sound, then compression murmurs, second tone, and disappearance of sounds" and he could not recognize the muffling which is phase II; these phases are frequently used in the everyday clinic practice. The phase I of Korotkoff sound is equal to the systolic pressure, which is the first stage of sound. During phases II and III of Korotkoff sounds, the quality of the sounds changes. In phase IV of Korotkoff sounds, the sound muffles, and in phase V, the sound disappears; in some pathologies like aortic regurgitation, Korotkoff sound would be never discontinued, and so, the final phase is phase IV which is considered as the diastolic pressure. It has been demonstrated that the Korotkoff sounds could be enhanced through a simple maneuver, i.e., "by elevating the arm overhead in a 30 s period then inflating the sphygmomanometer cuff, and finally returning the arm to the normal position for blood pressure measurement; we could listen Korotkoff sounds louder than normal without any bias of the measurement" (Riva-Rocci et al. 1996; Roguin 2006; Karamanou et al. 2015).

The indirect nature of noninvasive blood pressure measurement poses potential source of measurement errors. Three different sources for bias are possible in indirect blood pressure measurement: "observer bias, faulty equipment, and failure to standardize the techniques of measurement." Very rapid cuff deflation causes rapid "passage" over the Korotkoff sounds which would underestimate the blood pressure. If the sphygmomanometer cuff size is not appropriate, the measurements could be with error, especially when the cuff is undersized, though oversized cuffs do not create a significant error; the cuff is suggested to have a length of 80% and a width of 40% of the arm circumference. Also, the cuff should not be fastened so much tightly; otherwise, it would overmeasure the blood pressure (Bur et al. 2000; Drawz 2017).

5.1.1 Automated Blood Pressure Measurement

Automated noninvasive blood pressure measurement is clinically advantageous over manual measurement in such a way that some believe that "the conventional

Riva-Rocci/Korotkoff technique … with a mercury sphygmomanometer and stethoscope is now being relegated to the museum shelves" (O'Brien 2003).

So, this method has nowadays replaced the older manual control of blood pressure especially in some places like the intensive care units with which the healthcare personnel would be free to care for the patients. The most common technology used in these devices is the oscillometric technique; so, it has a considerable sensitivity for measuring the mean arterial pressure (MAP); however, the measurement of systolic and diastolic blood pressure is not as accurate as the MAP especially in some critical disease states or in some arrhythmias like atrial fibrillation or aortic regurgitation. Since most of the available cuffs for automated blood pressure measurement are made for the upper arm, their use in other parts like thigh or calf would result in errors of measurements. Other technologies for measurement of noninvasive blood pressure have been developed, but none had been able to replace the oscillometry technique (O'Brien 1998, 2003; O'Brien et al. 2001; Campbell et al. 2014; Papaioannou et al. 2016).

There are a number of complications due to the effects of noninvasive blood pressure measurement (including automated blood pressure monitoring); among them, the following could be mentioned:

Compartment syndrome: being the most drastic complication of noninvasive blood pressure monitoring, this syndrome is "a serious potential complication of trauma to the extremities." The following are quoted as predisposing patients at highest risk for the occurrence of compartment syndrome due to noninvasive blood pressure measurements: repeated measurements, fastening the cuff against a bony part or a joint, system errors causing repeated unyielding results, administration of thrombolytic therapy in coronary artery disease patients having "seizures, movement disorders, hyperactivity, or tremor" and finally, obtunded patients. Obtunded patients are those "having an altered level of consciousness, altered mental status or altered physical status secondary to injury, illness, or anesthesia, who are dulled, or have diminished or absent sensation in the upper extremity due to nerve injury or anesthesia; and finally, those patients in whom, the ability to communicate is impeded, like the mentally ill patients or the disabled patients or infants and young children". This syndrome will cause an increase in the tissue fluid leading to increased venous pressure and, at the same time, decreasing the arterial-venous pressure gradient, finally decreasing perfusion pressure of the tissues (Ouellette 1998; Myers and Godwin 2012; Campbell et al. 2014; Stergiou et al. 2016; Jegatheswaran et al. 2017; O'Brien and Stergiou 2017).

5.2 Invasive Blood Pressure Monitoring

"Invasive blood pressure (IBP) monitoring" or "direct blood pressure monitoring" is one of the most commonly used hemodynamic parameters both in operating room and intensive care unit; this fact is especially true in cardiac surgery patients who are exposed to sudden, frequent, and abrupt hemodynamic changes, both during the intraoperative and postoperative period; its feasibility, relatively simple equipment, and the ability for beat-to-beat readings and recordings are among the many favorable features of IBP monitoring. Also, IBP monitoring through arterial line cannula is usually safe with very *few* complications.

Usually, the systolic and diastolic measurements are displayed on the monitoring plane; however, most devices demonstrate the mean arterial pressure (MAP) value simultaneously. For MAP calculation, we use this formula:

MAP = [2(diastolic BP) + 1(systolic BP)]/3; (BP stands for blood pressure). MAP is a more accurate index of perfusion in nearly all body tissues except for the coronary perfusion bed in which the diastolic blood pressure is a more important index. However, in cardiac patients undergoing cardiopulmonary bypass, we usually use MAP to assess the overall tissue perfusion.

Although IBP measurement through the arterial line is the most familiar method, it is usually considered as an indirect indicator of the cardiovascular system, since "IBP measurement" depends on two main variables: cardiac output (CO) and systemic vascular resistance (SVR). However, in critical setting, IBP is more accurate than NIBP: when the patient is hypotensive, the blood pressure values measured with NIBP are usually higher than IBP; however, when the patient is hypertensive, NIBP is lower than IBP.

5.2.1 Common Indications and Contraindications for IBP Measurement and Arterial Line Cannulation

5.2.1.1 Indications

1. *Continuous, real-time blood pressure measurement* accompanied with *heart rate* monitoring, like those patients with "impaired hemodynamic status" due to "depressed function of the *left ventricle*," "severe myocardial *ischemia*," "*coronary ischemic syndromes*," "*septic or hypovolemic shock*," or "*severe right sided heart failure syndromes*," in which vigorous hemodynamic monitoring (including IBP) is essential.
2. *Repetitive measurement of BP* (while NIBP is not appropriate or not available, e.g., in patients with multiple, simultaneous *burn* or *fractures* in all extremities or compartment syndrome or in patients with morbid obesity in which NIBP monitoring is not possible).
3. *Need for assessment and evaluation of the BP curve and waveform*, including the components of the arterial waveform; in these cases, the waveform components are used for a number of clinical uses including the adjustment of intra-aortic balloon counterpulsation using the dicrotic notch or measuring the *cardiac output* through the arterial wave contour.
4. *Monitoring the effects of pharmacologic interventions or surgical manipulations* (e.g., those clinical states in which extensive blood pressure changes would happen, like administration of *inotropic* agents, manipulation of the heart, major blood vessels, or cardiopulmonary bypass "CPB").
5. *Severe and/or considerable blood loss* (e.g., in severe trauma with extensive *hemorrhage* or in *surgical* operations with massive bleeding).
6. *Induced hypotension* (due to the nature of the disease and its related surgical operation).

7. *Frequent blood sampling* (e.g., to perform *blood gas* analysis in acid-base or electrolyte disorders).

5.2.1.2 Contraindications

1. Local infection.
2. Proximal obstruction (like coarctation of the aorta) which would cause underestimation of blood pressure.
3. Coagulopathies and abnormalities associated with bleeding tendency; these mandate cannulation from more peripheral sites (*relative* contraindication).
4. Peripheral vascular disease like Raynaud's phenomenon and Buerger's disease (*relative* contraindication) which mandates more central arterial cannulation.

5.2.2 Sites of Measurement (Sites of Cannulation), Their Preferences, and Their Potential Complications

Ideally, the root of the ascending aorta is the ideal site for IBP measurement. However, in nearly all of the cases, this is not a practical approach. So, other arteries are used; usually, among all these arteries, radial, femoral, and axillary arteries are the most common sites for arterial line cannulation and IBP monitoring; in other words, radial artery is the first, femoral artery is the second, and axillary artery is the third most frequent site for arterial cannulation and IBP monitoring; however, among all of these sites, the radial artery of the nondominant hand (i.e., usually left radial artery) is more common than any other artery used for arterial cannulation.

Other common arteries include brachial, superficial temporal, dorsalis pedis, posterior tibialis, and ulnar artery; none of the above sites are as accurate as the aortic root pressure. In nearly all of these sites, the systolic measurement of BP is more, and the diastolic measurement of BP is lower than the aortic root pressure. However, the MAP amount is usually similar in all of these sites.

5.2.2.1 Radial Artery

Using radial artery for IBP measurement is the most common site among all the others, since it has a good collateral arterial flow. Also, percutaneous puncture method is the preferred method for insertion of the catheter. Regarding its anatomic features, it is superficial to the distal head of the radius bone, between flexor carpi radialis and brachioradialis tendons; also, it has a very rich collateral circulation through the ulnar artery and palmar arch. Since it is a peripheral artery, in hemodynamically unstable patients, its cannulation may not be as easy as the femoral artery (Miller and Bardin 2016).

Complications of radial artery cannulation:

- *Bleeding* (the most common complication).

Temporary occlusion and temporary *spasm* of radial artery (with about a 20% mean frequency in different studies) being a negligible and minor complication; "modified Allen's test" has not been proven to have predictive value for hand ischemia, though the controversy about this method still exists and some guidelines support doing this test for all the patients.

- *Permanent* occlusion which is a very rare complication.
- Other *mechanical* injuries of the artery rupture (like bleeding, hematoma formation, rupture, and pseudoaneurysm formation).
- *Discrepancy* between radial pressure and the real systolic pressure (especially after some clinical situations like post-CPB period, high-dose administration of vasoactive agents, etc.).
- *Thrombus* formation.
- *Sepsis* or local *infectious* complications (cellulitis, abscess, suppurative thromboarteritis).
- Local *injury* to other adjacent tissues (compartment syndrome, paralysis of the median nerve, air embolism, catheter fracture, and carpal tunnel syndrome).
- *Air embolization* to the cerebral arterial system after manual flushing (very rare).
- *Regional injuries* to the hand structures (embolization to the fingers, severe ischemia in the hand, or skin necrosis in a region proximal to the radial artery) (Fig. 5.1).

5.2.2.2 Femoral Artery

The femoral artery is located midway between the *anterior superior iliac spine* and *pubic symphysis*; using another anatomic landmark, it is lateral to the femoral vein and medial to the femoral nerve; it has one of the most accurate arterial waveforms similar to the aortic root (central) arterial wave, both regarding the shape of the wave and the measured values of blood pressure, *even in hypotensive and hypovolemic patients* (Fuda et al. 2016). Incidence of complications after femoral artery cannulation is equivalent to radial artery; however, some believe the complications, though infrequent, are more complicated to manage and could be listed as:

1. Pseudoaneurysm formation.
2. Bleeding and hematoma formation.
3. Infectious complications (including sepsis and systemic infection and also local infection); there is possibly no more risk of infectious complications for the femoral artery than the upper extremities.
4. Massive retroperitoneal bleeding (very *rare*).
5. *Minimal* thrombotic risk (due to the *large arterial lumen* compared with the catheter).
6. Temporary arterial occlusion (*very low* incidence).

5.2.2.3 Axillary Artery

The axillary artery provides IBP measurements very near to the aortic root pressure. Its anatomic location is between the triceps and coracobrachialis tendons, in the armpit; i.e., its landmarks are similar to the landmarks used for axillary block.

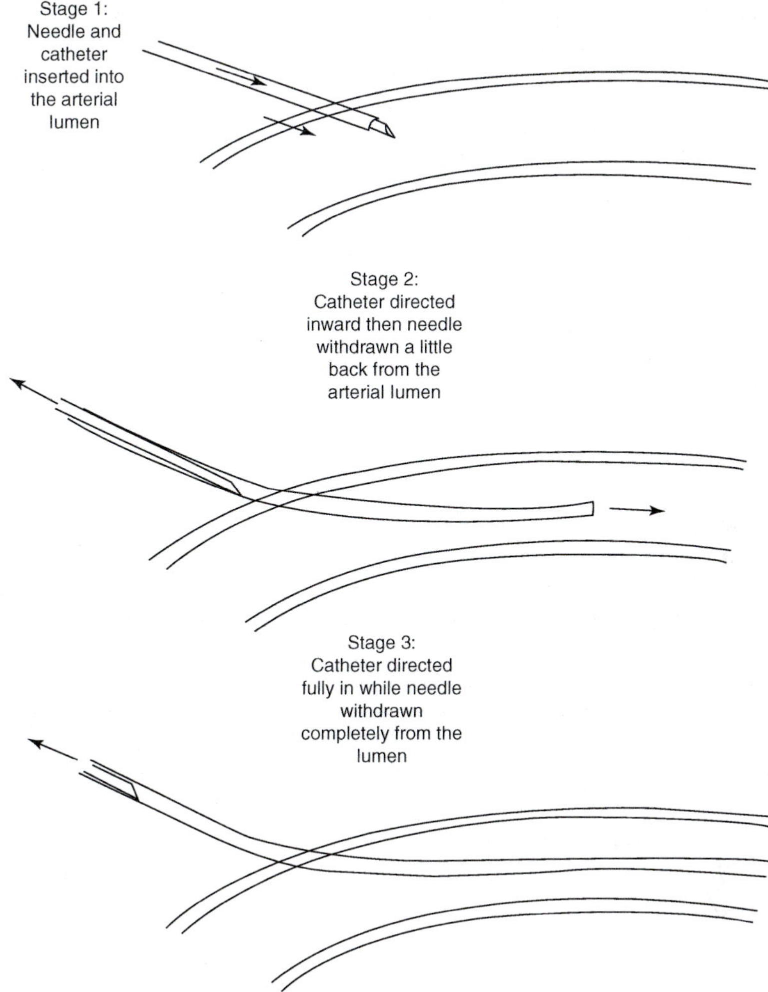

Fig. 5.1 Schematic presentation of needle through catheter technique in three stages; note that care must be taken not to withdraw the needle before the tip of the catheter lumen is entered into the arterial lumen (stage 2) (Dabbagh 2014)

However, performing this procedure is not technically easy, for those who are expert. This artery has also extensive collateral arterial flow. Its complications are:

- Permanent limb ischemia.
- Pseudoaneurysm.
- Sepsis.
- Paresthesia of the limb due to mechanical effects of the needle or the catheter.

- Some clinicians have the fear of cerebral air embolism due to retrograde flushing in the axillary artery; however, there is no evidence of such complication, and it is a safe approach (Htet et al. 2017).

5.2.2.4 Brachial Artery

The brachial artery is subject to inaccuracy, lacks *collateral* circulation, and is associated with the risk of *median nerve* injury and *compartment* syndrome (since it is located in the antecubital fossa); though the occurrence of compartment syndrome is not so much common, it is a *real danger*, since most of the patients are not fully conscious and also have been exposed to some anticoagulants. The complications of the brachial artery cannulation are:

- Injury
- Hematoma
- Local infection
- Arteriovenous fistula
- Pseudoaneurysm
- Paresthesia and median nerve injury

5.2.2.5 Ulnar Artery

Due to the location of the ulnar artery, its proximity and attachment to the ulnar nerve, and also the greater anatomical perfusion of the distal hand structures from the ulnar artery, some authors have claimed that ulnar artery cannulation might be associated with a higher risk of vascular and organ injury; however, complications of the ulnar artery cannulation are not so much higher than the radial artery, especially if modified Allen's test is done before arterial puncture and also the radial artery is not injured simultaneously.

5.2.2.6 Dorsalis Pedis

These are the main features of this site:

- Excellent collateral flow
- Easy cannulation
- Minimal patient discomfort
- A very low incidence of complications.

However, due to the relatively long distance of the artery with the aortic root, BP readings are not accurate with measurements being 5–20 mmHg higher than the radial arteryx.

5.2.2.7 Posterior Tibialis

Posterior tibialis artery cannulation is used mainly for the pediatric patients; however, there are not so many complications reported after cannulation of this artery.

5.2.2.8 Superficial Temporal Artery

The superficial temporal artery is one of the end arteries of the carotid; its cannulation has some "serious" complications; due to its disadvantages, this site is not recommended for IBP measurement.

5.2.3 Complications

5.2.3.1 Ischemic Complications

Risk factors for ischemic complications could be classified as:

- Female gender
- Preexisting hypertension
- Arteritis or other vascular diseases
- Size of catheter
- Composition of catheter
- Time duration for cannulation
- Simultaneous use of vasopressors

5.2.3.2 Thrombus Formation

The catheter used for the arterial line could injure the arterial bed and so lead to thrombus formation. There are a number of risk factors which increase the risk of thrombus formation:

- The percentage of the artery surface occupied by the catheter lumen; this occupation percentage is calculated according to the following proportion:
- (external diameter of the catheter/internal diameter of the artery); so, for radial artery, a 20 G catheter is recommended.
- Teflon catheters are claimed to **decrease** the risk for "thrombus formation," though this issue is controversial.
- Decreased cardiac output **increases** the risk of thrombus formation.
- Hematoma formation **increases** the risk for radial artery occlusion and thrombus formation.
- Systemic administration of aspirin or low-dose heparin **decreases** the chance for thrombus formation.
- Increased time for catheter preservation **increases** the risk of thrombus formation (the risk is especially increased after 48–72 h).

5.2.3.3 Infectious Complications

These include sepsis, local infections, infectious pseudoaneurysm, etc. The main issue in the prevention of these complications, devoid of the site of the arterial line, is to strictly adhere to aseptic techniques, both for the arterial puncture site and the related equipment (including the Luer locks and the connecting tubes). Also, any underlying inflammation or infection should be a warning against using the site for arterial blood pressure monitoring.

5.2.4 Technical Considerations in Arterial Line Cannulation

According to the *French Society of Anaesthesia and Intensive Care* (1995) guideline, the following steps should be followed in arterial line cannulation:

1. Use Teflon or polyurethane catheters (maximal size of 18 G for femoral or axillary arteries and 20 gauge for the other arteries).
2. Maximal length of catheter for small arteries (i.e., radial and dorsalis pedis arteries) is preferred to be 3–5 cm.
3. Heparin coating of catheters for prevention of complications is not proven.
4. Using salts for radiopacity is not useful and may even have thrombogenicity.
5. It is recommended to administer a flush device; the device should have a constant flow of 2 mL/h; at the same time, it is recommended to use a fast flush valve which is connected to normal saline under pressure.
6. Manual intermittent flushing with a syringe is contraindicated.
7. Addition of heparin (2500 IU.500 mL-1 of flush solution) increases the duration of catheter patency and is recommended for catheterizations of more than 24 h duration.
8. Ready for use devices are to be preferred.
9. Distortion of pressure wave may be minimized by employing low-volume, low-compliance, and low-resistance devices.
10. The number of connections should be as low as possible and all of Luer-lock type.
11. The stopcocks should be clearly identified to minimize the risk of accidental intra-arterial injection.
12. The device should be transparent for disclosure of bubbles, which lead to waveform distortion.
13. For catheter placement the operator should follow the usual preparation as for any aseptic surgical procedure with cap, mask, gloves, and sterile towel.
14. The insertion site should be prepped either with chlorhexidine or povidone-iodine.
15. In the conscious patient, local anesthesia by injection and/or topical application (EMLA) is recommended.
16. Direct arterial puncture should be preferred rather than transfixion method.
17. It is recommended to use percutaneous cannulation.
18. Needle-catheter assembly should be advanced as slowly as possible to prevent arterial transaction; blood return confirms arterial placement.
19. Resistance against needle advancing is a landmark of error.
20. Catheterization of deep vessels is facilitated by Seldinger technique, which is recommended whatever the site of placement when long-term monitoring and/or difficulties of insertion are foreseen.
21. The radial artery is the site of choice for elective cases. The nondominant hand should be preferred. Puncture must be preceded by assessment of adequacy of the collateral flow by the Allen test; also, in order to facilitate radial artery cannulation, we may use a 45° wrist angulation.
22. The femoral artery is a valuable site for emergency situations. Before catheterization, the artery should be auscultated for a murmur.

23. Puncture of a vascular prosthesis is contraindicated.
24. The dressing should be changed every 4 days only.
25. The dressing is recommended to be visible as much as possible to check for any possible leakage of blood; this issue mandates repeated checking of the catheter and its attachments and also minimal application of dressing material.
26. Whether peripheral or central arteries are used, the area distal to the puncture site should be checked for any possible signs or symptoms of ischemia, including change in color, temperature, or distal pulse; of course, it may even mandate Doppler assessment of distal flow.
27. Sites of blood withdrawal should be manipulated with compresses soaked with chlorhexidine or povidone-iodine.
28. The arterial catheter is only changed in case of evidence of local infection or ischemia.
29. The catheter removal should be considered as an aseptic surgical procedure, and the catheter completeness has to be checked.
30. A systematic culture of the catheter is not required.
31. Also, it has been demonstrated that *Doppler ultrasound-guided cannulation* may improve the results and decrease the rate of complications, especially in the elderly and pediatrics (Aouad-Maroun et al. 2016; Wanderer and Rathmell 2017).

5.2.5 Arterial Line Transducers and the "Coupling System"

The arterial line transducer and the "coupling system" is the name for the connections from the arterial line catheter connected up to the monitor. Its function is to change the mechanical data into the electrical data used for the monitor display screen. This system contains the following elements:

1. *Transducer*: the main "exchange system" which transforms mechanical data to electrical data through a delicate diaphragm usually made of silicon.
2. *Tubing*: the mediator between catheter and the transducer.
3. *Flushing system*: prevents clot formation throughout the catheter-transducer assembly by a continuous infusion of saline (usually 1–3 mL/h). This solution was used to be heparin-rinsed; however, recent studies discourage usage of heparin in such solutions for repetitive washing to prevent the real possibility of heparin-induced thrombocytopenia (see Chap. 6 "Postoperative Coagulation and Bleeding" for explanation of heparin-induced thrombocytopenia).

Zeroing: a very important technical consideration is frequent zeroing of the arterial line monitor in order to gain "real" zero readings and then to measure the blood pressure correctly. Each monitor has its recommendations for zeroing based on the manufacturer; however, considering the appropriate level, especially when the patient is in positions other than supine, is an important feature of zeroing. When the patient is in supine position, the level of the transducer should be positioned at the level of the fourth intercostal space which is approximately at the level of midaxillary line; frequent zeroing might increase the accuracy of readings.

Calibration: in order to prevent biased readings, calibration should be done in a timely fashion, especially after each episode of blood sampling, when there is a major change in arterial blood pressure or whenever the readings are doubtful (Mandel and Dauchot 1977; O'Rourke and Avolio 1980; O'Rourke and Yaginuma 1984; Moran 1990; Clark and Kruse 1992; Cockings et al. 1993; Klepper et al. 1993; 1995; Franklin 1995a; b; Horlocker and Bishop 1995; Anderson 1997; Kuhn 2001; O'Rourke et al. 2001; McGhee and Bridges 2002; Scheer et al. 2002; Cousins and O'Donnell 2004; Langesaeter et al. 2008; Nichols et al. 2008; Brzezinski et al. 2009; Wilcox 2009; Augusto et al. 2011; Chee et al. 2011; Ranganath and Hanumanthaiah 2011; Wax et al. 2011; Fuda et al. 2016; Melhuish and White 2016; Ahmad et al. 2017; Wanderer and Rathmell 2017).

5.3 Central Venous Pressure Monitoring

Since its first use in 1929 by Werner Forssmann, central venous pressure catheter (CVP catheter or CVC) has gained widespread use all over the world. CVP is the pressure of blood inside the central intrathoracic veins or the pressure of the right atrium. It is usually measured through a central venous catheter (most commonly known as CVP catheter or CVC). CVP is a very good surrogate for right ventricle pressure and is commonly used as an estimate of left ventricular preload; however, its use as an indicator of right ventricle pressure is not always correct, and many do not rely on the absolute CVP measurement as the index for preload due to many different factors affecting the exact CVP measurement. To compensate for this defect, a number of clinicians rely on the trend of its changes for assessment of the preload status of the patients, though this approach has its own "demerits"; nevertheless, CVP has its own many uses and is among the most commonly applicable devices for critical patients including cardiac surgery patients.

CVCs are used frequently not only for assessment of CVP but also for administration of drugs and fluids. Of course, CVCs are not considered as the primary route for urgent and rapid fluid replacement. Instead, peripheral large-bore catheters are considered for rapid fluid administration.

Many different indications have been cited for CVP; however, a number of them are mentioned here, and a detailed list could be found in Table 5.1.

5.3.1 Indications for CVC Insertion and Usage

1. *Fluid administration and management* (including assessment of loading status, patients with poor peripheral IV access, continuous renal replacement therapy, temporary hemodialysis), although usual multi-lumen 7 F, 20 cm catheters have a much lower capacity for fluid administration compared with usual peripheral IV access

Table 5.1 Indications and contraindications for central venous catheters (CVCs)

Indications
• Administration of pharmaceuticals (esp. the vasoactive or irritant drugs) • Monitoring the hemodynamic parameters (esp. loading status including CVP) • Transvenous pacing • Rapid fluid administration (in trauma or in procedures mandating large fluid shift or blood loss) • Poor peripheral IV access • Frequent or rapid aspiration (blood aspiration for frequent venous sampling or rapid air emboli aspiration in specific surgeries) • Total parenteral nutrition (TPN) • Continuous renal replacement therapy, temporary hemodialysis, plasmapheresis, or apheresis
Contraindications Absolute contraindications • SVC syndrome causes CVC to be useless and possibly increases the CVC risks for the patient Relative contraindications • Coagulopathies • Patients having pacemaker or ICD insertion in the 6 previous weeks • Anatomic abnormalities (due to coexisting pathologies or recent surgical manipulations disturbing the normal anatomy of the region) • Carotid disease especially in the presence of contralateral carotid involvement

2. *Diagnostic* measurements (pure values and changing trends of cardiac loading pressures)
3. *Pharmacologic interventions* (especially the vasoactive drugs or irritant drugs, plasmapheresis, or apheresis)
4. Other indications (like transvenous pacing)

5.3.2 Central Venous Pressure Curves

The CVP curve is composed of five main waves, namely, a, c, x, v, and y, which are the final result of interactions mainly occurring between the right atrium (RA), the right ventricle (RV), and the tricuspid valve (TV); however, among them a, c, and v are upward deflections, while x and y are downward deflections. These waves mainly demonstrate the right atrial pressure (RAP) as the following order (Fig. 5.2):

a: atrial contraction causes an increase in RAP; it appears just after P wave in electrocardiography.

c: isovolumetric contraction of RV increases RAP and creates c wave.

x: RV contraction pulls TV away from RA and decreases RAP; so we would have a downward deflection wave.

v: blood fills RA during late RV systole which increases RAP and again produces an upward deflection.

y: finally TV opens and causes emptying of RA; so, again we see a downward deflection.

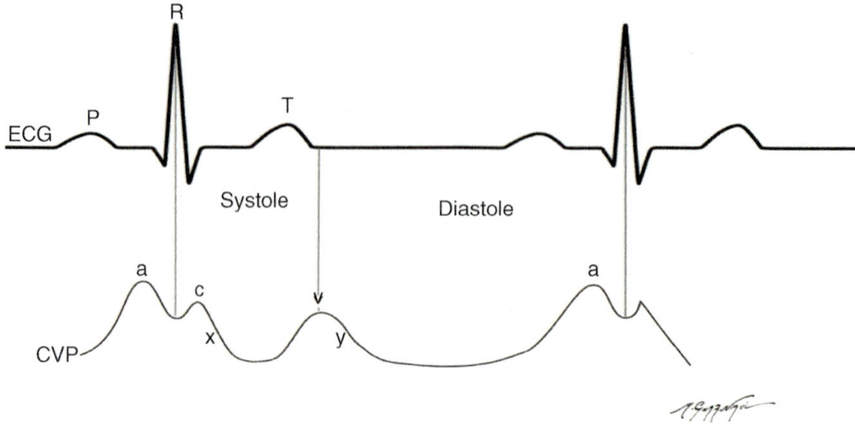

Fig. 5.2 CVP waves and the relation with ECG (Dabbagh 2014)

There are a number of well-recognized approaches for CVC insertion, "internal jugular vein" and "subclavian vein" being the two most common approaches, while the right internal jugular vein is more common than the left one, while some believe that left internal jugular vein approach is as easy as the right side.

5.3.2.1 Right Internal Jugular Vein Approach

The internal jugular vein (IJV) was first described by English in the 1960s and is the most frequently used approach for CVC insertion; it causes less complications, has a straight course to the RA, and has lower chance for thoracic duct and pleural dome puncture, both due to anatomic properties of right IJV, although some have claimed that the left IJV approach is as much easy. It also has a very high success rate (>90%) even in infants and children accompanied with very low rate of other mechanical complications like arterial puncture, pneumothorax, hematoma needing surgical intervention, etc. compared with all the other methods. Even in anatomically "difficult" patients, the IJV approach has a specific feasibility. The course of IJV, especially the right one, is straight, short, and with distinct anatomic landmarks; it is without venous valves until the superior vena cava and right atrium and could be reached by most anesthesiologist even during the operation time. Its most common and easiest "central approach" described in 1970 by Daily et al. is even the simplest one among all the right IJV access methods, in which the needle tip is inserted into the "apex of *Sedillot's triangle*, which is between the sternal and clavicular heads of sternocleidomastoid (SCM) and the related portion of the clavicle located between the two SCM muscle heads."

Correct sizing of the catheter length is a very challenging issue.

The following steps should be followed for insertion of CVC through right IJV:

1. Put the patient in supine position with a little leftward rotation of the head.
2. Gently extend the neck; excessive extension would distort the "favorable anatomy."

3. Check the anatomic landmark of the neck (*Sedillot's triangle*) once more before draping.
4. Use basic monitoring including electrocardiography (ECG), pulse oximetry (SpO_2), and noninvasive or invasive blood pressure measurement.
5. Use a "mild" degree of sedation if the patient is not anesthetized or not sedated accompanied with *supplemental oxygen.*
6. Administer strict aseptic techniques including handwashing, using sterile gown and gloves, and sterile preparation from the mastoid to the sternal notch (2% chlorhexidine is superior to others like 10% povidone-iodine).
7. Drape the patient with a *large* drape.
8. Put the patient slightly in head-down position except for patients with cardiovascular or respiratory disease.
9. In awake patients, use 1% lidocaine solution for local anesthesia using a 25G needle after another check of landmarks.
10. Use a 22G finder needle to find IJV.
11. Introduce the 18G needle from the apex of the *Sedillot's triangle* from between the two heads of SCM toward the ipsilateral nipple with a 30–45° angle from the skin plane.
12. If you could not draw dark blood, relocate the needle a bit laterally or medially in a fanwise model; beware of arterial puncture risk.
13. Check patency of the needle if there is no successful venous puncture yet; also, check the anatomic landmarks once more.
14. The two venous walls of a central vein are at times compressed against the needle; withdrawing the needle gently usually causes sudden filling of the syringe in such cases.
15. After appropriate backflow of relatively dark blood, insert the guidewire through the needle; there should not be any resistance in the course of guidewire insertion; otherwise the guidewire path is not correct; usually the guidewires used for adult CVCs are 0.032–0.035 mm; so, the guidewire passage should be never forceful.
16. The blood flow should be non-pulsatile except for cases of severe tricuspid regurgitation or high right ventricular pressure, in which the backflow of IJV would be pulsatile; if you are doubtful regarding the blood flow to be arterial or venous, attach a sterile stopcock to the 18G needle, which has an extension tube attached to one of its heads, and ask a colleague to attach the other head of the extension tube to the pressure monitoring to rule out potential arterial puncture.
17. The guidewire should be always in control, both regarding sterility of its distal end and potential arrhythmias of its proximal head, the former needs protection from contact with the unsterile adjacent objects, and the latter mandates careful ECG monitoring; in most adult cases, guidewire advancement below 20 cm prevents unwanted complications.
18. Withdraw the needle after guidewire installation; use a number 11 scalpel blade before advancing the dilator (especially when a pulmonary artery catheter

"PAC" introducer sheath or a large-bore CVC is used); care should be taken not to exert inappropriate force on the catheter; otherwise guidewire would easily be kinked; on the other hand, excessive dilator advancement would result in unwanted vascular or tissue trauma.

19. After dilator removal, while the guidewire is still in place, insert the catheter while caring to take the distal end of the guidewire out of the port of the CVC before the catheter is fully inserted; loss of control over the distal part of guidewire could result in catheter embolization, an unwanted complication discussed later.
20. Using this approach, CVC should be introduced no more than 15–17 cm in adult men and 13–15 cm in adult women to prevent CVC-induced cardiac tamponade (discussed later).
21. The CVC lines should be de-aired and washed to prevent clotting.
22. Sterile dressings (without any antibiotics) should be used in place.
23. Objective confirmation of the CVC tip which is done by CXR after catheter placement; the tip of the catheter should be above the carina which is approximately at the level of T3–T4 thoracic spines, which is also equal to the third rib or azygous vein.

5.3.2.2 Left Internal Jugular Vein Approach

The technique is similar to right IJV; however, the dome of the left pleura is higher than the right pleura, and also thoracic duct passes from the left; these two anatomic features increase the risk for two important complication: pneumothorax and chylothorax. Chylothorax is exclusive to the left hemithorax. The LIJV is shorter than the right IJV, but the venous path from the left side to the superior vena cava is longer than the right side. However, the chance for superior vena cava injury in left IJV is higher than right IJV since the path of right IJV is straightforward compared with left IJV.

5.3.2.3 Subclavian Approach

This approach has some specific features: more patient comfort, an easy approach, lower infection rate, and often used for long-term IV therapy but not monitoring purposes.

Method

1. Monitor the patient, accompanied with supplemental oxygen and mild sedation.
2. Head down the patient.
3. Rotate the head laterally.
4. Use a role beneath the two scapulae.
5. Use local anesthesia in a point just below the clavicle, between the lateral and middle thirds of the clavicle.
6. The 18G needle should be passed below the clavicle being directed to the sternal notch.
7. After appropriate backflow of relatively dark blood, insert the guidewire through the needle.

8. Other steps are similar to internal jugular vein approach.
9. Due to the potential risk of vascular injury or pneumothorax, one should keep in mind that a maximum of three tries from this approach is allowable and also bilateral (right and left subclavian) tries are forbidden since bilateral try would be potentially lethal.

5.3.2.4 External Jugular Vein

External jugular vein approach is a simple, really less risky approach, however, with lower chance for success; however, there are a few concerns for this approach.

1. Never use a dilator for these veins.
2. 90° abduction of the ipsilateral arm increases the success.
3. The vein course is sometimes tortuous, and the venous path could not be used for introduction of the catheter, in nearly 20% of patients (Fig. 5.3).

5.3.2.5 Femoral Vein

Usually used when IJV or subclavian approaches are not available (e.g., in neck injuries or thoracic involvements). The femoral vein is entered in a place just medial to the

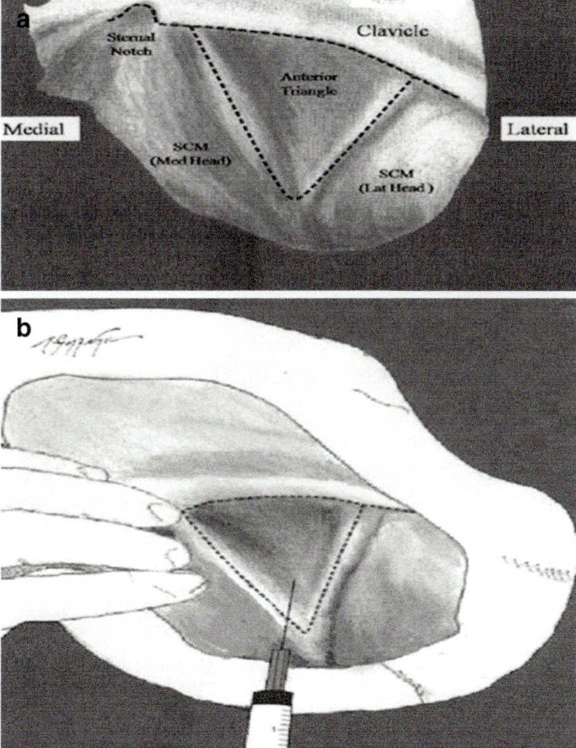

Fig. 5.3 Schematic presentation of the right anterior triangle (Sedillot's triangle) used for internal jugular vein cannulation when looking from above the patient's head. (**a**) The anatomic landmarks of the triangle, sternocleidomastoid muscle (SCM), Lat lateral, Med medial. (**b**) Anatomic location for needle punctures near the apex of triangle toward the ipsilateral nipple (Dabbagh 2014)

femoral artery pulse; however, the needle should be introduced to the vein distal to the inguinal ligament to prevent the risk of retroperitoneal bleeding. Besides femoral artery or femoral nerve injury, infectious complications and thromboembolic complications are the main other potential complications of this approach. Two different length catheters have been used in this approach: "40–70 cm" and "15–20 cm" catheters are used; both are near to SVC measurement but not exactly the same figures.

5.3.2.6 Peripheral CVC

Peripherally inserted catheters as CVC have been used to decrease complications of CVC; but, there is no difference between the two methods regarding infection rate. However, peripheral CVCs have more complications like "catheter tip malpositioning, thrombophlebitis and catheter dysfunction"; hence, central CVCs seem to be preferred over peripheral catheters.

5.3.3 Ultrasound-Guided CVC Insertion

This method was introduced for the first time in 1984 and could improve success and decrease the rate of complications, increasing patient safety, especially in IJV approach and in inexperienced hands. Though adult patients are more frequently said to benefit this method, ultrasound-guided CVC insertion has been shown efficacious in pediatric patients. A 7.5–10 MHz probe, covered by a sterile sheath , used by the nondominant hand, finds the transverse (short) axis at first in order to find the IJV lumen, which is larger, laterally located, and non-pulsatile compared with the medially located carotid artery; the transverse axis is also used for detection of the needle entry to the IJV lumen. Then, the longitudinal view (long axis) is used to confirm the appropriate passage of the guidewire into the lumen of IJV. However, in other approaches except for IJV, there is not much great utility for ultrasound-guided CVC insertion because of the sonographic "shadows and distances" between the skin and the vein lumen (Fig. 5.4).

5.3.4 Complications of CVCs

One of the very common topics in everyday practice of cardiac patients is the minor and major complications of CVCs; many complications have been attributed to CVCs, and too many studies have been published in this topic; the majority of these complications are not common; however, a few could potentially lead to major events and even death. These complications are categorized in four main categories, discussed more in the following paragraphs:

1. Mechanical (vascular injuries, tamponade, nerve injuries, pneumothorax, tissue trauma, etc.)
2. Thromboembolic
3. Infection
4. Other complications

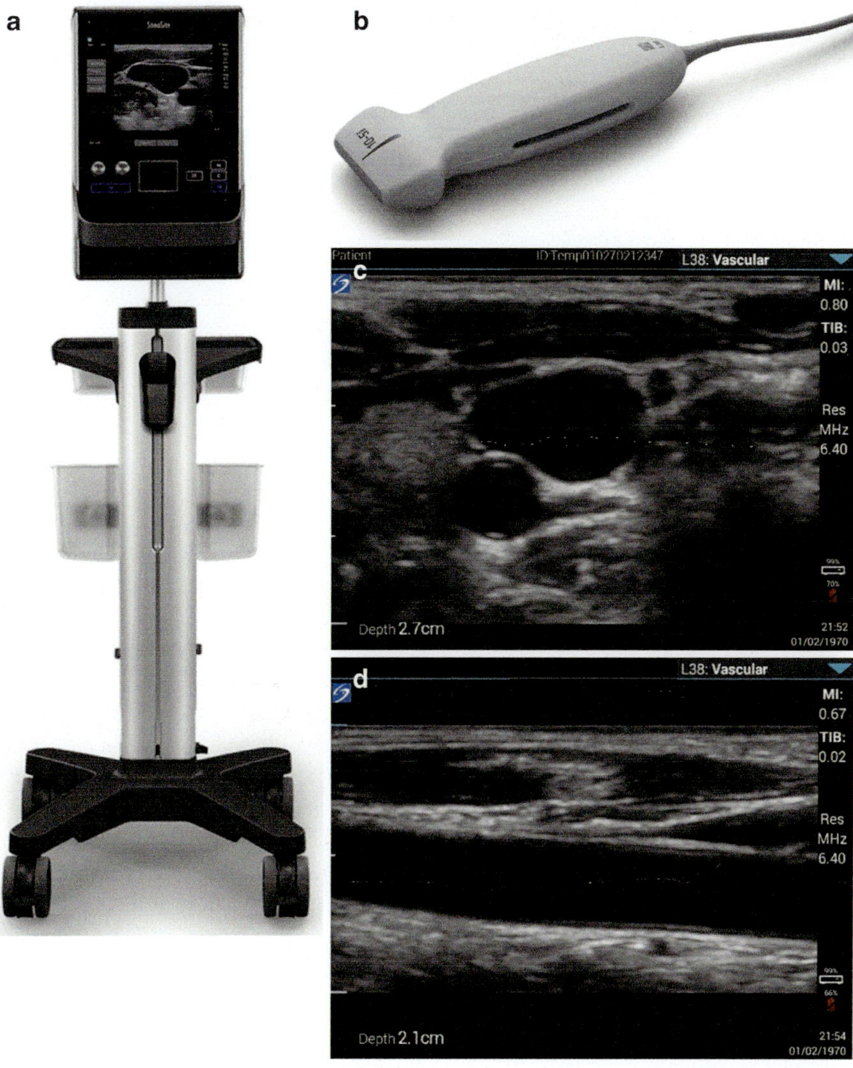

Fig. 5.4 (**a**) Portable sonography system for perioperative use; (**b**) specific vascular probe; (**c**) short axis of internal jugular vein lumen; (**d**) long axis of carotid artery lumen; (**e**) long axis of carotid artery lumen with color Doppler; The images are published with kind formal permission of FUJIFILM SonoSite, Inc.

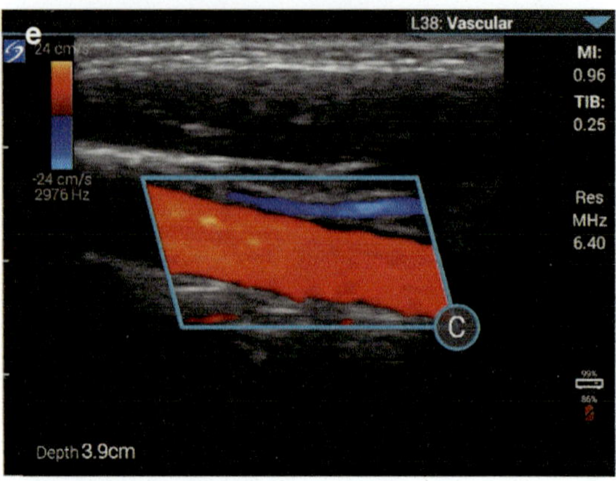

Fig. 5.4 (continued)

5.3.4.1 Mechanical Complications

Mechanical complications include mainly vascular injuries (arterial puncture, venous injuries), cardiac tamponade, vascular and neural injury, and pneumothorax. Vascular injuries could be arterial or venous.

Arterial puncture is the most frequent among all acute complications, often resulting in local hematoma, which usually resolves after a few minutes of local compression. Few numbers of the patients (especially when major arteries including aorta are injured) need more sophisticated care including emergent consult with a vascular surgeon. If arterial puncture is unintentionally used instead of central vein for catheter placement, the catheter should be removed urgently (except for very unusual circumstances) to prevent unwanted organ embolizations including CNS injuries. However, the risk of arterial bleeding at the puncture site is always potentially serious, needing more vigorous assessments and possible interventions by a vascular surgeon. If a central venous catheter is misplaced anatomically, the location of the catheter tip should be assessed. If it is not in a potentially risky place, we might withdraw the catheter; however, if the catheter tip is located in a risky organ which could not be compressed after catheter removal, or if the course of catheter passes through such an anatomic location, then the catheter should not be removed before an emergent consult with a vascular surgeon.

Other vascular injuries are frequent and diverse including minor venous injuries, hemomediastinum, hydromediastinum, hemothorax, hydrothorax, chylothorax, etc. And finally, *delayed* vascular injuries have been reported including different types of fistula between veins, arteries, bronchus, and other adjacent tissues, all being rare but needing vigorous attention and care.

Hemopericardium is the second common and the most lethal complication of CVC placement. It is usually due to perforation of the right ventricle, the right atrium, or the segment of the superior vena cava located inside the pericardium. The rupture would cause sudden cardiac tamponade blood or fluid tamponade. This is a delayed complication of CVC occurring usually in the first week after CVC placement and is usually preceded by arrhythmia unresponsive to anti-arrhythmia treatments. Mortality rates more than 80% are reported for this complication. Would the clinician perform objective documentation of the CVC tip location (i.e., by CXR), this lethal complication could be prevented in many cases.

Pneumothorax is another mechanical complication occurring more commonly after subclavian approach; however, the IJV approach (especially the left IJV) could also lead to pneumothorax though with a lower rate compared with subclavian approach. Minor cases are treated with supportive care, while others need chest tube insertion. Vigorous care should be devoted to high-risk patients especially those underlying mechanical ventilation or those in whom multiple or bilateral punctures have been done to prevent the occurrence of tension pneumothorax which is very lethal.

Nerve injuries could be seen mainly at the following sites: brachial plexus, stellate ganglion, and phrenic nerve. Chronic pain syndromes are also possible.

Tissue trauma: trauma due to needle, guidewire, dilator, or even the catheter had been reported. Dilator-induced tissue or vascular injuries are much more important since the dilators usually cause more harmful injuries than other items used in CVC kits. However, large-bore lumen catheters could lead to tissue injuries; catastrophic results should be anticipated if central vessels or cardiac chambers are injured or, in worst conditions, "*ruptured*" (see above).

Catheter or guidewire embolization usually mandates emergent consultation with an interventionist or a surgeon. During CVC placement, guidewire could be introduced inside the venous system unintentionally; so, it is necessary that the clinician take control of the distal end of the guidewire before introducing the whole catheter into the venous system. Also, there are reports of partial catheter fracture; both of these states could lead to catheter or guidewire embolization into the venous system, cardiac chambers, or even the pulmonary veins, being dislodged in between the lung tissues. The medical team should check any catheter fractures continually in patients admitted in intensive care wards, especially when the patients are awake and there is the possibility for spontaneous changes in body position. Another critical time for occurrence of this complication is at the time of CVC removal, which mandates careful examination of the whole CVC length and check for its tip to be intact after withdrawing from the patient.

5.3.4.2 Thromboembolic Complications

These complications are more common in patients with femoral CVC and are lowest in subclavian approach. The primary nidus can change to an infectious complication or may dislodge to the pulmonary vasculature; usually these complications need surgical removal.

5.3.4.3 Infectious Complications

Infectious complications are among the most common late complication of CVC, with 30–50% mortality. Strict adherence to aseptic techniques during catheter placement is the cornerstone of all preventing strategies for CVC infection. Using subclavian approach, catheters coated with chlorhexidine and silver sulfadiazine or rifampin and minocycline, and using single catheters have been demonstrated to decrease the rate of CVC-related infection. Also, the site of catheter insertion could affect the incidence of infectious complications being less in subclavian approach than other routes, though some controversies exist.

5.3.4.4 Other Complications

Arrhythmia is a very frequent and usually benign complication during CVC insertion especially in Seldinger technique (due to the guidewire); however, there are reported cases of malignant arrhythmias exactly at the time of CVC insertion; so, careful attention to patient's rhythm and hemodynamic status is a main concern during CVC insertion. However, the catheter itself could induce arrhythmias due to its physical effects if not in an appropriate location, which could happen intra- or postoperatively. Careful attention in the length of catheter entry is very important. Also, objective catheter tip confirmation by CXR is an essential job, confirming the CVC tip above the carina bifurcation; otherwise, the catheter should be a bit withdrawn in such a way that its tip is not far beyond carina.

Bleeding and air emboli are often related to CVCs with large-bore lumens, though other types of CVC may also have this side effect. Forgetting to secure the lumen ports could result in unnoticed bleeding. If the patient is hypovolemic, this complication would be manifested as air emboli entering the central venous circulation through the nonsecured lumen. Air embolism is also possible during two other situations besides unnoticed nonsecure ports: one is during catheter insertion, which is usually accompanied with small volumes of air going through the needle to the venous system, while the other situation is after CVC withdrawal which could be accompanied with air embolization through the skin lumen and subcutaneous tunnel created by after catheter removal. A compressed dressing with proper sealing could prevent both potential air embolism and CVC site bleeding after CVC removal.

Misinterpretation of data and errors in interpretation of data could lead to erroneous results and potential untoward clinical outcomes. For prevention of such erroneous judgments, the clinicians often do not rely only on the results of central venous pressure recordings; instead, the trend of CVP changes, curve of CVP, other measurements of filling pressures, jugular venous pressure figures, etc. are added to the online readings of CVP to prevent such unwanted events (Daily et al. 1970; Knopp and Dailey 1977; Berghella et al. 1979; Tyden 1982; Ferguson et al. 1988; Siradovic et al. 1988; Holmes et al. 1989; Kolodzik 1989; Meyer 1990; Heiss 1992; Mansfield et al. 1994; Tesio et al. 1994; English et al. 1995; Reed et al. 1995; Kuhn 2001; Merrer et al. 2001; Asheim et al. 2002; Keenan 2002; Woodrow 2002; Hind et al. 2003; Unal et al. 2003; Arai and Yamashita 2005; Botha et al. 2006; Di Iorio et al. 2006; Karakitsos et al. 2006; Ash 2007; Chen et al. 2007; Harrigan et al. 2007; Trieschmann et al. 2008; Brusasco et al. 2009; Kujur et al. 2009; Surov et al. 2009; Ishizuka et al. 2010; Kunizawa et al. 2010, 2010; Omar et al. 2010; Furuya et al. 2011; Kang et al. 2011; Kim et al. 2011, 2012; McGee et al. 2011; Uchida et al. 2011; Urban et al. 2011; Boyce 2012; Calabria et al. 2012; Chopra et al. 2012; Ge et al. 2012; Godoy et al. 2012; Guleri et al. 2012; Hewlett and Rupp 2012; Lee and Kamphuisen 2012; Liang et al. 2012; Linnemann and Lindhoff-Last 2012; Marik et al. 2012; Miller and Maragakis 2012; Parienti et al. 2012; Pikwer et al. 2012; Reems and Aumann 2012; Stone et al. 2012; Turi et al. 2012; Vats 2012; Walser 2012; Zhou et al. 2012; Gibson and Bodenham 2013).

5.4 Pulmonary Artery Pressure Monitoring

5.4.1 History

Pulmonary artery catheter (PAC) was reported first in 1970 by Dr Swan and Dr Ganz; hence the catheter is frequently known as the Swan-Ganz catheter. At that time, this catheter could introduce a new field of online cardiovascular monitoring, controlling the response to therapies and clinical data collection to the clinical world which was not accessible in such a novel way till that time. Due to its novel data, its use was rapidly increased during the following years both inside the operating rooms and intensive care units, for cardiac and non-cardiac patients. So, PAC could help us retrieve a number of useful data which are not retrievable by other monitoring devices like CVC-recorded pressure monitoring; these data are used for diagnostic and/or therapeutic uses, i.e., assessment of the effects of therapies.

5.4.2 Clinical Outcome of PAC Usage

During the recent years, there are an increasing number of evidence which question the clinical and final clinical outcome of using PAC, creating an overwhelming load of controversies in using this monitoring device, though some studies have confirm the usefulness of PAC in decreasing mortality in critical patients. Some results of these studies are discussed here briefly.

The negative studies claim that PAC could not decrease the overall mortality or hospital length of stay in critical care patients; also, right heart catheterization in ICU causes increased risk for severe end-organ complications, increased mortality, costs, and length of stay, in such a way that some studies have recommended withdrawal of PAC from current clinical practice in adult ICU patients as a cost-effective strategy; on the other hand, currently, many of the clinicians are seeking newer, less invasive monitoring to be validated and used in practice instead of PAC; among them, transesophageal echocardiography (TEE) could be named as one of the most useful devices for such an application that gives us the needed online data without potential risks of PAC; finally, these data at least recommend us not to use PAC as a routine monitoring, especially in low-risk patients; on the other hand, the positive studies confirm the beneficial role of PAC in decreasing mortality.

5.4.3 Indications for PAC Use

PAC is clinically indicated for assessment of these main variables and their response to therapeutic interventions during a wide range of different disease entities:

- Loading status, mainly including right heart failure, pulmonary dysfunction, pulmonary hypertension, severe left ventricular failure needing extra treatments like intra-aortic balloon pump, or shock (septic, cardiogenic, or non-cardiogenic)

- Main hemodynamic parameters of the right heart and the lung, including pulmonary artery pressure (PAP), pulmonary artery occlusion pressure (PAOP), pulmonary vascular resistance (PVR), and mixed venous oxygen saturation (SvO_2)
- Monitoring and assessment of cardiac output (CO)

However, risks and benefits of PAC insertion should be assessed before its utilization. Often in low- to moderate-risk cardiac patients, the risks outweigh the benefits, and it is not recommended to use PAC as a "routine" monitoring in such cardiac surgery patients, especially if there is not enough experience and sufficient skill in insertion of PAC and interpretation of its data. In other words, like many other diagnostic devices and technologies, "appropriate patient, sufficient skill in PAC insertion and data analysis and finally, appropriate setting" should be present before utilization of PAC.

5.4.4 Contraindications of PAC

These are usually due to anatomical causes and include:

- Tricuspid valve stenosis
- Pulmonary valve stenosis
- Previous mechanical prosthesis in any of the two above valves
- Current endocarditis in any of the two above valves
- Tumor and/or mass in the right atrium or right ventricle
- Thrombosis in the right atrium or right ventricle
- Tetralogy of Fallot due to the potential hyperreaction of the pulmonary artery in such patients to mechanical stimuli causing spasm and cyanotic spells
- Current underlying severe arrhythmia mandating full preparedness to treat any hemodynamic derangement
- Newly inserted pacemakers which could lead to displacement of the pacemaker wire
- Contraindications to insertion of CVC (see the previous section)

5.4.5 Technical Considerations for PAC Insertion

The basic principles for PAC insertion are in essence similar to CVC insertion; however, a few more points should be considered which are discussed here:

- The most preferred approach is right internal jugular vein, while subclavian and femoral veins are not routinely used especially for cardiac surgery patients.
- Guiding the catheter through its path in order to reach to pulmonary artery is used by three ways: the curve of the wave on monitor and its trend, fluoroscopic assessment of catheter tip, and electrocardiography (ECG)-guided approach;

however, in intensive care unit, usually the curve of the wave is used for catheter insertion and controlled by chest X ray.

- Changing the patient position to a head down and right lateral tilt helps the tip of the PAC to progress from the right atrium (RA) to the right ventricle (RV) and pulmonary artery (PA).
- An introducer sheath is inserted first, which is mainly like a CVC; this sheath is the conduit for passage of PAC and lets us move PAC back and forth; however, it is a relatively large-bore CVC, nearly 8.5–9 Fr. and so mandates vigorous caution during its insertion.
- The catheter is 110 cm length and usually 7–8 Fr. having length markers at 10 cm intervals for accurate and careful back and forth movements of the catheter.
- There is a sterile plastic cover on the catheter; this plastic cover should be attached firmly to the distal head of the introducer sheath to prevent contamination, though it is not fully protective and mandates strict adherence to infection

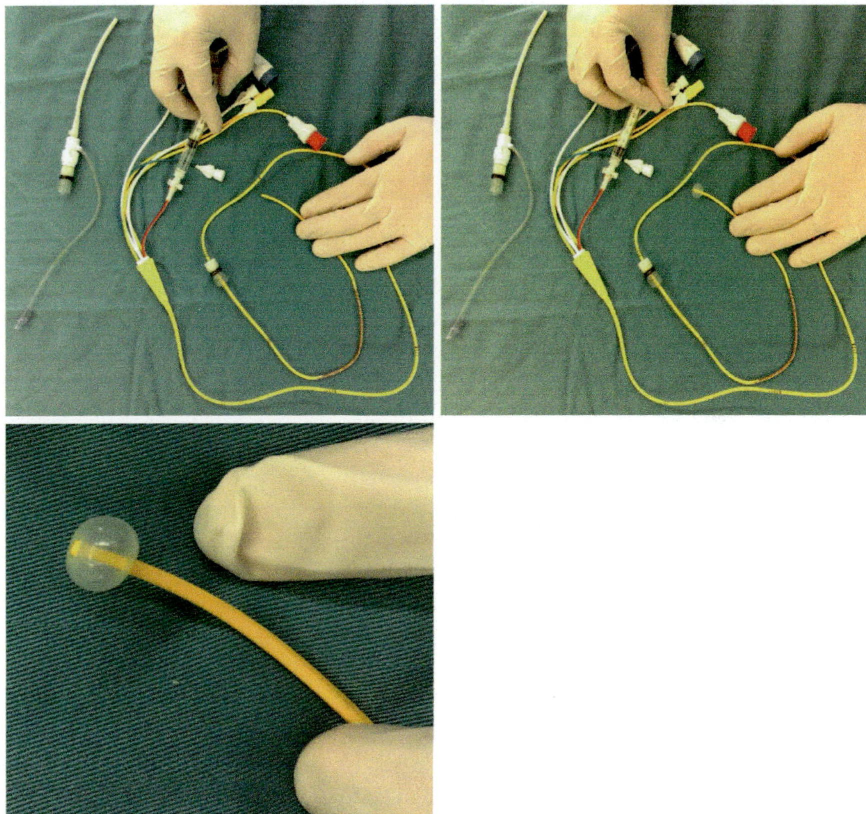

Fig. 5.5 PAC ingredients: note the tip of the balloon in three subsequent figures to be inflated; the third figure demonstrates a filled balloon in large view (Dabbagh 2014)

prevention methods and, more importantly, avoidance of unnecessary back and forth movements.

- Before passing the catheter tip through the introducer sheath and advancing it to the right heart, zeroing of the catheter with the monitoring system at the level of the right atrium should be done, while the patient is at supine position; also, the tip of PAC should be raised about 30 cm, and the pressure should be checked with the monitor which equals 22 mmHg.
- PAC has usually 4–5 lumens for the following purposes (demonstrated in Fig. 5.5):
  1. The distal lumen near the tip of catheter for the measurement of pulmonary artery pressure.
  2. A balloon located 4–5 cm proximal to the tip of catheter and 1.5 mL volume which should be filled for "flow directed movement of the catheter"; its related lumen should be attached to a specific 2 mL syringe, and the balloon should be checked for symmetrical filling before insertion of PAC; also, the balloon should not be filled when PAC tip is in wedge position to prevent unwanted injuries in lung tissue and pulmonary arterial branches.
  3. The most proximal lumen opening nearly 30 cm proximal to the tip of catheter used for measurement of central venous pressure or RA pressure.
  4. The fourth lumen having a thermistor for measurement of cardiac output using thermodilution method.
  5. Often the fifth lumen being used for assessment of mixed venous blood oxygen saturation (SvO_2).

When advancing PAC through introducer sheath from right internal jugular vein approach, we should have different related curve patterns at related distance intervals, i.e., for CVP (10–15 cm), RA pressure (15–25 cm), RV pressure (30–35 cm), PA pressure (40–45 cm), and wedge pressure (45–55 cm) as described below and demonstrated in Fig. 5.6:

1. Central venous pressure curve; demonstrating the tip of the catheter being located in central veins and/or RA, for CVP at 10–15 cm and for RA pressure at about 15–25 cm.
2. The catheter tip passes through the tricuspid valve, to go to the right ventricle (RV); a significant increase in systolic deflection is seen, and the diastolic deflection does not change so much; this part of the curve belongs to RV when PAC tip goes in as much as 30–35 cm.
3. With catheter progress through the course of pulmonary valve to the end of the pulmonary artery (PA), a dicrotic notch is seen in the point just after the peak of systole; however, the bottom of the increases suddenly showing the diastolic pressure of PA which is higher than the diastole of RV and resembles the wave contour of the systemic arterial pressure, of course in a smaller scale; so, PA pressure appears when PAC tip goes in for about 40–45 cm.
4. Afterwards, catheter progression for about 5 cm would be located nearly at 45–55 cm from PAC tip; here, there would be another change in the wave contour which indicates pulmonary artery wedge pressure (PAWP) or pulmonary artery occlusion pressure (PAOP); this would be demonstrated on the monitor screenplay

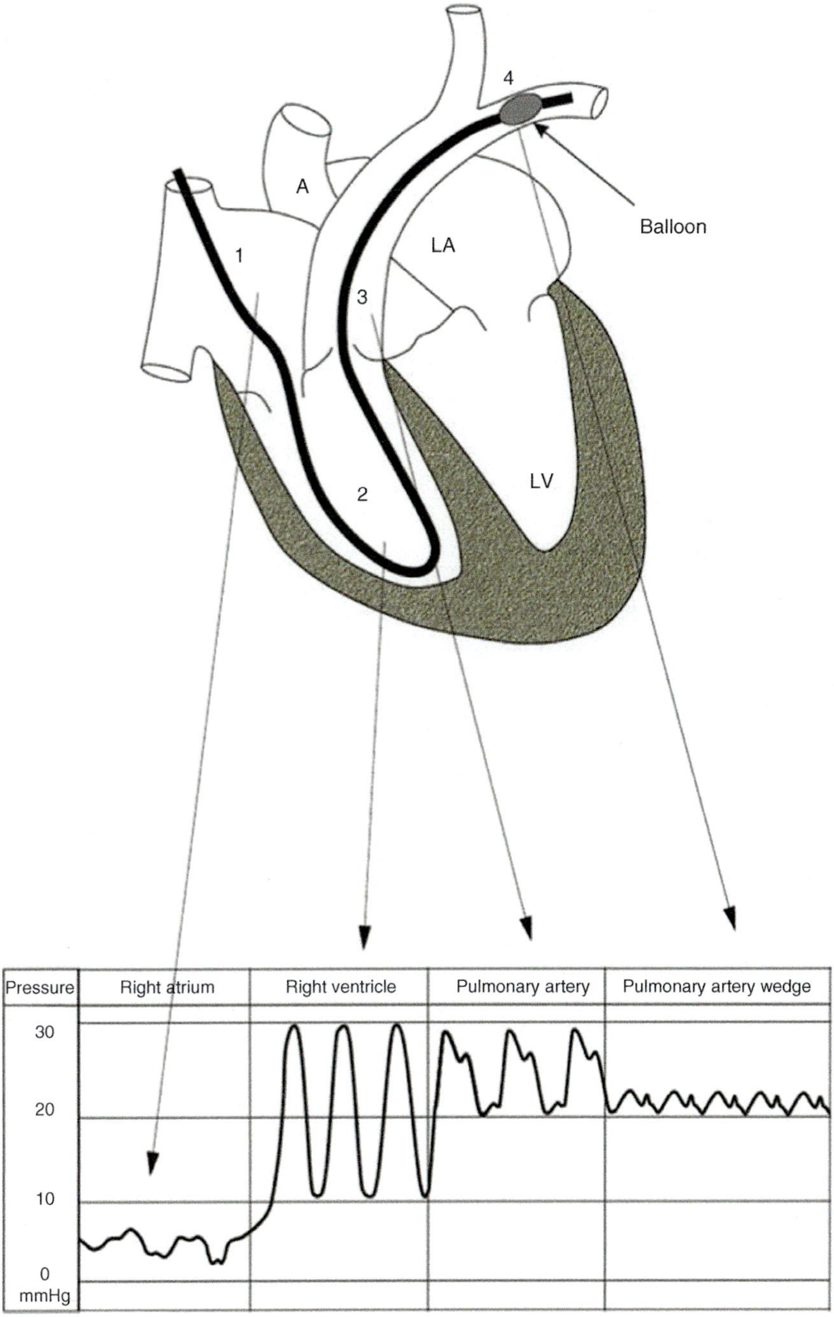

Fig. 5.6 A schematic presentation of the PAC course and its related pressure waveforms in cardiac chambers, pulmonary artery, and main left pulmonary artery (Dabbagh 2014)

after PAC balloon dilatation leading to wedge location of the tip of catheter; of course, PAC tip should not stay in wedge position for more than a few minutes to prevent unwanted complications like rupture of the pulmonary arterial branches or segmental necrosis of lung tissue; frequent withdrawal of PAC as much as 3–5 cm prevents PAC tip lodging, hence preventing such problems.
5. If these curves are not seen in the above length intervals, there is a real chance of catheter coiling, a dangerous complication of PAC discussed in the next paragraph; for prevention of such an event, strictly following the curves is a useful preventive strategy.

5.4.6 Complications of PAC

In 2003, the American Society of Anesthesiologists Task Force on PAC stated that "overall deaths attributable to PAC are 0.02–1.5%" and also classified PAC complications in three main categories:

1. PAC complications due to complications of CVC, i.e., "arterial puncture, postoperative neuropathy (pain and sensation deficit), air embolism (air in blood vessels) and pneumothorax (air outside the lungs), reported in less than 3.6%"
2. The complications mainly related to the mechanical effects of the catheter itself, i.e., "severe dysrhythmias, right bundle branch block and complete heart block, seen in 0.3% to 3.8%"
3. The complications related to persisting catheter in place, i.e., "rupture of the pulmonary artery and its attributed death, infarction of the pulmonary tissue, catheter related sepsis, positive catheter tip culture, valvular/endocardial vegetation, thrombophlebitis, mural thrombosis and thrombosis of the veins, i.e. clots in vein, occurring between 0.03% to 3%"

Sufficient skill, enough experience, having a high index of suspicion, and vigilance in detection of any complication may help the clinician prevent these potentially deadly complications or diagnose them as early as possible. The following comments should be remembered regarding the complications of PAC:

- Atrial or ventricular arrhythmias, often in the form of ventricular premature contractions, are seen during catheter passage from RV; these arrhythmias are usually benign; head-up and right lateral position might decrease the incidence of this complication.
- PAC could lead to right bundle branch block (RBBB); so, in patients with underlying left bundle branch block (LBBB), complete atrioventricular block (AV block) would be possible; though not frequent, it could be lethal.
- Pulmonary artery injuries might cause lethal pulmonary artery perforation or rupture mandating emergent surgery or stenting of the rupture; late pulmonary artery false aneurysm is also reported.

- Pulmonary infarction due to catheter dislodgement in segmental or bronchial pulmonary arterial branches is another potential complication.
- Right ventricle rupture is a highly morbid complication, needing extreme vigilance for prevention; once occurred; rigorous and prompt surgical treatment in the first minutes is mandatory.
- Endobronchial hemorrhage is a highly morbid complication especially in patients receiving anticoagulants.
- Catheter coiling due to excessive and repetitive back and forth movements of the catheter, which might even mandate surgical catheter removal.
- Catheter tip balloon rupture.
- Catheter tip entrapment is RV trabeculae leading to mechanical injury of RV wall, if the balloon is not filled.
- Tricuspid or pulmonary valve mechanical injuries if the catheter is withdrawn without deflation of the catheter tip balloon (Taylor and Tiede 1952; Swan et al. 1970; Swan and Ganz 1974, 1975; Elliott et al. 1979; Swan and Ganz 1979; Kelly et al. 1981; Sise et al. 1981; Hardy et al. 1983; Mohr et al. 1987; Matthay and Chatterjee 1988; Durbin 1990; Himpe 1990; Ikeda et al. 1991; Urschel and Myerowitz 1993; Westenskow and Silva 1993; Shevde et al. 1994; Zarshenas and Sparschu 1994; Poelaert et al. 1995; Sumita et al. 1995; Connors et al. 1996; Mueller et al. 1998; Rhodes et al. 2002; 2003; Cotter et al. 2003; Gibson and Francis 2003; Masugata et al. 2003; Richard et al. 2003; Sandham et al. 2003; Yu et al. 2003; Domino et al. 2004; Monnet et al. 2004; Uzun et al. 2004; Binanay et al. 2005; Harvey et al. 2005; Oransky 2005; Shah et al. 2005; Stevens et al. 2005; Summerhill and Baram 2005; Swan 2005; Harvey et al. 2006; Heresi et al. 2006; Lavine and Lavine 2006; Vender 2006; Wheeler et al. 2006; Williams and Frenneaux 2006; Akima et al. 2007; Bussieres 2007; Leibowitz and Oropello 2007; Mielniczuk et al. 2007; Pirracchio et al. 2007; Frazier and Skinner 2008; Langesaeter et al. 2008; Mathews and Singh 2008; Vincent et al. 2008; de Waal et al. 2009; Katsikis et al. 2009; Ramaswamykanive and Bihari 2009; Renner et al. 2009; Schramm et al. 2009; Hida et al. 2010; Nossaman et al. 2010; Reuter et al. 2010; Takada et al. 2010; Zuffi et al. 2010; Alhashemi et al. 2011; Barmparas et al. 2011; Gurgel and do Nascimento 2011; Hessel and Apostolidou 2011; Richard et al. 2011; Schwann et al. 2011; Trof et al. 2011; Trzebicki et al. 2011; Booth et al. 2012; Godoy et al. 2012; Gologorsky et al. 2012; Pipanmekaporn et al. 2012; Truijen et al. 2012; Kalra et al. 2013; Rajaram et al. 2013; Satler 2013).

5.5 Cardiac Output Monitoring

Cardiac output monitoring is performed using a number of invasive and noninvasive approaches. Also, it is a very determining issue in cardiovascular monitoring, especially in critical patients including cardiac surgery patients. A brief discussion of the currently used methods for cardiac output assessment is presented here, though the interested reader could find detailed discussion in the related textbooks. Also, a great number of clinical and laboratory studies have been performed on this topic due to the importance of this variable especially in critically ill patients to define the benefits and weaknesses of each method (Fick 1870; Figueiredo et al. 2011; Fanari et al. 2016; West 2017).

Fick principle was described in 1870 by the German physiologist and physicist, Adolf Eugen Fick, who developed this principle to be used for a number of applications including direct cardiac output measurement. The Fick principle assumes that the amount of oxygen taken up by the lungs (i.e., O_2 consumption) is taken up from the air, entirely transferred through the lungs, and transported in blood flow (circulation). Based on this fact, we use the Fick principle and calculate how much oxygen is taken from the air and is then transported to the tissues by pulmonary circulation. So, if we calculate the amount of oxygen transferred from the air to the lungs, we could assume it as the amount of oxygen transported from the lungs to the tissues; hence we could consider "consumed oxygen" instead of "transported oxygen" to calculate "cardiac output." In other words, we can simply express Fick principle as follows:

$$\mathrm{O_2\ uptake\left(by\ the\ lungs\right) = O_2\ consumption\left(by\ total\ body\right) = VO_2}.$$

We could calculate arterial oxygen content (CaO_2) and venous oxygen content (CvO_2) and then subtract them (CaO_2–CvO_2); finally we multiply the result in cardiac output (CO); so we will have the Fick formula:

$$\mathrm{VO_2 = CO \times \left(CaO_2 - CvO_2\right)}.$$

And then we resolve the above formula for cardiac output:

$$\mathrm{CO = VO_2 / \left(CaO_2 - CvO_2\right)}.$$

Although the Fick principle seems basically simple and is still considered as the most accurate method of cardiac output measurement, in clinical practice its calculation is very difficult and mandates sophisticated technical procedures, being used more commonly in experimental labs than the clinical setting.

Other less sophisticated and more practical methods have been developed based on Fick principle with some modifications in practice. One of these is the "partial carbon dioxide rebreathing" method which uses carbon dioxide instead of O_2 for calculations discussed here (Fick 1870; Lategola and Rahn 1953; Freed and Keane 1978; Valtier et al. 1998; Haryadi et al. 2000; Mathews and Singh 2008; Raval et al. 2008; Geerts et al. 2011; Li 2012; Fanari et al. 2016; Opotowsky et al. 2017, 2017; West 2017).

5.5.1 Indicator Dilution Techniques

Today, mainly two indicators are used for calculation of cardiac output in the clinical setting and include *lithium* and *cold water*; these methods use an indicator

Table 5.2 Commonly used cardiac output monitoring devices (Alhashemi et al. 2011; Laher et al. 2017; Saugel et al. 2017)

Techniques
Techniques using cold water and its temperature change including: • Thermodilution using PAC (PAC-TD) with application of a bolus of cold water and measurement of cardiac output based on this injection • Continuous thermodilution using PAC (continuous thermodilution with PAC) • Transpulmonary bolus thermodilution (often using a CVC and an arterial catheter like femoral or radial arterial catheters)
Transpulmonary lithium indicator dilution
Partial carbon dioxide (CO_2) rebreathing
Esophageal Doppler
Pulse contour analysis
Bioimpedance and bioreactance
Ultrasonic cardiac output monitor
Other noninvasive systems

(thermal or chemical) and calculate its passage time and/or passage dilution model after passing downstream the blood flow circulation; based on the indicator, the cardiac output measurement techniques are classified as follows (Table 5.2).

5.5.1.1 Techniques Using Cold Water and its Temperature Change

- *Thermodilution using PAC (PAC-TD)* with application of a bolus of cold water and measurement of cardiac output based on this injection. Thermodilution method is usually done using a pulmonary artery catheter (i.e., PAC-TD) and is considered the gold standard for cardiac output monitoring, though the technique needs many points to be considered and also is invasive and relatively expensive and needs experience and enough training. Although PAC-TD method has been defined as the superior method for cardiac output assessment, there are studies considering its accuracy and invasiveness, suggesting other methods including less invasive thermodilution methods, pulse contour cardiac output assessment methods, respirator-based estimates, esophageal Doppler monitoring, flow probe, and transcutaneous Doppler for cardiac output monitoring.
- *Continuous thermodilution using PAC* (continuous thermodilution with PAC).
- *Transpulmonary thermodilution*: conventional thermodilution method mandates using a PAC with a thermistor in its tip; this system has a thermistor inside the CVC and calculates the variables using the curve of arterial line (usually from femoral, axillary, or brachial arteries); so, in this system, a bolus dose of cold water is injected in the right atrium, and at the same time, the temperature fluctuations are recorded in the next seconds and measured using a central arterial line. CO is calculated based on these temperature changes to decrease measurement errors; usually three different measurements are done and the average CO is calculated. Also, the measurements are done in 3–10 min to have more accurate data. The "PiCCO" system (Pulsion Medical Systems, Munich, Germany) uses this technology accompanied with "pulse contour analysis" and estimates

these variables: "CO, cardiac output"; "ITBV, intrathoracic blood volume"; "GEDV, global end-diastolic volume"; and "EVLW, extravascular lung water"; the use of transpulmonary thermodilution at bedside is relatively easy; GEDV is a good index of ventricular preload.

5.5.2 Transpulmonary Lithium Indicator Dilution

This invasive method involves using a bolus dose of isotonic lithium chloride (150–300 mmol LiCl; 1–2 mL) which is injected inside the right atrium (often through a central venous catheter); then, the arterial concentration of lithium is calculated by the machine. The lithium dose does not have any clinical significant effect.

This method is usually not used in:

- Patients below 40 kg (88 lb).
- Patients in the first trimester of pregnancy.
- Patients receiving high doses of neuromuscular blocking agents since they may interfere with the sensor readings of lithium.
- Caution should be taken in patients under lithium therapy.

After injection of lithium dose, the concentration-time curve of lithium dilution in the arterial system is drawn by machine, and cardiac output (CO) is often calculated through a central arterial line, and the "Stewart-Hamilton" equation is used to calculate cardiac output:

$$\mathrm{CO} = \mathrm{LiD} \times 60 / \left[\mathrm{AUC} \times \left(1 - \mathrm{PCV}\right)\right]$$

in which:

CO = calculated cardiac output

LiD = lithium dose (mmol) = the amount of injected lithium

AUC = area under curve for concentration-time curve of lithium

PCV = packed cell volume based on hemoglobin concentration calculated as g/dl; this correction is due to the lack of lithium entry into red blood cells (RBCs) and white blood cells (WBCs) in its first pass. This method is used in LiDCO® system, LiDCO® Group plc, London, UK.

5.5.3 Partial Carbon Dioxide (CO_2) Rebreathing

This method is based on Fick principle; however, instead of calculating oxygen transport, it calculates cardiac output based on CO_2 transport from tissues to the lungs and its excretion, which is done based on 3 min rebreathing intervals. In fact, CO_2 is the marker of choice in this method for calculating cardiac output. For this purpose, a disposable rebreathing loop is added to the mechanical ventilation circuit. This rebreathing loop contains three items:

- Airflow measurement device
- Pulse oximeter
- CO_2 infrared light absorption sensor

For this method, we could consider the following modification as "Fick formula for calculation of cardiac output using CO_2":

$$CO = \Delta VCO_2 / (S \times \Delta etCO_2)$$

in which:
CO = cardiac output
ΔVCO_2 = changes in CO_2 elimination
S = correction index
$\Delta etCO_2$ = changes in partial pressure of end-tidal CO_2 between normal breathing and CO_2 rebreathing

The rebreathing cycles are used in 3 min intervals to calculate the amount of change in CO_2 during rebreathing episodes. The noninvasive cardiac output (NICO) monitor (Novametrix Medical Systems Inc., Wallingford, CT, USA) uses a minimally invasive partial rebreathing method in order to measure cardiac output through a distinctive mode of the Fick equation, utilizing CO_2 rebreathing technology. The method is applicable to adults above 40 kg. This method is more appropriate for ICU and operating room patients with clinically stable conditions and under full mechanical ventilatory support. But in patients with intrapulmonary shunt, the accuracy of this method is decreased. Using NICO for cardiac output measurement mandates strict control of ventilation through full mechanical ventilatory support; meanwhile, there should not be any intrapulmonary shunts, and minimal aberrations in gas exchange are a prerequisite for measurement of cardiac output in this system; these are the main limitations of this system, though the speed of measurement is much higher and the application is easier than conventional PAC when appropriate patient selection is performed (Haryadi et al. 2000; van Heerden et al. 2000; Maxwell et al. 2001; Nilsson et al. 2001; Gueret et al. 2006; Raval et al. 2008; Alhashemi et al. 2011; Litton and Morgan 2012; Sangkum et al. 2016).

5.5.4 Esophageal Doppler

The application of this method was first introduced in the 1970s and then developed in the 1980s; it is usually administered through the "esophageal Doppler monitoring" or simply "EDM" which uses ultrasound for calculation of cardiac output. It is noninvasive and uses the pulsatile flow through the ascending thoracic

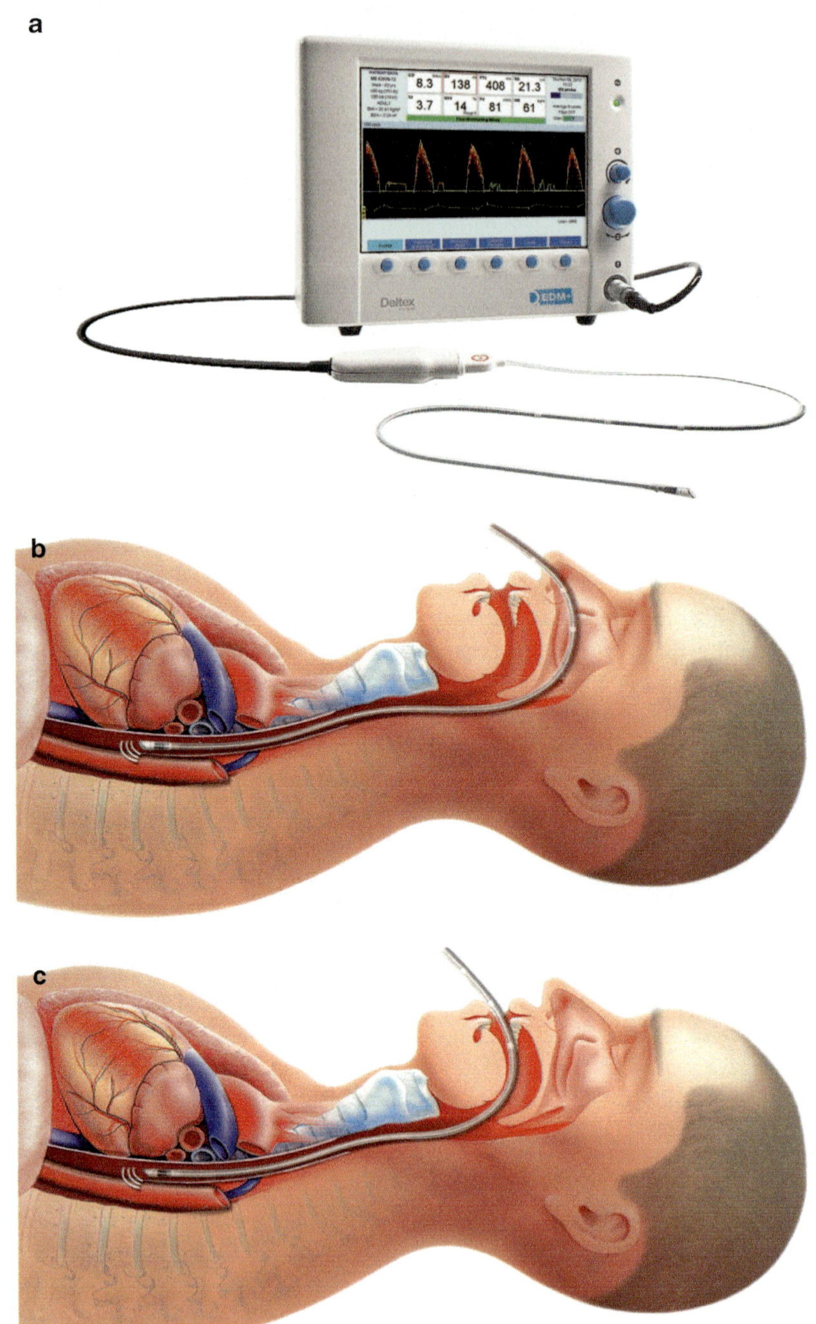

Fig. 5.7 (**a**) Esophageal Doppler monitoring and the probe. (**b**) Nasal probe placement. (**c**) Oral probe placement. With kind permission from Deltex Medical Limited, Terminus Road, Chichester, West Sussex, UK

aorta for calculation of cardiac output. The ultrasound transducer is attached to the tip of a flexible probe; this probe is introduced into the esophagus through the mouth; nasal passage, while not routine, is possible. However, for oral use, it may be more comfortable if the patient is anesthetized or sedated; however there are probes available for awake patients. Also, in patients with esophageal disease, EDM probe should not be used unless extreme caution is applied to prevent any possible injury; even the least resistance should prevent further advancement. Usually a depth inside the esophagus of 30–35 cm from the incisors, or 35–40 cm from the nostril, is acceptable (mid-thoracic level). Then transducer often uses pulsed wave Doppler (5 MHz) or continuous wave Doppler (4 MHz); less frequently, M-mode Doppler is used by some manufacturers (Fig. 5.7). EDM calculates the cross-sectional area of the aorta based on age, sex, weight, and height according to the machine software. EDM needs some training before use; about 10–12 probe placements is often enough; however, maintenance of the probe in its place needs care in order to prevent "probe displacement" out of the esophagus (e.g., during routine ICU nursing care).

In some of esophageal monitors, there is a need for a 70/30 correction: the blood passing through the lumen of the aorta in each heartbeat is about 70% of stroke volume, while 30% of the stroke volume goes to head and neck arteries and the coronary vascular bed; so the calculated cardiac output by the machine should be multiplied by a constant of 1.4 to compensate for cerebral and coronary perfusion; some machines automatically compensate this ratio and demonstrate the final figure. However, in esophageal Doppler monitoring and the probe belonging to Deltex Medical Limited, West Sussex, UK, Deltex does not need this calculation. The results of CO assessments with EDM are more useful when the trend of change is considered rather than the punctual readings of CO.

There are a number of limitations for EDM use including:

- In hypovolemic states, cerebral and coronary blood flow is increased compared to total body flow; so, the calculated cardiac output may be underestimated; however, based on a number of studies, hypovolemia is not a limitation, and ultimate outcome might benefit using the device even when hypovolemia is present.
- The situation is conversed in patients with lower limb vasodilation (like post-cardiopulmonary bypass interval or pregnancy); on the other hand, there are studies demonstrating that vasodilation is not a limitation, although there may be some issues with the nomogram when there is extreme vasodilation, for example, following spinal anesthesia.
- Also, surgeries with aortic cross clamping or intra-aortic balloon pump (IABP) disturbs the turbulent flow of the thoracic aorta, so the calculations of EDM in these states are not quite exact.
- There are some concerns when the patients have underlying thoracic aortic disease, aortic stenosis (AS), or aortic insufficiency (AI); however, studies have demonstrated that the monitor is used successfully in AS and AI; while regurgitation shows reversed flow during diastole and only the forward flow is measured, it can be used for trends; besides, with aortic stenosis, depending on where the

patient is in the disease process, the Doppler monitor can clearly see whether there is ventricular dysfunction and or afterload changes.

- Personal training and abilities in correct positioning of the probe are certainly among the prerequisites of the device for correct CO assessments; inappropriate positioning due to inadequate training might give incorrect readings.

Finally, EDM is noninvasive and needs minimal training; though it has a few limitations, its efficacy is comparable with PAC-TD technique, both for cardiac output monitoring and also for assessment of fluid response in critical patients (Singer et al. 1989; Gan and Arrowsmith 1997; Valtier et al. 1998; Berton and Cholley 2002; Dark and Singer 2004; Feldman et al. 2004; Bajorat et al. 2006; Gueret et al. 2006; Schubert et al. 2008; Chatti et al. 2009; Phan et al. 2011; Lechner et al. 2012; Litton and Morgan 2012; Waldron et al. 2014; Broch et al. 2016; Vakily et al. 2017).

5.5.5 Pulse Contour Analysis

Maybe the simplest method for calculation of cardiac output is "pulse contour analysis or PCA." The arterial wave contour is a function of the "interaction between each individual stroke volume and the physical and anatomical characteristics of the arterial tree." There are a number of devices using this method for cardiac output assessment; in all of them, the main basic principle for these methods is analysis of "the systolic portion of curve in the arterial line curve." This analysis is based on "Windkessel model" described first by Otto Frank in 1899 which describes the interaction between the stroke volume and the compliance of the aorta and large elastic arteries, known as "Windkessel vessels"—Windkessel is a German name which means "air chamber"—and uses the following formula for estimation of cardiac output (Hayashi et al. 2006; Goepfert et al. 2013; Schloglhofer et al. 2014; Sangkum et al. 2016; Reshetnik et al. 2017):

$$\mathrm{CO} = \left(\mathrm{SAUC} / \text{aortic impedance}\right) \times \mathrm{HR}$$

in which:
CO: cardiac output
SAUC: systolic portion of area under curve of arterial line
HR: heart rate

Currently the following devices or systems use this method for CO, based on an alphabetical order.

FloTrac/Vigileo (Edwards Lifesciences, Irvine, CA, USA) was first introduced in 2005 and calculates cardiac output based on the following equation:

$$\mathrm{CO} = \mathrm{HR} \times \mathrm{SV}$$

in which:

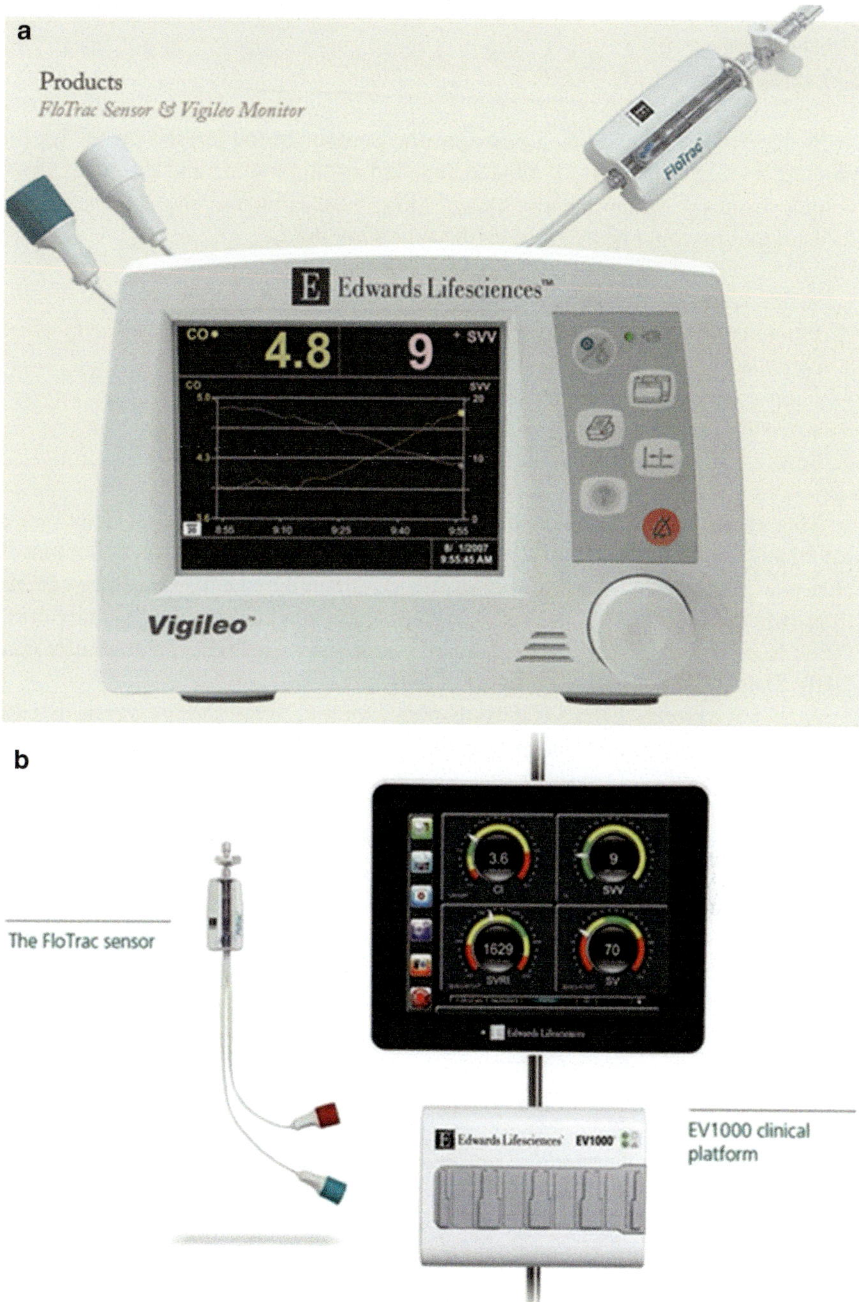

Fig. 5.8 FloTrac/Vigileo system. (**a**) Portable monitor with sensors demonstrating cardiac output and stroke volume variation. (**b**) The EV1000 clinical platform demonstrating physiologic variables with FloTrac sensor. With kind permission from Edwards Lifesciences, Irvine, CA 92614, USA

CO: cardiac output
HR: heart rate
SV: stroke volume

Stroke volume is estimated based on the contour of the arterial pulse. So, this method calculates CO based on heart rate and stroke volume and estimates stroke volume from the "arterial pulse curve" (Fig. 5.8). However, the accuracy of the measurements would be affected by the following items:

1. Artifacts of the arterial wave
2. Problems in the catheter of arterial line
3. Patients with aortic insufficiency
4. Intense peripheral vasoconstriction
5. Arrhythmias causing irregular pulse
6. Severe left ventricular dysfunction

This system *does not need* calibration like the other two systems. This system calculates the blood flow based on "arterial curve signal and arterial compliance"; also, age, gender, and body surface area are considered in the final machine calculations (Manecke 2005; Compton et al. 2008b; Kapoor et al. 2008; Mayer and Suttner 2009; Jo et al. 2011; Phan et al. 2011; Litton and Morgan 2012; Schloglhofer et al. 2014; Sangkum et al. 2016; Lamia et al. 2018).

LiDCO® system (LiDCO® Group plc, London, UK) and its versions (i.e., LiDCOrapid®/PulseCO®) transform pressure wave to volume wave using its algorithm; like PiCCO system, this device uses indicator dilution technique and calculates cardiac output based on the Wesseling algorithm by pulse contour analysis (Fig. 5.9); so, it calculates cardiac output based on pulse contour and calibrates the results after comparing them with the measured amounts of cardiac output calculated in each beat by *lithium dilution* methods; this calibration should be done each in 8 h (Pearse et al. 2004; Mayer and Suttner 2009; Phan et al. 2011; Litton and Morgan 2012; Schloglhofer et al. 2014; Sangkum et al. 2016; Lamia et al. 2018).

PiCCO® system: "pulse index continuous cardiac output" system (Pulsion Medical Systems, Munich, Germany); this system combines two techniques for cardiac output measurement (Fig. 5.10):

1. *Transpulmonary thermodilution (invasive method):* this is the invasive mode of measurement which is based on indicator dilution technique through transpulmonary thermodilution.
2. *Pulse contour analysis (noninvasive method):* calculates cardiac output using the Wesseling algorithm by pulse contour analysis through an arterial line catheter, femoral, axillary, brachial, or radial arteries. Cardiac output and stroke volume could be monitored throughout their beat-to-beat variations with varying conditions of preload using "pulse contour analysis"; at the same time, the noninvasive measurement is calibrated using the invasive module of PiCCO® through

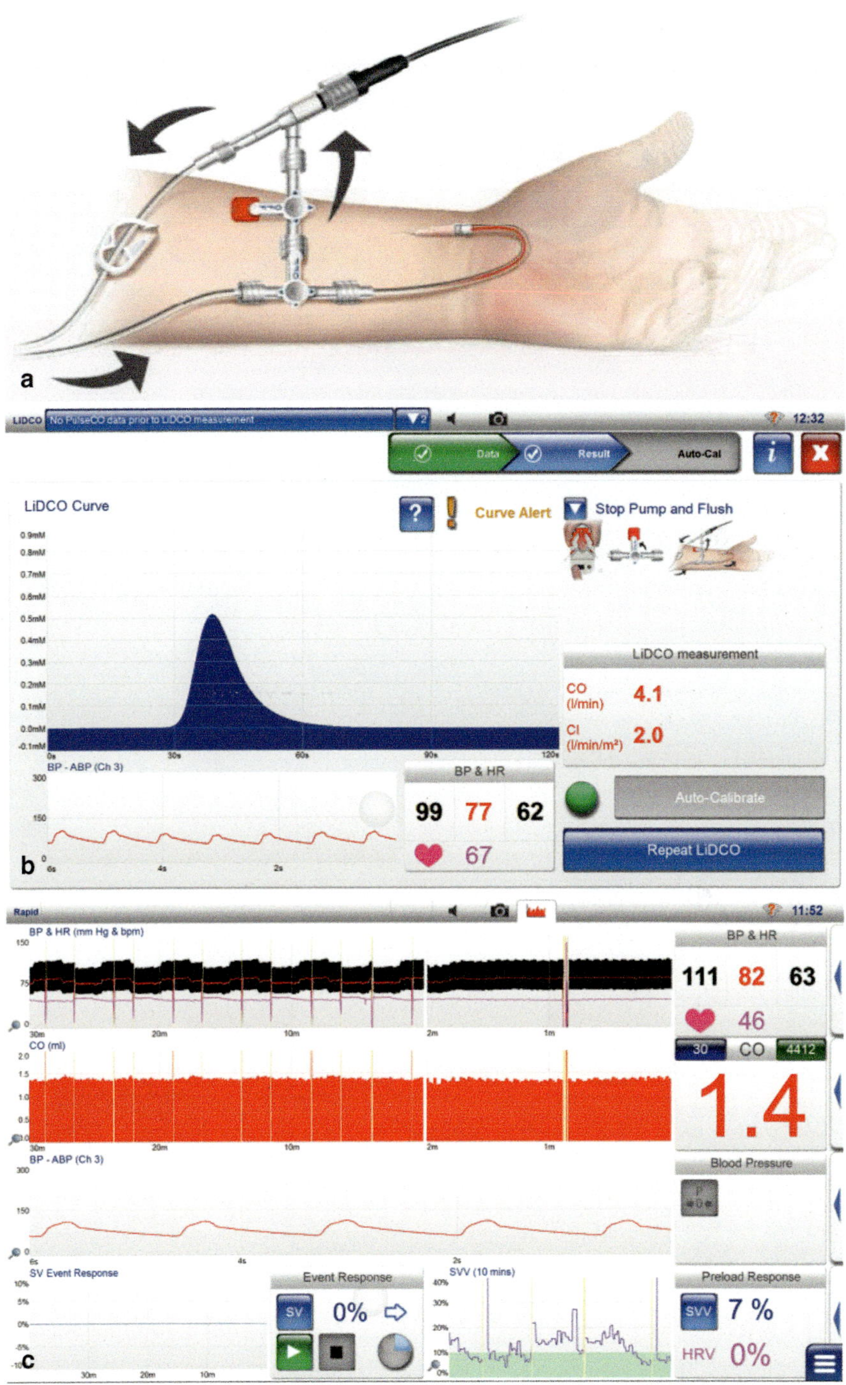

Fig. 5.9 (**a**) LiDCO® lithium sensor attached to the patient; (**b**) LiDCOPlus® system; (**c**) LiDCOrapid® system. With kind permission from LiDCO® Ltd. London, UK

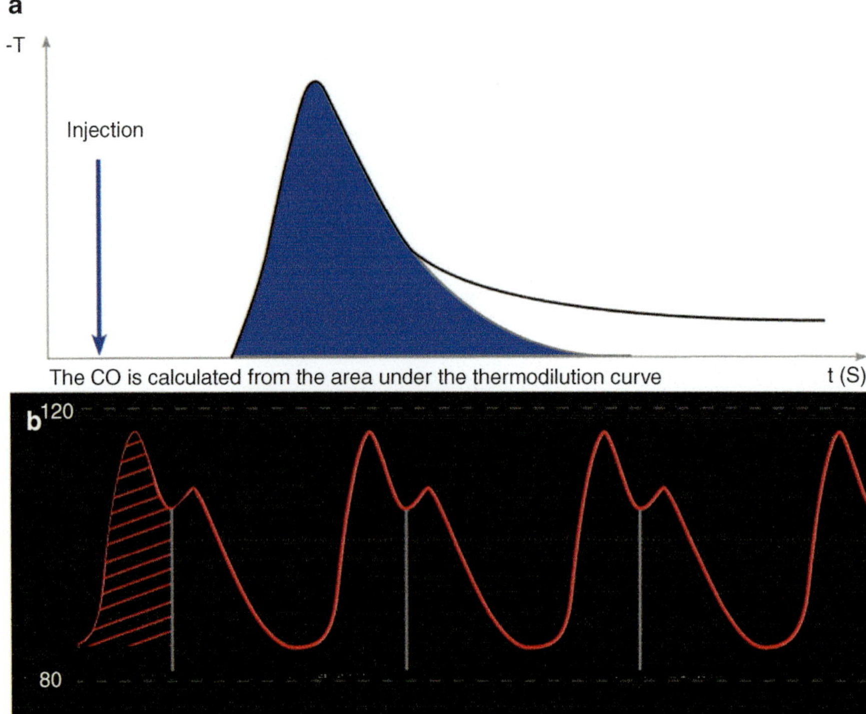

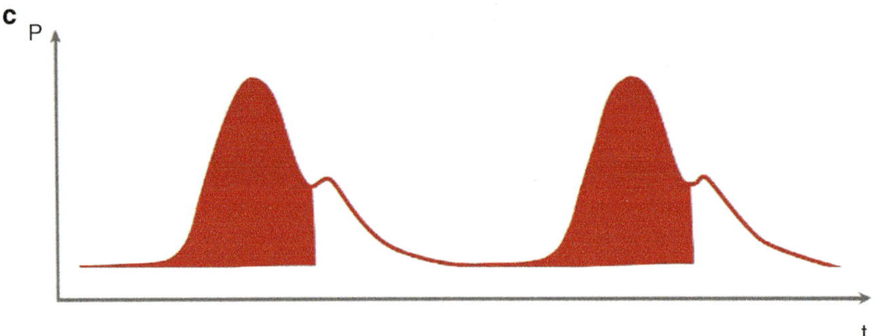

Fig. 5.10 (**a**) PiCCO® transpulmonary thermodilution method for calculation of cardiac output (CO); (**b**) calculation of stroke volume by pulse contour analysis by PiCCO®; (**c**) calculation of cardiac output by pulse contour analysis by PiCCO®; (**d**) graphic setup of PiCCO®. With kind permission from Pulsion Medical Systems SE, Germany

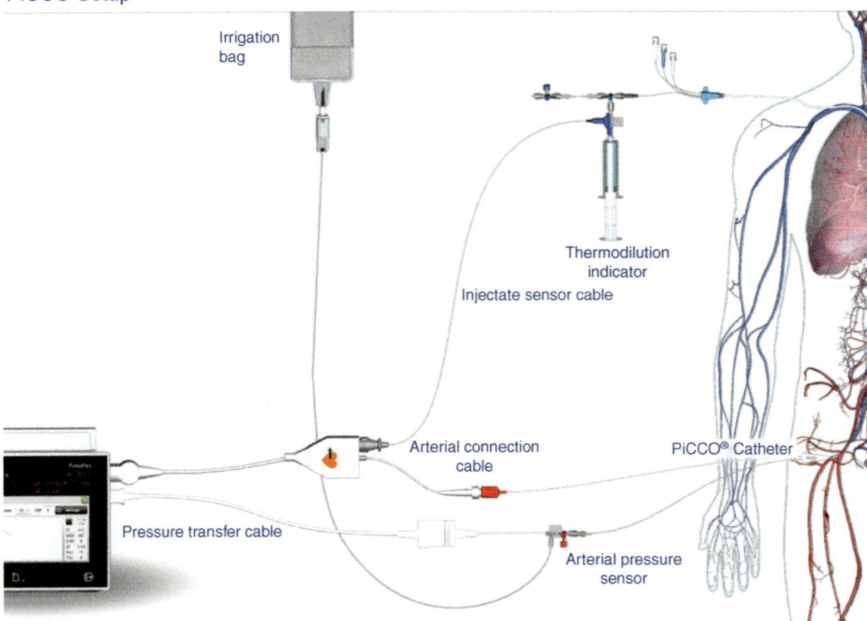

Fig. 5.10 (continued)

transpulmonary thermodilution. Noninvasive mode of PiCCO® needs to be calibrated at least two to three times a day.

In brief, PiCCO® integrates both static and dynamic hemodynamic data through both invasive (transpulmonary thermodilution) and noninvasive (pulse contour analysis) measurements and calibrates the data combining the two techniques of cardiac output measurement. At the start of measurements, PiCCO® asks for patient data like age, sex, weight, and height. PiCCO® is indicated for complex states like septic, cardiogenic, or traumatic shock or other high-risk patients in the perioperative period (Sander et al. 2005; Bajorat et al. 2006; Fakler et al. 2007; Compton et al. 2008a, 2008b; Mayer and Suttner 2009; Alhashemi et al. 2011; Kiefer et al. 2012; Litton and Morgan 2012; Donati et al. 2014; Schloglhofer et al. 2014; Sangkum et al. 2016; Lamia et al. 2018; Reshetnik et al. 2017).

PRAM system: Pressure recording analytical method "PRAM" used in "MostCare" system (Vytech Health, Padova, Italy) is an invasive method which measures cardiac indices based on a continuous and beat-to-beat method designed on the basis of "morphologic analysis of both the pulsatile and continuous components of the arterial pressure waveform"; this analysis is performed by the system at a higher sampling frequency, compared with other pulse contour analysis technologies (Scolletta et al. 2005; Mayer and Suttner 2009; Alhashemi et al. 2011; Litton and Morgan 2012; Donati et al. 2014; Alonso-Inigo et al. 2016; Huygh et al. 2016;

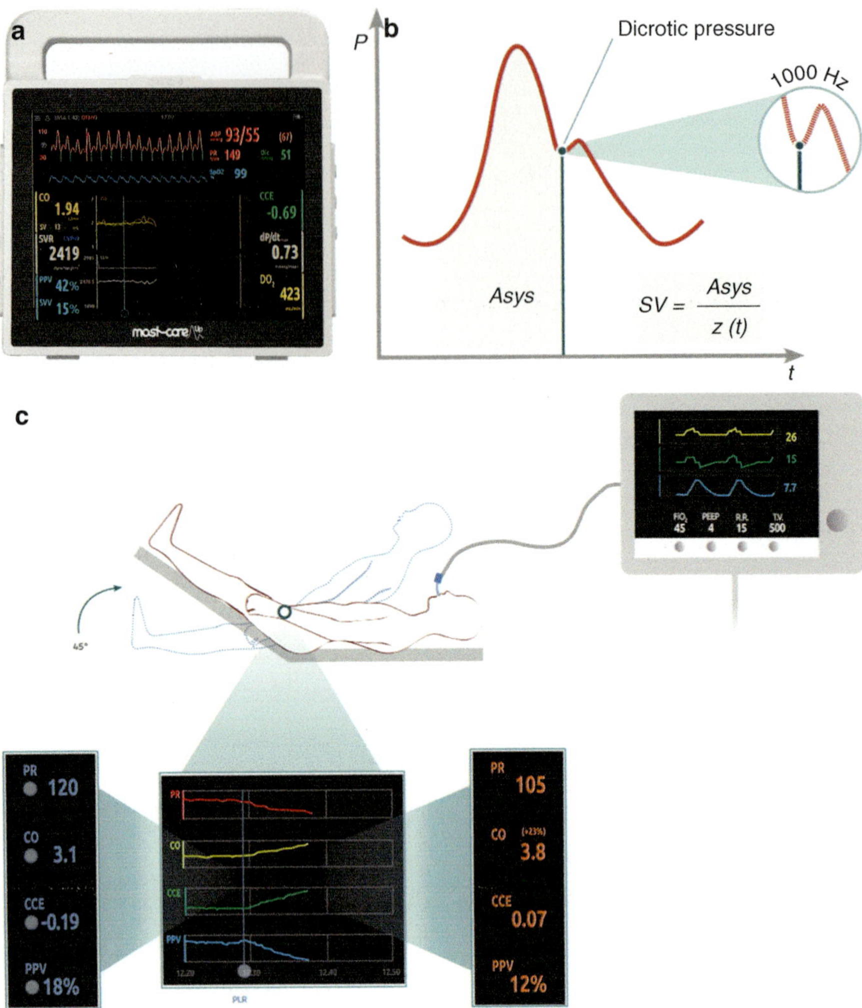

Fig. 5.11 Pressure recording analytical method "PRAM" used in "MostCare" system; (**a**) monitor panel; (**b**) basic principle of calculations in the system; (**c**) effects of passive leg raising demonstrated by the MostCare system. With kind permission from Vytech Health, Division of Vygon Italia Srl, Vygon Group, Padova, Italy

Sangkum et al. 2016; Urbano et al. 2016); also, the method is not "calibration dependent" and calculates cardiac output based on the curve of the arterial line pressure (Fig. 5.11).

In all cardiac output assessment methods based on "arterial pressure contour" analysis, the following entities could disturb the results of assessments:

- Aortic insufficiency or aortic regurgitation
- Under-damping or overdamping of the arterial line curve

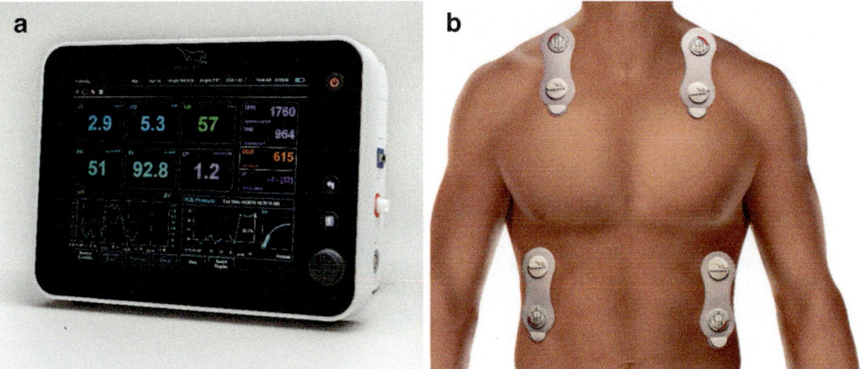

Fig. 5.12 (**a**) Cheetah NICOM system; (**b**) location of sensors on torso. With kind permission from Cheetah Medical, Inc., MA, USA

- Patients with considerable arrhythmia which could disturb the readings
- Vascular leakage syndromes leading to decreased arterial wall compliance

5.5.6 Bioimpedance and Bioreactance®

These two approaches are "nearly totally" noninvasive methods using physical effects of blood flow on transthoracic variables; for this purpose, by using chest leads attached to the chest wall, this method assesses the physical effects of blood flow inside the thorax, including the changes in impedance of the chest (i.e., bio-impedance system) or "blood flow-dependent changes in electrical currents across the thorax" which could be named as the changes in electrical frequencies of the chest (i.e., bioreactance). These systems are noninvasive; however, some believe that their measurements are not yet as accurate as some invasive methods, though their use as devices for "tracking the cardiovascular system responses to treatment in clinical practice" could be much more reliable; also, the noise (especially electrical noise) produced in ICU environment could affect their calculations, and the estimated cardiac output could be affected; two systems that are based on Bioreactance® are the CHEETAH NICOM and Starling SV hemodynamic systems (Fig. 5.12); they can assess stroke volume index (SVI), cardiac index (CI), and total peripheral resistance index (TPRI), being a measure of the vascular tone as a continuous mode of hemodynamic monitoring (de Waal et al. 2009; Maurer et al. 2009; Alhashemi et al. 2011; Fagnoul et al. 2012; Jakovljevic et al. 2012; Litton and Morgan 2012; Marik et al. 2013; Waldron et al. 2014; Sangkum et al. 2016; Doherty et al. 2017; Laher et al. 2017; Lamia et al. 2018).

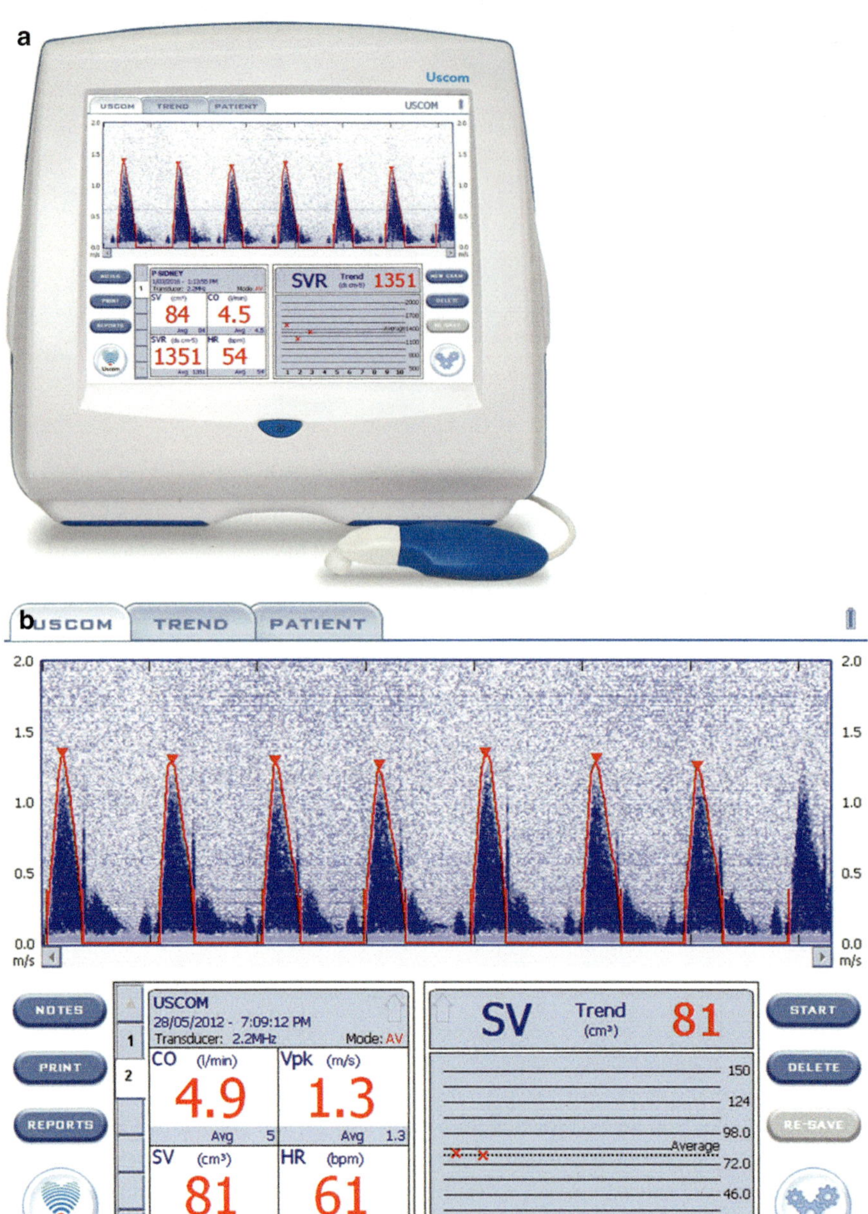

Fig. 5.13 (**a**) The monitor and its probe. (**b**) Stroke volume (SV) measurement. (**c**) Stroke volume index (SVI) measurement. (**d**) Trend of measured parameters over time. (**e**) Suprasternal approach for using USCOM. With kind permission from USCOM Ltd., Sydney NSW 2000, Australia

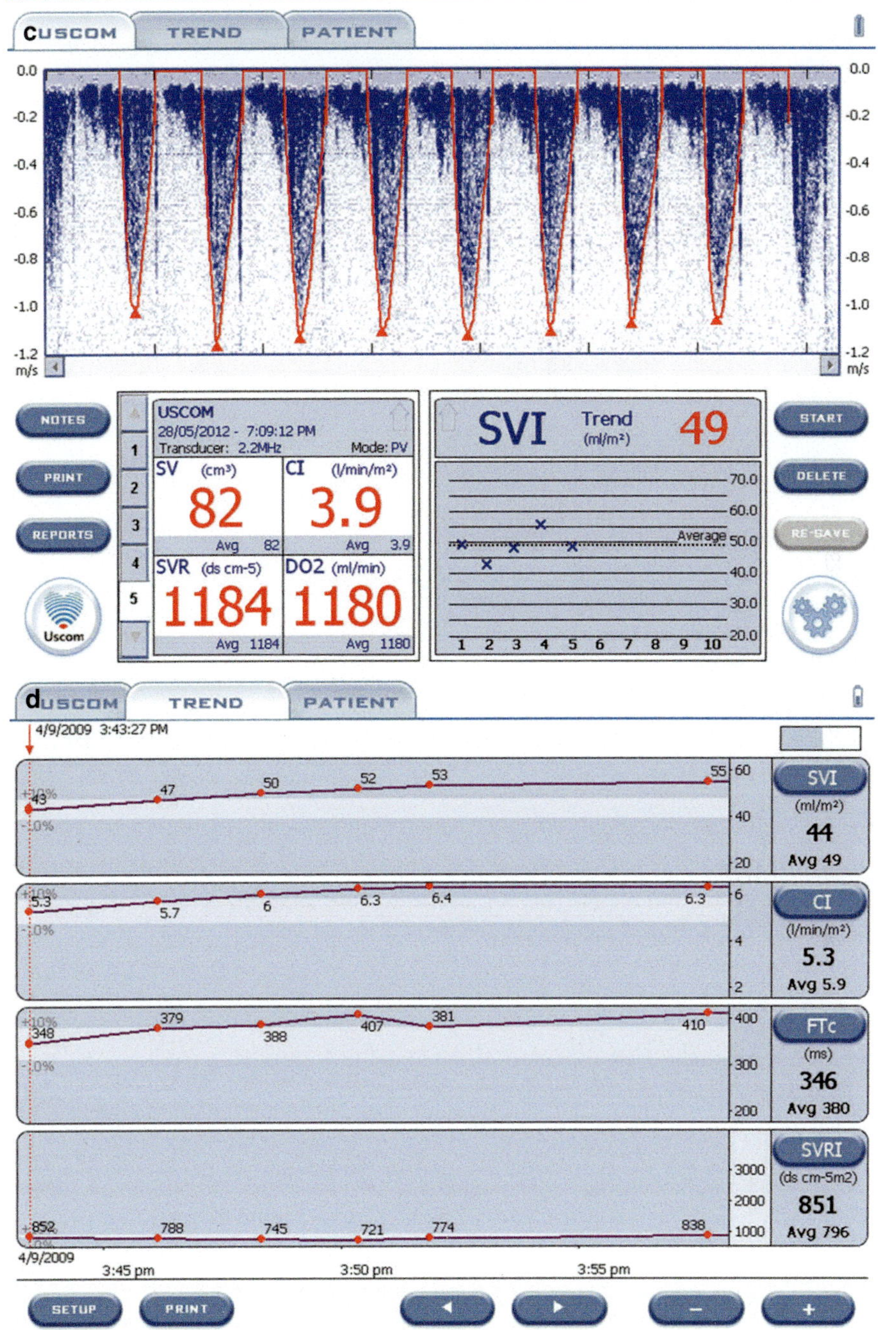

Fig. 5.13 (continued)

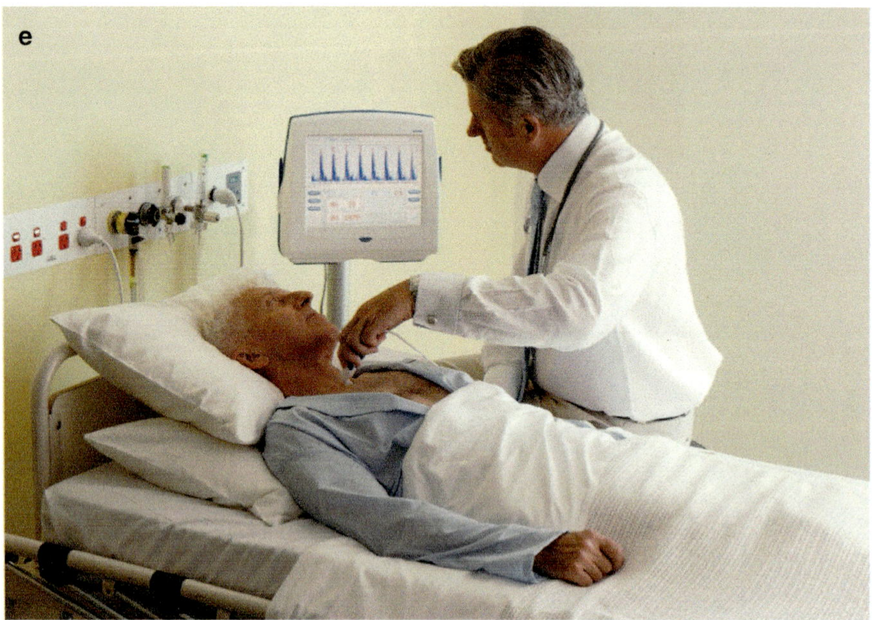

Fig. 5.13 (continued)

5.5.7 Ultrasonic Cardiac Output Monitor (USCOM, USCOM Ltd., Sydney, Australia)

This system is a completely noninvasive one, which permits serial assessments of cardiac output and is based on "continuous wave Doppler, CWD" technology, using a Doppler probe to "calculate velocity-time interval." The probe could be placed in one of the two following anatomic positions (Fig. 5.13):

- Suprasternal notch, which measures the blood flow through the aortic outflow tract, hence the trans-aortic flow
- Left sternal edge, which measures the blood flow through the pulmonary artery outflow tract, hence the transpulmonary flow

This is why appropriate alignment of the probe has an essential role in taking appropriate results; also, this issue mandates time spending for gaining an "appropriate window." Calculation of cardiac output is done by the following equation:

$$\text{CO} = \text{CSA} \times \text{VTI}$$

in which:
CO: cardiac output
CSA: cross-sectional area of the main arterial system which is used for measurement of cardiac output (aorta or pulmonary artery)
VTI: velocity-time integral, which is calculated by the machine

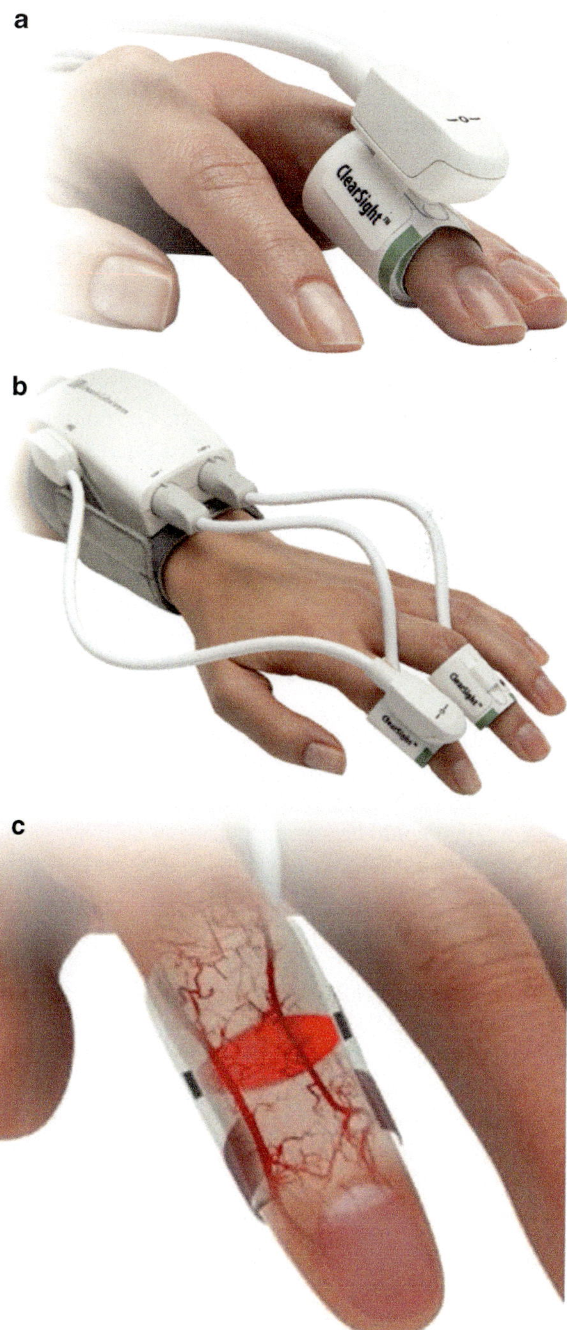

Fig. 5.14 ClearSight system; Edwards Lifesciences. (**a**) Finger Clip of ClearSight. (**b**) ClearSight finger cuff. (**c**) Brief demonstration of ClearSight system technology. With kind permission from Edwards Lifesciences, Irvine, CA, USA

This system may have a useful role in cardiac output estimation based on clinical studies; also, it estimates cardiac output in a real-time model and is also noninvasive; however, the personal training has a main role in the results (Compton et al. 2008a, b; Compton and Schafer 2009; Chong and Peyton 2012; Critchley and Huang 2014; Hodgson et al. 2016; Elgendy et al. 2017; Elwan et al. 2017; Razavi et al. 2017; Reshetnik et al. 2017).

5.5.8 The Noninvasive Monitoring of Cardiac Output

The noninvasive monitoring of cardiac output is has an continual improvement pattern; this modality has been introduced a few years ago and has been a useful monitor in a number of studies, though not all studies confirm its precision; especially in low cardiac output patients. However, the trend of cardiac output measured by this device seems much more useful. ClearSight system, Edwards Lifesciences, Irvine, CA, USA, could be mentioned as one of the systems under this classification and is demonstrated in Fig. 5.14 (Alhashemi et al. 2011; Maguire et al. 2011; Vincent et al. 2011; Monnet et al. 2012; Bubenek-Turconi et al. 2013; Imhoff 2013; Alonso-Inigo et al. 2016; Sangkum et al. 2016).

5.6 Selection of Cardiac Output Monitoring Modality

Though a detailed list of different monitoring devices are available clinically, none could be nominated as the "best." However, a few criteria could be used to select the appropriate cardiac output monitoring device. There are a number of conclusive reviews that could be summated as guideline for cardiac output monitoring, though the majority of them are not meta-analysis or consensus-based; however, they could be considered as useful approaches for selection of cardiac output monitoring device; a briefing of these reviews is presented here (Monnet et al. 2004; Alhashemi et al. 2011; Vincent et al. 2011; Chong and Peyton 2012; Monnet and Teboul 2015; Fanari et al. 2016; Sangkum et al. 2016):

- None of the hemodynamic monitoring devices are able to "improve outcome by itself."
- "Device availability" and "training" could affect the selection process based on the individual user.
- None of the monitoring could be "the only best" for all the patients; monitoring each patient should be "tailored" specifically.
- Integrating different data from different sources could help us improve the quality of data used for monitoring.
- Mixed venous oxygen saturation (SvO_2) is a very useful and decisive indicator; though its measurement is through PAC, using the amount of mixed venous oxygen saturation ($ScvO_2$) from superior vena cava sampling (using a CVC) could be considered as a useful surrogate for SvO_2.

- Though many patients benefit from increased cardiac output, this is not always the rule, since increased cardiac output using any possible treatment could at times be associated with detrimental effects; the same might be true for SvO_2 as its increase in critical patients might occur due to maldistribution of perfusion and not necessarily due to improved clinical condition.
- None of the cardiac output monitoring devices could measure the real values of "CO"; instead, they all estimate cardiac output, though "intermittent thermodilution technique" is usually considered as the "technique of reference" with its own limitations. Maybe using a less invasive monitoring to track "the trend of CO estimations" could be as valuable as directly using PAC-TD method.
- Ability to respond as fast as possible to pathologic changes is very important; this is why we need "very rapid response" monitoring devices which show the changes as fast as possible to help the clinician, and the clinical team respond as fast as possible; increasing the number of appropriate monitoring may also increase our speed of response.

Table 5.3 Normal range for the main pressures in the cardiovascular system (Dabbagh 2014)

	Variable	Normal range
1	Heart rate (HR)	60–100
2	Central venous pressure (CVP)	3–8 mmHg
3	Right atrial pressure (RAP)	2–10 mmHg
4	Right ventricular pressure (RVP)	Systolic: 15–30 mmHg Diastolic: 3–8 mmHg
5	Pulmonary artery pressure (PAP)	Systolic: 15–30 mmHg Diastolic: 6–12 mmHg
6	Pulmonary artery wedge pressure (PAWP); pulmonary capillary wedge pressure (PCWP)	6–12 mmHg
7	Left atrial pressure (LAP)	4–12 mmHg
8	Left ventricular end-systolic pressure (LVESP)	90–140 mmHg
9	Left ventricular end-diastolic pressure (LVEDP)	4–12 mmHg
10	Aortic pressure	Systolic: 90–140 mmHg Diastolic: 60–90 mmHg

Table 5.4 Calculation formulas and normal range of main physiologic variables in the cardiovascular system (Dabbagh 2014)

	Variable	Formula	Normal range
1	Cardiac output (CO)	CO = SV × HR	4–6 L/min
2	Cardiac index (CI)	CI = CO/BSA	3–5 L/min/m^2
3	Stroke volume (SV)	SV = (CO × 1000)/HR	50–100 mL
4	Mean arterial pressure (MAP)	MAP = (2DBP + SBP)/3	70–100 mmHg
5	Systemic vascular resistance (SVR)	SVR = [(MAP - CVP) × 80]/CO	800–1200 dynes/s/cm^5
6	Pulmonary vascular resistance (PVR)	PVR = [(PAP - PAWP) × 80] CO	35–250 dynes/s/cm^5

HR heart rate (beats/min), *BSA* body surface area (m^2), *DBP* diastolic blood pressure, *SBP* systolic blood pressure

Taylor and Tiede (1952), Mohr et al. (1987), Himpe (1990), Cotter et al. (2003), Gibson and Francis (2003), Masugata et al. (2003), Uzun et al. (2004), Lavine and Lavine (2006), Williams and Frenneaux (2006), Akima et al. (2007), Mielniczuk et al. (2007), Pirracchio et al. (2007), Renner et al. (2009), and Trof et al. (2011)

- Real-time (beat-to-beat) CO assessments could guide us in a much better pattern than delayed, intermittent measurements; these real-time results seem superior to methods with delayed measurements in their technique.
- Although noninvasiveness is a very important issue for selection of monitoring devices, it is not the only determinant factor, as invasive blood pressure monitoring could not be replaced in some patients with indirect blood pressure monitoring (measuring with blood pressure cuff) especially in cardiac surgery patients; also, noninvasive cardiac output monitoring systems using "pulse contour analysis, CO_2 rebreathing and trans-thoracic bioimpedance" are not as accurate as more invasive methods; this is why we should believe in "noninvasiveness" as one of the many factors and not "the only determining factor" for selection of monitoring.

5.7 Normal Values for Hemodynamic Parameters

There are a number of different studies which have assessed and calculated the normal variables of hemodynamic parameters. The following two tables demonstrate a number of the most important hemodynamic variables (Tables 5.3 and 5.4).

5.8 Transesophageal Echocardiography (TEE)

TEE is a noninvasive real-time monitoring used extensively especially for cardiac patients during perioperative period; its application has increased very wide acceptance with the increasing experience and familiarity of anesthesiologists and intensivists in perioperative fields; however, its description needs a separate discussion beyond the scope of this book, and the readers are suggested to refer to perioperative TEE books.

5.9 Electrocardiography (EEG)

This monitoring is described in more detail in a separate chapter of the book. Please refer to the related chapter.

5.10 Near-Infrared Spectroscopy and Cerebral Oximetry

The full description of this monitoring device is presented in the chapter titled "Central Nervous System Monitoring." Please refer to the related chapter.

References

ANON. French Society of Anesthesia and Intensive Care. Arterial catheterization and invasive measurement of blood pressure in anesthesia and intensive care in adults. Ann Fr Anesth Reanim. 1995;14:444–53.

American Society of Anesthesiologists Task Force on Pulmonary Artery Catheterization. Practice guidelines for pulmonary artery catheterization: an updated report by the American Society of Anesthesiologists Task Force on Pulmonary Artery Catheterization. Anesthesiology. 2003;99:988–1014.

Ahmad RA, Ahmad S, Naveed A, Baig MAR. Peripheral arterial blood pressure versus central arterial blood pressure monitoring in critically ill patients after cardio-pulmonary bypass. Pak J Med Sci. 2017;33:310–4.

Akima T, Takase B, Kosuda S, Ohsuzu F, Kawai T, Ishihara M, Akira K. Systemic peripheral vascular resistance as a determinant of functional cardiac reserve in response to exercise in patients with heart disease. Angiology. 2007;58:463–71.

Alhashemi JA, Cecconi M, Hofer CK. Cardiac output monitoring: an integrative perspective. Crit Care. 2011;15:214.

Alonso-Inigo JM, Escriba FJ, Carrasco JI, Fas MJ, Argente P, Galvis JM, Llopis JE. Measuring cardiac output in children undergoing cardiac catheterization: comparison between the Fick method and PRAM (pressure recording analytical method). Paediatr Anaesth. 2016;26:1097–105.

Anderson JS. Arterial cannulation: how to do it. Br J Hosp Med. 1997;57:497–9.

Aouad-Maroun M, Raphael CK, Sayyid SK, Farah F, Akl EA. Ultrasound-guided arterial cannulation for paediatrics. Cochrane Database Syst Rev. 2016;9:Cd011364.

Arai T, Yamashita M. Central venous catheterization in infants and children—small caliber audio-Doppler probe versus ultrasound scanner. Paediatr Anaesth. 2005;15:858–61.

Ash SR. Fluid mechanics and clinical success of central venous catheters for dialysis—answers to simple but persisting problems. Semin Dial. 2007;20:237–56.

Asheim P, Mostad U, Aadahl P. Ultrasound-guided central venous cannulation in infants and children. Acta Anaesthesiol Scand. 2002;46:390–2.

Augusto JF, Teboul JL, Radermacher P, Asfar P. Interpretation of blood pressure signal: physiological bases, clinical relevance, and objectives during shock states. Intensive Care Med. 2011;37:411–9.

Bajorat J, Hofmockel R, Vagts DA, Janda M, Pohl B, Beck C, Noeldge-Schomburg G. Comparison of invasive and less-invasive techniques of cardiac output measurement under different haemodynamic conditions in a pig model. Eur J Anaesthesiol. 2006;23:23–30.

Barmparas G, Inaba K, Georgiou C, Hadjizacharia P, Chan LS, Demetriades D, Friese R, Rhee P. Swan-Ganz catheter use in trauma patients can be reduced without negatively affecting outcomes. World J Surg. 2011;35:1809–17.

Berghella S, Tempo B, Bernocco A, Neri G, Fiorucci G. Indications, methods and results of bacteriological examinations of central venous catheters in patients admitted to a polyvalent resuscitation center. Minerva Anestesiol. 1979;45:379–86.

Berton C, Cholley B. Equipment review: new techniques for cardiac output measurement—oesophageal Doppler, Fick principle using carbon dioxide, and pulse contour analysis. Crit Care. 2002;6:216–21.

Binanay C, Califf RM, Hasselblad V, O'Connor CM, Shah MR, Sopko G, Stevenson LW, Francis GS, Leier CV, Miller LW. Evaluation study of congestive heart failure and pulmonary artery catheterization effectiveness: the ESCAPE trial. JAMA. 2005;294:1625–33.

Booth KL, Mercer-Smith G, McConkey C, Parissis H. Catheter-induced pulmonary artery rupture: haemodynamic compromise necessitates surgical repair. Interact Cardiovasc Thorac Surg. 2012;15:531–3.

Botha R, van Schoor AN, Boon JM, Becker JH, Meiring JH. Anatomical considerations of the anterior approach for central venous catheter placement. Clin Anat. 2006;19:101–5.

Boyce JM. Prevention of central line-associated bloodstream infections in hemodialysis patients. Infect Control Hosp Epidemiol. 2012;33:936–44.

Broch O, Bein B, Gruenewald M, Masing S, Huenges K, Haneya A, Steinfath M, Renner J. Accuracy of cardiac output by nine different pulse contour algorithms in cardiac surgery patients: a comparison with transpulmonary thermodilution. Biomed Res Int. 2016;2016:3468015.
Brusasco C, Corradi F, Zattoni PL, Launo C, Leykin Y, Palermo S. Ultrasound-guided central venous cannulation in bariatric patients. Obes Surg. 2009;19:1365–70.
Brzezinski M, Luisetti T, London MJ. Radial artery cannulation: a comprehensive review of recent anatomic and physiologic investigations. Anesth Analg. 2009;109:1763–81.
Bubenek-Turconi SI, Craciun M, Miclea I, Perel A. Noninvasive continuous cardiac output by the Nexfin before and after preload-modifying maneuvers: a comparison with intermittent thermodilution cardiac output. Anesth Analg. 2013;117:366–72.
Bur A, Hirschl MM, Herkner H, Oschatz E, Kofler J, Woisetschlager C, Laggner AN. Accuracy of oscillometric blood pressure measurement according to the relation between cuff size and upper-arm circumference in critically ill patients. Crit Care Med. 2000;28:371–6.
Bussieres JS. Iatrogenic pulmonary artery rupture. Curr Opin Anaesthesiol. 2007;20:48–52.
Calabria M, Zamboli P, D'Amelio A, Granata A, Di Lullo L, Floccari F, Logias F, Fiorini F. Use of ECG-EC in the positioning of central venous catheters. G Ital Nefrol. 2012;29:49–57.
Campbell NR, Berbari AE, Cloutier L, Gelfer M, Kenerson JG, Khalsa TK, Lackland DT, Lemogoum D, Mangat BK, Mohan S, Myers MG, Niebylski ML, O'Brien E, Stergiou GS, VeIga EV, Zhang XH. Policy statement of the world hypertension league on noninvasive blood pressure measurement devices and blood pressure measurement in the clinical or community setting. J Clin Hypertens (Greenwich). 2014;16:320–2.
Chatti R, de Rudniki S, Marque S, Dumenil AS, Descorps-Declere A, Cariou A, Duranteau J, Aout M, Vicaut E, Cholley BP. Comparison of two versions of the Vigileo-FloTrac system (1.03 and 1.07) for stroke volume estimation: a multicentre, blinded comparison with oesophageal Doppler measurements. Br J Anaesth. 2009;102:463–9.
Chee BC, Baldwin IC, Shahwan-Akl L, Fealy NG, Heland MJ, Rogan JJ. Evaluation of a radial artery cannulation training program for intensive care nurses: a descriptive, explorative study. Aust Crit Care. 2011;24:117–25.
Chen CK, Tan PP, Lee HC. Sternocleidomastoid muscle length predicts depth of central venous catheter insertion. Acta Anaesthesiol Taiwanica. 2007;45:211–5.
Chong SW, Peyton PJ. A meta-analysis of the accuracy and precision of the ultrasonic cardiac output monitor (USCOM). Anaesthesia. 2012;67:1266–71.
Chopra V, Anand S, Krein SL, Chenoweth C, Saint S. Bloodstream infection, venous thrombosis, and peripherally inserted central catheters: reappraising the evidence. Am J Med. 2012;125:733–41.
Clark VL, Kruse JA. Arterial catheterization. Crit Care Clin. 1992;8:687–97.
Cockings JG, Webb RK, Klepper ID, Currie M, Morgan C. The Australian Incident Monitoring Study. Blood pressure monitoring—applications and limitations: an analysis of 2000 incident reports. Anaesth Intensive Care. 1993;21:565–9.
Compton F, Schafer JH. Noninvasive cardiac output determination: broadening the applicability of hemodynamic monitoring. Semin Cardiothorac Vasc Anesth. 2009;13:44–55.
Compton F, Wittrock M, Schaefer JH, Zidek W, Tepel M, Scholze A. Noninvasive cardiac output determination using applanation tonometry-derived radial artery pulse contour analysis in critically ill patients. Anesth Analg. 2008a;106:171–4; table of contents.
Compton FD, Zukunft B, Hoffmann C, Zidek W, Schaefer JH. Performance of a minimally invasive uncalibrated cardiac output monitoring system (Flotrac/Vigileo) in haemodynamically unstable patients. Br J Anaesth. 2008b;100:451–6.
Connors AF Jr, Speroff T, Dawson NV, Thomas C, Harrell FE Jr, Wagner D, Desbiens N, Goldman L, Wu AW, Califf RM, Fulkerson WJ Jr, Vidaillet H, Broste S, Bellamy P, Lynn J, Knaus WA. The effectiveness of right heart catheterization in the initial care of critically ill patients. SUPPORT Investigators. JAMA. 1996;276:889–97.
Cotter G, Williams SG, Vered Z, Tan LB. Role of cardiac power in heart failure. Curr Opin Cardiol. 2003;18:215–22.
Cousins TR, O'Donnell JM. Arterial cannulation: a critical review. AANA J. 2004;72:267–71.

Critchley LA, Huang L. USCOM-window to the circulation: utility of supra-sternal Doppler in an elderly anaesthetized patient for a robotic cystectomy. J Clin Monit Comput. 2014;28: 83–93.

Dabbagh A. Cardiovascular monitoring. In: Dabbagh A, Esmailian F, Aranki S, editors. Postoperative critical care for cardiac surgical patients. 1st ed. Berlin: Springer; 2014. p. 77–127.

Daily PO, Griepp RB, Shumway NE. Percutaneous internal jugular vein cannulation. Arch Surg. 1970;101:534–6.

Dark PM, Singer M. The validity of trans-esophageal Doppler ultrasonography as a measure of cardiac output in critically ill adults. Intensive Care Med. 2004;30:2060–6.

de Waal EE, Wappler F, Buhre WF. Cardiac output monitoring. Curr Opin Anaesthesiol. 2009;22:71–7.

Di Iorio BR, Mondillo F, Bortone S, Nargi P, Capozzi M, Spagnuolo T, Cucciniello E, Bellizzi V. Fourteen years of hemodialysis with a central venous catheter: mechanical long-term complications. J Vasc Access. 2006;7:60–5.

Doherty A, El-Khuffash A, Monteith C, McSweeney L, Breatnach C, Kent E, Tully E, Malone F, Thornton P. Comparison of bioreactance and echocardiographic non-invasive cardiac output monitoring and myocardial function assessment in primagravida women. Br J Anaesth. 2017;118:527–32.

Domino KB, Bowdle TA, Posner KL, Spitellie PH, Lee LA, Cheney FW. Injuries and liability related to central vascular catheters: a closed claims analysis. Anesthesiology. 2004;100:1411–8.

Donati A, Carsetti A, Tondi S, Scorcella C, Domizi R, Damiani E, Gabbanelli V, Munch C, Adrario E, Pelaia P, Cecconi M. Thermodilution vs pressure recording analytical method in hemodynamic stabilized patients. J Crit Care. 2014;29:260–4.

Drawz P. Clinical implications of different blood pressure measurement techniques. Curr Hypertens Rep. 2017;19:54.

Durbin CG Jr. The range of pulmonary artery catheter balloon inflation pressures. J Cardiothorac Anesth. 1990;4:39–42.

Elgendy A, Seppelt IM, Lane AS. Comparison of continuous-wave Doppler ultrasound monitor and echocardiography to assess cardiac output in intensive care patients. Crit Care Resusc. 2017;19:222–9.

Elliott CG, Zimmerman GA, Clemmer TP. Complications of pulmonary artery catheterization in the care of critically ill patients. A prospective study. Chest. 1979;76:647–52.

Elwan MH, Hue J, Green SJ, Eltahan SM, Sims MR, Coats TJ. Thoracic electrical bioimpedance versus suprasternal Doppler in emergency care. Emerg Med Australas. 2017;29:391–3.

English IC, Frew RM, Pigott JF, Zaki M. Percutaneous catheterisation of the internal jugular vein. 1969. Anaesthesia. 1995;50:1071–6; discussion 1070.

Fagnoul D, Vincent JL, Backer DD. Cardiac output measurements using the bioreactance technique in critically ill patients. Crit Care. 2012;16:460.

Fakler U, Pauli C, Balling G, Lorenz HP, Eicken A, Hennig M, Hess J. Cardiac index monitoring by pulse contour analysis and thermodilution after pediatric cardiac surgery. J Thorac Cardiovasc Surg. 2007;133:224–8.

Fanari Z, Grove M, Rajamanickam A, Hammami S, Walls C, Kolm P, Saltzberg M, Weintraub WS, Doorey AJ. Cardiac output determination using a widely available direct continuous oxygen consumption measuring device: a practical way to get back to the gold standard. Cardiovasc Revasc Med. 2016;17:256–61.

Feldman LS, Anidjar M, Metrakos P, Stanbridge D, Fried GM, Carli F. Optimization of cardiac preload during laparoscopic donor nephrectomy: a preliminary study of central venous pressure versus esophageal Doppler monitoring. Surg Endosc. 2004;18:412–6.

Ferguson M, Max MH, Marshall W. Emergency department infraclavicular subclavian vein catheterization in patients with multiple injuries and burns. South Med J. 1988;81:433–5.

Fick A. Über die Messung des Blutquantums in der Herzventrikeln. Stahelschen Universitats-Buch Kunsthandlung: Sitzungsberichte der physikalisch-medicinischen Gesellschaftzu Würzburg; 1870. p. XVI–XVII.

Figueiredo A, Germano N, Guedes P, Marcelino P. The evolving concepts of haemodynamic support: from pulmonary artery catheter to echocardiography and theragnostics. Curr Cardiol Rev. 2011;7:136–45.
Franklin C. The technique of radial artery cannulation. Tips for maximizing results while minimizing the risk of complications. J Crit Illn. 1995a;10:424–32.
Franklin CM. The technique of dorsalis pedis cannulation. An overlooked option when the radial artery cannot be used. J Crit Illn. 1995b;10:493–8.
Frazier SK, Skinner GJ. Pulmonary artery catheters: state of the controversy. J Cardiovasc Nurs. 2008;23:113–21; quiz 122-113.
Freed MD, Keane JF. Cardiac output measured by thermodilution in infants and children. J Pediatr. 1978;92:39–42.
Fuda G, Denault A, Deschamps A, Bouchard D, Fortier A, Lambert J, Couture P. Risk factors involved in central-to-radial arterial pressure gradient during cardiac surgery. Anesth Analg. 2016;122:624–32.
Furuya EY, Dick A, Perencevich EN, Pogorzelska M, Goldmann D, Stone PW. Central line bundle implementation in US intensive care units and impact on bloodstream infections. PLoS One. 2011;6:e15452.
Gan TJ, Arrowsmith JE. The oesophageal Doppler monitor. BMJ. 1997;315:893–4.
Ge X, Cavallazzi R, Li C, Pan SM, Wang YW, Wang FL. Central venous access sites for the prevention of venous thrombosis, stenosis and infection. Cochrane Database Syst Rev. 2012;3:CD004084.
Geerts BF, Aarts LP, Jansen JR. Methods in pharmacology: measurement of cardiac output. Br J Clin Pharmacol. 2011;71:316–30.
Gibson DG, Francis DP. Clinical assessment of left ventricular diastolic function. Heart. 2003;89:231–8.
Gibson F, Bodenham A. Misplaced central venous catheters: applied anatomy and practical management. Br J Anaesth. 2013;110:333–46.
Godoy MC, Leitman BS, de Groot PM, Vlahos I, Naidich DP. Chest radiography in the ICU: Part 2: Evaluation of cardiovascular lines and other devices. AJR Am J Roentgenol. 2012;198:572–81.
Goepfert MS, Richter HP, Zu Eulenburg C, Gruetzmacher J, Rafflenbeul E, Roeher K, von Sandersleben A, Diedrichs S, Reichenspurner H, Goetz AE, Reuter DA. Individually optimized hemodynamic therapy reduces complications and length of stay in the intensive care unit: a prospective, randomized controlled trial. Anesthesiology. 2013;119:824–36.
Gologorsky E, Gologorsky A, Barron ME. Pulmonary artery catheter in cardiac surgery revisited. Anesth Analg. 2012;114:1368; author reply 1369.
Gueret G, Kiss G, Rossignol B, Bezon E, Wargnier JP, Miossec A, Corre O, Arvieux CC. Cardiac output measurements in off-pump coronary surgery: comparison between NICO and the swan-Ganz catheter. Eur J Anaesthesiol. 2006;23:848–54.
Guleri A, Kumar A, Morgan RJ, Hartley M, Roberts DH. Anaphylaxis to chlorhexidine-coated central venous catheters: a case series and review of the literature. Surg Infect. 2012;13:171–4.
Gurgel ST, do Nascimento P Jr. Maintaining tissue perfusion in high-risk surgical patients: a systematic review of randomized clinical trials. Anesth Analg. 2011;112:1384–91.
Hardy JF, Morissette M, Taillefer J, Vauclair R. Pathophysiology of rupture of the pulmonary artery by pulmonary artery balloon-tipped catheters. Anesth Analg. 1983;62:925–30.
Harrigan RA, Chan TC, Moonblatt S, Vilke GM, Ufberg JW. Temporary transvenous pacemaker placement in the emergency department. J Emerg Med. 2007;32:105–11.
Harvey S, Harrison DA, Singer M, Ashcroft J, Jones CM, Elbourne D, Brampton W, Williams D, Young D, Rowan K. Assessment of the clinical effectiveness of pulmonary artery catheters in management of patients in intensive care (PAC-Man): a randomised controlled trial. Lancet. 2005;366:472–7.
Harvey S, Stevens K, Harrison D, Young D, Brampton W, McCabe C, Singer M, Rowan K. An evaluation of the clinical and cost-effectiveness of pulmonary artery catheters in patient management in intensive care: a systematic review and a randomised controlled trial. Health Technol Assess. 2006;10:1–133; iii–iv, ix–xi.

Haryadi DG, Orr JA, Kuck K, McJames S, Westenskow DR. Partial CO_2 rebreathing indirect Fick technique for non-invasive measurement of cardiac output. J Clin Monit Comput. 2000;16:361–74.

Hayashi S, Hayase T, Shirai A, Maruyama M. Numerical simulation of noninvasive blood pressure measurement. J Biomech Eng. 2006;128:680–7.

Heiss HW. Werner Forssmann: a German problem with the Nobel Prize. Clin Cardiol. 1992;15:547–9.

Heresi GA, Arroliga AC, Wiedemann HP, Matthay MA. Pulmonary artery catheter and fluid management in acute lung injury and the acute respiratory distress syndrome. Clin Chest Med. 2006;27:627–35; abstract ix.

Hessel EA, Apostolidou I. Pulmonary artery catheter for coronary artery bypass graft: does it harm our patients? Primum non nocere. Anesth Analg. 2011;113:987–9.

Hewlett AL, Rupp ME. New developments in the prevention of intravascular catheter associated infections. Infect Dis Clin N Am. 2012;26:1–11.

Hida S, Ohashi S, Kinoshita H, Honda T, Yamamoto S, Kazama J, Endoh H. Knotting of two central venous catheters: a rare complication of pulmonary artery catheterization. J Anesth. 2010;24:486–7.

Himpe D. New approach to systemic vascular resistance calculation and clinical decision making. Acta Anaesthesiol Belg. 1990;41:291–5.

Hind D, Calvert N, McWilliams R, Davidson A, Paisley S, Beverley C, Thomas S. Ultrasonic locating devices for central venous cannulation: meta-analysis. BMJ. 2003;327:361.

Hodgson LE, Forni LG, Venn R, Samuels TL, Wakeling HG. A comparison of the non-invasive ultrasonic cardiac output monitor (USCOM) with the oesophageal Doppler monitor during major abdominal surgery. J Intensive Care Soc. 2016;17:103–10.

Holmes SJ, Kiely EM, Spitz L. Vascular access. Prog Pediatr Surg. 1989;22:133–9.

Horlocker TT, Bishop AT. Compartment syndrome of the forearm and hand after brachial artery cannulation. Anesth Analg. 1995;81:1092–4.

Htet N, Vaughn J, Adigopula S, Hennessey E, Mihm F. Needle-guided ultrasound technique for axillary artery catheter placement in critically ill patients: a case series and technique description. J Crit Care. 2017;41:194–7.

Huygh J, Peeters Y, Bernards J, Malbrain ML. Hemodynamic monitoring in the critically ill: an overview of current cardiac output monitoring methods. F1000Res. 2016;5:F1000 Faculty Rev-2855.

Ikeda S, Yagi K, Schweiss JF, Homan SM. In vitro reappraisal of the pulmonary artery catheter balloon volume-pressure relationship: comparison of four different catheters. Can J Anaesth. 1991;38:648–53.

Imhoff M. Alea iacta est: a new approach to cardiac output monitoring? Anesth Analg. 2013;117:295–6.

Ishizuka M, Nagata H, Takagi K, Kubota K. Right internal jugular vein is recommended for central venous catheterization. J Investig Surg. 2010;23:110–4.

Jakovljevic DG, Moore S, Hallsworth K, Fattakhova G, Thoma C, Trenell MI. Comparison of cardiac output determined by bioimpedance and bioreactance methods at rest and during exercise. J Clin Monit Comput. 2012;26:63–8.

Jegatheswaran J, Ruzicka M, Hiremath S, Edwards C. Are automated blood pressure monitors comparable to ambulatory blood pressure monitors? A systematic review and meta-analysis. Can J Cardiol. 2017;33:644–52.

Jo YY, Song JW, Yoo YC, Park JY, Shim JK, Kwak YL. The uncalibrated pulse contour cardiac output during off-pump coronary bypass surgery: performance in patients with a low cardiac output status and a reduced left ventricular function. Korean J Anesthesiol. 2011;60:237–43.

Kalra A, Heitner S, Topalian S. Iatrogenic pulmonary artery rupture during swan-Ganz catheter placement—a novel therapeutic approach. Catheter Cardiovasc Interv. 2013;81:57–9.

Kang M, Ryu HG, Son IS, Bahk JH. Influence of shoulder position on central venous catheter tip location during infraclavicular subclavian approach. Br J Anaesth. 2011;106:344–7.

Kapoor PM, Kakani M, Chowdhury U, Choudhury M, Lakshmy KU. Early goal-directed therapy in moderate to high-risk cardiac surgery patients. Ann Card Anaesth. 2008;11:27–34.
Karakitsos D, Labropoulos N, De Groot E, Patrianakos AP, Kouraklis G, Poularas J, Samonis G, Tsoutsos DA, Konstadoulakis MM, Karabinis A. Real-time ultrasound-guided catheterisation of the internal jugular vein: a prospective comparison with the landmark technique in critical care patients. Crit Care. 2006;10:R162.
Karamanou M, Papaioannou TG, Tsoucalas G, Tousoulis D, Stefanadis C, Androutsos G. Blood pressure measurement: lessons learned from our ancestors. Curr Pharm Des. 2015;21:700–4.
Katsikis A, Karavolias G, Voudris V. Transfemoral percutaneous removal of a knotted swan-Ganz catheter. Catheter Cardiovasc Interv. 2009;74:802–4.
Keenan SP. Use of ultrasound to place central lines. J Crit Care. 2002;17:126–37.
Kelly TF Jr, Morris GC Jr, Crawford ES, Espada R, Howell JF. Perforation of the pulmonary artery with Swan-Ganz catheters: diagnosis and surgical management. Ann Surg. 1981;193:686–92.
Kiefer N, Hofer CK, Marx G, Geisen M, Giraud R, Siegenthaler N, Hoeft A, Bendjelid K, Rex S. Clinical validation of a new thermodilution system for the assessment of cardiac output and volumetric parameters. Crit Care. 2012;16:R98.
Kim MC, Kim KS, Choi YK, Kim DS, Kwon MI, Sung JK, Moon JY, Kang JM. An estimation of right- and left-sided central venous catheter insertion depth using measurement of surface landmarks along the course of central veins. Anesth Analg. 2011;112:1371–4.
Kim WY, Lee CW, Sohn CH, Seo DW, Yoon JC, Koh JW, Kim W, Lim KS, Hong SB, Lim CM, Koh Y. Optimal insertion depth of central venous catheters—is a formula required? A prospective cohort study. Injury. 2012;43:38–41.
Klepper ID, Webb RK, Van der Walt JH, Ludbrook GL, Cockings J. The Australian incident monitoring study. The stethoscope: applications and limitations—an analysis of 2000 incident reports. Anaesth Intensive Care. 1993;21:575–8.
Knopp R, Dailey RH. Central venous cannulation and pressure monitoring. JACEP. 1977;6:358–66.
Kolodzik PW. Guide wire embolization as a potential complication of central line placement. J Emerg Med. 1989;7:291.
Kuhn CWK. Hemodynamic monitoring. In: Holzheimer RG, Mannick JA, editors. Surgical treatment: evidence-based and problem-oriented. Munich: Zuckschwerdt; 2001.
Kujur R, Rao MS, Mrinal M. How correct is the correct length for central venous catheter insertion. Indian J Crit Care Med. 2009;13:159–62.
Kunizawa A, Fujioka M, Mink S, Keller E. Central venous catheter-induced delayed hydrothorax via progressive erosion of central venous wall. Minerva Anestesiol. 2010;76:868–71.
Laher AE, Watermeyer MJ, Buchanan SK, Dippenaar N, Simo NCT, Motara F, Moolla M. A review of hemodynamic monitoring techniques, methods and devices for the emergency physician. Am J Emerg Med. 2017;35:1335–47.
Lamia B, Kim HK, Severyn DA, Pinsky MR. Cross-comparisons of trending accuracies of continuous cardiac-output measurements: pulse contour analysis, bioreactance, and pulmonary-artery catheter. J Clin Monit Comput. 2018;32(1):33–43.
Langesaeter E, Rosseland LA, Stubhaug A. Continuous invasive blood pressure and cardiac output monitoring during cesarean delivery: a randomized, double-blind comparison of low-dose versus high-dose spinal anesthesia with intravenous phenylephrine or placebo infusion. Anesthesiology. 2008;109:856–63.
Lategola M, Rahn H. A self-guiding catheter for cardiac and pulmonary arterial catheterization and occlusion. Proc Soc Exp Biol Med. 1953;84:667–8.
Lavine SJ, Lavine JA. The effect of acute hypertension on left ventricular diastolic pressures in a canine model of left ventricular dysfunction with a preserved ejection fraction and elevated left ventricular filling pressures. J Am Soc Echocardiogr. 2006;19:1350–8.
Lechner E, Hofer A, Leitner-Peneder G, Freynschlag R, Mair R, Weinzettel R, Rehak P, Gombotz H. Levosimendan versus milrinone in neonates and infants after corrective open-heart surgery: a pilot study. Pediatr Crit Care Med. 2012;13:542–8.
Lee AY, Kamphuisen PW. Epidemiology and prevention of catheter-related thrombosis in patients with cancer. J Thromb Haemost. 2012;10:1491–9.

Leibowitz AB, Oropello JM. The pulmonary artery catheter in anesthesia practice in 2007: an historical overview with emphasis on the past 6 years. Semin Cardiothorac Vasc Anesth. 2007;11:162–76.
Li J. Systemic oxygen transport derived by using continuous measured oxygen consumption after the Norwood procedure-an interim review. Interact Cardiovasc Thorac Surg. 2012;15:93–101.
Liang SY, Khair H, Durkin MJ, Marschall J. Prevention and management of central line-associated bloodstream infections in hospital practice. Hosp Pract (Minneap). 2012;40:106–18.
Linnemann B, Lindhoff-Last E. Risk factors, management and primary prevention of thrombotic complications related to the use of central venous catheters. Vasa. 2012;41:319–32.
Litton E, Morgan M. The PiCCO monitor: a review. Anaesth Intensive Care. 2012;40:393–409.
Maguire S, Rinehart J, Vakharia S, Cannesson M. Technical communication: respiratory variation in pulse pressure and plethysmographic waveforms: intraoperative applicability in a North American academic center. Anesth Analg. 2011;112:94–6.
Mandel MA, Dauchot PJ. Radial artery cannulation in 1,000 patients: precautions and complications. J Hand Surg [Am]. 1977;2:482–5.
Manecke GR. Edwards FloTrac sensor and Vigileo monitor: easy, accurate, reliable cardiac output assessment using the arterial pulse wave. Expert Rev Med Devices. 2005;2:523–7.
Mansfield PF, Hohn DC, Fornage BD, Gregurich MA, Ota DM. Complications and failures of subclavian-vein catheterization. N Engl J Med. 1994;331:1735–8.
Marik PE, Flemmer M, Harrison W. The risk of catheter-related bloodstream infection with femoral venous catheters as compared to subclavian and internal jugular venous catheters: a systematic review of the literature and meta-analysis. Crit Care Med. 2012;40:2479–85.
Marik PE, Levitov A, Young A, Andrews L. The use of bioreactance and carotid Doppler to determine volume responsiveness and blood flow redistribution following passive leg raising in hemodynamically unstable patients. Chest. 2013;143:364–70.
Masugata H, Peters B, Lafitte S, Strachan GM, Ohmori K, Mizushige K, Kohno M. Assessment of adenosine-induced coronary steal in the setting of coronary occlusion based on the extent of opacification defects by myocardial contrast echocardiography. Angiology. 2003;54:443–8.
Mathews L, Singh RK. Cardiac output monitoring. Ann Card Anaesth. 2008;11:56–68.
Matthay MA, Chatterjee K. Bedside catheterization of the pulmonary artery: risks compared with benefits. Ann Intern Med. 1988;109:826–34.
Maurer MM, Burkhoff D, Maybaum S, Franco V, Vittorio TJ, Williams P, White L, Kamalakkannan G, Myers J, Mancini DM. A multicenter study of noninvasive cardiac output by bioreactance during symptom-limited exercise. J Card Fail. 2009;15:689–99.
Maxwell RA, Gibson JB, Slade JB, Fabian TC, Proctor KG. Noninvasive cardiac output by partial CO_2 rebreathing after severe chest trauma. J Trauma. 2001;51:849–53.
Mayer J, Suttner S. Cardiac output derived from arterial pressure waveform. Curr Opin Anaesthesiol. 2009;22:804–8.
McGee WT, Mailloux PT, Martin RT. Safe placement of central venous catheters: a measured approach. J Intensive Care Med. 2011;26:392–6.
McGhee BH, Bridges EJ. Monitoring arterial blood pressure: what you may not know. Crit Care Nurse. 2002;22:60–4, 66–70, 73 passim.
Melhuish TM, White LD. Optimal wrist positioning for radial arterial cannulation in adults: a systematic review and meta-analysis. Am J Emerg Med. 2016;34:2372–8.
Merrer J, De Jonghe B, Golliot F, Lefrant JY, Raffy B, Barre E, Rigaud JP, Casciani D, Misset B, Bosquet C, Outin H, Brun-Buisson C, Nitenberg G. Complications of femoral and subclavian venous catheterization in critically ill patients: a randomized controlled trial. JAMA. 2001;286:700–7.
Meyer JA. Werner Forssmann and catheterization of the heart, 1929. Ann Thorac Surg. 1990;49:497–9.
Mielniczuk LM, Lamas GA, Flaker GC, Mitchell G, Smith SC, Gersh BJ, Solomon SD, Moye LA, Rouleau JL, Rutherford JD, Pfeffer MA. Left ventricular end-diastolic pressure and risk of subsequent heart failure in patients following an acute myocardial infarction. Congest Heart Fail. 2007;13:209–14.

Miller AG, Bardin AJ. Review of ultrasound-guided radial artery catheter placement. Respir Care. 2016;61:383–8.

Miller SE, Maragakis LL. Central line-associated bloodstream infection prevention. Curr Opin Infect Dis. 2012;25:412–22.

Mohr R, Meir O, Smolinsky A, Goor DA. A method for continuous on-line monitoring of systemic vascular resistance (COMS) after open heart procedures. J Cardiovasc Surg. 1987;28:558–65.

Monnet X, Picard F, Lidzborski E, Mesnil M, Duranteau J, Richard C, Teboul JL. The estimation of cardiac output by the Nexfin device is of poor reliability for tracking the effects of a fluid challenge. Crit Care. 2012;16:R212.

Monnet X, Richard C, Teboul JL. The pulmonary artery catheter in critically ill patients. Does it change outcome? Minerva Anestesiol. 2004;70:219–24.

Monnet X, Teboul JL. Minimally invasive monitoring. Crit Care Clin. 2015;31:25–42.

Moran J. Pulse. In: Walker HK, Hall WD, Hurst JW, editors. Clinical methods: the history, physical, and laboratory examinations. 3rd ed. Boston: Butterworths; 1990. Chapter 17. http://www.ncbi.nlm.nih.gov/books/NBK278/.

Mueller HS, Chatterjee K, Davis KB, Fifer MA, Franklin C, Greenberg MA, Labovitz AJ, Shah PK, Tuman KJ, Weil MH, Weintraub WS. ACC expert consensus document. Present use of bedside right heart catheterization in patients with cardiac disease. J Am Coll Cardiol. 1998;32: 840–64.

Myers MG, Godwin M. Automated office blood pressure. Can J Cardiol. 2012;28:341–6.

Nichols WW, Denardo SJ, Wilkinson IB, McEniery CM, Cockcroft J, O'Rourke MF. Effects of arterial stiffness, pulse wave velocity, and wave reflections on the central aortic pressure waveform. J Clin Hypertens (Greenwich). 2008;10:295–303.

Nilsson LB, Eldrup N, Berthelsen PG. Lack of agreement between thermodilution and carbon dioxide-rebreathing cardiac output. Acta Anaesthesiol Scand. 2001;45:680–5.

Nossaman BD, Scruggs BA, Nossaman VE, Murthy SN, Kadowitz PJ. History of right heart catheterization: 100 years of experimentation and methodology development. Cardiol Rev. 2010;18:94–101.

O'Brien E. Automated blood pressure measurement: state of the market in 1998 and the need for an international validation protocol for blood pressure measuring devices. Blood Press Monit. 1998;3:205–11.

O'Brien E. Demise of the mercury sphygmomanometer and the dawning of a new era in blood pressure measurement. Blood Press Monit. 2003;8:19–21.

O'Brien E, Stergiou GS. The pursuit of accurate blood pressure measurement: a 35-year travail. J Clin Hypertens (Greenwich). 2017;19:746–52.

O'Brien E, van Montfrans G, Palatini P, Tochikubo O, Staessen J, Shirasaki O, Lipicky R, Myers M. Task force I: methodological aspects of blood pressure measurement. Blood Press Monit. 2001;6:313–5.

O'Rourke MF, Avolio AP. Pulsatile flow and pressure in human systemic arteries. Studies in man and in a multibranched model of the human systemic arterial tree. Circ Res. 1980;46:363–72.

O'Rourke MF, Pauca A, Jiang XJ. Pulse wave analysis. Br J Clin Pharmacol. 2001;51:507–22.

O'Rourke MF, Yaginuma T. Wave reflections and the arterial pulse. Arch Intern Med. 1984;144:366–71.

Omar HR, Fathy A, Mangar D, Camporesi E. Missing the guidewire: an avoidable complication. Int Arch Med. 2010;3:21.

Opotowsky AR, Hess E, Maron BA, Brittain EL, Baron AE, Maddox TM, Alshawabkeh LI, Wertheim BM, Xu M, Assad TR, Rich JD, Choudhary G, Tedford RJ. Thermodilution vs estimated Fick cardiac output measurement in clinical practice: an analysis of mortality from the veterans affairs clinical assessment, reporting, and tracking (VA CART) program and Vanderbilt University. JAMA Cardiol. 2017;2:1090–9.

Oransky I. H. Jeremy C. Swan. Lancet. 2005;365:1132.

Ouellette EA. Compartment syndromes in obtunded patients. Hand Clin. 1998;14:431–50.

Papaioannou TG, Karageorgopoulou TD, Sergentanis TN, Protogerou AD, Psaltopoulou T, Sharman JE, Weber T, Blacher J, Daskalopoulou SS, Wassertheurer S, Khir AW, Vlachopoulos

C, Stergiopulos N, Stefanadis C, Nichols WW, Tousoulis D. Accuracy of commercial devices and methods for noninvasive estimation of aortic systolic blood pressure a systematic review and meta-analysis of invasive validation studies. J Hypertens. 2016;34:1237–48.

Parienti JJ, du Cheyron D, Timsit JF, Traore O, Kalfon P, Mimoz O, Mermel LA. Meta-analysis of subclavian insertion and nontunneled central venous catheter-associated infection risk reduction in critically ill adults. Crit Care Med. 2012;40:1627–34.

Pearse RM, Ikram K, Barry J. Equipment review: an appraisal of the LiDCO plus method of measuring cardiac output. Crit Care. 2004;8:190–5.

Phan TD, Kluger R, Wan C, Wong D, Padayachee A. A comparison of three minimally invasive cardiac output devices with thermodilution in elective cardiac surgery. Anaesth Intensive Care. 2011;39:1014–21.

Pikwer A, Akeson J, Lindgren S. Complications associated with peripheral or central routes for central venous cannulation. Anaesthesia. 2012;67:65–71.

Pipanmekaporn T, Bunchungmongkol N, Pin on P, Punjasawadwong Y. Impact of patients' positions on the incidence of arrhythmias during pulmonary artery catheterization. J Cardiothorac Vasc Anesth. 2012;26:391–4.

Pirracchio R, Cholley B, De Hert S, Solal AC, Mebazaa A. Diastolic heart failure in anaesthesia and critical care. Br J Anaesth. 2007;98:707–21.

Poelaert JI, Trouerbach J, De Buyzere M, Everaert J, Colardyn FA. Evaluation of transesophageal echocardiography as a diagnostic and therapeutic aid in a critical care setting. Chest. 1995;107:774–9.

Rajaram SS, Desai NK, Kalra A, Gajera M, Cavanaugh SK, Brampton W, Young D, Harvey S, Rowan K. Pulmonary artery catheters for adult patients in intensive care. Cochrane Database Syst Rev. 2013;2:CD003408.

Ramaswamykanive H, Bihari DJ. Entrapment of the introducing sheath of a pulmonary artery catheter. Anaesth Intensive Care. 2009;37:1025–6.

Ranganath A, Hanumanthaiah D. Radial artery pseudo aneurysm after percutaneous cannulation using Seldinger technique. Indian J Anaesth. 2011;55:274–6.

Raval NY, Squara P, Cleman M, Yalamanchili K, Winklmaier M, Burkhoff D. Multicenter evaluation of noninvasive cardiac output measurement by bioreactance technique. J Clin Monit Comput. 2008;22:113–9.

Razavi A, Newth CJL, Khemani RG, Beltramo F, Ross PA. Cardiac output and systemic vascular resistance: clinical assessment compared with a noninvasive objective measurement in children with shock. J Crit Care. 2017;39:6–10.

Reed CR, Sessler CN, Glauser FL, Phelan BA. Central venous catheter infections: concepts and controversies. Intensive Care Med. 1995;21:177–83.

Reems MM, Aumann M. Central venous pressure: principles, measurement, and interpretation. Compend Contin Educ Vet. 2012;34:E1–E10.

Renner J, Scholz J, Bein B. Monitoring fluid therapy. Best Pract Res Clin Anaesthesiol. 2009;23:159–71.

Reshetnik A, Compton F, Scholzel A, Tolle M, Zidek W, Giet MV. Noninvasive oscillometric cardiac output determination in the intensive care unit - comparison with invasive transpulmonary thermodilution. Sci Rep. 2017;7:9997.

Reuter DA, Huang C, Edrich T, Shernan SK, Eltzschig HK. Cardiac output monitoring using indicator-dilution techniques: basics, limits, and perspectives. Anesth Analg. 2010;110: 799–811.

Rhodes A, Cusack RJ, Newman PJ, Grounds RM, Bennett ED. A randomised, controlled trial of the pulmonary artery catheter in critically ill patients. Intensive Care Med. 2002;28:256–64.

Richard C, Monnet X, Teboul JL. Pulmonary artery catheter monitoring in 2011. Curr Opin Crit Care. 2011;17:296–302.

Richard C, Warszawski J, Anguel N, Deye N, Combes A, Barnoud D, Boulain T, Lefort Y, Fartoukh M, Baud F, Boyer A, Brochard L, Teboul JL. Early use of the pulmonary artery catheter and outcomes in patients with shock and acute respiratory distress syndrome: a randomized controlled trial. JAMA. 2003;290:2713–20.

Riva-Rocci S, Zanchetti A, Mancia G. A new sphygmomanometer. Sphygmomanometric technique. J Hypertens. 1996;14:1–12.

Roguin A. Scipione Riva-Rocci and the men behind the mercury sphygmomanometer. Int J Clin Pract. 2006;60:73–9.

Sander M, von Heymann C, Foer A, von Dossow V, Grosse J, Dushe S, Konertz WF, Spies CD. Pulse contour analysis after normothermic cardiopulmonary bypass in cardiac surgery patients. Crit Care. 2005;9:R729–34.

Sandham JD, Hull RD, Brant RF, Knox L, Pineo GF, Doig CJ, Laporta DP, Viner S, Passerini L, Devitt H, Kirby A, Jacka M. A randomized, controlled trial of the use of pulmonary-artery catheters in high-risk surgical patients. N Engl J Med. 2003;348:5–14.

Sangkum L, Liu GL, Yu L, Yan H, Kaye AD, Liu H. Minimally invasive or noninvasive cardiac output measurement: an update. J Anesth. 2016;30:461–80.

Satler LF. Iatrogenic pulmonary artery rupture: the realities of management. Catheter Cardiovasc Interv. 2013;81:60–1.

Saugel B, Bendjelid K, Critchley LA, Rex S, Scheeren TW. Journal of clinical monitoring and computing 2016 end of year summary: cardiovascular and hemodynamic monitoring. J Clin Monit Comput. 2017;31:5–17.

Scheer B, Perel A, Pfeiffer UJ. Clinical review: complications and risk factors of peripheral arterial catheters used for haemodynamic monitoring in anaesthesia and intensive care medicine. Crit Care. 2002;6:199–204.

Schloglhofer T, Gilly H, Schima H. Semi-invasive measurement of cardiac output based on pulse contour: a review and analysis. Can J Anaesth. 2014;61:452–79.

Schramm R, Abugameh A, Tscholl D, Schafers HJ. Managing pulmonary artery catheter-induced pulmonary hemorrhage by bronchial occlusion. Ann Thorac Surg. 2009;88:284–7.

Schubert S, Schmitz T, Weiss M, Nagdyman N, Huebler M, Alexi-Meskishvili V, Berger F, Stiller B. Continuous, non-invasive techniques to determine cardiac output in children after cardiac surgery: evaluation of transesophageal Doppler and electric velocimetry. J Clin Monit Comput. 2008;22:299–307.

Schwann NM, Hillel Z, Hoeft A, Barash P, Mohnle P, Miao Y, Mangano DT. Lack of effectiveness of the pulmonary artery catheter in cardiac surgery. Anesth Analg. 2011;113:994–1002.

Scolletta S, Romano SM, Biagioli B, Capannini G, Giomarelli P. Pressure recording analytical method (PRAM) for measurement of cardiac output during various haemodynamic states. Br J Anaesth. 2005;95:159–65.

Shah MR, Hasselblad V, Stevenson LW, Binanay C, O'Connor CM, Sopko G, Califf RM. Impact of the pulmonary artery catheter in critically ill patients: meta-analysis of randomized clinical trials. JAMA. 2005;294:1664–70.

Shevde K, Raab R, Lee P. Decreasing the risk of pulmonary artery rupture with a pressure relief balloon. J Cardiothorac Vasc Anesth. 1994;8:30–4.

Singer M, Clarke J, Bennett ED. Continuous hemodynamic monitoring by esophageal Doppler. Crit Care Med. 1989;17:447–52.

Siradovic A, Stoll R, Kern F, Haertel M. Optimizing puncture of the internal jugular vein. Effects and advantages of the Valsalva maneuver in catheterization. Anaesthesist. 1988;37:387–91.

Sise MJ, Hollingsworth P, Brimm JE, Peters RM, Virgilio RW, Shackford SR. Complications of the flow-directed pulmonary artery catheter: a prospective analysis in 219 patients. Crit Care Med. 1981;9:315–8.

Stergiou GS, Parati G, Vlachopoulos C, Achimastos A, Andreadis E, Asmar R, Avolio A, Benetos A, Bilo G, Boubouchairopoulou N, Boutouyrie P, Castiglioni P, de la Sierra A, Dolan E, Head G, Imai Y, Kario K, Kollias A, Kotsis V, Manios E, McManus R, Mengden T, Mihailidou A, Myers M, Niiranen T, Ochoa JE, Ohkubo T, Omboni S, Padfield P, Palatini P, Papaioannou T, Protogerou A, Redon J, Verdecchia P, Wang J, Zanchetti A, Mancia G, O'Brien E. Methodology and technology for peripheral and central blood pressure and blood pressure variability measurement: current status and future directions—Position statement of the European Society of Hypertension Working Group on blood pressure monitoring and cardiovascular variability. J Hypertens. 2016;34:1665–77.

Stevens K, McCabe C, Jones C, Ashcroft J, Harvey S, Rowan K. The incremental cost effectiveness of withdrawing pulmonary artery catheters from routine use in critical care. Appl Health Econ Health Policy. 2005;4:257–64.

Stone PA, Hass SM, Knackstedt KS, Jagannath P. Malposition of a central venous catheter into the right internal mammary vein: review of complications of catheter misplacement. Vasc Endovasc Surg. 2012;46:187–9.

Sumita S, Ujike Y, Namiki A, Watanabe H, Watanabe A, Satoh O. Rupture of pulmonary artery induced by balloon occlusion pulmonary angiography. Intensive Care Med. 1995;21:79–81.

Summerhill EM, Baram M. Principles of pulmonary artery catheterization in the critically ill. Lung. 2005;183:209–19.

Surov A, Wienke A, Carter JM, Stoevesandt D, Behrmann C, Spielmann RP, Werdan K, Buerke M. Intravascular embolization of venous catheter—causes, clinical signs, and management: a systematic review. JPEN J Parenter Enteral Nutr. 2009;33:677–85.

Swan HJ. The pulmonary artery catheter in anesthesia practice. 1970. Anesthesiology. 2005;103:890–3.

Swan HJ, Ganz W. Letter: guidelines for use of balloon-tipped catheter. Am J Cardiol. 1974;34:119–20.

Swan HJ, Ganz W. Use of balloon flotation catheters in critically ill patients. Surg Clin North Am. 1975;55:501–9.

Swan HJ, Ganz W. Complications with flow-directed balloon-tipped catheters. Ann Intern Med. 1979;91:494.

Swan HJ, Ganz W, Forrester J, Marcus H, Diamond G, Chonette D. Catheterization of the heart in man with use of a flow-directed balloon-tipped catheter. N Engl J Med. 1970;283:447–51.

Takada M, Minami K, Murata T, Inoue C, Sudani T, Suzuki A, Yamamoto T. Anesthetic management using the arterial pressure-based cardiac output monitor and a central venous oximetry catheter for tricuspid valve replacement in a patient receiving hemodialysis. Masui. 2010;59:1016–20.

Taylor HL, Tiede K. A comparison of the estimation of the basal cardiac output from a linear formula and the cardiac index. J Clin Invest. 1952;31:209–16.

Tesio F, De Baz H, Panarello G, Calianno G, Quaia P, Raimondi A, Schinella D. Double catheterization of the internal jugular vein for hemodialysis: indications, techniques, and clinical results. Artif Organs. 1994;18:301–4.

Trieschmann U, Kruessell M, Cate UT, Sreeram N. Central venous catheters in children and neonates (Part 2)—Access via the internal jugular vein. Images Paediatr Cardiol. 2008;10:1–7.

Trof RJ, Danad I, Reilingh MW, Breukers RM, Groeneveld AB. Cardiac filling volumes versus pressures for predicting fluid responsiveness after cardiovascular surgery: the role of systolic cardiac function. Crit Care. 2011;15:R73.

Truijen J, van Lieshout JJ, Wesselink WA, Westerhof BE. Noninvasive continuous hemodynamic monitoring. J Clin Monit Comput. 2012;26:267–78.

Trzebicki J, Lisik W, Blaszczyk B, Pacholczyk M, Fudalej M, Chmura A, Lazowski T. Unexpected fatal right ventricular rupture during liver transplantation: case report. Ann Transplant. 2011;16:70–4.

Turi G, Tordiglione P, Araimo F. Anterior mediastinal central line malposition. Anesth Analg. 2012;117(1):123–5.

Tyden H. Cannulation of the internal jugular vein—500 cases. Acta Anaesthesiol Scand. 1982;26:485–8.

Uchida Y, Sakamoto M, Takahashi H, Matsuo Y, Funahashi H, Sasano H, Sobue K, Takeyama H. Optimal prediction of the central venous catheter insertion depth on a routine chest x-ray. Nutrition. 2011;27:557–60.

Unal AE, Bayar S, Arat M, Ilhan O. Malpositioning of Hickman catheters, left versus right sided attempts. Transfus Apher Sci. 2003;28:9–12.

Urban T, Wappler F, Sakka SG. Intra-arterial ECG leads of a positive P-wave potential during central venous catheterization. Anasthesiol Intensivmed Notfallmed Schmerzther. 2011;46:94–7.

Urbano J, Lopez J, Gonzalez R, Fernandez SN, Solana MJ, Toledo B, Carrillo A, Lopez-Herce J. Comparison between pressure-recording analytical method (PRAM) and femoral arterial thermodilution method (FATD) cardiac output monitoring in an infant animal model of cardiac arrest. Intensive Care Med Exp. 2016;4:13.

Urschel JD, Myerowitz PD. Catheter-induced pulmonary artery rupture in the setting of cardiopulmonary bypass. Ann Thorac Surg. 1993;56:585–9.

Uzun M, Erinc K, Kirilmaz A, Baysan O, Sag C, Kilicarslan F, Genc C, Karaeren H, Demirtas E. A novel method to estimate pulmonary artery wedge pressure using the downslope of the Doppler mitral regurgitant velocity profile. Echocardiography. 2004;21:673–9.
Vakily A, Parsaei H, Movahhedi MM, Sahmeddini MA. A system for continuous estimating and monitoring cardiac output via arterial waveform analysis. J Biomed Phys Eng. 2017;7:181–90.
Valtier B, Cholley BP, Belot JP, de la Coussaye JE, Mateo J, Payen DM. Noninvasive monitoring of cardiac output in critically ill patients using transesophageal Doppler. Am J Respir Crit Care Med. 1998;158:77–83.
van Heerden PV, Baker S, Lim SI, Weidman C, Bulsara M. Clinical evaluation of the non-invasive cardiac output (NICO) monitor in the intensive care unit. Anaesth Intensive Care. 2000;28:427–30.
Vats HS. Complications of catheters: tunneled and nontunneled. Adv Chronic Kidney Dis. 2012;19:188–94.
Vender JS. Pulmonary artery catheter utilization: the use, misuse, or abuse. J Cardiothorac Vasc Anesth. 2006;20:295–9.
Vincent JL, Pinsky MR, Sprung CL, Levy M, Marini JJ, Payen D, Rhodes A, Takala J. The pulmonary artery catheter: in medio virtus. Crit Care Med. 2008;36:3093–6.
Vincent JL, Rhodes A, Perel A, Martin GS, Della Rocca G, Vallet B, Pinsky MR, Hofer CK, Teboul JL, de Boode WP, Scolletta S, Vieillard-Baron A, De Backer D, Walley KR, Maggiorini M, Singer M. Clinical review: update on hemodynamic monitoring—a consensus of 16. Crit Care. 2011;15:229.
Waldron NH, Miller TE, Thacker JK, Manchester AK, White WD, Nardiello J, Elgasim MA, Moon RE, Gan TJ. A prospective comparison of a noninvasive cardiac output monitor versus esophageal Doppler monitor for goal-directed fluid therapy in colorectal surgery patients. Anesth Analg. 2014;118:966–75.
Walser EM. Venous access ports: indications, implantation technique, follow-up, and complications. Cardiovasc Intervent Radiol. 2012;35:751–64.
Wanderer JP, Rathmell JP. Utilizing ultrasound: let us help you with that arterial line! Anesthesiology. 2017;127:A15.
Wax DB, Lin HM, Leibowitz AB. Invasive and concomitant noninvasive intraoperative blood pressure monitoring: observed differences in measurements and associated therapeutic interventions. Anesthesiology. 2011;115:973–8.
West JB. The beginnings of cardiac catheterization and the resulting impact on pulmonary medicine. Am J Phys Lung Cell Mol Phys. 2017;313:L651–l658.
Westenskow DR, Silva FH. Device to limit inflation of a pulmonary artery catheter balloon. Crit Care Med. 1993;21:1365–8.
Wheeler AP, Bernard GR, Thompson BT, Schoenfeld D, Wiedemann HP, deBoisblanc B, Connors AF Jr, Hite RD, Harabin AL. Pulmonary-artery versus central venous catheter to guide treatment of acute lung injury. N Engl J Med. 2006;354:2213–24.
Wilcox TA. Catheter-related bloodstream infections. Semin Interv Radiol. 2009;26:139–43.
Williams L, Frenneaux M. Diastolic ventricular interaction: from physiology to clinical practice. Nat Clin Pract Cardiovasc Med. 2006;3:368–76.
Woodrow P. Central venous catheters and central venous pressure. Nurs Stand. 2002;16:45–51; quiz 52.
Yu DT, Platt R, Lanken PN, Black E, Sands KE, Schwartz JS, Hibberd PL, Graman PS, Kahn KL, Snydman DR, Parsonnet J, Moore R, Bates DW. Relationship of pulmonary artery catheter use to mortality and resource utilization in patients with severe sepsis. Crit Care Med. 2003;31:2734–41.
Zarshenas Z, Sparschu RA. Catheter placement and misplacement. Crit Care Clin. 1994;10:417–36.
Zhou Q, Xiao W, An E, Zhou H, Yan M. Effects of four different positive airway pressures on right internal jugular vein catheterisation. Eur J Anaesthesiol. 2012;29:223–8.
Zuffi A, Biondi-Zoccai G, Colombo F. Swan-Ganz-induced pulmonary artery rupture: management with stent graft implantation. Catheter Cardiovasc Interv. 2010;76:578–81.

Postoperative Central Nervous System Monitoring in Adult Cardiac Surgery

6

Ali Dabbagh

Abstract

The central nervous system (CNS) has the highest rank of priority in all medical interventions including cardiac surgery. Optimal care of the CNS in postoperative period of cardiac surgery mandates appropriate cerebral monitoring to ensure safe course of postoperative care especially when the patient is not fully awake due to residual anesthetics or ongoing effects of sedatives and analgesics.

Implementing CNS monitoring includes a battery of tests from clinical assessments and scoring systems to sophisticated and high-technology invasive and noninvasive monitors. Though for some of these monitors their use is not a common practice for all patients in cardiac surgery ICU, there is a trend to increase using more objective CNS monitoring in these patients especially when considering the ever-increasing rate of higher-risk patients, especially the aging population on one side and the wondrous developments in microprocessor technology and their widespread use in medicine on the other side.

There are some cardiac surgery patients in whom using even more than one modality is suggested, hence using "multimodal CNS monitoring." A number of standard guidelines and statements for CNS modalities are nowadays available; some are discussed here in the chapter.

Keywords

Richmond Agitation-Sedation Scale (RASS) · Sedation-Agitation Scale (SAS) · Ramsay Sedation Scale (Ramsay) · Electroencephalography (EEG) including multichannel or uni-channel EEG · Electroencephalography (EEG) including

A. Dabbagh, M.D.
Cardiac Anesthesiology Department, Anesthesiology Research Center, Faculty of Medicine, Shahid Beheshti University of Medical Sciences, Tehran, Iran
e-mail: alidabbagh@sbmu.ac.ir

A. Dabbagh et al. (eds.), *Postoperative Critical Care for Adult Cardiac Surgical Patients*, https://doi.org/10.1007/978-3-319-75747-6_6

traditional EEG · qEEG and CCEEG · Cerebral oximetry · Jugular venous oxygen saturation (SjVO2) · Monitoring depth of anesthesia · Evoked potentials: somatosensory-evoked potential (SSEP) · Motor-evoked potential (MEP) · Visual-evoked potential (VEP) · Auditory-evoked potential (AEP) · Gamma rhythm · Beta rhythm · Alpha rhythm · Theta rhythm · Delta rhythm · Normal and abnormal EEG · EEG spectrogram · Bispectral index · Cerebral oximetry · Near-infrared spectroscopy (NIRS) · Jugular venous oxygen saturation (SjvO2) · Transcranial Doppler (TCD)

6.1 Role of Central Nervous System (CNS) Monitoring in Postoperative Care of Adult Surgery

CNS is among the highest priorities for oxygen supplementation in health and disease. However, during the perioperative period, prevention of CNS ischemia would depend on appropriate cerebral oxygen delivery, which in turn is directly dependent on appropriate cardiac output, appropriate cerebral oxygen delivery, and prevention of cerebral hyperactivity causing extraordinary oxygen demand.

CNS monitoring is mainly a matter of concern during the operation; however, there are a number of patients who need more sophisticated postoperative CNS assessments; among them, cardiac surgery patients should be mentioned.

The concept of fast-track cardiac surgery has gained much concern during the last decade; however, CNS monitoring has received increased attention and an important role because of its effects on quality outcomes, making the different techniques used for CNS monitoring an essential part of "anesthesia arsenal"; at the same time, CNS monitoring is advised to be applied as *multimodal monitoring* especially for high-risk patients; this *multimodal* approach includes a number of CNS monitoring devices currently available like (Johansen and Sebel 2000; Shaaban Ali et al. 2001; White and Baker 2002; Moppett and Mahajan 2004; Wright 2007; Palanca et al. 2009; Fedorow and Grocott 2010; Rohlwink and Figaji 2010; Ghosh et al. 2012):

- Clinical assessment of CNS status and of sedation in postoperative period (intensive care unit)
- Classic electroencephalogram (EEG) including multichannel or uni-channel EEG
- Monitoring depth of anesthesia
- Evoked potentials (including motor-evoked potential, somatosensory-evoked potential, and auditory-evoked potential)
- Regional cerebral oximetry (rSO2) by near-infrared spectroscopy technique (NIRS)
- Jugular vein oxygen saturation (SjvO2)
- Transcranial Doppler (TCD)
- Other modes for assessment of cerebral blood flow

Among the above options, the more common devices are discussed in the next pages of this chapter. Multimodal CNS monitoring is demonstrated to improve patient outcome, especially neurologic measures of outcome.

For cardiac surgery patients, the early postoperative period is a critical time interval since these patients have the following characteristics:

1. There are frequent episodes of hemodynamic instabilities in a considerable proportion of these patients.
2. Postoperative hyperthermia is a common unwanted event in many of those undergoing cardiopulmonary bypass (CPB).
3. Usually the anesthetic drugs causing decreased level of consciousness are discontinued causing CNS arousal and increasing oxygen demand.
4. Postoperative pain is usually undertreated; this is also seen in cardiac surgery patients, making the use of analgesics mandatory in such patients.
5. Cardiac surgery patients often have a number of important CNS comorbidities like cerebral vascular or carotid artery diseases which mandate preoperative and postoperative CNS care.
6. Aortic manipulations might dislodge embolic particles mainly into the CNS arterial system which is usually composed of end arteries; such potential ischemic events are presented clinically in the postoperative period.
7. Inflammatory process induced by CPB or the process of surgery is usually continued throughout the early postoperative days.
8. Very high doses of anticoagulants are administered for cardiac surgery patients undergoing CPB; also, many patients receive preoperative anticoagulants; these events might cause postoperative hemorrhagic events, though postoperative CNS dysfunctions are mainly ischemic and not hemorrhagic.
9. Nowadays, an increasing number of patients undergoing cardiac procedures receive hemodynamic support using extracorporeal membrane oxygenation (ECMO); some of them should also be supported by right or left ventricular assist devices (RVAD or LVAD); a number of these patients are at risk of postoperative CNS complications, like ischemia or hemorrhage or indirectly due to hemodynamic instability affecting the CNS; all of these states mandate vigorous postoperative CNS monitoring (Cengiz et al. 2005; Dalton et al. 2005; Nelson et al. 2008; Brogan et al. 2009; Isley et al. 2009; Cogan 2010; Fedorow and Grocott 2010; Edmonds et al. 2011; Hervey-Jumper et al. 2011; 2012; Rollins et al. 2012; Chiarelli et al. 2017; Dabbagh 2014a, b; Dabbagh and Ramsay 2017a, b).

6.2 Clinical Assessment of CNS Status and of Sedation in Postoperative Period (Especially Cardiac ICU)

A number of sedation assessment scales have been introduced for use in the clinical setting of ICU. All of these scales are based on clinical assessment of patient arousal state and responsiveness; the response could be to vocal stimulation (simple patient calling) up to mechanical stimulation; also, the agitation level of response is often incorporated in these scales. It is "strongly recommended" to frequently assess the "level of consciousness using a sedation scale," according to Sessler et al. and other related studies (Sessler et al. 2002, 2008; Burk et al. 2014a, b; Halpern et al. 2014; Grap et al. 2016; Ouellette et al. 2017).

The American College of Critical Care Medicine has published the "Clinical practice guidelines for the management of pain, agitation, and delirium in adult patients in the intensive care unit". This guideline has incorporated an "evidence-based, integrated, and interdisciplinary approach" for management of agitation, pain, sedation, and delirium in ICU patients (Barr et al. 2013a, b).

The guideline is based on the "ABCDE bundle" concept abbreviated for:

- Awakening
- Breathing
- Coordination
- Delirium
- Early mobility

This concept leads to "significant improvements in ICU patient care" (Barr and Pandharipande 2013; Carrothers et al. 2013).

The ACCM guideline has assessed ten subjective sedation scales which include:

1. Observer's Assessment of Alertness/Sedation Scale (OAA/S)
2. Ramsay Sedation Scale (Ramsay)
3. New Sheffield Sedation Scale (Sheffield)
4. Sedation Intensive Care Score (SEDIC)
5. Motor Activity Assessment Scale (MAAS)
6. Adaptation to the Intensive Care Environment (ATICE)
7. Minnesota Sedation Assessment Tool (MSAT)
8. Vancouver Interaction and Calmness Scale (VICS)
9. Sedation-Agitation Scale (SAS)
10. Richmond Agitation-Sedation Scale (RASS)

The guideline declares that "RASS and SAS yielded the highest psychometric scores." Also, the guideline announces that "moderate to high correlations were found between the sedation scores and either EEG or BIS values." Also, the guideline stresses on the feasibility of RASS. Moreover, the guideline adds "RASS and SAS to be the most valid and reliable for use in critically ill patients; whereas ATICE, MSAT, and VICS are moderately valid and reliable." Meanwhile, it enunciates that "MAAS, SEDIC, Sheffield, Ramsay, and OAA/S scales had a lower quality of evidence." Based on this newly published guideline, here, the three scales, i.e., RASS, SAS, and Ramsay, are described in brief. The interested reader could find the others as needed (Carrasco 2000; De Jonghe et al. 2000; Young and Prielipp 2001; Watson and Kane-Gill 2004; Olson et al. 2007; Sessler et al. 2008; Thuong 2008; Brush and Kress 2009; Barr et al. 2013a, b; Barr and Pandharipande 2013).

6.2.1 Richmond Agitation-Sedation Scale (RASS)

This scale has ten grades:

- Four positive scores (+4 to +1) which stand for combative to restless stages
- One zero score which stands for an "alert and calm" patient
- Five minus scores (−1 to −5) which stand for drowsy to unarousable patient

A very important practical point for application of RASS is to determine in the first step of visit if the patient is "alert and calm" which would be scored "zero." If the patient is agitated, the scoring would be above zero (i.e., from +4 to +1); however, if the patient is sedated or drowsy, the score would be negative (i.e., from −1 to −5).

A full grading is presented here based on the studies of Sessler and others. The full description of the scale is described in Table 6.1 and could be found in Sessler et al. study (Sessler et al. 2002; Barr et al. 2013a, b; Barr and Pandharipande 2013; Benitez-Rosario et al. 2013).

6.2.2 Sedation-Agitation Scale (SAS)

SAS is much easier than RASS; in other words, it is a seven-step scale without negative scores. The "calm and cooperative patient" in SAS gets a score of 4. However, SAS is graded as in Table 6.2.

Table 6.1 A summary of the Richmond Agitation-Sedation Scale (RASS)

Score	Clinical term
+4	Combative
+3	Very agitated
+2	Agitated
+1	Restless
0	Alert and calm
−1	Drowsy
−2	Light sedation
−3	Moderate sedation
−4	Deep sedation
−5	Unarousable

Table 6.2 A summary of the Sedation-Agitation Scale (SAS) (Dabbagh 2014b; Dabbagh and Ramsay 2017b)

Score	Clinical term
7	Dangerous agitation
6	Very agitated
5	Agitated
4	Calm and cooperative
3	Sedated
2	Very sedated
1	Unarousable

Table 6.3 A summary of Ramsay Sedation Scale

Score	Clinical description
1	Patient anxious and agitated or restless or both
2	Patient cooperative, orientated, and tranquil
3	Patient asleep, *responds* to commands
4	Patient asleep, with *brisk* response to light glabellar tap or loud auditory stimulus
5	Patient asleep, with *sluggish* response to light glabellar tap or loud auditory stimulus
6	*Unresponsive* to any stimulus

SAS is demonstrated as a valid and reliable scale for assessment of sedation status in postoperative period of adult patients in intensive care unit (Riker et al. 1999, 2001; Brandl et al. 2001; Barr et al. 2013a, b; Barr and Pandharipande 2013; Benitez-Rosario et al. 2013).

6.2.3 Ramsay Sedation Scale (Ramsay)

It was in the early 1970s that Ramsay introduced a sedation scale known as Ramsay Sedation Scale thereafter. This scale has been widely used in critical care setting. This scale is composed of six scores from 1 to 6 (Table 6.3). Score 2 is designated for the "cooperative, orientated, and tranquil" patient (Ramsay et al. 1974; Dabbagh 2014b; Dabbagh and Ramsay 2017b).

6.3 Electroencephalography (EEG) Including Multichannel or Uni-channel EEG

The oxygen supply to CNS is divided into two main categories; the majority (i.e., about 60%) is provided for specialized neuronal activity including axonal and synaptic transmission; this section is suppressed after administration of anesthetic. Another 40% of the energy supply is assigned to the maintenance of cellular integrity; usually, anesthetics do not affect the latter, while hypothermia could depress it. Usually CNS neurons adjust themselves in the ischemic state to be able to continue their basal function, i.e., the portion of their activity related to the 40% energy requirements for basal homeostasis.

When monitoring the CNS using EEG, we should always consider EEG as a "good" CNS monitoring but not a "perfect" one, since:

- The EEG electrodes record the electrical activity of the neurons just under the scalp (i.e., the cortical neurons); however, these electrodes could not record the electrical activity of thalamus or the subcortical nuclei; this is why EEG electrodes, even if located directly on the cortical tissue, just record the neurologic activity of the cortex and do not assure ischemia prevention in the subcortical brain nuclei.

- Though the EEG presentations in ischemic insult are often similar, it is not always the same; at times, the ischemic neurons are those which have inhibitory function, and their ischemic presentation would be as overactivity of CNS.
- EEG could demonstrate the ischemic events; however, its role as a CNS monitoring is not to demonstrate the site of ischemia, the etiologic mechanism responsible for ischemia, or the anatomic location of injury.
- EEG is a "biorhythm" that affected a number of factors like age, environment, and circadian variations, as cited by Constant et al.
- EEG has not been widely used for cardiac operations; due to its technical limitations.

In 2009, the American Society of Neurophysiological Monitoring (ASNM) has published the "Guidelines for intraoperative neuromonitoring using raw and quantitative electroencephalography" prepared by Isley et al.; the recommendations presented in this guideline are direct and decisive regarding perioperative EEG monitoring.

In patients undergoing cardiac surgery, especially those with higher risk of CNS injury (including the older patients), perioperative EEG could help in detection, monitoring, and prevention of CNS-related problems. The following are among the most common uses of perioperative EEG in cardiac surgery patients according to Isley et al. and Gugino et al.:

1. Detection and documentation of any preoperative baseline CNS disorder and documentation of any possible new event in the perioperative period (including postoperative period).
2. Baseline EEG (i.e., before anesthesia induction) should be documented as the baseline data especially in those at increased risk of CNS injury for comparison with later findings.
3. Intraoperative EEG monitoring and postoperative EEG records both discover new findings and differentiate them from baseline abnormalities while detecting new findings; intraoperative or postoperative new findings should be assessed carefully and cautiously to find potentially treatable new findings.
4. EEG could help us tailor the dosage of anesthetics and sedatives during intraoperative and postoperative period.
5. Monitoring the efficacy of anticonvulsant therapies in patients having seizure in postoperative period.
6. Acute hemodilution due to rapid postoperative bleeding (necessitating volume replacement with large volumes of crystalloids) and hemodilution during cardiopulmonary bypass are examples of states in which cardiac surgery patients are exposed to acute hemodilution; this hematocrit drop needs CNS monitoring to detect any possible regional or global ischemic insult associated with microcirculatory collapse, especially in patients at risk of CNS injury; these patients benefit from EEG monitoring.
7. During the early period after rewarming from CPB, the brain neurons return to the normal temperature, while the CNS perfusion arteries remain partially in

some degrees of spam; it means that during early rewarming period, brain oxygen demands would be more than oxygen supply which causes some degrees of brain ischemia; also, this phenomenon could be extended to the postoperative period in which EEG monitoring could help detect these ischemic periods.

8. When hypothermia is administered during the perioperative period as a method of cerebral protection, EEG could help us monitor the efficacy of hypothermia presented as EEG silence.
9. Hyperventilation in postoperative period causes hypocapnia which would in turn lead to cerebral arterial vasoconstriction and reduced CNS perfusion; monitoring the potential ischemic effects of this phenomenon could be done using EEG whenever the patient needs more vigorous care.

6.3.1 How EEG Works

EEG is the indicator for CNS activity, mainly the cortex and especially the postsynaptic activity of the cortical neurons; usually, the total brain electrical activity is recorded using the standard 10–20 electrodes placed on different parts of the scalp. EEG electrodes record the electrical activities of those cortical neurons located in the brain cortex just under the scalp; these neurons are "pyramids" with their direction being perpendicular to the scalp; in fact, the cortical neurons are long ones with elongated axons located vertical to the scalp.

EEG is the summative activity of cortical neurons' functions (both excitatory and inhibitory functions); in other words, *postsynaptic* electrical currents of millions of cortical neurons (called pyramidal cortical cells or Betz cells) are summated and accumulated together to create EEG waves; however, the axonal activity of the cortex does not contribute an important role in EEG wave production.

EEG waves have three main electrical characteristics:

1. Frequency: the number of times in each second that a wave recurs, presented as waves per second, i.e., Hz; each EEG wave is usually consisted of at least two basic waves which are overlapped together and compose the final waves; the composing waves could be analyzed by Fourier analysis detailed description could be found in Table 6.3. "GBATD" is the mnemonics used in this Table 6.3 for memorizing EEG waves.
2. Amplitude: amplitude of waves is decreased with increasing age as a result of aging; the electrical amplitude of EEG waves is in the range of 10–100 μV, about 100 times less than electrical amplitude of electrocardiography.
3. Time: the horizontal axis of EEG is always time.
4. Symmetry is an index of normality; even when the patients are anesthetized, the hemispheres present symmetric EEG changes, while pathologic states disturb symmetry.
5. Voltage: the summative difference between two EEG electrodes across the time scale is called voltage; in other words, the deflections above or below the horizontal scale are the result; the following pattern is created:

- If the difference between the first and the second electrodes is negative, it would appear as *above the scale deflection* (i.e., up deflection) on EEG.
- If this difference between the first and the second electrodes is positive, it would appear as *below the scale deflection* (i.e., down deflection) on EEG.

The EEG electrodes could be metal discs called "cup" electrodes made of "tin, silver, or gold." Also, needle electrodes are availably used when sterile application of EEG electrodes is mandatory like neurosurgical operations, though their use should be limited to "obligatory" conditions. The third type of electrodes is called "silver-silver chloride" electrodes. Whatever type of electrode is used, the electrode montage should be from a constant type, with appropriate quality to prevent artifacts and, also, enough gel to guarantee low amount of impedance. We also should be sure that electrodes be well attached.

Another important point is that EEG connection wires and cables should not be in contact or in the vicinity of other cables to improve EEG signal quality. Also, it is recommended to use EEG leads as shielded leads.

Usually, 2–8 channels are used for intraoperative or postoperative CNS recording; even at times, three electrodes are used on the frontal area, two of them for recording the neuronal electrical activity as "differential amplifier with voltage difference" and the third electrode used as the "mandatory reference signal" electrode.

The function of EEG is divided into "few-second" interval; this is why EEG waves are taken in defined time periods called *epochs*. These time periods are usually 2–4 s. The electrical activity waves are taken during these time epochs and are then analyzed by the device microprocessor to be demonstrated as final EEG waves on a time-based scale.

EEG electrode attachment order on the scalp is named "montage" of electrodes. In the standard system of the electrodes, there are four main anatomic landmarks used for electrode attachment over the scalp in different directions:

1. One nasion (anterior)
2. One inion (posterior)
3. Two preauricular points

The location of electrodes is named according to the above anatomic locations and, also, the standard coding system which uses anatomic, alphabetic, and numeric items (i.e., anatomic and alphanumeric recording); this standard system helps us differentiate the location of any abnormal wave and, also, to compare similar locations on two hemispheres:

1. F for frontal electrodes.
2. T for temporal electrodes.
3. O for occipital electrodes.
4. P for parietal electrodes.
5. C for central electrodes.

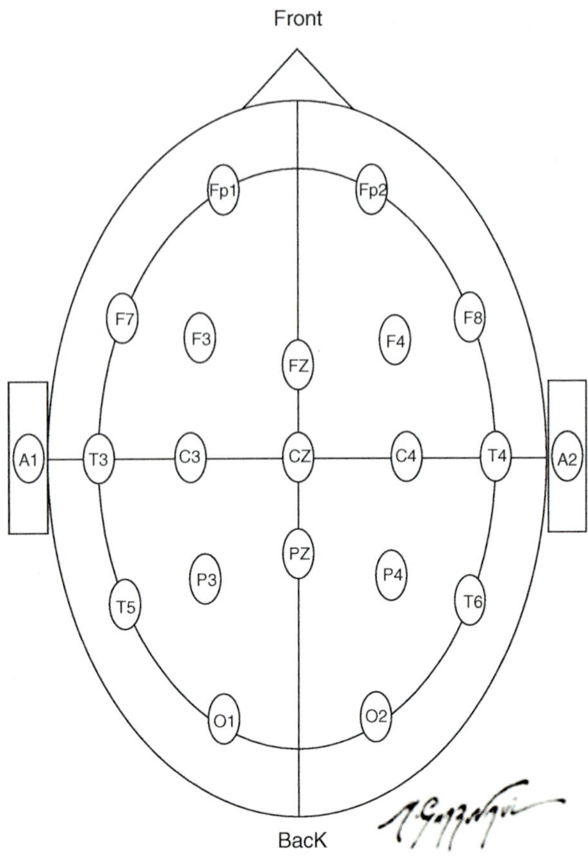

Fig. 6.1 The standard 10/20 electrode system (Dabbagh 2014b; Dabbagh and Ramsay 2017b)

6. A for auricular electrodes.
7. M for mastoid electrodes.
8. Even numbers as subscripts demonstrate right hemisphere.
9. Odd numbers as subscripts demonstrate left hemisphere.
10. Z as subscript demonstrates midline electrodes (z: zero) (Fig. 6.1).

6.3.2 Frequency of EEG Waves and the Changes During Wakefulness, Sleep, and Anesthesia

EEG rhythms during wakefulness, sleep, and anesthesia are the result of balance between cortex and thalamus, depending on the level of consciousness or the stage of anesthesia. However, EEG waves are classified as the five frequency bands; their frequencies are a bit different between different authors; however, according to Gugino et al., the frequencies are classified as demonstrated in Table 6.3 and, also, described in the following paragraphs.

6.3.3 Normal and Abnormal EEG

Normal and Abnormal EEG in normal EEG, symmetry between hemispheres is clearly evident; also, the EEG waves are according to the category mentioned above without any spike waves; the spike waves suggest epileptic activity.

However, abnormal EEG may be mainly due to ischemia, infarct, epilepsy, or tumor. For example, these are a number of well-known findings in pathologic EEG:

- Asymmetric patterns between hemispheres (could be sign of ischemia or arterial occlusion).
- Spikes.
- Decreased frequency.
- Decreased voltage.
- Also, if normal waves are seen in abnormal states, it would be suggestive of a pathologic state (like abnormal appearance of delta waves which could be suggestive for a brain lesion).

6.3.4 EEG in Cardiac Surgery Patients

The role of EEG in cardiac surgery ICU could be among the following:

- As a continuous monitoring device and a real-time neurologic assessment tool and, at the same time, to monitor CNS like the other major organ systems which should be monitored in the perioperative period; this is especially important when the hemodynamic status is not stable and there is a risk for impaired CNS perfusion.
- As a diagnostic tool, for example, in detection of epilepsy, ischemic or hemorrhagic CNS events, coma, brain death, and drug toxicities or to rule out decreased level of consciousness due to residual anesthetic effects from other etiologies of decreased consciousness.
- As a therapy-tailoring method, dosage titration tool, or drug adjustment scale, for example, as a tool in clinical approval of the anticonvulsant drugs' efficacy or making any needed change in their dose or in barbiturate-induced or hypothermia- induced coma, for objective approval of their efficacy and confirmation of barbiturate- or hypothermia-induced cortical silence.

Also, as discussed in other chapters of this book, cardiac surgery patients tolerate a considerable effect on their CNS due to the process of the disease and the therapeutic approaches. For example, in cardiac surgery patients, postoperative cerebral edema and decreased CNS oxygen delivery due to edema is often seen in the early postoperative days. This finding is seen in nearly all cardiac procedures, though the frequency is not always the same, with the following characteristics:

- EEG findings in cardiac surgery patients are similar to findings in those affected with organic brain syndrome.

- The postoperative changes are more frequent in the left hemisphere.
- These EEG findings are more common after more invasive, complex procedures; so, the prevalence is higher in valve replacement compared with valve repair or CABG.
- More common in on-pump CABG's compared with off-pump CABG's; however, seen even in off-pump patients.
- During periods of postoperative CNS ischemia, EEG waves change to ischemic pattern whenever cerebral blood flow (CBF) is <22 mL/100 g/min.
- During early stages of ischemia, frequency of waves decreases, while the voltage is preserved.
- If more severe ischemia occurs, both wave frequency and voltage are depressed.
- These changes are especially seen as significant decrease "in the beta and the alpha 2 bands."
- EEG amplitude drop >30% or duration of EEG changes >30 s have been cited as important indicators of ischemia by Florence et al.
- The effects of anesthetics, analgesic agents, temperature variations, and blood pressure fluctuations in postoperative period should be considered (Table 6.4).

6.3.5 Normal and Abnormal EEG

In normal EEG, symmetry between hemispheres is clearly evident; also, the EEG waves are according to the category mentioned above without any spike waves; the spike waves suggest epileptic activity.

However, abnormal EEG may be mainly due to ischemia, infarct, epilepsy, or tumor. Asymmetric patterns between hemispheres, spikes, and decreased frequency or voltage are the main findings in pathologic EEG.

In cardiac surgery patients, postoperative cerebral edema and decreased CNS oxygen delivery due to edema are often seen in the early postoperative days. This finding is seen in nearly all cardiac procedures, though the frequency is not always the same; the following are the characteristics:

- EEG findings in cardiac surgery patients are similar to findings in those affected with organic brain syndrome.
- The postoperative changes are more frequent in the left hemisphere.
- These EEG findings are more common after more invasive, complex procedures; so, the prevalence is higher in valve replacement compared with valve repair or CABG.
- More common in on-pump CABG's compared with off-pump CABG's; however, seen even in off-pump patients.
- During periods of postoperative CNS ischemia, EEG waves change to ischemic pattern whenever cerebral blood flow (CBF) is <22 mL/100 g/min.
- During early stages of ischemia, frequency of waves decreases, while the voltage is preserved.
- If more severe ischemia occurs, both wave frequency and voltage are depressed.

Table 6.4 Normal EEG waves standing for GBATD mnemonics (Gugino et al. 1999, 2001, 2004); Dabbagh 2014b; Dabbagh and Ramsay 2017b)

Wave category	Symbol	Frequency	Amplitude and/or voltage	Related activity	Clinical equivalent
Gamma rhythm	γ	25.1–55 Hz	High voltage and amplitude	Corticothalamic perception. both during wakefulness and sleep	Engaged in: • Sensory-processing activities • Perception process
Beta rhythm	β	12.6–25 Hz	In adults 10–20 μV	Cortico-cortical network	Fully awake patient with: • Open eyes • Mental activity
Alpha rhythm	α	8–12.5 Hz	Relatively high voltage and amplitude In adults 10–20 μV	Mainly composed of electrical activity emerged from parietal and occipital lobes of the corticothalamic network	• Awake, but relaxed individual with closed eyes • Equals drowsy state
Theta rhythm	θ	4–8 Hz	In adults 10–20 μV	• Often seen in temporal lobes in the awake state but sleepy and relaxed • Corticothalamic activity and limbic activity	• Equals stage 2 of sleep (i.e., light sleep) or drowsy state • Also, frequently seen in young children
Delta rhythm	δ	1–4 Hz	High amplitude 100–200 μV	Corticothalamic dissociation	• Equals deep dreamless sleep (stage 3 of non-REM sleep); so helps defining the depth of sleep • Another name is slow-wave sleep • Also, seen during coma or other brain disorders

- These changes are especially seen as significant decrease "in the beta and the alpha 2 bands."
- EEG amplitude drop >30% and duration of EEG changes >30 s have been cited as important indicators of ischemia by Florence et al.
- The effects of anesthetics, analgesic agents, temperature variations, and blood pressure fluctuations in postoperative period should be considered (Zeitlhofer et al. 1988; Chabot and Gugino 1993; Hauser et al. 1993; Newburger et al. 1993; Chabot et al. 1997; Nuwer 1997; Pua and Bissonnette 1998; Sebel 1998; Gugino et al. 1999, 2001, 2004; Jacobson and Jerrier 2000; Johansen and Sebel 2000; Rasmussen et al. 2002; Zimpfer et al. 2002; Grimm et al. 2003; Florence et al. 2004; Jameson and Sloan 2006; Markowitz et al. 2007; Williams and

Ramamoorthy 2007; Nelson et al. 2008; Isley et al. 2009; Palanca et al. 2009; Brown et al. 2010; Chakravarthy et al. 2010; Golukhova et al. 2010, 2011; Poe et al. 2010; Constant and Sabourdin 2012; Futier et al. 2012).

6.3.6 EEG Spectrogram

Being introduced as a relatively novel method for CNS assessment, EEG spectrogram describes the effects of different anesthetics on the brain as a three-dimensional model of EEG using power, amplitude, and frequency of EEG waves as the three vectors of the spectrogram. In this spectrogram, power is calculated as 10 log10 (amplitude). The 3D graph known as compressed spectral array (CSA) is transformed as a 2D color graph, with 3 s consecutive intervals, and each two adjacent spectra have 0.5 s overlaps (Purdon et al. 2013, 2015; Hudetz and Mashour 2016; Akeju and Brown 2017).

6.4 Monitoring Depth of Anesthesia (Including Bispectral Analysis Index)

Bispectral index (BIS) could help us deliver an appropriate level of anesthesia and/or sedation. During postoperative period, during the time interval from patient transfer to ICU until tracheal extubation, the overall patient status (including hemodynamic, pulmonary, hematologic, consciousness, etc.) is not yet prepared for extubation. Meanwhile, the residual effects of anesthetics are usually vanished in this time, and the patient needs some degree of sedation. Besides, frequently it happens in a number of patients that some invasive procedures are needed (like intubation, orotracheal suctioning, central line insertion, chest tube change, etc.), or, less frequently, it happens that more time is needed for full recovery: some need prolonged intubation and mechanical ventilatory support or hemodynamic support, mandating additional sedation/analgesia. Level of sedation/analgesia should be monitored to deliver adequate analgesic agents while preventing over-administration. BIS monitor could help us in such cases to improve sedation/analgesia level; in these clinical states during ICU care, BIS monitoring may improve analgesia (Brocas et al. 2002; Faritous et al. 2016).

Depth of anesthesia scoring for bispectral analysis index is defined as Table 6.5.

In some studies, BIS is considered as the "most widely used method at the present time" for monitoring sedation as part of an integrated monitoring approach for

Table 6.5 Level of bispectral index and clinically relevant state (Dabbagh 2014b; Dabbagh and Ramsay 2017b)

Level of bispectral index	Clinically relevant state
>80	Awake
60–80	Sedation
40–60	Surgical anesthesia
<40	Deep anesthesia

assessment of sedation/analgesia in critical patients; however, some studies have failed to demonstrate the effect of using BIS in improving fast-track extubation in adult cardiac surgery. Another important issue is the legal aspects of delivering appropriate level of sedation/analgesia to create both patient satisfaction and amnesia and, so, prevent patient recall (Simmons et al. 1999; Drummond 2000; Brocas et al. 2002; Frenzel et al. 2002; Courtman et al. 2003; Deogaonkar et al. 2004; Watson and Kane-Gill 2004; Fraser and Riker 2005; Hernandez-Gancedo et al. 2006; Payen et al. 2007; Lamas and Lopez-Herce 2010; Vance et al. 2014).

6.5 Evoked Potentials

Evoked potentials are used as monitoring devices to check the functional integrity of the central and peripheral nervous system, especially the different neural circuits and pathways. Although both EEG and evoked potentials assess the electrical activity of the nervous system, there are some differences between these two neural monitoring, discriminating evoked potentials from EEG:

- Evoked potentials have lower-voltage amplitude compared to EEG.
- Evoked potentials assess the neurologic response to a stimulus (sensory or motor).
- Evoked potentials are not limited to the cortical areas of the nervous system; in other words, evoked potentials monitor cortical areas, deeper neural structures of the CNS, spine, and also peripheral nervous system.
- In periods when EEG is flat (like therapeutic hypothermia), evoked potentials could still work and monitor the functional integrity of the nervous system.

Evoked potentials are divided into three main categories:

1. Somatosensory-evoked potential (SSEP): Somatosensory-evoked potential (SSEP) which monitors the functional integrity of the ascending pathways, from the peripheral receptors (median or ulnar nerve for upper extremity and posterior tibial nerve or peroneal nerve for lower extremity) up to the multiple spinal segments and then to the contralateral thalamus, reaching finally to the cortex; a subtype of this monitoring modality is called visual-evoked potential (VEP) which incorporates visual stimuli as the sensory input.
2. Motor-evoked potential (MEP): Motor-evoked potential (MEP) which monitors the motor pathway activated in response to electrical stimulus, from the cortical areas down to the related nuclei and corticospinal tracts and finally to motor units.
3. Auditory-evoked potential (AEP): Auditory-evoked potential (AEP) which objectively monitors the neural pathway involved in hearing from the cochlea in the ear to the auditory (eighth cranial) nerve to the brainstem then related brain ganglia and finally to the related cortical areas; the first milliseconds of this monitoring controls the brainstem function involved in auditory pathway and is called brainstem auditory-evoked response (BAEP).

The above modes have a relatively wide application in perioperative care, including cardiac surgical procedures. Their application in the postoperative period of cardiac surgery patients could be very useful and help us gather important objective data; however, this is not a common practice; one could stress on the following as the main indications of evoked potentials in postoperative period:

During periods of postoperative-controlled (therapeutic) hypothermia, EEG becomes flat; however, evoked potentials could monitor functional integrity of the nervous system even at such states.

Monitoring the physiologic integrity of the neural system while the patient is hemodynamically unstable, is deeply sedated, has altered consciousness state, or is comatose; possibly other nervous system monitoring could not assess the functional status of the patients in these periods of time.

In summary, evoked potentials could help the clinicians in assessment of neural system integrity with objective and reproducible data which are a new window besides the routine CNS monitoring; possibly, their postoperative application in cardiac surgery patients would be more common in future years.

6.6 Cerebral Oximetry

Cerebral oximetry is a relatively new technology for cerebral monitoring though it has passed more than 35 years from the first publication regarding the in vivo application of the technique; however, it has been used in a number of procedures including cardiac surgery. Successful previous studies have shown the use of this monitoring both in animal models and in human studies involving some high-risk procedures like cardiac and vascular surgery and in patients with underlying acute cerebral events though there are still some controversies.

The technology of "near-infrared spectroscopy" (NIRS) was described for this purpose in 1977 by Professor "Frans Jöbsis." NIR light has a specific characteristic which is the power to penetrate a wide range of body tissues (including bone) and, unlike pulse oximetry, utilizes the reflection phenomenon of light rather than the process used in pulse oximetry; transmission of light from a small part of the body (e.g., a finger) is the technology used in pulse oximetry; in other words, this technology utilizes passage of near-infrared (NIR) light in the range of 700–1000 nm, through skull and underlying tissues; part of the NIR light is absorbed by biologic chromophores, especially two main chromophores oxyhemoglobin (OHb) and deoxyhemoglobin (HHb) and cytochrome oxidase; and the rest of the light is returned back; the returned portion of NIR light is used for data collection, processing, calculation, and demonstration of the absorbed fraction of light in each of the above chromophores; finally these data are processed by the machine software to demonstrate the figures of rSO2 on the monitor screen. NIR light is produced by "light-emitting diodes" (LEDs) and absorbed by silicon photodiodes. In summary, its mechanism is by differential absorption of near-infrared spectroscopy "NIRS" in the range of 700–1000 nm, through the skin and bone (Fig. 6.2).

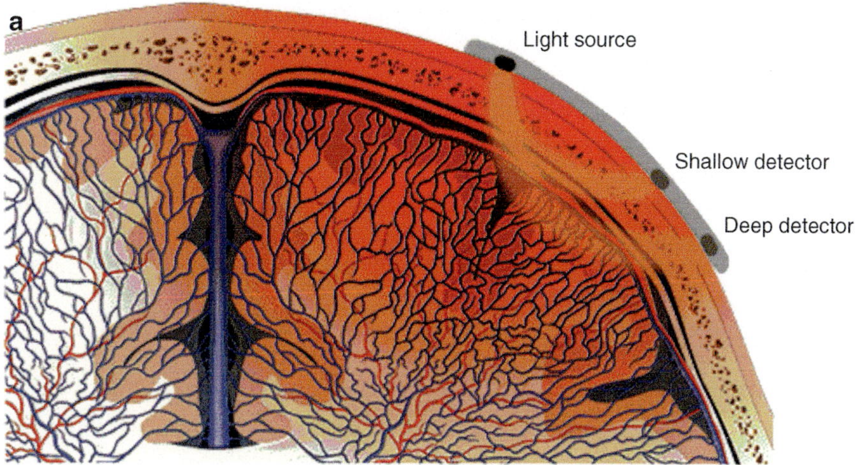

The INVOS™ system uses two depths of light penetration to subtract out surface data, resulting in a regional oxygenation value for deeper tissues.

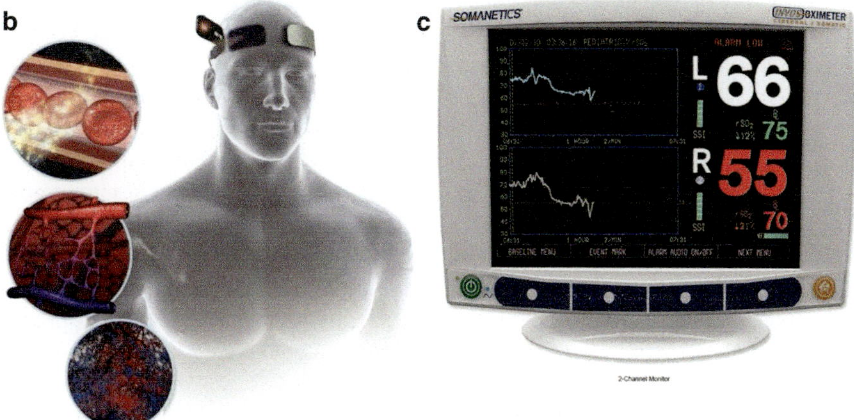

Fig. 6.2 Cerebral oximetry; (**a**) schematic presentation of NIRS mechanism in brain tissue; (**b**) schematic presentation of NIRS mechanism in brain vasculature; (**c**) monitor panel (© 2017 Medtronic. All rights reserved. Used with the permission of Medtronic", Mansfield, MA, USA)

One of the key features of cerebral oximetry by NIRS is that rSO2 figures are in appropriate range only if the brain tissue receives adequate oxygenated blood, which mandates not only adequate *cerebral oxygenation* but also appropriate state of *cerebral hemodynamic*, patency of *cerebral arteries*, and efficient cerebral *venous drainage*. Possibly this is why in some high-risk patients like cardiac surgeries (including CABG patients), regional cerebral oxygen saturation monitoring (rSO2) prevents episodes of severe cortical hypoxia; so, application of this monitoring has the potential to significantly reduce the "incidence of major organ dysfunction" and "improve outcome," though some controversies exist yet.

A number of practical notes for utilization of this monitoring are:

- Monitors the in vivo state of the CNS.
- Monitoring is noninvasive, real time, and portable.
- Measures both oxygenation and perfusion of the CNS (i.e., mandates appropriate hemodynamic of the CNS).
- Monitors not only the CNS status but also the hemodynamic status since it monitors both oxygenation and perfusion of the CNS.
- A drop more than 20% from baseline or an absolute decrease below 50% in measured rSco2 values is considered as cerebral hypoxia.
- Could be used for preoperative, intraoperative, or postoperative monitoring (all over the perioperative period).
- Does not need pulsatile flow like pulse oximetry for monitoring during CPB.
- Is an important member of the "multimodal CNS monitoring" in cardiac surgery.
- Fine attachment and correct positioning of the probes are very important for its application, and this is a very important application point which could bias the measurements.
- For patients receiving hemodynamic support by ECMO, cerebral oximetry is a very useful and promising CNS monitoring; also, if the patient would be under non-pulsatile flow with ECMO, this device could be more practical than many other CNS monitors.
- Could be used as a predictor for successfulness of extubation in cardiac surgery patients.
- Its application in high-risk patients (like the elderly and the patients undergoing surgery with underlying cerebral vascular disorders) is recommended more than the others.
- Underlying diseases like decreased cardiac output, pulmonary problems, anemia, and underlying disorders of the cerebral vessels are considered as confounders which could decrease the rSco2 readings and create bias.

If a decrease in rSco2 is observed, the following steps are suggested by Murkin et al. and Denault et al. as a useful approach for relieving the etiologic disorder causing cerebral ischemia:

1. Control head position: if head is rotated extensively, turn it to normal position.
2. Check the possibility of arterial or venous occlusion due to arterial or venous cannula physical effects.
3. Check for mean arterial pressure (MAP), and treat it if it is low.
4. Control arterial saturation (by pulse oximeter or blood gas analysis); if it is low, rule out possible causes of systemic desaturation.
5. Treat possible hyperventilation which could decrease arterial PaCO2, especially if it is below 35 mmHg.
6. Treat possible anemia to increase hematocrit above 30%.

7. Assess the cardiac function including the situation of the heart using methods like echocardiography and also SjvO2; relieve potential underlying etiologies including treatment of failing heart.
8. Check cerebral oxygen consumption; if it is increased, rule out and treat "convulsions" and/or "hyperthermia."
9. But if cerebral oxygen consumption is normal, rule out increased "intracerebral hypertension" and/or "cerebral edema"; for this purpose, use the help of imaging modalities (Rolfe 2000; Casati et al. 2005, 2006; Hoshi 2007, 2011; Murkin et al. 2007; Wolf et al. 2007; Wright 2007; Fischer et al. 2009; Hasegawa and Okita 2009; Huppert et al. 2009; Slater et al. 2009; Vohra et al. 2009; Brady et al. 2010; Erickson and Cole 2010; Fedorow and Grocott 2010; Green and Paklet 2010; La Monaca et al. 2010; Palombo et al. 2010; Sellmann et al. 2010; Svyatets et al. 2010; Veel et al. 2010; Andritsos et al. 2011; Bronicki and Chang 2011; Lampe and Becker 2011; Lima et al. 2011; Radovanovic and Radovanovic 2011; Rao and Durga 2011; Roggenbach and Rauch 2011; Smith 2011; Cyrous et al. 2012; Ghosh et al. 2012; Hankey 2012; Kertai et al. 2012; Li 2012; Scheeren et al. 2012; Tsygan 2012; Hampton and Schreiber 2013; Seule et al. 2013).

6.7 Jugular Venous Oxygen Saturation (SjvO2)

Monitoring the CNS oxygenation status has been used for more than 60 years: Gibbs et al. first in 1942 and then Datsur et al. in 1963. Assessment of the jugular venous oxygen saturation (SjvO2) is an "indirect surrogate indicator for global oxygenation of the cortex" and, also, is an indicator of the balance between cerebral blood flow (CBF) and cerebral metabolism rate of oxygen (CMRO2) (Hu et al. 2016). SjvO2 monitoring could be used to monitor the trend of change in the following items:

- Oxygen uptake by the brain tissue (i.e., the difference between brain arterial and venous difference which equals CNS oxygen uptake).
- Arterial and venous difference of CNS blood gases and their related parameters.
- Arterial and venous difference of CNS blood glucose levels.
- Arterial and venous difference of CNS blood lactate levels; impaired CNS perfusion leads to decreased cerebral oxygenation which would activate anaerobic metabolism leading to increased lactate level in the jugular venous bulb blood samples.

The normal values for SjvO2 are lower than the normal values for global mixed venous oxygen saturation (which is usually measured by pulmonary artery catheter). This is due to the fact that oxygen uptake and consumption in the cerebral tissue is much higher than the global body oxygen uptake and consumption (Weigl et al. 2016).

Table 6.6 Absolute and relative contraindications for SjvO2 catheter insertion (Shaaban Ali et al. 2001; Dabbagh 2014b; Dabbagh and Ramsay 2017b)

Absolute contraindications	Relative contraindications
• Injuries in the cervical spine • Bleeding diathesis • Local neck trauma • Local infection	• Compromised drainage of the cerebral venous system • Patients having tracheostomy

6.7.1 Contraindications for SjvO2 Catheter Insertion

These could be found in Table 6.6.

6.7.2 Method of SjvO2 Measurement

This is done through either using the *conventional technique* with serial measurements of SjvO2 and other factors or using a fiber-optic catheter with near-infrared light in the catheter tip; however, this conventional technique has the limitation of being "point assessment" needing serial measurements but could not provide real-time data. On the other hand, malpositioning of the catheter tip could cause reading errors, or the near-infrared light of the fiber-optic catheter may be out of its defined range, and hence, misreading would occur. Also, rotation of the head to either side could affect the venous return and distort the measurements. The technology used in fiber-optic SjVO2 monitor is similar to the oximetry technology used for some types of pulmonary artery catheters.

6.7.3 Technique of Catheter Insertion

SjvO2 is assessed through a catheter introduced to the internal jugular vein using the following technique (Shaaban Ali et al. 2001; Le Roux et al. 2014):

- The technique is through the internal jugular vein, usually the right side.
- Usually, the right IJV is the dominant vein for cerebral venous drainage; however, the mixing pattern between right and left hemispheres is not always the same.
- SjVO2 catheter insertion is exactly the same as central venous catheter (CVC) insertion; the anterior triangle approach is the preferred one; however, the needle and guidewire direction should be a cephalic one (compared to CVC direction).
- Seldinger technique is used for guidewire insertion.
- After guidewire insertion, the catheter should be inserted and conducted upward until resistance is sensed, or in the awake patient, a sense of pressure in skull base is noted by the patient or Doppler sonography or sizing the inserted length of the catheter by an external sizer.

- The catheter is sent from the right internal jugular vein over the guidewire to the cephalic direction.
- The catheter tip is sent cephalad to the "common facial vein outlet"; from there, it is sent to the jugular bulb; the jugular bulb is the dilated portion of the internal jugular vein; it is located distal to the jugular foramen (i.e., the anatomic opening in the bony skull from which the jugular vein exits).
- Inside the jugular bulb, the catheter tip should be positioned in the roof of the bulb; this is the site for SjVO2 measurements.
- The location of the catheter tip should be documented by lateral or anteroposterior neck X-ray; it should be located at the level of the mastoid process; in lateral neck X-ray, this location is equal to the lower border of the first cervical spine or the inferior margin of the orbital rim; also, if we draw an line between the two mastoid processes, the tip of the catheter should be just cephalad to this line.
- Another way is the surface landmarks: the surface landmark for jugular vein bulb is 1 cm anterior and 1 cm below the mastoid process.
- The measurements made by the catheter should be calibrated, in vivo or in vitro, per information provided by the manufacturer.
- If the catheter tip is misplaced and attached to the vessel wall or if the catheter tip has moved in either direction (cephalic or caudal) more than 2 cm from the bulb of jugular vein, the readings would be biased due to venous sample "contamination" and would fall in the biased range of measurement.
- Also, the speed of sampling should be less than 2 mL/min, to prevent mixing of cerebral venous blood with the venous blood from extra cranial veins; otherwise, mixing of these two samples would result in erroneous over-readings, falsely above the real normal values

6.7.4 Complications of SjvO2 Catheter

Complications of SjvO2 catheter insertion are similar to the complications of central venous catheter insertion and could be classified as those related to catheter insertion (like tissue or arterial injuries) and those related to the presence of catheter (like possible increased risk of catheter infection or thrombosis).

6.7.5 Data Collection by SjvO2 Catheter

Normal values for SjvO2 are between 55–85%; however, most studies have declared the normal value for SjvO2 in the range of 55–75%. Anyway, values lower than 50% are considered abnormal and accompanied with poor outcome in the majority of studies (Kadoi et al. 2002; Kadoi and Fujita 2003; Kawahara et al. 2003; Weigl et al. 2016).

As mentioned above, SjvO2 is an indirect surrogate index of global cerebral perfusion; so, it has a high specificity, but its sensitivity is low; in other words, SjvO2 could detect global cerebral ischemia but cannot detect exactly the location of the ischemic region in cerebral hemispheres. Also, as mentioned by White and Baker, the following factors could affect the accuracy of SjvO2 readings (White and Baker 2002):

- Simultaneous hemoglobin concentration
- Saturation of the systemic arterial blood
- Core body temperature
- Level of CO2 in the arterial blood

6.7.6 Arterial-Jugular Vein Oxygen Gradient (AjvDO2)

Another important index measured by calculating SjvO2 is the gradient between arterial and jugular vein oxygen content, abbreviated as AjvDO2. Schell and Cole have done this calculation using the sequence of following formulas (Shaaban Ali et al. 2001; Kadoi et al. 2002; Kadoi and Fujita 2003; Kawahara et al. 2003; Weigl et al. 2016):

$$\mathrm{DO2} = \mathrm{CBF} \times \mathrm{CaO2}$$

$$\mathrm{CMRO2} = \mathrm{CBF} \times (\mathrm{CaO2} - \mathrm{CjvO2})$$

$$\mathrm{AjvDO2} = \mathrm{CaO2} - \mathrm{CjvO2}$$

in which
DO2: Cerebral O2 delivery
CBF: Cerebral blood flow
CaO2: Arterial O2 content
CMRO2: Cerebral O2 consumption
CjvO2: Jugular Vein O2 content
AjvDO2: Arterial-jugular vein oxygen gradient

Considering the above equations, AjvDO2 could be calculated by solving the above formulas:

$$\mathrm{AjvDO2} = \mathrm{CMRO2} / \mathrm{CBF}$$

Schell and Cole have declared that normal AjvDO2 values are between 4–8 mL O2/100 mL of blood. Values less than 4 denote that O2 delivery is more than O2 consumption (i.e., luxury O2 delivery), while values above 8 demonstrate O2 shortage in brain tissue which could be due to increased cerebral metabolic rate (CMRO2) or decreased CBF (desaturation state). CMRO2 is normally 3.0–3.8 mL O2/100 g brain/min. According to Schell and Cole, each of the above ranges for AjvDO2 is associated with a number of differential diagnoses discussed here.

SjvO2 > 75 or AjvDO2 < 4 (luxury O2 delivery): this is due to decreased CMRO2 (like hypothermia, administration of sedatives), increased CBF (like

Table 6.7 The main determinants of cerebral perfusion and the absolute value of SjVO2 and AjvDO2 (Schell and Cole 2000; Shaaban Ali et al. 2001)

Desaturated state (SjVO2 < 50% or AjvDO2 > 8)	Versus	Luxuriant state (SjVO2 > 80% or AjvDO2 < 4)
Decreases CBF	Versus	Increased CBF
Increased CMRO2	Versus	Decreased CMRO2

Table 6.8 Differential diagnosis of desaturated SjvO2 (Schell and Cole 2000; Shaaban Ali et al. 2001)

Desaturated state (SjVO2 < 50% or AjvDO2 > 8)
Decreases cerebral blood flow (CBF) • Increased ICP (e.g., brain edema/impaired cerebral venous return) • Head injury • Arterial vasospasm/vasoconstriction • Hyperventilation/hypocapnia • Thromboembolism • Systemic hypotension • Arterial hypoxia (e.g., due to impaired ventilation after lung pathology or ventilator problems/ due to impaired hemoglobin oxygenation or impaired transfer and delivery of oxygen to tissues including brain)
Increased cerebral metabolic rate (CMRO2) • Increased brain tissue metabolism and oxygen demand (fever/hyperthermia) • Abnormal electrical activity of brain (seizure/convulsion) • Inadequate anesthesia/sedation level

Table 6.9 Differential diagnosis of luxuriant SjvO2 (Schell and Cole 2000; Shaaban Ali et al. 2001)

Luxuriant state (SjVO2 > 80% or AjvDO2 < 4)
Increased CBF • Hyperemia • Arteriovenous shunts
Decreased CMRO2 • Anesthetic drugs which depress the level of brain function • Hypothermia • Brain death

hypothermia), increased arterial oxygen content, or other causes like bran death (Tables 6.7, 6.8, and 6.9).

SjvO2 < 50 or AjvDO2 > 8 (desaturation state): this is due to the following etiologies which should be considered and ruled out in the postoperative period for patients undergoing cardiac surgery (Tables 6.7, 6.8, and 6.9):

- Increased CMRO2 (like fever, hyperthermia or seizure)
- Decreased CBF (like systemic hypotension, cerebral arterial vasospasm, hyperventilation-induced hypocapnia)
- Increased intracranial pressure (like brain edema or impaired cerebral venous return)

- Arterial hypoxia (impaired ventilation due to lung pathology or ventilator problems, impaired hemoglobin oxygenation, or impaired transfer and delivery of oxygen to tissues including brain)

According to White and Baker, in cardiac surgery patients, low systemic perfusion pressure during cardiopulmonary bypass, low hematocrit values, and rapid rewarming are the three main causes of intraoperative low SjvO2 (Hatiboglu and Anil 1992; Sheinberg et al. 1992; Dearden and Midgley 1993; Croughwell et al. 1995; von Knobelsdorff et al. 1997; Gupta et al. 1999; Ip-Yam et al. 2000; Nandate et al. 2000; Schell and Cole 2000; Shaaban Ali et al. 2001; Kadoi et al. 2002; Smythe and Samra 2002; White and Baker 2002; Chieregato et al. 2003; Kadoi and Fujita 2003; Kawahara et al. 2003; Perez et al. 2003; Sarrafzadeh et al. 2003; Oh et al. 2004; Stocchetti et al. 2004; Alten and Mariscalco 2005; Shimizu et al. 2005; Wright 2007; Rohlwink and Figaji 2010; Le Roux et al. 2014).

6.8 Transcranial Doppler (TCD)

TCD was presented to the clinical practice for the first time by Rune Aaslid in 1982 in order to assess blood flow velocities in cerebral arteries. TCD is a noninvasive monitor applicable to either operating room or intensive care unit patients, both in adult or pediatric patients. TCD is used to assess CNS vascular status through measurement of *cerebral blood flow velocity* (*of course not the blood flow*); usually the mean flow velocity (*FV mean*) is used for assessments. This device is based on using ultrasonic Doppler signal, in the low-frequency (1–2 MHz) pulse-waved range; the Doppler shift in signals gained during passage of red blood cells through the cerebral arteries is calculated by the device to demonstrate the blood flow velocity in the arteries under assessment (Aaslid et al. 1982; D'Andrea et al. 2016a, b).

Although electroencephalography (EEG) could assess the integrity of physiologic function in the cortical regions of the brain, the subcortical areas are usually neglected by EEG; this is while the cognitive functions are mainly affected by the latter nuclei, while the blood flow to such regions is assessed more effectively by TCD; however, these two technologies assess different aspects of CNS integrity and function; this is why their complementary use is more justified in higher-risk patients than their competitive comparison. Such high-risk patients may benefit their CNS outcome when both devices are used in the perioperative period. In fact, TCD has an integral role as a tool for detecting cerebral emboli during surgery; in other words, TCD is considered as a "stethoscope of the brain" (Patel et al. 2016; Robba et al. 2017). The main features of transcranial Doppler in assessment of cerebral blood flow are named in Table 6.10.

Table 6.10 Main features of transcranial Doppler in assessing cerebral blood flow

• Noninvasiveness
• Real-time assessment of cerebral blood flow
• Relatively low price
• Continuous monitoring
• The possibility for repeated assessments
• Indirect information from CNS arteries
• Applicability in perioperative care, i.e., before operation, in the operating theater, and in postoperative care (including the intensive care unit)
• Application to all age ranges

6.8.1 What Is the Mechanism of TCD?

Low-frequency (1–2 MHz) ultrasonic Doppler signal used, through pulse-waved Doppler, is the mechanism of TCD. Blood flow velocity is calculated based on the "Doppler shift" in the Doppler beam; the movement of RBC's inside arterial lumen causes the Doppler shift. There are piezoelectric crystals located in TCD probe which project Doppler waves toward the tissue; these waves after being reflected back to the crystal. In this process, the insonation angle is a determining factor.

In perioperative care of cardiac surgery patients, the main index measured by TCD is *Blood flow velocity in the middle cerebral artery (VMCA).*

TCD calculates blood flow velocity in different CNS arteries, including anterior, middle, and posterior cerebral arteries (i.e., ACA, MCA, and PCA) and, also, internal carotid arteries (ICA). There are a number of factors affecting arterial blood flow velocity which could be found in Table 6.11.

TCD has been used for cardiac surgery patients mainly during the intraoperative period to detect and prevent sandblasting events, microemboli and macroemboli caused by aortic clamping and manipulations; if there is severe aortic atherosclerosis, preventive surgical methods should be used to prevent stroke in high risk of stroke; even, it may lead to an important change in the surgical strategy to prevent unwanted postoperative CNS insults. However, the main applications of TCD in postoperative care of adult cardiac patients are named in Table 6.12.

6.8.2 Windows Used for TCD

For gaining the Doppler data, one needs appropriate acoustic (or insonation) window; this window is usually an anatomic area in which the bone plate of the skull is thin or there is a normal anatomic window in the skull; the following locations are the main appropriate acoustic (or insonation) windows in the skull for performing TCD:

Table 6.11 Factors affecting blood flow velocity in TCD (Alexandrov et al. 2012; Robba et al. 2017)

Factors determining *arterial flow velocity*: • Cerebral blood flow (CBF) • The inherent vascular anatomy • The anatomy of the collateral circulation and their perfusion ratio • The insonation window and hence insonation angle • The anatomical diameter of the artery
Confounding factors affecting reliability of TCD • Underlying hemodynamic status especially blood pressure (including systolic, diastolic, and mean arterial blood pressure) • Arterial pressure of CO2 • Gender, i.e., female has a bit higher arterial velocity, possibly to compensate for lower hematocrit values than male • Age (cerebral blood flow has the lowest values after birth, i.e., 25 cm/s, reaching to its peak at the age of 4–6 years, i.e., 100 cm/s, and then decreasing gradually with a steady velocity, to reach 40 cm/s at the 7th decade of life) • Diurnal time pattern of blood pressure and CNS perfusion (blood velocity remains the lowest at 11 AM) • Patient posture (i.e., the arterial flow is different, while the patient is seated compared to supine position) • Intracranial pressure (ICP) • Level of consciousness, including administration or discontinuation of analgesic regimens

Table 6.12 Applications of TCD in postoperative care (D'Andrea et al. 2016a, b; Robba et al. 2017)

• Adequacy of CBF and arterial blood flow through the cerebral arteries
• Assessment of the CNS arterial patency (e.g., to rule out cerebral arterial vasospasm)
• Noninvasive monitoring of intracranial pressure (ICP)
• Assessment of brain death
• Assessment of CNS autoregulatory response (i.e., CNS cardiovascular response to a spectrum of stimuli like hypercapnia or blood pressure changes)
• Assessment of postoperative CNS perfusion in patients undergoing cardiac surgery (with or without cardiopulmonary bypass) with underlying borderline carotid stenosis
• Assessing the efficacy of antithrombotic therapies in reducing the platelet embolic load sent to CNS
• Measurement of effective downstream pressure

1. *Transtemporal* window (the supra-zygomatic portion of the temporal bone) usually used for assessment of anterior, middle, and posterior cerebral arteries (ACA, MCA and PCA); this is the most commonly used approach for TCD and is shown in Fig. 6.3.
2. *Transorbital* window (through the eye globe) usually used for assessment of the ophthalmic arteries and, also, some cavernous portions of the internal carotid artery (i.e., the carotid siphon) which is shown in Fig. 6.4.
3. *Suboccipital* window used for assessment of the posterior cerebral circulation, mainly the basilar and vertebral arteries, and used for anterior cerebral artery "ACA" and posterior cerebral artery "PCA" which is shown in Fig. 6.5.

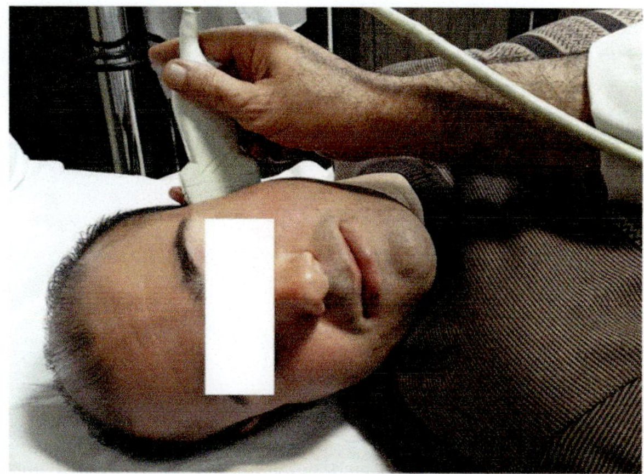

Fig. 6.3 Transtemporal window

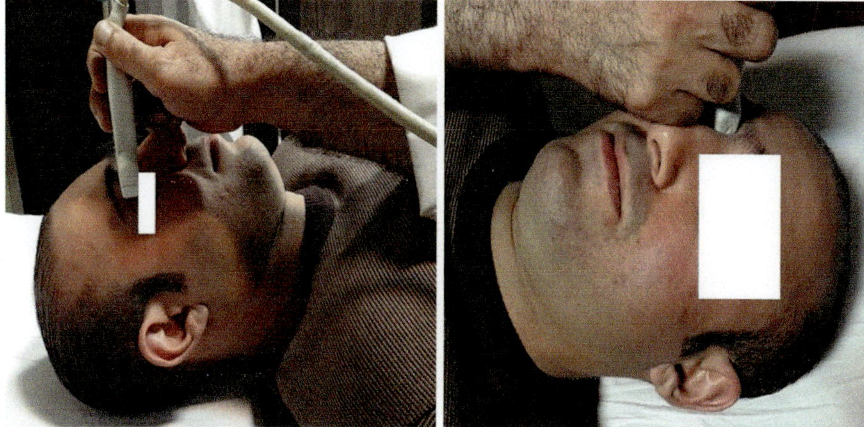

Fig. 6.4 Transorbital window

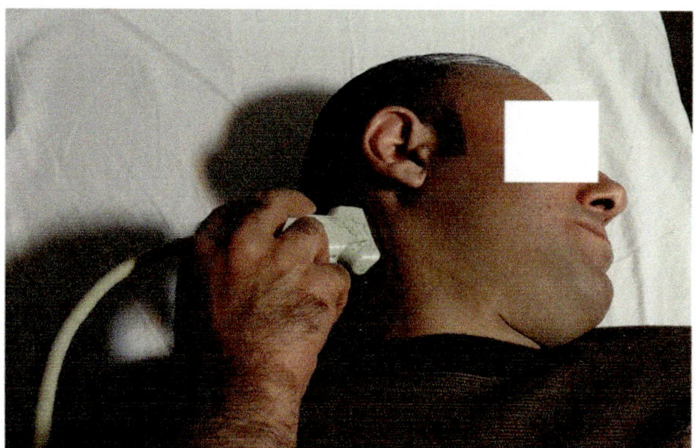

Fig. 6.5 Suboccipital window

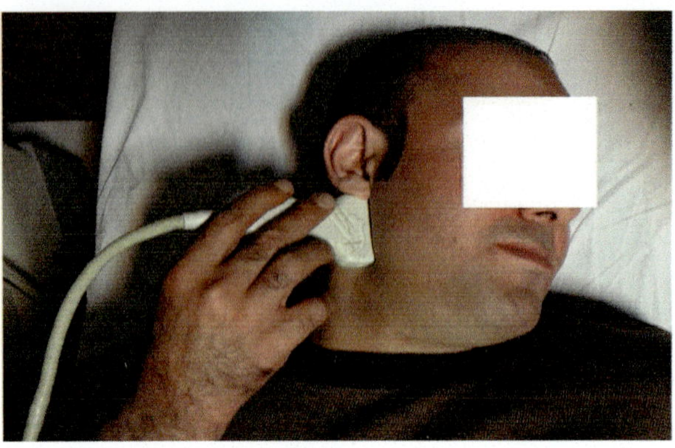

Fig. 6.6 Retromandibular window

4. *Retromandibular* which is shown in Fig. 6.6.

However, the application of this device needs the following items as its prerequisites by the user:

- Having appropriate training and experience by the user; albeit all tries, 5–10% of patients remain "poor window" with inadequate access.
- The main cerebral perfusion arteries should be used for assessments.
- Having appropriate Doppler window.
- The probe should be in a fixed position during assessment.
- Stable clinical condition for the patient should be prepared, either in the operating room or inside the intensive care unit, including constant blood pressure and other hemodynamic measurements and, also, a constant level of sedation or anesthesia (Aaslid et al. 1982; Sturzenegger et al. 1995; Zurynski et al. 1995; Schmidt et al. 1997; Soustiel et al. 1998; Kaposzta et al. 1999; Markus 1999; Markus and Reid 1999; Fearn et al. 2001; Kumral et al. 2001; Costin et al. 2002; Kral et al. 2003; Moppett and Mahajan 2004; Radvany and Wholey 2008; Rasulo et al. 2008; Enninful-Eghan et al. 2010; Mok et al. 2012; Horsfield et al. 2013; McDonnell et al. 2013; Mills et al. 2013; D'Andrea et al. 2016a, b) (Fig. 6.7).

6.9 Other Modes for Assessment of Cerebral Blood Flow (besides TCD)

Positron emission tomography (PET): is one of the latest imaging techniques based on nuclear medicine technology; in this method, positron-emitting radionuclides are administered to assess the fate of their metabolism in normal and abnormal tissues. PET could demonstrate us many of CNS variables; like cerebral blood flow (CBF) and cerebral oxygen uptake (CMRO2). However, the main disadvantage of PET is its invasiveness (Abraham and Feng 2011; Portnow et al. 2013).

a

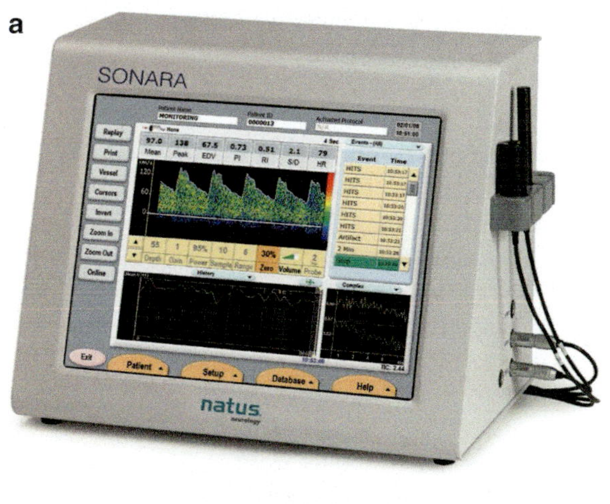

b

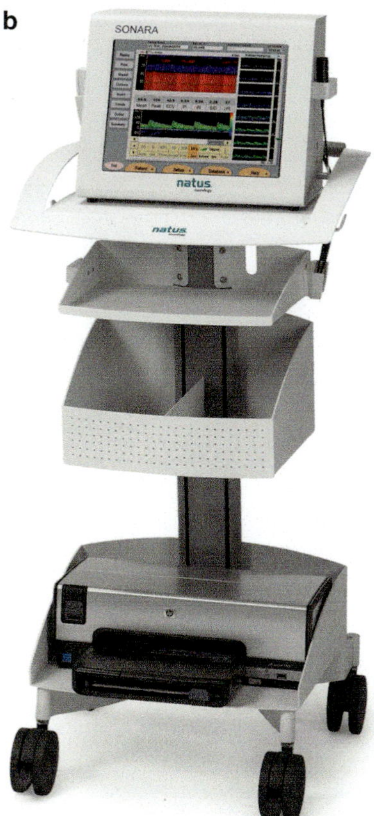

Fig. 6.7 (**a**) TCD screen display SONARA; (**b**) portable TCD set for perioperative use purposes (With kind permission of Natus Neurology, Natus Medical Incorporated, CA, USA)

Dynamic CT scanning: is a method of imaging used for measurement of regional cerebral blood flow (rCBF) based on the clearance of inhaled xenon or intravenous radionuclide contrast (O'Connor et al. 2011; Hochberg and Young 2012).

Magnetic resonance angiography (MRA): was first introduced in 1986, is noninvasive, and has many applications in the detection of cerebral vascular disease states like stenosis, occlusion, or aneurysm; some believe that in patients with peripheral vascular disease or history of previous cerebral disease undergoing cardiac surgery, preoperative assessment of cranial arteries using MRA has an effective role in preventing postoperative unwanted cerebral events (Uehara et al. 2001).

Functional magnetic resonance imaging (fMRI): this technology is based on the fact that cerebral blood flow and cortical activity level are parallel phenomenon; this technology is noninvasive and is a very potent method for CBF assessment, both in research and clinic (Stern and Silbersweig 2001).

Laser Doppler flowmetry: is used clinically to assess "microvascular blood flow" and in brain for "brain blood flow"; this technique is continuous and real time; however, there are a number of limitations in this technique including choice of bandwidth, patient motion artifact, calibration of the probe, the type of the laser, and its invasiveness; also, it monitors a small sample of the total brain tissue and, finally, is not a routine monitor in cardiac postoperative care (Obeid et al. 1990; Leahy et al. 1999; Alvarez del Castillo 2001; Stevens 2004; De Georgia and Deogaonkar 2005).

Thermal diffusion flowmetry: measures cerebral blood flow based on the thermal conductivity of the brain tissue; however, this method is invasive and has nearly no application in cardiac surgery ICU (Carter 1996; Vajkoczy et al. 2003).

Intracranial pressure (ICP) monitoring: an invasive technique usually used for neurosurgical intensive care; this technique is rarely used in cardiac surgery ICU.

References

Aaslid R, Markwalder TM, Nornes H. Noninvasive transcranial Doppler ultrasound recording of flow velocity in basal cerebral arteries. J Neurosurg. 1982;57:769–74.

Abraham T, Feng J. Evolution of brain imaging instrumentation. Semin Nucl Med. 2011;41:202–19.

Akeju O, Brown EN. Neural oscillations demonstrate that general anesthesia and sedative states are neurophysiologically distinct from sleep. Curr Opin Neurobiol. 2017;44:178–85.

Alexandrov AV, Sloan MA, Tegeler CH, Newell DN, Lumsden A, Garami Z, Levy CR, Wong LK, Douville C, Kaps M, Tsivgoulis G. Practice standards for transcranial Doppler (TCD) ultrasound. Part II. Clinical indications and expected outcomes. J Neuroimaging. 2012;22:215–24.

Alten J, Mariscalco MM. Critical appraisal of Perez et al: jugular venous oxygen saturation or arteriovenous difference of lactate content and outcome in children with severe traumatic brain injury. Pediatr Crit Care Med. 2005;6:480–2.

Alvarez del Castillo M. Monitoring neurologic patients in intensive care. Curr Opin Crit Care. 2001;7:49–60.

Andritsos M, Singh N, Patel P, Sinha A, Fassl J, Wyckoff T, Riha H, Roscher C, Subramaniam B, Ramakrishna H, Augoustides JG. The year in cardiothoracic and vascular anesthesia: selected highlights from 2010. J Cardiothorac Vasc Anesth. 2011;25:6–15.

Barr J, Fraser GL, Puntillo K, Ely EW, Gelinas C, Dasta JF, Davidson JE, Devlin JW, Kress JP, Joffe AM, Coursin DB, Herr DL, Tung A, Robinson BR, Fontaine DK, Ramsay MA, Riker RR, Sessler CN, Pun B, Skrobik Y, Jaeschke R. Clinical practice guidelines for the management of pain, agitation, and delirium in adult patients in the intensive care unit. Crit Care Med. 2013a;41:263–306.

Barr J, Kishman CP Jr, Jaeschke R. The methodological approach used to develop the 2013 pain, agitation, and delirium clinical practice guidelines for adult ICU patients. Crit Care Med. 2013b;41:S1–15.

Barr J, Pandharipande PP. The pain, agitation, and delirium care bundle: synergistic benefits of implementing the 2013 pain, agitation, and delirium guidelines in an integrated and interdisciplinary fashion. Crit Care Med. 2013;41:S99–115.

Benitez-Rosario MA, Castillo-Padros M, Garrido-Bernet B, Gonzalez-Guillermo T, Martinez-Castillo LP, Gonzalez A. Appropriateness and reliability testing of the modified richmond agitation-sedation scale in spanish patients with advanced cancer. J Pain Symptom Manag. 2013;45:1112–9.

Brady KM, Mytar JO, Kibler KK, Hogue CW Jr, Lee JK, Czosnyka M, Smielewski P, Easley RB. Noninvasive autoregulation monitoring with and without intracranial pressure in the naive piglet brain. Anesth Analg. 2010;111:191–5.

Brandl KM, Langley KA, Riker RR, Dork LA, Quails CR, Levy H. Confirming the reliability of the sedation-agitation scale administered by ICU nurses without experience in its use. Pharmacotherapy. 2001;21:431–6.

Brocas E, Dupont H, Paugam-Burtz C, Servin F, Mantz J, Desmonts JM. Bispectral index variations during tracheal suction in mechanically ventilated critically ill patients: effect of an alfentanil bolus. Intensive Care Med. 2002;28:211–3.

Brogan TV, Thiagarajan RR, Rycus PT, Bartlett RH, Bratton SL. Extracorporeal membrane oxygenation in adults with severe respiratory failure: a multi-center database. Intensive Care Med. 2009;35:2105–14.

Bronicki RA, Chang AC. Management of the postoperative pediatric cardiac surgical patient. Crit Care Med. 2011;39:1974–84.

Brown EN, Lydic R, Schiff ND. General anesthesia, sleep, and coma. N Engl J Med. 2010;363:2638–50.

Brush DR, Kress JP. Sedation and analgesia for the mechanically ventilated patient. Clin Chest Med. 2009;30:131–41, ix.

Burk RS, Grap MJ, Munro CL, Schubert CM, Sessler CN. Agitation onset, frequency, and associated temporal factors in critically ill adults. Am J Crit Care. 2014a;23:296–304.

Burk RS, Grap MJ, Munro CL, Schubert CM, Sessler CN. Predictors of agitation in critically ill adults. Am J Crit Care. 2014b;23:414–23.

Carrasco G. Instruments for monitoring intensive care unit sedation. Crit Care. 2000;4:217–25.

Carrothers KM, Barr J, Spurlock B, Ridgely MS, Damberg CL, Ely EW. Contextual issues influencing implementation and outcomes associated with an integrated approach to managing pain, agitation, and delirium in adult ICUs. Crit Care Med. 2013;41:S128–35.

Carter LP. Thermal diffusion flowmetry. Neurosurg Clin N Am. 1996;7:749–54.

Casati A, Fanelli G, Pietropaoli P, Proietti R, Tufano R, Danelli G, Fierro G, De Cosmo G, Servillo G. Continuous monitoring of cerebral oxygen saturation in elderly patients undergoing major abdominal surgery minimizes brain exposure to potential hypoxia. Anesth Analg. 2005;101:740–7, table of contents.

Casati A, Spreafico E, Putzu M, Fanelli G. New technology for noninvasive brain monitoring: continuous cerebral oximetry. Minerva Anestesiol. 2006;72:605–25.

Cengiz P, Seidel K, Rycus PT, Brogan TV, Roberts JS. Central nervous system complications during pediatric extracorporeal life support: incidence and risk factors. Crit Care Med. 2005;33:2817–24.

Chabot RJ, Gugino LD, Aglio LS, Maddi R, Cote W. QEEG and neuropsychological profiles of patients after undergoing cardiopulmonary bypass surgical procedures. Clin Electroencephalogr. 1997;28:98–105.

Chabot RJ, Gugino VD. Quantitative electroencephalographic monitoring during cardiopulmonary bypass. Anesthesiology. 1993;78:209–11.
Chakravarthy M, Holla S, Jawali V. Index of consciousness and bispectral index values are interchangeable during normotension and hypotension but not during non pulsatile flow state during cardiac surgical procedures: a prospective study. J Clin Monit Comput. 2010;24:83–91.
Chiarelli AM, Zappasodi F, Di Pompeo F, Merla A. Simultaneous functional near-infrared spectroscopy and electroencephalography for monitoring of human brain activity and oxygenation: a review. Neurophotonics. 2017;4:041411.
Chieregato A, Calzolari F, Trasforini G, Targa L, Latronico N. Normal jugular bulb oxygen saturation. J Neurol Neurosurg Psychiatry. 2003;74:784–6.
Cogan J. Pain management after cardiac surgery. Semin Cardiothorac Vasc Anesth. 2010;14:201–4.
Constant I, Sabourdin N. The EEG signal: a window on the cortical brain activity. Paediatr Anaesth. 2012;22:539–52.
Costin M, Rampersad A, Solomon RA, Connolly ES, Heyer EJ. Cerebral injury predicted by transcranial Doppler ultrasonography but not electroencephalography during carotid endarterectomy. J Neurosurg Anesthesiol. 2002;14:287–92.
Courtman SP, Wardurgh A, Petros AJ. Comparison of the bispectral index monitor with the comfort score in assessing level of sedation of critically ill children. Intensive Care Med. 2003;29:2239–46.
Croughwell ND, White WD, Smith LR, Davis RD, Glower DD Jr, Reves JG, Newman MF. Jugular bulb saturation and mixed venous saturation during cardiopulmonary bypass. J Card Surg. 1995;10:503–8.
Cyrous A, O'Neal B, Freeman WD. New approaches to bedside monitoring in stroke. Expert Rev Neurother. 2012;12:915–28.
D'Andrea A, Conte M, Cavallaro M, Scarafile R, Riegler L, Cocchia R, Pezzullo E, Carbone A, Natale F, Santoro G, Caso P, Russo MG, Bossone E, Calabro R. Transcranial Doppler ultrasonography: from methodology to major clinical applications. World J Cardiol. 2016a;8:383–400.
D'Andrea A, Conte M, Scarafile R, Riegler L, Cocchia R, Pezzullo E, Cavallaro M, Carbone A, Natale F, Russo MG, Gregorio G, Calabro R. Transcranial Doppler ultrasound: physical principles and principal applications in neurocritical care unit. J Cardiovasc Echogr. 2016b;26:28–41.
Dabbagh A. Postoperative CNS care. In: Dabbagh A, Esmailian F, Aranki S, editors. Postoperative critical care for cardiac surgical patients. 1st ed. New York: Springer; 2014a. p. 245–56.
Dabbagh A. Postoperative central nervous system monitoring. In: Dabbagh A, Esmailian F, Aranki S, editors. Postoperative critical care for cardiac surgical patients. 1st ed. New York: Springer; 2014b. p. 129–59.
Dabbagh A, Ramsay MAE. Postoperative central nervous system management in patients with congenital heart disease. In: Dabbagh A, Conte AH, Lubin L, editors. Congenital heart disease in pediatric and adult patients: anesthetic and perioperative management. 1st ed. New York: Springer; 2017a. p. 829–50.
Dabbagh A, Ramsay MAE. Central nervous system monitoring in pediatric cardiac surgery. In: Dabbagh A, Conte AH, Lubin L, editors. Congenital heart disease in pediatric and adult patients: anesthetic and perioperative management. 1st ed. New York: Springer; 2017b. p. 279–316.
Dalton HJ, Rycus PT, Conrad SA. Update on extracorporeal life support 2004. Semin Perinatol. 2005;29:24–33.
De Georgia MA, Deogaonkar A. Multimodal monitoring in the neurological intensive care unit. Neurologist. 2005;11:45–54.
De Jonghe B, Cook D, Appere-De-Vecchi C, Guyatt G, Meade M, Outin H. Using and understanding sedation scoring systems: a systematic review. Intensive Care Med. 2000;26:275–85.
Dearden NM, Midgley S. Technical considerations in continuous jugular venous oxygen saturation measurement. Acta Neurochir Suppl (Wien). 1993;59:91–7.
Deogaonkar A, Gupta R, DeGeorgia M, Sabharwal V, Gopakumaran B, Schubert A, Provencio JJ. Bispectral index monitoring correlates with sedation scales in brain-injured patients. Crit Care Med. 2004;32:2403–6.

Drummond JC. Monitoring depth of anesthesia: with emphasis on the application of the bispectral index and the middle latency auditory evoked response to the prevention of recall. Anesthesiology. 2000;93:876–82.

Edmonds HL Jr, Isley MR, Sloan TB, Alexandrov AV, Razumovsky AY. American Society of Neurophysiologic Monitoring and American Society of Neuroimaging joint guidelines for transcranial doppler ultrasonic monitoring. J Neuroimaging. 2011;21:177–83.

Enninful-Eghan H, Moore RH, Ichord R, Smith-Whitley K, Kwiatkowski JL. Transcranial Doppler ultrasonography and prophylactic transfusion program is effective in preventing overt stroke in children with sickle cell disease. J Pediatr. 2010;157:479–84.

Erickson KM, Cole DJ. Carotid artery disease: stenting vs endarterectomy. Br J Anaesth. 2010;105(Suppl 1):i34–49.

Faritous Z, Barzanji A, Azarfarin R, Ghadrdoost B, Ziyaeifard M, Aghdaei N, Alavi M. Comparison of bispectral index monitoring with the critical-care pain observation tool in the pain assessment of intubated adult patients after cardiac surgery. Anesth Pain Med. 2016;6:e38334.

Fearn SJ, Pole R, Wesnes K, Faragher EB, Hooper TL, McCollum CN. Cerebral injury during cardiopulmonary bypass: emboli impair memory. J Thorac Cardiovasc Surg. 2001;121: 1150–60.

Fedorow C, Grocott HP. Cerebral monitoring to optimize outcomes after cardiac surgery. Curr Opin Anaesthesiol. 2010;23:89–94.

Fischer GW, Torrillo TM, Weiner MM, Rosenblatt MA. The use of cerebral oximetry as a monitor of the adequacy of cerebral perfusion in a patient undergoing shoulder surgery in the beach chair position. Pain Pract. 2009;9:304–7.

Florence G, Guerit JM, Gueguen B. Electroencephalography (EEG) and somatosensory evoked potentials (SEP) to prevent cerebral ischaemia in the operating room. Neurophysiol Clin. 2004;34:17–32.

Fraser GL, Riker RR. Bispectral index monitoring in the intensive care unit provides more signal than noise. Pharmacotherapy. 2005;25:19S–27S.

Frenzel D, Greim CA, Sommer C, Bauerle K, Roewer N. Is the bispectral index appropriate for monitoring the sedation level of mechanically ventilated surgical ICU patients? Intensive Care Med. 2002;28:178–83.

Futier E, Chanques G, Cayot Constantin S, Vernis L, Barres A, Guerin R, Chartier C, Perbet S, Petit A, Jabaudon M, Bazin JE, Constantin JM. Influence of opioid choice on mechanical ventilation duration and ICU length of stay. Minerva Anestesiol. 2012;78:46–53.

Ghosh A, Elwell C, Smith M. Review article: cerebral near-infrared spectroscopy in adults: a work in progress. Anesth Analg. 2012;115:1373–83.

Golukhova EZ, Polunina AG, Lefterova NP, Begachev AV. Electroencephalography as a tool for assessment of brain ischemic alterations after open heart operations. Stroke Res Treat. 2011;2011:980873.

Golukhova EZ, Polunina AG, Zhuravleva SV, Lefterova NP, Begachev AV. Size of left cardiac chambers correlates with cerebral microembolic load in open heart operations. Cardiol Res Pract. 2010;2010:143679.

Grap MJ, Munro CL, Wetzel PA, Ketchum JM, Ketchum JS 3rd, Anderson WL, Best AM, Hamilton VA, Arief NY, Burk R, Bottoms T, Sessler CN. Stimulation of critically ill patients: relationship to sedation. Am J Crit Care. 2016;25:e48–55.

Green D, Paklet L. Latest developments in peri-operative monitoring of the high-risk major surgery patient. Int J Surg. 2010;8:90–9.

Grimm M, Zimpfer D, Czerny M, Kilo J, Kasimir MT, Kramer L, Krokovay A, Wolner E. Neurocognitive deficit following mitral valve surgery. Eur J Cardiothorac Surg. 2003;23:265–71.

Gugino LD, Aglio LS, Yli-Hankala A. Monitoring the electroencephalogram during bypass procedures. Semin Cardiothorac Vasc Anesth. 2004;8:61–83.

Gugino LD, Chabot RJ, Aglio LS, Aranki S, Dekkers R, Maddi R. QEEG changes during cardiopulmonary bypass: relationship to postoperative neuropsychological function. Clin Electroencephalogr. 1999;30:53–63.

Gugino LD, Chabot RJ, Prichep LS, John ER, Formanek V, Aglio LS. Quantitative EEG changes associated with loss and return of consciousness in healthy adult volunteers anaesthetized with propofol or sevoflurane. Br J Anaesth. 2001;87:421–8.

Gupta AK, Hutchinson PJ, Al-Rawi P, Gupta S, Swart M, Kirkpatrick PJ, Menon DK, Datta AK. Measuring brain tissue oxygenation compared with jugular venous oxygen saturation for monitoring cerebral oxygenation after traumatic brain injury. Anesth Analg. 1999;88:549–53.

Halpern SD, Becker D, Curtis JR, Fowler R, Hyzy R, Kaplan LJ, Rawat N, Sessler CN, Wunsch H, Kahn JM. An official American Thoracic Society/American Association of Critical-Care Nurses/American College of Chest Physicians/Society of Critical Care Medicine policy statement: the choosing wisely(R) top 5 list in critical care medicine. Am J Respir Crit Care Med. 2014;190:818–26.

Hampton DA, Schreiber MA. Near infrared spectroscopy: clinical and research uses. Transfusion. 2013;53(Suppl 1):52S–8S.

Hankey GJ. Anticoagulant therapy for patients with ischaemic stroke. Nat Rev Neurol. 2012;8:319–28.

Hasegawa T, Okita Y. Intraoperative monitoring of the brain and spinal cord ischemia during thoracic aortic surgery. Kyobu Geka. 2009;62:655–60.

Hatiboglu MT, Anil A. Structural variations in the jugular foramen of the human skull. J Anat. 1992;180(Pt 1):191–6.

Hauser E, Seidl R, Rohrbach D, Hartl I, Marx M, Wimmer M. Quantitative EEG before and after open heart surgery in children. A significant decrease in the beta and alpha 2 bands postoperatively. Electroencephalogr Clin Neurophysiol. 1993;87:284–90.

Hernandez-Gancedo C, Pestana D, Pena N, Royo C, Perez-Chrzanowska H, Criado A. Monitoring sedation in critically ill patients: bispectral index, Ramsay and observer scales. Eur J Anaesthesiol. 2006;23:649–53.

Hervey-Jumper SL, Annich GM, Yancon AR, Garton HJ, Muraszko KM, Maher CO. Neurological complications of extracorporeal membrane oxygenation in children. J Neurosurg Pediatr. 2011;7:338–44.

Hochberg AR, Young GS. Cerebral perfusion imaging. Semin Neurol. 2012;32:454–65.

Horsfield MA, Jara JL, Saeed NP, Panerai RB, Robinson TG. Regional differences in dynamic cerebral autoregulation in the healthy brain assessed by magnetic resonance imaging. PLoS One. 2013;8:e62588.

Hoshi Y. Functional near-infrared spectroscopy: current status and future prospects. J Biomed Opt. 2007;12:062106.

Hoshi Y. Towards the next generation of near-infrared spectroscopy. Philos Transact A Math Phys Eng Sci. 2011;369:4425–39.

Hu Z, Xu L, Zhu Z, Seal R, McQuillan PM. Effects of hypothermic cardiopulmonary bypass on internal jugular bulb venous oxygen saturation, cerebral oxygen saturation, and bispectral index in pediatric patients undergoing cardiac surgery: a prospective study. Medicine. 2016;95:e2483.

Hudetz AG, Mashour GA. Disconnecting consciousness: is there a common anesthetic end point? Anesth Analg. 2016;123:1228–40.

Huppert TJ, Diamond SG, Franceschini MA, Boas DA. HomER: a review of time-series analysis methods for near-infrared spectroscopy of the brain. Appl Opt. 2009;48:D280–98.

Ip-Yam PC, Thomas SD, Jackson M, Rashid A, Behl S. Effects of temperature strategy during cardiopulmonary bypass on cerebral oxygen balance. J Cardiovasc Surg. 2000;41:1–6.

Isley MR, Edmonds HL Jr, Stecker M. Guidelines for intraoperative neuromonitoring using raw (analog or digital waveforms) and quantitative electroencephalography: a position statement by the American Society of Neurophysiological Monitoring. J Clin Monit Comput. 2009;23:369–90.

Jacobson S, Jerrier H. EEG in delirium. Semin Clin Neuropsychiatry. 2000;5:86–92.

Jameson LC, Sloan TB. Using EEG to monitor anesthesia drug effects during surgery. J Clin Monit Comput. 2006;20:445–72.

Johansen JW, Sebel PS. Development and clinical application of electroencephalographic bispectrum monitoring. Anesthesiology. 2000;93:1336–44.
Kadoi Y, Fujita N. Increasing mean arterial pressure improves jugular venous oxygen saturation in patients with and without preexisting stroke during normothermic cardiopulmonary bypass. J Clin Anesth. 2003;15:339–44.
Kadoi Y, Saito S, Goto F, Fujita N. Slow rewarming has no effects on the decrease in jugular venous oxygen hemoglobin saturation and long-term cognitive outcome in diabetic patients. Anesth Analg. 2002;94:1395–401, table of contents.
Kaposzta Z, Young E, Bath PM, Markus HS. Clinical application of asymptomatic embolic signal detection in acute stroke: a prospective study. Stroke. 1999;30:1814–8.
Kawahara F, Kadoi Y, Saito S, Goto F, Fujita N. Slow rewarming improves jugular venous oxygen saturation during rewarming. Acta Anaesthesiol Scand. 2003;47:419–24.
Kertai MD, Whitlock EL, Avidan MS. Brain monitoring with electroencephalography and the electroencephalogram-derived bispectral index during cardiac surgery. Anesth Analg. 2012;114:533–46.
Kral MC, Brown RT, Nietert PJ, Abboud MR, Jackson SM, Hynd GW. Transcranial Doppler ultrasonography and neurocognitive functioning in children with sickle cell disease. Pediatrics. 2003;112:324–31.
Kumral E, Balkir K, Yagdi T, Kara E, Evyapan D, Bilkay O. Microembolic signals in patients undergoing coronary artery bypass grafting. Effect of aortic atherosclerosis. Tex Heart Inst J. 2001;28:16–20.
La Monaca M, David A, Gaeta R, Lentini S. Near infrared spectroscopy for cerebral monitoring during cardiovascular surgery. Clin Ter. 2010;161:549–53.
Lamas A, Lopez-Herce J. Monitoring sedation in the critically ill child. Anaesthesia. 2010;65:516–24.
Lampe JW, Becker LB. State of the art in therapeutic hypothermia. Annu Rev Med. 2011;62:79–93.
Le Roux P, Menon DK, Citerio G, Vespa P, Bader MK, Brophy G, Diringer MN, Stocchetti N, Videtta W, Armonda R, Badjatia N, Bosel J, Chesnut R, Chou S, Claassen J, Czosnyka M, De Georgia M, Figaji A, Fugate J, Helbok R, Horowitz D, Hutchinson P, Kumar M, McNett M, Miller C, Naidech A, Oddo M, Olson D, O'Phelan K, Provencio JJ, Puppo C, Riker R, Roberson C, Schmidt M, Taccone F. The international multidisciplinary consensus conference on multimodality monitoring in Neurocritical care: a list of recommendations and additional conclusions: a statement for healthcare professionals from the Neurocritical care society and the European Society of Intensive Care Medicine. Neurocrit Care. 2014;21(Suppl 2):S282–96.
Leahy MJ, de Mul FF, Nilsson GE, Maniewski R. Principles and practice of the laser-Doppler perfusion technique. Technol Health Care. 1999;7:143–62.
Li J. Systemic oxygen transport derived by using continuous measured oxygen consumption after the Norwood procedure-an interim review. Interact Cardiovasc Thorac Surg. 2012;15:93–101.
Lima A, van Bommel J, Sikorska K, van Genderen M, Klijn E, Lesaffre E, Ince C, Bakker J. The relation of near-infrared spectroscopy with changes in peripheral circulation in critically ill patients. Crit Care Med. 2011;39:1649–54.
Markowitz SD, Ichord RN, Wernovsky G, Gaynor JW, Nicolson SC. Surrogate markers for neurological outcome in children after deep hypothermic circulatory arrest. Semin Cardiothorac Vasc Anesth. 2007;11:59–65.
Markus HS. Transcranial Doppler ultrasound. J Neurol Neurosurg Psychiatry. 1999;67:135–7.
Markus HS, Reid G. Frequency filtering improves ultrasonic embolic signal detection. Ultrasound Med Biol. 1999;25:857–60.
McDonnell MN, Berry NM, Cutting MA, Keage HA, Buckley JD, Howe PR. Transcranial Doppler ultrasound to assess cerebrovascular reactivity: reliability, reproducibility and effect of posture. PeerJ. 2013;1:e65.
Mills JN, Mehta V, Russin J, Amar AP, Rajamohan A, Mack WJ. Advanced imaging modalities in the detection of cerebral vasospasm. Neurol Res Int. 2013;2013:415960.

Mok V, Ding D, Fu J, Xiong Y, Chu WW, Wang D, Abrigo JM, Yang J, Wong A, Zhao Q, Guo Q, Hong Z, Wong KS. Transcranial Doppler ultrasound for screening cerebral small vessel disease: a community study. Stroke. 2012;43:2791–3.

Moppett IK, Mahajan RP. Transcranial Doppler ultrasonography in anaesthesia and intensive care. Br J Anaesth. 2004;93:710–24.

Murkin JM, Adams SJ, Novick RJ, Quantz M, Bainbridge D, Iglesias I, Cleland A, Schaefer B, Irwin B, Fox S. Monitoring brain oxygen saturation during coronary bypass surgery: a randomized, prospective study. Anesth Analg. 2007;104:51–8.

Nandate K, Vuylsteke A, Ratsep I, Messahel S, Oduro-Dominah A, Menon DK, Matta BF. Effects of isoflurane, sevoflurane and propofol anaesthesia on jugular venous oxygen saturation in patients undergoing coronary artery bypass surgery. Br J Anaesth. 2000;84:631–3.

Nelson DP, Andropoulos DB, Fraser CD Jr. Perioperative neuroprotective strategies. Semin Thorac Cardiovasc Surg Pediatr Card Surg Annu. 2008:49–56.

Newburger JW, Jonas RA, Wernovsky G, Wypij D, Hickey PR, Kuban KC, Farrell DM, Holmes GL, Helmers SL, Constantinou J, et al. A comparison of the perioperative neurologic effects of hypothermic circulatory arrest versus low-flow cardiopulmonary bypass in infant heart surgery. N Engl J Med. 1993;329:1057–64.

Nuwer M. Assessment of digital EEG, quantitative EEG, and EEG brain mapping: report of the American Academy of Neurology and the American Clinical Neurophysiology Society. Neurology. 1997;49:277–92.

O'Connor JP, Tofts PS, Miles KA, Parkes LM, Thompson G, Jackson A. Dynamic contrast-enhanced imaging techniques: CT and MRI. Br J Radiol. 2011;84(2):S112–20.

Obeid AN, Barnett NJ, Dougherty G, Ward G. A critical review of laser Doppler flowmetry. J Med Eng Technol. 1990;14:178–81.

Oh YJ, Kim SH, Shinn HK, Lee CS, Hong YW, Kwak YL. Effects of milrinone on jugular bulb oxygen saturation and cerebrovascular carbon dioxide reactivity in patients undergoing coronary artery bypass graft surgery. Br J Anaesth. 2004;93:634–8.

Olson DM, Thoyre SM, Auyong DB. Perspectives on sedation assessment in critical care. AACN Adv Crit Care. 2007;18:380–95.

Ouellette DR, Patel S, Girard TD, Morris PE, Schmidt GA, Truwit JD, Alhazzani W, Burns SM, Epstein SK, Esteban A, Fan E, Ferrer M, Fraser GL, Gong MN, Hough CL, Mehta S, Nanchal R, Pawlik AJ, Schweickert WD, Sessler CN, Strom T, Kress JP. Liberation from mechanical ventilation in critically ill adults: an official American College of Chest Physicians/American Thoracic Society clinical practice guideline: inspiratory pressure augmentation during spontaneous breathing trials, protocols minimizing sedation, and noninvasive ventilation immediately after Extubation. Chest. 2017;151:166–80.

Palanca BJ, Mashour GA, Avidan MS. Processed electroencephalogram in depth of anesthesia monitoring. Curr Opin Anaesthesiol. 2009;22:553–9.

Palombo G, Stella N, Faraglia V, Taurino M. Aortic arch catheterization during transfemoral carotid artery stenting: an underestimated source of cerebral emboli. Acta Chir Belg. 2010;110:165–8.

Patel N, Minhas JS, Chung EM. Intraoperative embolization and cognitive decline after cardiac surgery: a systematic review. Semin Cardiothorac Vasc Anesth. 2016;20:225–31.

Payen JF, Chanques G, Mantz J, Hercule C, Auriant I, Leguillou JL, Binhas M, Genty C, Rolland C, Bosson JL. Current practices in sedation and analgesia for mechanically ventilated critically ill patients: a prospective multicenter patient-based study. Anesthesiology. 2007;106:687–95; quiz 891-682.

Perez A, Minces PG, Schnitzler EJ, Agosta GE, Medina SA, Ciraolo CA. Jugular venous oxygen saturation or arteriovenous difference of lactate content and outcome in children with severe traumatic brain injury. Pediatr Crit Care Med. 2003;4:33–8.

Poe GR, Walsh CM, Bjorness TE. Cognitive neuroscience of sleep. Prog Brain Res. 2010;185:1–19.

Portnow LH, Vaillancourt DE, Okun MS. The history of cerebral PET scanning: from physiology to cutting-edge technology. Neurology. 2013;80:952–6.

Pua HL, Bissonnette B. Cerebral physiology in paediatric cardiopulmonary bypass. Can J Anaesth. 1998;45:960–78.

Purdon PL, Pierce ET, Mukamel EA, Prerau MJ, Walsh JL, Wong KF, Salazar-Gomez AF, Harrell PG, Sampson AL, Cimenser A, Ching S, Kopell NJ, Tavares-Stoeckel C, Habeeb K, Merhar R, Brown EN. Electroencephalogram signatures of loss and recovery of consciousness from propofol. Proc Natl Acad Sci U S A. 2013;110:E1142–51.

Purdon PL, Sampson A, Pavone KJ, Brown EN. Clinical electroencephalography for anesthesiologists: Part I: background and basic signatures. Anesthesiology. 2015;123:937–60.

Radovanovic D, Radovanovic Z. Awareness during general anaesthesia—implications of explicit intraoperative recall. Eur Rev Med Pharmacol Sci. 2011;15:1085–9.

Radvany MG, Wholey M. Expanding use of embolic protection devices. Semin Interv Radiol. 2008;25:27–36.

Ramsay MA, Savege TM, Simpson BR, Goodwin R. Controlled sedation with alphaxalone-alphadolone. Br Med J. 1974;2:656–9.

Rao GS, Durga P. Changing trends in monitoring brain ischemia: from intracranial pressure to cerebral oximetry. Curr Opin Anaesthesiol. 2011;24:487–94.

Rasmussen LS, Sperling B, Abildstrom HH, Moller JT. Neuron loss after coronary artery bypass detected by SPECT estimation of benzodiazepine receptors. Ann Thorac Surg. 2002;74:1576–80.

Rasulo FA, De Peri E, Lavinio A. Transcranial Doppler ultrasonography in intensive care. Eur J Anaesthesiol Suppl. 2008;42:167–73.

Riker RR, Fraser GL, Simmons LE, Wilkins ML. Validating the sedation-agitation scale with the bispectral index and visual analog scale in adult ICU patients after cardiac surgery. Intensive Care Med. 2001;27:853–8.

Riker RR, Picard JT, Fraser GL. Prospective evaluation of the sedation-agitation scale for adult critically ill patients. Crit Care Med. 1999;27:1325–9.

Robba C, Cardim D, Sekhon M, Budohoski K, Czosnyka M. Transcranial Doppler: a stethoscope for the brain-neurocritical care use. J Neurosci Res. 2017. https://doi.org/10.1002/jnr.24148.

Roggenbach J, Rauch H. Type a dissection. Principles of anesthesiological management. Anaesthesist. 2011;60:139–51.

Rohlwink UK, Figaji AA. Methods of monitoring brain oxygenation. Childs Nerv Syst. 2010;26:453–64.

Rolfe P. In vivo near-infrared spectroscopy. Annu Rev Biomed Eng. 2000;2:715–54.

Rollins MD, Hubbard A, Zabrocki L, Barnhart DC, Bratton SL. Extracorporeal membrane oxygenation cannulation trends for pediatric respiratory failure and central nervous system injury. J Pediatr Surg. 2012;47:68–75.

Sarrafzadeh AS, Kiening KL, Unterberg AW. Neuromonitoring: brain oxygenation and microdialysis. Curr Neurol Neurosci Rep. 2003;3:517–23.

Scheeren TW, Schober P, Schwarte LA. Monitoring tissue oxygenation by near infrared spectroscopy (NIRS): background and current applications. J Clin Monit Comput. 2012;26:279–87.

Schell RM, Cole DJ. Cerebral monitoring: jugular venous oximetry. Anesth Analg. 2000;90:559–66.

Schmidt B, Klingelhofer J, Schwarze JJ, Sander D, Wittich I. Noninvasive prediction of intracranial pressure curves using transcranial Doppler ultrasonography and blood pressure curves. Stroke. 1997;28:2465–72.

Sebel PS. Central nervous system monitoring during open heart surgery: an update. J Cardiothorac Vasc Anesth. 1998;12:3–8.

Sellmann T, Winterhalter M, Herold U, Kienbaum P. Implantation of cardioverter-defibrillators. How much anesthesia is necessary? Anaesthesist. 2010;59:507–18.

Sessler CN, Gosnell MS, Grap MJ, Brophy GM, O'Neal PV, Keane KA, Tesoro EP, Elswick RK. The Richmond agitation-sedation scale: validity and reliability in adult intensive care unit patients. Am J Respir Crit Care Med. 2002;166:1338–44.

Sessler CN, Grap MJ, Ramsay MA. Evaluating and monitoring analgesia and sedation in the intensive care unit. Crit Care. 2008;12(Suppl 3):S2.

Seule M, Muroi C, Sikorski C, Keller E. Monitoring of cerebral hemodynamics and oxygenation to detect delayed ischemic neurological deficit after aneurysmal subarachnoid hemorrhage. Acta Neurochir Suppl. 2013;115:57–61.

Shaaban Ali M, Harmer M, Latto I. Jugular bulb oximetry during cardiac surgery. Anaesthesia. 2001;56:24–37.

Sheinberg M, Kanter MJ, Robertson CS, Contant CF, Narayan RK, Grossman RG. Continuous monitoring of jugular venous oxygen saturation in head-injured patients. J Neurosurg. 1992;76:212–7.

Shimizu N, Gilder F, Bissonnette B, Coles J, Bohn D, Miyasaka K. Brain tissue oxygenation index measured by near infrared spatially resolved spectroscopy agreed with jugular bulb oxygen saturation in normal pediatric brain: a pilot study. Childs Nerv Syst. 2005;21:181–4.

Simmons LE, Riker RR, Prato BS, Fraser GL. Assessing sedation during intensive care unit mechanical ventilation with the Bispectral index and the sedation-agitation scale. Crit Care Med. 1999;27:1499–504.

Slater JP, Guarino T, Stack J, Vinod K, Bustami RT, Brown JM 3rd, Rodriguez AL, Magovern CJ, Zaubler T, Freundlich K, Parr GV. Cerebral oxygen desaturation predicts cognitive decline and longer hospital stay after cardiac surgery. Ann Thorac Surg. 2009;87:36–44; discussion 44-35.

Smith M. Shedding light on the adult brain: a review of the clinical applications of near-infrared spectroscopy. Philos Transact A Math Phys Eng Sci. 2011;369:4452–69.

Smythe PR, Samra SK. Monitors of cerebral oxygenation. Anesthesiol Clin North Am. 2002;20:293–313.

Soustiel JF, Bruk B, Shik B, Hadani M, Feinsod M. Transcranial Doppler in vertebrobasilar vasospasm after subarachnoid hemorrhage. Neurosurgery. 1998;43:282–91; discussion 291-283.

Stern E, Silbersweig DA. Advances in functional neuroimaging methodology for the study of brain systems underlying human neuropsychological function and dysfunction. J Clin Exp Neuropsychol. 2001;23:3–18.

Stevens WJ. Multimodal monitoring: head injury management using SjvO2 and LICOX. J Neurosci Nurs. 2004;36:332–9.

Stocchetti N, Canavesi K, Magnoni S, Valeriani V, Conte V, Rossi S, Longhi L, Zanier ER, Colombo A. Arterio-jugular difference of oxygen content and outcome after head injury. Anesth Analg. 2004;99:230–4.

Sturzenegger M, Mattle HP, Rivoir A, Baumgartner RW. Ultrasound findings in carotid artery dissection: analysis of 43 patients. Neurology. 1995;45:691–8.

Svyatets M, Tolani K, Zhang M, Tulman G, Charchaflieh J. Perioperative management of deep hypothermic circulatory arrest. J Cardiothorac Vasc Anesth. 2010;24:644–55.

Thuong M. Sedation and analgesia assessment tools in ICU patients. Ann Fr Anesth Reanim. 2008;27:581–95.

Tsygan NV. The algorithm of the comprehensive assessment of the brain during cardiac surgery with cardiopulmonary bypass. Voen Med Zh. 2012;333:42–6.

Uehara T, Tabuchi M, Kozawa S, Mori E. MR angiographic evaluation of carotid and intracranial arteries in Japanese patients scheduled for coronary artery bypass grafting. Cerebrovasc Dis. 2001;11:341–5.

Vajkoczy P, Horn P, Thome C, Munch E, Schmiedek P. Regional cerebral blood flow monitoring in the diagnosis of delayed ischemia following aneurysmal subarachnoid hemorrhage. J Neurosurg. 2003;98:1227–34.

Vance JL, Shanks AM, Woodrum DT. Intraoperative bispectral index monitoring and time to extubation after cardiac surgery: secondary analysis of a randomized controlled trial. BMC Anesthesiol. 2014;14:79.

Veel T, Bugge JF, Kirkeboen KA, Pleym H. Anaesthesia for open-heart surgery in adults. Tidsskr Nor Laegeforen. 2010;130:618–22.

Vohra HA, Modi A, Ohri SK. Does use of intra-operative cerebral regional oxygen saturation monitoring during cardiac surgery lead to improved clinical outcomes? Interact Cardiovasc Thorac Surg. 2009;9:318–22.

von Knobelsdorff G, Hanel F, Werner C, Schulte am Esch J. Jugular bulb oxygen saturation and middle cerebral blood flow velocity during cardiopulmonary bypass. J Neurosurg Anesthesiol. 1997;9:128–33.

Watson BD, Kane-Gill SL. Sedation assessment in critically ill adults: 2001-2004 update. Ann Pharmacother. 2004;38:1898–906.

Weigl W, Milej D, Janusek D, Wojtkiewicz S, Sawosz P, Kacprzak M, Gerega A, Maniewski R, Liebert A. Application of optical methods in the monitoring of traumatic brain injury: a review. J Cereb Blood Flow Metab. 2016;36:1825–43.

White H, Baker A. Continuous jugular venous oximetry in the neurointensive care unit—a brief review. Can J Anaesth. 2002;49:623–9.

Williams GD, Ramamoorthy C. Brain monitoring and protection during pediatric cardiac surgery. Semin Cardiothorac Vasc Anesth. 2007;11:23–33.

Wolf M, Ferrari M, Quaresima V. Progress of near-infrared spectroscopy and topography for brain and muscle clinical applications. J Biomed Opt. 2007;12:062104.

Wright WL. Multimodal monitoring in the ICU: when could it be useful? J Neurol Sci. 2007;261:10–5.

Young CC, Prielipp RC. Benzodiazepines in the intensive care unit. Crit Care Clin. 2001;17:843–62.

Zeitlhofer J, Saletu B, Anderer P, Asenbaum S, Spiss C, Mohl W, Kasall H, Wolner E, Deecke L. Topographic brain mapping of EEG before and after open-heart surgery. Neuropsychobiology. 1988;20:51–6.

Zimpfer D, Czerny M, Kilo J, Kasimir MT, Madl C, Kramer L, Wieselthaler GM, Wolner E, Grimm M. Cognitive deficit after aortic valve replacement. Ann Thorac Surg. 2002;74:407–12; discussion 412.

Zurynski YA, Dorsch NW, Fearnside MR. Incidence and effects of increased cerebral blood flow velocity after severe head injury: a transcranial Doppler ultrasound study II. Effect of vasospasm and hyperemia on outcome. J Neurol Sci. 1995;134:41–6.

Postoperative Coagulation and Bleeding: Monitoring and Hematologic Management After Adult Cardiac Surgery

7

Dominic Emerson and Ali Dabbagh

Abstract

There is a never-ending physiologic balance between thrombotic and antithrombotic factors in vivo. However, this balance changes to a major challenge in cardiac surgery which is a potential dilemma for postoperative care: what is the ideal goal in postoperative management of bleeding and hemostasis in these patients, especially when considering the importance of preoperative, intraoperative, and postoperative factors on the thrombosis and coagulation cascade?

The postoperative management of coagulation in adult cardiac surgery patients follows the rules of medicine with a specific focus on medication history, all coexisting diseases or comorbidities, including but not limited to previous events in the coagulation system. Postoperative test especially point-of-care battery of tests has an important role in the diagnosis of underlying conditions, TEG® and ROTEM® being part of these tests. Treatment includes pharmaceutical agents, blood component therapy, and surgical management, each of them with specific benefits, merits, and potential disadvantages which are discussed in detail in this chapter.

Keywords

Physiology of coagulation and bleeding · Oral anticoagulants/antiplatelet agents Parenteral anticoagulants/antiplatelet agents · Prothrombin time (PT)

D. Emerson, M.D.
Cardiothoracic Surgery, Department of Surgery, Cedars Sinai Medical Center, Los Angeles, CA, USA
e-mail: Dominic.Emerson@cshs.org

A. Dabbagh, M.D. (✉)
Faculty of Medicine, Cardiac Anesthesiology Department, Anesthesiology Research Center, Shahid Beheshti University of Medical Sciences, Tehran, Iran

Cardiac Anesthesiology Fellowship Program, Shahid Beheshti University of Medical Sciences, Tehran, Iran
e-mail: alidabbagh@sbmu.ac.ir

A. Dabbagh et al. (eds.), *Postoperative Critical Care for Adult Cardiac Surgical Patients*, https://doi.org/10.1007/978-3-319-75747-6_7

International normalized ratio (INR) · Partial thromboplastin time (PTT) Platelet count · Fibrinogen level · Thromboelastography (TEG) · Rotational thromboelastography (ROTEM) · Heparin-induced thrombocytopenia (HIT) Antifibrinolytic agents · Cryoprecipitate · Fibrinogen · Human prothrombin complex (PCC) · Activated recombinant factor 7 (rFVIIa) · Factor eight inhibitor bypass activity (FEIBA) · Surgical management of bleeding

7.1 Overview of Postoperative Bleeding in Adult Cardiac Surgery Patients

Cardiac surgery presents unique challenges with regard to the presence and management of postoperative bleeding. Management of the postoperative cardiac surgical patient is often complicated by acquired hemostatic derangements, which arise from multiple factors primarily stemming from the use of cardiopulmonary bypass (CPB). These changes in hemostatic pathways derive from a multitude of factors, including hemodilution, fibrinolysis, acquired platelet dysfunction, and loss of coagulation factors. Most bleeding and blood utilization occur in patients who can be determined to be high risk preoperatively, and a detailed assessment of preoperative risk is essential. Factors that contribute include advanced age, preoperative anemia, small body size, urgent/emergent operation, planned noncoronary artery bypass graft operation, preoperative antithrombotic drugs, acquired or congenital coagulation/clotting abnormalities, and multiple patient comorbidities (Ferraris et al. 2007). Most patients who present today for cardiac surgery have at least one of these factors, and even in cases where the patient is of lower risk, the potential for postoperative bleeding is always present. An understanding of the hemostatic process, derangements to this process, and how to evaluate them, as well as interventions taken to correct such derangements, is key to good outcomes within this population. The following chapter presents an overview of these elements for the postoperative cardiac surgery patient.

7.1.1 Physiology of Coagulation and Bleeding

The physiology of human coagulation is a complex process that is beyond the scope of this chapter. However, a brief overview of the essential components follows.

The coagulation cascade involves multiple actors functioning as a combination of coagulation activating and inhibiting forces that serve to, in the normal physiologic state, rapidly provide cessation of bleeding when needed while preserving normal blood flow elsewhere. The procoagulant system is divided into two parts, the intrinsic and extrinsic pathways, with both pathways culminating in the formation of cross-linked fibrin. In normal physiology, the extrinsic pathway predominates, with the inciting event here being the exposure of blood to tissue factor (TF) due to trauma (this pathway is also known as the tissue factor pathway). TF is then exposed to circulating factor VII, which converts to VIIa in a TF-VIIa complex. This

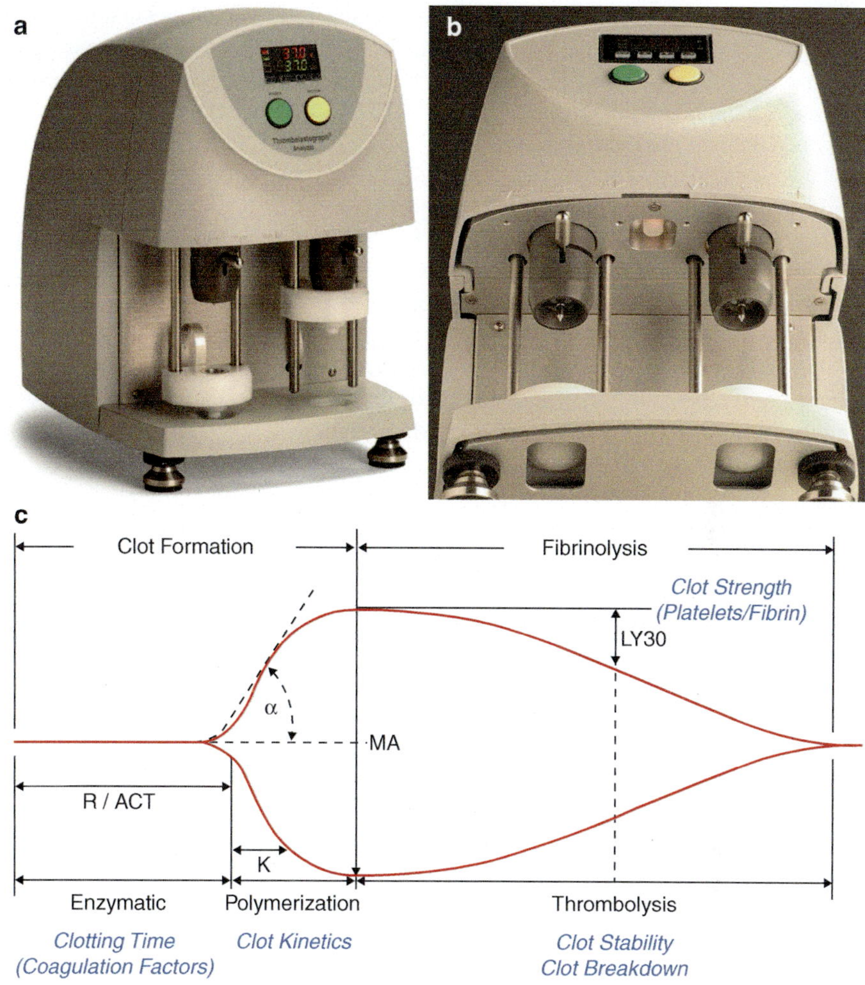

Fig. 7.1 (**a**) TEG front viewed from left middle. (**b**) TEG closeup pins. (**c**) Analytic graph of TEG. With kind permission of Haemonetics Corporation S.A. Suisse

complex is an extremely potent activator of factors IX and X, which in turn have downstream effects leading to prothrombin's conversion to thrombin. Thrombin rapidly converts fibrinogen to the active fibrin, as well as activates other factors, leading to clot formation (Fig. 7.1).

The intrinsic pathway appears to be less important in normal physiology but becomes more significant when the blood is exposed to foreign material, such as during CPB or in patients with ventricular assist devices. The initiating steps here involve blood interaction with foreign material and exposed collagen, which activates factor XII and leads to downstream activation of other factors. This culminates with the activation of factor X, resulting in downstream effects that are identical to the extrinsic pathway detailed above after the activation of factor X. The pathway following the activation of factor X is dubbed the common pathway, as it is shared by both. In vivo, the two pathways act in concert with each other, and the designation of different "pathways" is somewhat of a false division; however, this nomenclature is standard within the medical literature and serves to help with discrimination between the two groups.

At every step noted above, the fibrinolytic system is working to balance the onset and advancement of the coagulation cascade. Multiple actors, including tissue plasminogen activator (tPA; degrades fibrin), heparin-like glycosaminoglycans (stimulate antithrombin which inactivates thrombin), tissue factor pathway inhibitor (TFPI; inhibits factor Xa and the TF-VIIa complex), and thrombomodulin (activates protein C), among others, serve to keep coagulation in check.

Under normal circumstances, these multiple components act in concert to maintain a normal physiologic coagulation and fibrinolytic system. This system is significantly affected by the use of CPB and experiences derangements that can lead to postoperative coagulopathy and bleeding.

7.2 Preoperative Medication-Related Risk Factors

Alterations in the patient's coagulation system that are related to preoperative medications are a significant factor in intraoperative and postoperative bleeding. A brief discussion regarding common medication that may contribute is detailed below.

7.2.1 Oral Anticoagulants/Antiplatelet Agents

Patients are frequently on home doses of oral anticoagulants or antiplatelet agents. These agents can be a significant cause for bleeding and may be problematic as the duration of effects after cessation is often variable. Special consideration must be made to patients with impaired renal or hepatic function. Recommendations for some common medication are as follows.

7.2.1.1 Warfarin

Warfarin (Coumadin) is one of the most widely prescribed anticoagulants worldwide and is a common preoperative medication for this population. It acts by inhibiting the production of vitamin K-dependent factors in the liver, resulting in a reduction of factors II, VII, IX, and X as well as protein C and S and a measurable elevation in the INR. Cessation of warfarin is required for at least 4 days to allow these factors to replenish; if more urgent surgery is required, vitamin K may be given to accelerate the natural replacement of factors or factors replaced directly with FFP.

7.2.1.2 Aspirin

Aspirin is the most common antiplatelet drug given worldwide. It irreversibly binds and inhibits thromboxane A2, limiting platelet aggregation and function. Bleeding risk may be slightly increased with platelet dysfunction, but aspirin is often continued up until the time of surgery as survival has been demonstrated to be improved in CABG with continuation of aspirin (Dacey et al. 2000). If it is to be discontinued, cessation should occur at least 3–4 days prior to surgery due to the irreversible inhibition of platelet function (resolving the platelet inhibition requires creation of new platelets). More rapid reversal requires the administration of platelets. To evaluate the effect of aspirin, a TEG should be performed as platelet count is not an effective indicator.

7.2.1.3 Clopidogrel (Plavix)

Clopidogrel is an irreversible platelet inhibitor that acts by inhibiting the P2Y12 ADP receptor. Due to the irreversible effect of the drug, current STS guidelines indicate that discontinuation should occur at least 3 days before surgery (level I recommendation) (Ferraris et al. 2007), with most surgeons allowing 5–7 days before surgery. Reversal is not possible, and administration of platelets may be required if operative intervention is required earlier.

7.2.1.4 Rivaroxaban (Xarelto) and Apixaban (Eliquis)

Rivaroxaban and apixaban are highly selective factor Xa inhibitors that have gained popularity as dosing does not require routine monitoring of labs. With a half-life of between 5 and 9 h for rivaroxaban and 9 and 14 h for apixaban, cessation of the medication should occur at least 24 and 48 h before the planned operation for rivaroxaban and apixaban, respectively. More urgent reversal may be accomplished with prothrombin complex concentrates (Eerenberg et al. 2011); however, this strategy appears to be more effective with rivaroxaban than apixaban.

7.2.1.5 Dabigatran (Pradaxa)

Dabigatran is a direct thrombin inhibitor that, like the direct Xa inhibitors above, may be taken without routine monitoring. Drug activity can be assessed with PTT. Cessation should occur at least 2–3 days before surgery is planned. In cases where urgent reversal is needed, a reversal agent (idarucizumab (Praxbind)) is available and effective.

7.2.2 Parenteral Anticoagulants/Antiplatelet Agents

7.2.2.1 Heparin

Both unfractionated (UFH) and low-molecular-weight (LMWH) heparin act to increase the activity of antithrombin III, with resultant inactivation of thrombin, factor Xa, and other proteases. Measurement of heparin effect with the PTT is effective only for UFH. Reversal is often not required for UFH as the half-life is short, though urgent reversal with protamine is effective when required. LMWH should be stopped 24 h before surgery when possible, and reversal with protamine is less effective but possible (Kincaid et al. 2003).

7.2.2.2 Eptifibatide (Integrilin) and Tirofiban (Aggrastat)

Both eptifibatide and tirofiban are short-acting reversible platelet inhibitors that function by inhibition of glycoprotein IIb/IIa. These medications serve as a good option for bridging patients on clopidogrel who cannot come off platelet inhibitors. Current recommendations indicate that stopping infusions at least 4 h before surgery is sufficient to restore around 80% of function (Ferraris et al. 2007).

7.2.2.3 Abciximab (ReoPro)

Abciximab also acts to inhibit IIb/IIIa in a reversible fashion; however, it has a much longer half-life than eptifibatide or tirofiban, at around 12 h. Surgery should be delayed by at least 12 and ideally 24 h to reduce the risk of bleeding. More urgent operations will require administration of platelets.

7.2.2.4 Argatroban

Argatroban is a short-acting direct thrombin inhibitor with a half-life of less than 1 h. Due to the rapid elimination, cessation of the medication can occur between 3 and 4 h before the time of surgery. No specific reversal agent exists.

7.2.3 Supplements

Nutritional supplement usage is on the rise, with up to 20–30% of patients in the United States using some form of supplement, typically without any physician oversight. These supplements are often unregulated in terms of quality and substance and are potential sources for drug-induced coagulopathy. Common supplements that are known to have anticoagulant effects include arnica, garlic, ginseng, kelp extract, and licorice (platelet dysfunction), among others. As the effects are variable, it is our practice to have patients stop all supplements at least a week prior to surgery.

7.3 Monitoring

Upon arriving to the ICU and serially thereafter, patients should undergo an assessment of their bleeding status, including monitoring chest tube output, hemodynamics, and laboratory values. The initial assessment of the patient in the ICU should take place with both the surgical team and ICU team present, to facilitate a comprehensive handoff of care. Monitoring of chest tube output should occur at frequent intervals, at least hourly, while in the ICU, and this evaluation should include both quantity of fluid and the quality (bloody, serous, etc.). Tubes should also be frequently checked for patency, to ensure no clot has obstructed the lumen. Sudden changes in output should be brought to the attention of the surgical team immediately, with the caveat that patients may "dump" from chest tubes when turned or when ambulating for the first time and that this fluid is merely volume that had accumulated in the chest over time rather than a new onset of bleeding.

Laboratory values should be obtained serially, and a brief description of the most commonly obtained studies to evaluate coagulopathy in this population follows.

7.3.1 Prothrombin Time (PT)/International Normalized Ratio (INR)

This test evaluates the extrinsic coagulation cascade (factors I (fibrinogen) , II (prothrombin), V, VII, X), with the raw PT value normalized to the institution and reported as the INR. The INR is commonly elevated following CPB due to depletion of factors, and elevations in the setting of bleeding can be corrected with FFP. A mild to moderately elevated INR without evidence of ongoing bleeding does not warrant correction with FFP (Dacey et al. 2000).

7.3.2 Partial Thromboplastin Time (PTT)

The PTT assesses the intrinsic arm of the coagulation cascade (factors I, II, V, VIII, IX, X, XI, XII). It is notably affected by heparin, whereas the INR is not. An elevated PTT in the setting of bleeding in the postoperative patient is concerning for continued heparin effect and may be addressed with an additional protamine dose (see below).

7.3.3 Platelet Count

The use of CPB causes a reduction in platelet counts, as well as some degree of platelet dysfunction, which is variable. It is our practice to transfuse platelets when the level drops below 100,000 in the bleeding patient, but in those without evidence of bleeding, this value should be simply monitored unless it drops below 50,000. It is important to remember that many agents contribute to platelet dysfunction (aspirin and clopidogrel being the most common) and that the administration of platelets in the setting of dysfunction is often required in cases of ongoing bleeding, even with a normal platelet count. Assessment of platelet function requires additional testing (see TEG below).

7.3.4 Fibrinogen Level

Fibrinogen (also known as factor I) serves to help with platelet aggregation and platelet-platelet binding. Circulating fibrinogen is decreased by CPB, and intervention is typically required in cases where the level drops below 100 and bleeding is ongoing. Cryoprecipitate contains high levels of fibrinogen (as well as factors VIII and XIII) and is used as a replacement when needed.

7.3.5 TEG and ROTEM

Thromboelastography (TEG) and rotational thromboelastography (ROTEM) are two tests of whole blood coagulation that use activated blood to measure coagulation in multiple different parameters. They maintain several advantages over standard lab values such as PT/PTT, but the tests themselves are more difficult to perform, require special blood handling, and are not available at all centers. These costs come with the advantage of a more complete analysis of the entire coagulation cascade, including the effects of specific factors and both thrombosis and fibrinolysis effects. The TEG and ROTEM performed today are computer controlled and generally result in a set of values alongside the expected normal ranges for the individual center. A brief discussion of their mechanism and the resultant values follows which is accompanied by Figs. 7.1, 7.2, 7.3, 7.4, and 7.5.

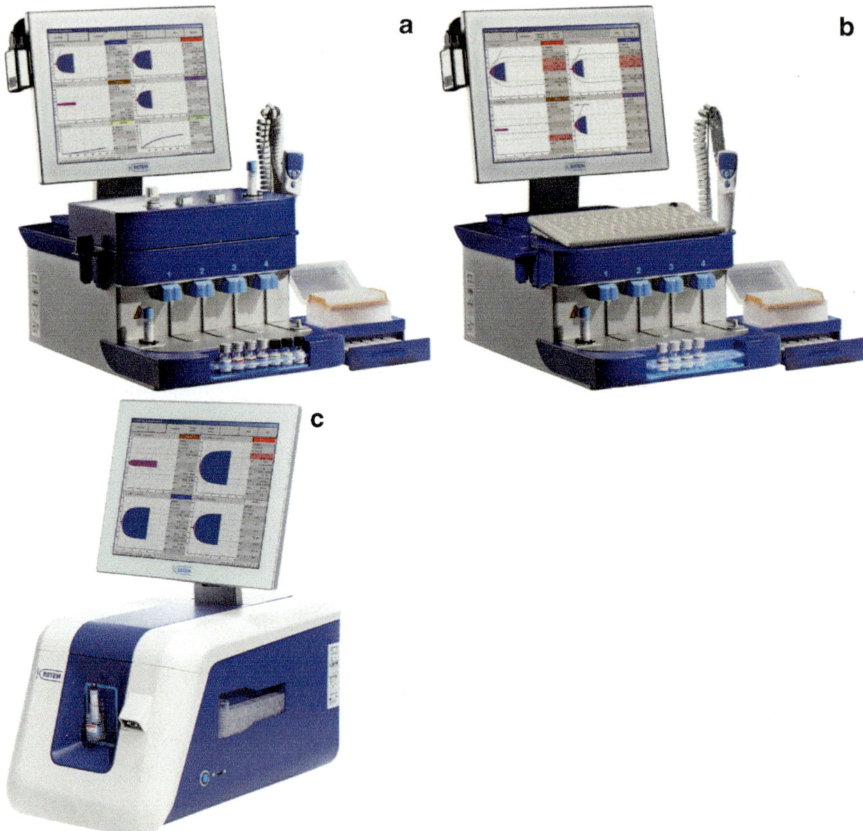

Fig. 7.2 Different versions of the monitor. (**a**) ROTEM delta platelet. (**b**) ROTEM delta. (**c**) ROTEM sigma. With kind permission of and by courtesy of Instrumentation Laboratory, ROTEM®, Tem International GmbH, Munich, Germany

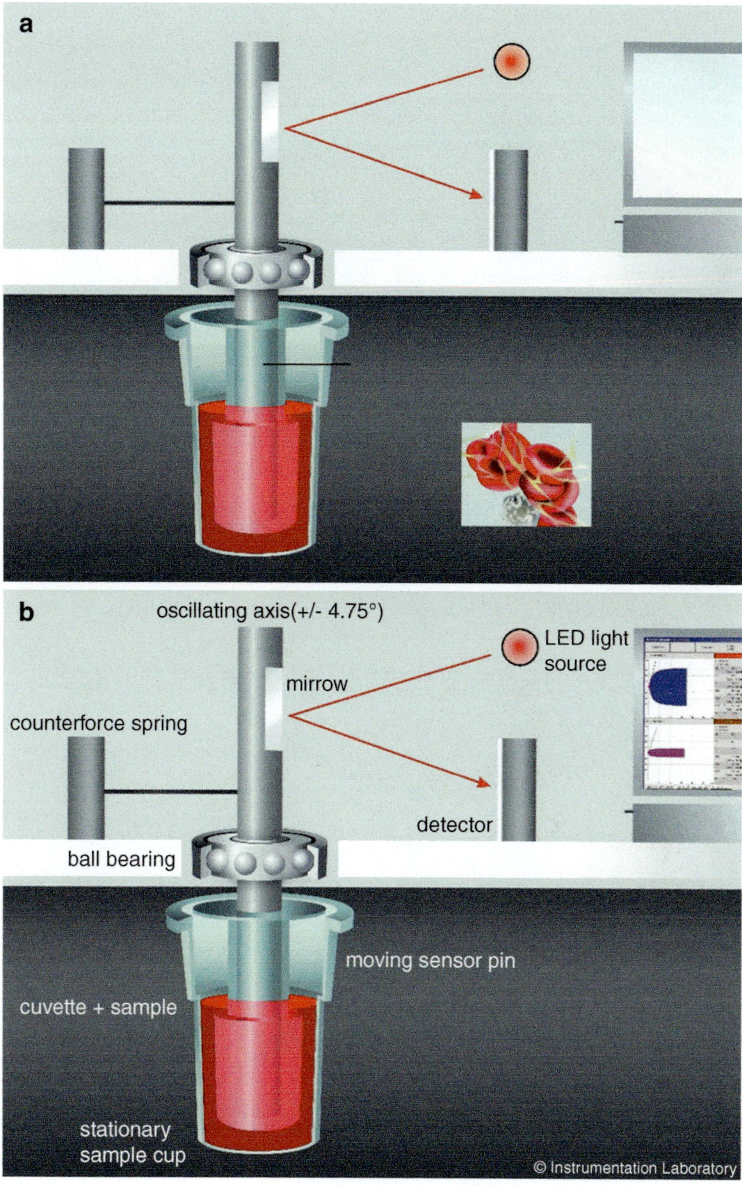

Fig. 7.3 Mechanism of function and measurement principles of ROTEM. A cuvette is used for sampling whole blood; then, the cylindrical pin is inserted and put down well the blood sample. There is a 1 mm gap between the cuvette and the pin which is filled with blood sample. The pin has a continuous rotational movement right and left. As long as the viscosity of blood permits, this rotational left-right-sided movement continues; however, whenever the blood clots, there is more and more hindrance against movement until the movement is stopped at all. This process, which is simplified, is transformed by an internal computer and its software program to the demonstrated graphs and clotting indices. With kind permission of and by courtesy of Instrumentation Laboratory, ROTEM®, Tem International GmbH, Munich, Germany

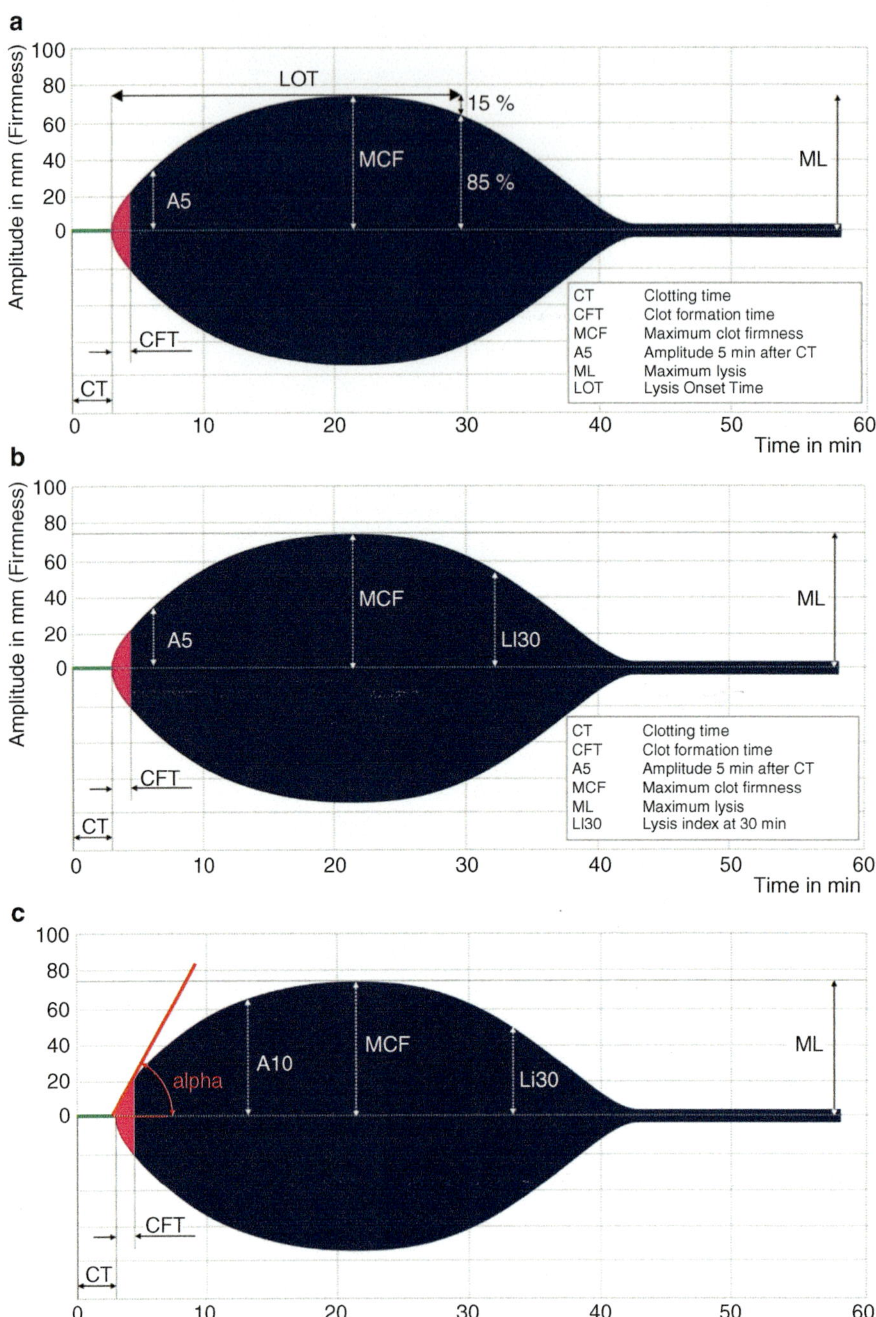

Fig. 7.3 (continued)

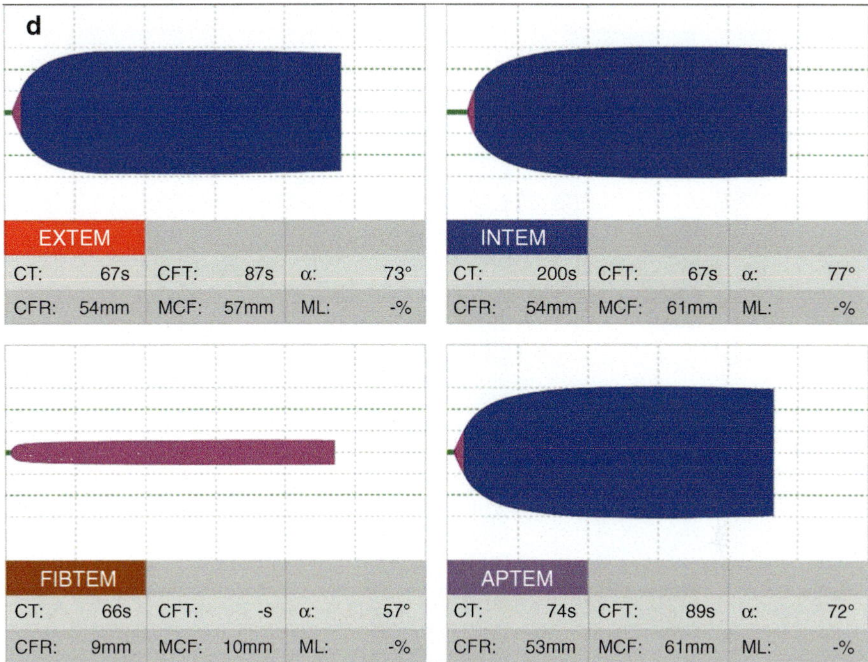

Fig. 7.4 Interpretation of normal graphs in ROTEM. (**a**) Lysis onset time (LOT). (**b**) Amplitude 4 min after clotting time (A5). (**c**) Alpha angle of the starting clot. (**d**) Normal graph sample, demonstrating EXTEM, INTEM, FIBTEM, and APTEM. With kind permission of and by courtesy of Instrumentation Laboratory, ROTEM®, Tem International GmbH, Munich, Germany

The working principles for both devices are similar: the viscosity of blood sample used in the device and its change over time when it is changed to polymerized fibrin are the basis for operation in both devices. There is just an operational difference summarized in Table 7.1:

- TEG®: the tray rotates right to left longitudinally for ±4.75°, and the pin has no movement; the pin checks whenever the range of motion of the tray is decreased to make the graph based on the trend of movement.
- ROTEM®: the pin rotates while the tray is fixed with no movements; whenever fibrin production starts, pin movements are restricted, sensed, and traced by the tray resulting in electronic graph.

7.3.6 Parameter Definition in TEG®

R time: Activation of the clotting cascade is initiated in the sample with the addition of kaolin, which induces the intrinsic pathway. The R time is the reaction time to initial fibrin formation; this is a representation of the intrinsic pathway function.

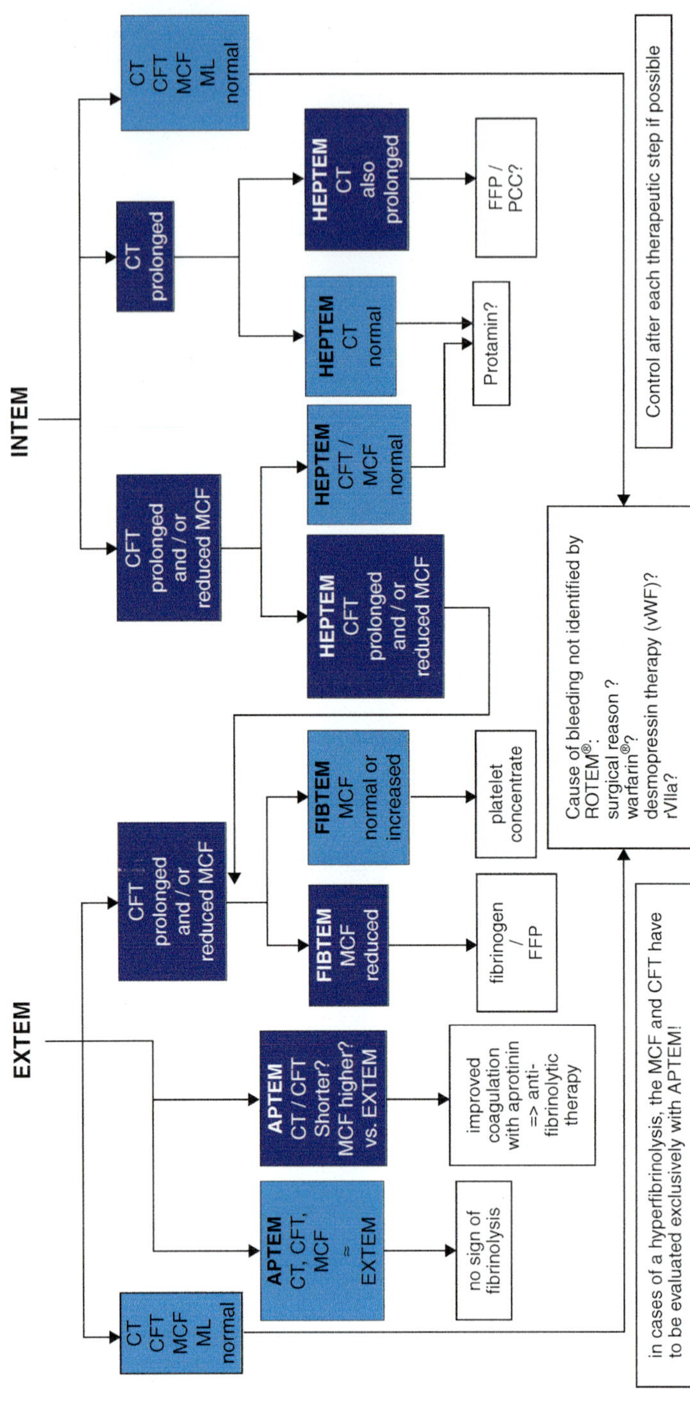

Fig. 7.5 Differential diagnosis of coagulation disorders based on ROTEM results. Find the two different pathways indicated as INTEM and EXTEM with their resulting algorithm. With kind permission of and by courtesy of Instrumentation Laboratory, ROTEM®, Tem International GmbH, Munich, Germany

Table 7.1 Parameters and operational difference in TEG® and ROTEM®; see also Figs. 7.1, 7.2, 7.3, 7.4, and 7.5

Parameter name in TEG®	Parameter name in ROTEM®	Definition of the time interval	Which part of graph is composed of this variable?	The measured variable outcome	Factors affecting this parameter
R time (reaction time)	CT (clotting time)	Time measured in seconds from the start of measurement till the beginning of clot formation	The part of graph from its beginning until the graph reaches an amplitude of 2 mm in terms of seconds	The speed in fibrin formation	• Coagulation factors in plasma • Anticoagulants in circulation
α angle	CFT (clot formation time)	Time after clotting until interaction between a number of factors is done for clot formation and is known as clot kinetics (K)	Part of graph in seconds that the width of graph increases from 2–20 mm	Affected by many variables; so it is a nonspecific parameter	• Anticoagulants • Coagulating factors • Polymerization of fibrin • Stability of the clot (platelets, fibrin, and FXIII)
MA: Maximal graph amplitude	MCF: Maximum clot firmness	The measurement in mm of the graph that demonstrates maximal graph firmness	The thickest part of the normal graph	During the process of fibrin polymerization, the increased polymerization between fibrin, platelets, and FXIII is translated as this parameter; hence it indicates "the maximal clot firmness" and is one of the most important parameters	The cumulative result of all coagulation parameters creating the most strong segment of clot firmness

TEG-ACT (rapid TEG®): The TEG-ACT is a variation on the traditional TEG®, in that the activating agent for clot formation (kaolin) is supplemented with tissue factor (TF). This addition activates both the intrinsic and extrinsic pathways. The resultant activation time is analogous to the R time, with a shorter normal time to activation (80–140 s) and with a value that represents the function of both intrinsic and extrinsic pathways.

K time: The kinetic time (K time) represents the time required for fibrin cross-linking to reach a specified strength. This value is dependent on fibrinogen and platelet count.

α angle: The angle created between the x-axis and a line drawn between the baseline and the curve of the clot formation plot (see diagram below). Depicts fibrinogen and platelet count effects.

Maximum amplitude (MA): It is the widest point on the clot formation plot, depicting effects of platelet function and count.

A30 or LY30: It represents the rate of fibrinolysis at 30 min. High values here demonstrate excessive fibrinolysis.

Interventions for derangements in TEG values are typically managed with FFP for elevated R time or TEG-ACT time, cryoprecipitate alone for elevated K times, cryoprecipitate with or without platelets in the setting of a narrow α angle, platelets alone for low MA, and TXA for rapid fibrinolysis (elevated A30/LY30).

7.3.7 Parameter Definition in ROTEM®

ROTEM® has four channels for selecting among the below; EXTEM and INTEM are the first tests to be done; other tests including FIBTEM, HAPTEM, APTEM, and NATEM are done with comparison to the two former tests (Table 7.2).

7.4 Postoperative Factors

Multiple postoperative factors may ultimately effect bleeding in the postoperative cardiac surgery patient. An adequate understanding of these factors is essential to assessment and management of bleeding in the cardiac surgery patient.

7.4.1 Medications

Multiple medications administered in the perioperative and postoperative period can have effects on bleeding. The most significant effects are seen from medications that cause direct effects, such as medication-induced thrombocytopenia or the effects of residual heparin, but important consideration should also be paid to drug interactions, such as the potentiation of warfarin with the concomitant administration of amiodarone. Careful review of medications administered should be performed frequently by pharmacy staff to avoid complications.

Heparin: Cardiac surgery requires large doses of heparin, which are reversed with protamine at the end of the case. This reversal can be assessed by the ACT and heparin levels, typically obtained at the end of the case while still in the operating room. While the initial reversal may be effective, a "heparin rebound" effect is often seen as residual heparin redistributes and may be significant in up to 50% of patients

Table 7.2 The six different tests used in ROTEM®

Specific tests of ROTEM®	Definition in brief	Factors assessed
EXTEM	• An in vitro semiquantitative measurement • Uses citrated blood • Monitors the process of coagulation from the start of the coagulation pathway till formation of clot and then fibrinolysis	• Factors VII, X, V, II, I • Platelets • Fibrinolytic system
INTEM	• An in vitro semiquantitative measurement • Uses citrated blood • Measures from the beginning of coagulation pathway until formation of the clot formation and finally, fibrinolysis	• Factors XII, XI, IX, VII, X, V, II, I • Platelets • Fibrinolytic system
FIBTEM	• An in vitro specific measurement of fibrinogen • Similar to EXTEM but inactivating platelets • When platelets are excluded from the clot, fibrinogen measurement is the net resultant measurement; so, we compare EXTEM with FIBTEM for final measurement	• Specific measurement of fibrinogen
HEPTEM	• Similar to INTEM but has heparinase in the reactant; comparing HEPTEM and INTEM<, we can reach to the role of remaining heparin and, so, correct it with protamine	• Remaining heparin
APTEM	• Similar to EXTEM, except for having aprotinin in the reagent, inactivating fibrinolysis in vitro; the final comparison between EXTEM and APTEM shows us if bleeding could be improved based on this comparison	• Fibrinolysis has role in remaining bleeding
NATEM	• An in vitro semiquantitative measurement • Uses citrated blood • No coagulation activator is used; but the contact between tray and pin activates the test	• No significant superiority to traditional coagulation tests

Koch et al. (2012), Lee et al. (2012), Momeni et al. (2013), Wikkelso et al. (2016), Dotsch et al. (2017), Prat et al. (2017a, b), Schmidt et al. (2017), Wikkelso et al. (2017)

(Pifarre et al. 1981). The etiology of this rebound is likely a liberation of previously bound heparin back into the circulation after the initial protamine dosing (Teoh et al. 2004). A reduction of this rebound effect can be abated with additional protamine dosing (typically around 1/4th–1/5th the initial dose).

Aspirin: Current recommendations strongly indicate that aspirin should be administered to post-CABG patients in the immediate postoperative period to improve outcomes (level 1A) (Patrono et al. 2004). The associated antiplatelet effects of aspirin do not usually cause bleeding issues; however, in patients where an underlying thrombocytopenia is present, aspirin dose should be reduced or held to avoid an increase in bleeding risk.

Medication-induced thrombocytopenia: Multiple medications that are administered commonly in the cardiac ICU are known to cause thrombocytopenia. These include multiple antibiotic agents, ranitidine, amiodarone, and several psychiatric drugs. In addition, heparin-induced thrombocytopenia is a potential source for significant derangements in platelet counts (see below).

7.4.2 Heparin-Induced Thrombocytopenia: HIT

7.4.2.1 Definition and Mechanism of HIT

Heparin-induced thrombocytopenia is among the rare but potentially lethal thrombotic complications of heparin therapy. It occurs typically with the use of unfractionated heparin or, less commonly, low-molecular-weight heparin and is mediated through immunologic mechanisms which are discussed below (Greinacher 2015; Salter et al. 2016; Favaloro et al. 2017).

High intravenous heparin doses are among the main risk factors for HIT, a risk factor that is common to all cardiac surgery patients. Additionally, it is not uncommon for cardiac surgery patients to experience low platelet counts due to the effects of cardiopulmonary bypass. Typically, non-HIT-related decreases in platelet counts after cardiac surgery continue for 1–2 days, which serves as a distinguishing feature between HIT and non-HIT decreases in platelet counts. According to an older nomenclature, there were two types of HIT:

Type I: a mild decrease in platelet count during the first 2 days after heparin administration and a relatively benign course

Type II: a significant (more than 50%) drop in platelet count, usually occurring 4–10 days after high-dose heparin, with diagnosis based on a number of criteria including platelet count, clinical signs, and specific laboratory tests, which are discussed below

The usual clinical picture includes onset in a patient exposed to high doses of heparin 5–10 days earlier (e.g., after cardiac surgery), increased levels of "PF4/heparin/antibody" complexes in the blood, platelet decrease of more than 50%, and a prothrombotic state. This combination of clinical manifestations results in a 20–30% rate of potentially lethal complications including vascular limb thrombosis.

The mechanism of HIT is simplified as Table 7.3. A key component to this mechanism is platelet factor 4 (PF4), which is briefly discussed here:

- PF4 is a factor that is released from alpha granules of activated platelets.
- PF4 has a very high affinity for heparin and other negatively charged proteoglycans, including heparin-like molecules, and acts to neutralize them.
- PF4 promotes coagulation through binding to antithrombin III and advancing coagulation (Sandset 2012; Prechel and Walenga 2015).

Clinical manifestations: Though a considerable number of cardiac surgery patients develop antibodies against PF4/heparin complex, the incidence of clinically significant disease is much lower. Both the antibody titer and the molecular size of PF4 complexes affect the clinical incidence. Common clinical presentations of HIT include myocardial infarction, thrombotic CNS complications like stroke, limb embolism due to thrombosis of the aorta or iliofemoral arteries, deep venous thrombosis (DVT) and pulmonary embolism (PE), hemorrhage or infarction in the adrenal glands, skin lesions (from erythematous plaques to necrosis), and a number of

Table 7.3 Mechanism of HIT (Salter et al. 2016; Farm et al. 2017; Favaloro et al. 2017)

1. Platelets are activated after contact with heparin
2. Activated platelets release platelet factor 4 (PF4) which is a small cytokine on the platelet surface
3. immunologic response is provoked to this complex; immunoglobulins bind to the heparin/PF4 compound
4. IgG antibodies are the most common antibody in HIT, as well as other possible antibodies against platelets, including IgG, IgM, and IgA
5. The "heparin-PF4-IgG" complex binds to the Fcϒ receptor IIa located on platelets, monocytes, and other cell surfaces
6. Binding of "heparin-PF4-IgG" to Fcϒ receptor IIa leads to vigorous activation of platelets
7. The result of platelet activation is the release of procoagulant microparticles from platelets and monocytes, which offer a negatively charged phospholipid surface
8. The negatively charged phospholipid surface enhances procoagulant activity and generation of thrombin
9. In addition to the generation of thrombin, the release of tissue factor, which attaches to factor VIIa, subsequently activates the coagulation cascade, leading to activation of factors IX and X
10. Thrombin is attached to antithrombin, creating thrombin-antithrombin (TAT) complexes
11. Increase in TAT and D-dimer levels, which are a marker of a hypercoagulable state
12. Further release of PF4 enhances the neutralization of heparin's anticoagulant activity

general signs and symptoms that may occur after re-administration of heparin including dyspnea, tachycardia, hypertension, fever and chills, and very rarely cardiopulmonary arrest.

Clinical diagnosis: The diagnosis of HIT is based on a number of clinical and laboratory findings. For early detection and active management of the disease, an algorithm and scoring system has been developed by Warkentin and colleagues, in Hamilton Health Sciences, McMaster University, known as 4 Ts which is discussed in brief in Table 7.4. This scoring system has been widely used for more than a decade (Lo et al. 2006; Pouplard et al. 2007; Cuker et al. 2012; Crowther et al. 2014; Greinacher 2015; Salter et al. 2016; Farm et al. 2017). Due to the clinicopathological elements of diagnosis, early suspicion should result in requesting specific laboratory tests, including an ELISA and serotonin-release assay (SRA) to detect PF4 as soon as possible and start treatment.

ELISA for PF4 is a highly sensitive, but not specific test, which detects "PF4/heparin/antibody" complexes. This includes IgG, IgM, and IgA antibodies; however, only IgG results are related to HIT, and as such there is a high rate of false-positive results. As such the role of ELISA for HIT is primarily as an early screening tool.

SRA specifically detects the PF4 complexes involved in HIT, and as such positive results are conclusive and should lead to treatment.

ELISA for PF4 is a highly sensitive but not a specific test and detects "PF4/heparin/antibody" complexes; these antibodies include IgG, IgM and IgA. Only IgG results are related to HIT, and this is why there is a high rate of false-positive results in ELISA for PF4. So, the role of ELISA for HIT is an early screening one.

Table 7.4 The 4 T pretest scoring system for evaluating HIT (Lo et al. 2006; Greinacher 2015; Salter et al. 2016; Farm et al. 2017)

4 T variables	Scoring		
	2 points	1 point	0 point
Thrombocytopenia	Platelet count decrease of >50% and nadir ≥20,000/mm³	Platelet count decrease of 30–50% or nadir 10,000–19,000/mm³	Platelet count decrease of <30% or nadir ≤10,000/mm³
Timing of onset of platelet count fall	• Days 5–10 • Or ≤1 day with prior heparin exposure within 30 days	• Day 10 • Or timing unclear • Or day 1 with prior heparin exposure 30–100 days ago	Platelet count fall <4 days (no recent heparin exposure)
Thrombosis	• Confirmed new thrombosis • Or skin necrosis at heparin injection sites • Or acute systemic reaction after intravenous heparin bolus	• Progressive or recurrent thrombosis • Or non-necrotizing (erythematous) skin lesions • Or suspected nonproven thrombosis	None
OTher causes of thrombocytopenia	None apparent	Possible	Definite
Interpretation of probability of HIT • Maximum score = 8 • High probability of HIT = 6–8 points (20–100%) • Intermediate probability of HIT = 4–5 points: a minority of patients are involved (10–30%) • Low probability of HIT = 0–3 points: HIT is unlikely (<2%)			

Treatment includes the following general principles:

- Prompt cessation of all forms of heparin.
- Avoiding warfarin.
- Starting an alternative anticoagulant with intravenous DTIs such as argatroban, danaparoid, fondaparinux, lepirudin, or bivalirudin.
- A follow-up protocol should be established if an ELISA test is positive and SRA is negative, as this may require a repeated SRA test.
- Management of complications including limb ischemia or ischemia/thrombosis in other organs especially major organs (Lee and Arepally 2013; Bakchoul et al. 2014; Greinacher 2015).

7.5 Medical Management of Bleeding

Initial management of bleeding in the postoperative cardiac patient should be managed medically, provided there are no indications for urgent surgical intervention (see Surgical Management below). For the modern cardiac surgery patient, an extensive toolbox exists for the nonsurgical management of bleeding, which is detailed below. With proper intervention, the majority of these patients will be successfully managed in this manor, without the need for reoperation. Despite the anticipated success of medical management in most cases, frequent reevaluation of the clinical situation should be performed to assess for changes that may require surgical intervention. Patients who appear to be amenable to medical therapy alone may cross into the surgical bleeding path at any time, and prompt intervention is essential.

7.5.1 Antifibrinolytic Agents

7.5.1.1 Desmopressin

Desmopressin (DDAVP; 1-deamino-8-D-arginine-vasopressin) is an analog of antidiuretic hormone, which enhances release of von Willebrand factor (vWF) from Weibel–Palade bodies (storage granules in endothelial cells). Due to this primary effect, factor VIII is also increased due to the increased level of vWF. The ultimate effect is augmented platelet adhesion, which augments the quantitative function of platelets and improves coagulation at sites of injury. The routine dose is 0.3 μg/kg IV. However, there is rapid tachyphylaxis to effects of desmopressin since it leads to augmented release of vWF but does not change the rate of production of the factor. Routine use of desmopressin in cardiac surgery patients is not recommended to control bleeding; however, the following selection of patients may benefit from desmopressin administration:

- Patients with inherited platelet disorders
- Patients who have received aspirin within 7 days before surgery
- Patients who have CPB times more than 140 min
- Patients who have platelet dysfunction which is demonstrable by TEG analysis (with an MA value <50 mm) or platelet function assays (Wademan and Galvin 2014; Bignami et al. 2016; Mirmansoori et al. 2016; Desborough et al. 2017a, b; Orsini et al. 2017)

7.5.1.2 Tranexamic Acid and Epsilon-Aminocaproic Acid (EACA)

Currently there are two available antifibrinolytic agents:

- Tranexamic acid
- ε-Aminocaproic acid (EACA)

Both are recommended for use in pediatric and adult cardiac patients in order to reduce perioperative bleeding, chest tube drainage, and transfusion requirements. Both are synthetic lysine analogs, and their mechanism of action is primarily a competitive binding to the lysine binding location of plasminogen, resulting in competitive prevention of plasma binding to fibrin, which inhibits fibrinolysis. The potency of tranexamic acid is ten times greater than EACA, and it has a significantly longer half-life. Additionally, some studies suggest using topical application of tranexamic acid diluted in normal saline into the pericardium, leading to less chest tube drainage after cardiac surgery. There are some concerns about proposed adverse effects

Table 7.5 Dosing antifibrinolytic agents: tranexamic acid and epsilon-aminocaproic acid used for prevention of perioperative bleeding in adult cardiac surgery (Koster et al. 2015)

Pharmaceutical compound	Dose regimen	Elimination route	Half-life in plasma
Tranexamic acid (Cyklokapron®)	Loading dose: 10–30 mg/kg through IV route plus 1–2 mg/kg on CPB Infusion dose: 10–15 mg/kg/h	Renal	3 h
Epsilon-aminocaproic acid (Amicar®)	First hour: 100 mg/kg or 3 g/m^2 of body surface area Follow up infusion: 33.3 mg/h or 1/g/m^2/h Upper limit of the total dose: 18 g/m^2/day	Renal	2 h

of tranexamic acid including the risk of seizure or other neurologic effects and the risk of thromboembolic events, though these are not well established. Where concern for an individual patient exists, a "low-dose protocol" may be appropriate. A brief review is presented in Table 7.5 (Eaton 2008; Abrishami et al. 2009; Schouten et al. 2009; Bojko et al. 2012; Sharma et al. 2012; Faraoni and Goobie 2014; Koster et al. 2015; Ng et al. 2015).

7.5.1.3 Factor Concentrates

Cryoprecipitate

General indications for administration of cryoprecipitate are:

1. Hypofibrinogenemia or afibrinogenemia, which is associated with a bleeding event including an invasive procedure
2. Before surgery in one of the following preexisting conditions: von Willebrand disease not responding to desmopressin, dysfibrinogenemias, or hemophilia A
3. In patients with factor XIII deficiency who are bleeding
4. In uremic patients when other modalities are ineffective

Dose of administration and the perioperative considerations are described in Table 7.6 (Sorensen and Bevan 2010; Ferraris et al. 2011; Levy et al. 2014; Carvalho et al. 2016; McQuilten et al. 2018).

Fibrinogen

Fibrinogen is a key protein in the coagulation cascade, forming a fibrin plug when activated and transformed to insoluble fibrin and adhered to platelets. Fibrinogen is an alternative to cryoprecipitate. A frequent factor in impaired coagulation in patients after cardiac surgery, especially during the post bypass period, is low levels of circulating fibrinogen, and this deficit often mandates supplementation. Normal plasma levels of fibrinogen are between 150 and 400 g/dL, and supplementation is typically indicated when levels drop below 150–200 in the setting of bleeding. It should be noted that although fibrinogen is one of the cornerstones of the

Table 7.6 Exogenous coagulation factors

Product	Dose and considerations in administration	Considerations
Cryoprecipitate contains: • 15–30 mL of plasma • Factor VIII (80–150 units) • von Willebrand factor (100–150 units) • Factor XIII (50–75 units) • Fibrinogen (150–250 mg) • Fibronectin	• The initial dose in adults is "1 unit of whole blood derived cryo"/5–10 kg of body weight; so, in a standard adult, the recommended dose of cryoprecipitate would be ten whole blood cryoprecipitate units or five apheresis units • For fibrinogen replacement, one cryoprecipitate unit /5 kg usually increases the concentration of fibrinogen by 100 mg/dL (fibrinogen concentration of 100 mg/dL is the goal) • The needed dose should be repeated each 12 h or based on the coagulation tests	• Risk of pathogen transmission is a potential one • Volume overload is less than FFP but more than fibrinogen • Needs ABO matching • The dose of factors is varying from each unit to the other • Thawing is needed before administration • There is chance of pooling with cryoprecipitate; so, transfusion should be done using a standard blood filter
Fibrinogen concentrate	• Initial dose is 30–60 mg/kg • Next doses should be adjusted based on fibrinogen level measurement (Clauss method) or TEG/ROTEM parameters (especially FIBTEM)	• No risk of pathogen transmission, volume overload, or ABO mismatching • No thawing is needed before administration
PCC (human prothrombin complex)	• **PCC** (human prothrombin complex): Which has factor IX with varying doses of other coagulation factors (II, VII, and X); some forms of PCC may also contain protein C and S, heparin, and antithrombin • **PCC** dose is 20–40 IU/kg based on INR and point-of-care tests (including TEG®/ROTEM®)	• When bleeding is uncontrollable, selective replacement of coagulation factors results in rapid and direct replacement of factor deficiencies • Potential risk of thromboembolic events and acute kidney injury have been proposed
Activated recombinant factor 7 (rFVIIa)	• 40–80 µg/kg (off-label dose in cardiac patients) when there is intractable bleeding as the final option • Risk of arterial and venous thrombotic and thromboembolic events is about 10%	• Half-life about 3 h • Available as 1, 2 , 5, and 8 mg vial sizes
FEIBA: Factor eight inhibitor bypass activity	• FEIBA contains all factors of PCC except for prothrombin and factor Xa • Produced as a lyophilized powder (single-use vials) • Available as 500, 1000, or 2500 units per vial • Leads to decreased use of blood product and diminished chest tube drainage especially in refractory postoperative bleeding • Routine dose is 50–100 IU/kg • Could be repeated each 6–12 h	• Risk of pathogen transmission is a potential one • There is potential risk of hypersensitivity reactions and thromboembolic events • Some studies suggest similar efficacy and adverse event profiles for both rFVIIa and FEIBA controlling postoperative bleeding in cardiac surgical patients (Rao et al. 2014)

Groom et al. (1996), Turecek et al. (2004), Balsam et al. (2008), Solomon et al. (2010), Sorensen and Bevan (2010), Ferraris et al. (2011), Yang et al. (2012), Curley et al. (2014), Dietrich et al. (2014), Levy et al. (2014), Rao et al. (2014), Song et al. (2014), Tanaka et al. (2014), Durandy (2015), Jobes et al. (2015), Lei and Xiong (2015), Payani et al. (2015), Remy et al. (2015), Cappabianca et al. (2016), Carvalho et al. (2016), Ghadimi et al. (2016), McQuilten et al. (2018)

coagulation cascade, it is often not monitored routinely in many critical care settings. In cardiac surgery patients, three factors are the primary drivers of decreased fibrinogen level:

- Increased consumption
- Volume resuscitation-related hemodilution
- Increased fibrinogen breakdown related to acidosis

Though being one of the cornerstones of coagulation pathway, fibrinogen is not monitored as a routine practice in many critical care settings for perioperative bleeding. However, normal plasma levels of fibrinogen are between 150 and 400 g/dL. There are three sources for administration of fibrinogen:

- **FFP**: has low concentration of fibrinogen with resultant need for large doses of fibrinogen to reach acceptable plasma levels, which carries a risk of volume overload. Infection risk and ABO mismatching are a risk as well.
- **Cryoprecipitate**: the amount of fibrinogen in each unit of cryoprecipitate is variable, but it is higher than in FFP. The product requires thawing, and also there carries a risk of pathogen infection and ABO mismatching.
- **Fibrinogen concentrate**: which is in the form of lyophilized fibrinogen, does not impose risk of pathogen contamination or ABO incompatibility and delivers a known amount of fibrinogen, without risk of volume overload.

If plasma fibrinogen level falls below 150–200 g/dL and the patient has active bleeding, fibrinogen supplementation is indicated, with an initial dose of 30–60 mg/kg. Additional doses should be adjusted based on fibrinogen level measurement (Clauss method) or TEG/ROTEM parameters (especially assessment of fibrin-based maximum clot amplitude in FIBTEM). Fibrinogen concentrate has led to a reduction or even total avoidance of blood product transfusion in several studies and is a good adjunct when available. A good rule of thumb is for a standard 70 kg adult, 3 g of lyophilized fibrinogen is needed to increase the plasma level of fibrinogen 100 mg/dL. Studies have demonstrated that concomitant administration of both fibrinogen and tranexamic acid may lead to decreased chest tube drainage and decreased need for blood transfusion. Table 7.6 addresses these items in brief (Solomon et al. 2010; Sorensen and Bevan 2010; Theusinger et al. 2011; Warmuth et al. 2012; Yang et al. 2012; Momeni et al. 2013; Dietrich et al. 2014; Levy et al. 2014; Zhu et al. 2014; Payani et al. 2015, 2016; Carvalho et al. 2016).

Human Prothrombin Complex (PCC)

Human prothrombin complex is isolated from human plasma and includes vitamin K-dependent clotting factors: factor IX with varying doses of factors II, VII, and X. PCC is available as two different formulations based on the concentration of factor VII included:

- 3-factor PCC formulation
- 4-factor PCC formulation

Some forms of PCC may also contain protein C and S, heparin, and antithrombin III. The amount of the latter items depends on the formulation of PCC. The recommended dose of PCC is 20–40 IU/kg, which is adjusted based on INR and depends on the patient's underlying coagulation profile. In a patient with uncontrollable bleeding, selective replacement of coagulation factors results in rapid and direct replacement of factor deficiencies. In an observational study from 2005 to 2013 on 3454 cardiac surgery patients, it was demonstrated that PCC leads to decreased postoperative bleeding and reduced RBC transfusion, though there also may be an increased risk of postoperative acute kidney injury. Point-of-care testing (especially TEG®/ROTEM®) should be used to decrease the chance of unwanted complications including thromboembolic events with administration of PCC. Table 7.6 addresses these items in brief (Tanaka et al. 2014; Cappabianca et al. 2016; Ghadimi et al. 2016).

Activated Recombinant Factor 7 (rFVIIa)

rFVIIa has been introduced as a measure to control intractable bleeding primarily through activation of the external pathway in the coagulation cascade. There are a number of well-defined indications for the drug; however, use for control of bleeding postoperatively is not FDA-approved and is technically an "off-label" use. In cardiothoracic surgery (both adult and pediatric), rFVIIa can lead to significant reduction in blood transfusion and may control intractable bleeding; however, its use should be reserved for those patients where bleeding is intractable. The following should be optimized before administration of rFVIIa:

- Fibrinogen concentration
- Platelet count
- Temperature
- pH
- Hyperfibrinolysis

There is risk of arterial and venous thrombotic and thromboembolic events (including stroke and MI) in approximately one tenth of patients where rFVIIa is used. Usually, a single intravenous dose of 40 μg/kg rFVIIa is sufficient; however, higher doses from 60–80 μg/kg to 90–120 μg/kg have been reported. Table 7.6 addresses these items in brief (Ranucci et al. 2008; Yank et al. 2011; Guzzetta et al. 2012; Omar et al. 2015; Carvalho et al. 2016; Cooper and Ritchey 2017).

Factor Eight Inhibitor Bypass Activity (FEIBA)

FEIBA contains all factors of PCC except for prothrombin and factor Xa and is prepared as a lyophilized powder in single-use vials which are available as 500, 1000, or 2500 unit doses (per vial). Studies have demonstrated that in postoperative bleeding, use of FEIBA leads to the decreased use of blood product and diminished chest tube drainage, especially in the postoperative patient that is refractory to other drugs and compounds and has continued bleeding after surgery. In such cases, the routine dose of FEIBA is 50–100 IU/kg which may be repeated each 6–12 h as needed. FEIBA has the potential risk of thromboembolic events, hypersensitivity reactions, and pathogen transmission. It should be noted that a number of clinical studies have demonstrated similar efficacy and adverse event profiles for both rFVIIa and FEIBA regarding postoperative bleeding in cardiac surgical patients. Table 7.6 addresses these items in brief (Turecek et al. 2004; Balsam et al. 2008; Rao et al. 2014; Song et al. 2014).

7.6 Blood Products

The utilization of blood products, including packed red blood cells, fresh frozen plasma, pooled platelets, and cryoprecipitate, is commonplace within cardiac surgery patients, with around 50% of these patients receiving blood products (Mehta et al. 2009). The high rate of blood product use within this population is reflected on the fact that up to 10–15% of all blood products consumed in the United States are used in cardiac surgery patients, a fraction that continues to grow due to the increasing complexity of cardiac surgical procedures (Ferraris et al. 2007). While this utilization of blood products is undeniably essential in most cases, data would indicate that there is a relationship between the use of blood products and worse short- and long-term outcomes (Engoren et al. 2002; Koch et al. 2008). To help guide the use of blood products in the cardiac surgical patient, the Society of Thoracic Surgeons and the Society of Cardiovascular Anesthesiologists have developed a consensus guideline statement, which should serve as a data-driven guide for blood product use and conservation in this population and should be considered essential reading for anyone caring for this population. These guidelines indicate that while PRBC transfusion triggers vary patient to patient, transfusion to a hemoglobin concentration >10 g/dL does not improve oxygen transport and is not recommended (class III, level C). If the hemoglobin level falls below 7 g/dL in the postoperative patient, transfusion is reasonable, though no high-level evidence exists for this (class IIa, level C). While transfusion between the levels of 7–10 g/dL remains somewhat controversial, a recent randomized trial evaluating a liberal vs. restrictive trigger for PRBC transfusion (Hb < 9 vs. Hb < 7.5) demonstrated a slight increase in all-cause mortality among the restrictive group (Murphy et al. 2015). Consequentially, it is our practice to transfuse patients when Hb levels fall below 8–9 g/dL but to no greater than 10 g/dL. This narrow window is maintained more aggressively in the immediate postoperative period, with lower levels tolerated in the floor patient who is otherwise doing well.

The use of other blood products (FFP, platelets, or cryoprecipitate) is appropriate to correct individual deficits (including functional deficits in cases of platelet inhibition) in patients who are bleeding. FFP administration is typically utilized when the INR rises above 1.4–1.6 in the setting of ongoing bleeding. Administration of FFP for patients without bleeding or in those with normal coagulation studies is not indicated (class III, level A), though adding FFP to a massive transfusion protocol is reasonable (class IIb, level B). Platelet transfusion is typically indicated when levels fall below 100,000/μL in the setting of bleeding or where significant inhibition is known and bleeding ongoing. One unit typically will increase the platelet count by

7–10,000/μL, and administration of two units is often required in the setting of significant functional derangement. Cryoprecipitate use is most often reserved for patients with ongoing persistent bleeding, with low levels of fibrinogen.

It should be noted that transfusion rates are a tracked metric in the Society of Thoracic Surgeons public reporting dataset (see https://www.sts.org/adult-public-reporting-module). This database tracks outcomes for isolated CABG, isolated AVR, and AVR + CABG and is publically available/searchable to evaluate individual centers. While significant attention is often paid to the outcomes represented here, it is important to remember that data-driven care for the individual patient is truly what matters.

7.7 Surgical Management of Bleeding

As mentioned above, the single most important branch point in the decision tree for management of bleeding in the postoperative cardiac surgery patient is the need for surgical intervention. Postoperative bleeding may be either surgical, medical (due to coagulopathies or platelet dysfunction), or a combination of both. Bleeding that cannot be adequately managed with medical means, is rapidly changing, or is associated with hemodynamic collapse requires urgent surgical intervention. The urgency of the intervention cannot be overstated in some cases, and the surgical team should always be prepared to reopen the chest of a fresh postoperative patient at the bedside in the ICU when hemodynamic collapse occurs. When safe, patients should be moved to the operating room for re-exploration in a sterile environment, something that is more likely to be an option when signs of hemodynamic instability are identified early.

7.7.1 Risk Factors for Rebleeding

There are a number of items which increase the risk of postoperative bleeding in adult patients undergoing cardiac surgery (Table 7.7).

7.7.2 Clinical Management of Rebleeding

It is difficult to identify strict criteria that dictate the need for a patient to undergo a re-exploration, and most will fall to a patient-by-patient evaluation. Some general rules of thumb have been quoted and are summarized in Table 7.8.

In the case of tamponade, early identification is key, and it is far better to return a stable patient to the operating room for very early tamponade physiology than to emergently open a chest of a hemodynamically unstable patient in the ICU. Consequently, if significant concern exists, waiting for a bedside echocardiogram to confirm the diagnosis is not warranted and could be potentially catastrophic.

Table 7.7 Risk factors associated with increased risk of postoperative bleeding

Platelet status: • Preoperative administration of antiplatelet drugs • Prolonged CPB time • Quantitative abnormalities in platelets (low preoperative platelet count, decreased platelet count after cardiopulmonary bypass, low early postoperative platelet count) • Qualitative abnormalities in platelets (abnormalities in platelet function)
Changes in the profile of coagulation factors
Increased fibrinolytic activity by cardiopulmonary bypass
Surgical damage to blood vessels: • Cannulation site bleeding • Incomplete control of internal mammary artery bed and its anastomosis • Failures in saphenous vein graft branches • Bleeding from arterial anastomoses • Bleeding from sternal wire sites • Raw surface bleeding in reoperative surgery
Patient risk factors: • Advanced age • Left ventricular dysfunction • Lower body mass index (BMI) • Urgent/emergent operation: nonelective cases • Five or more distal anastomoses • Chronic renal failure

Karthik et al. (2004), Tettey et al. (2009), Pompilio et al. (2011), Stone et al. (2012), Tokushige et al. (2014), Biancari et al. (2016), Alfredsson et al. (2017), Brascia et al. (2017), Kinnunen et al. (2017)

Table 7.8 The primary indications for returning to the operating room for bleeding after cardiac surgery (Karthik et al. 2004; Pompilio et al. 2011; Colson et al. 2016)

The amount of continuous chest tube drainage: 1. >500 mL in the first hour postoperatively 2. >400 mL during each of the first 2 h postoperatively 3. >300 mL during each of the first 3 h postoperatively 4. >1000 mL (total bleeding) during the first 4 h postoperatively
Sudden massive bleeding at any time in postoperative period
Evidence of a large pericardial or pleural effusion on imaging (by chest X-ray or echocardiography at the bedside) in the setting of hemodynamic changes
Any evidence of tamponade physiology with varying combinations of: • Increased central venous pressure (CVP) • Decreased urinary output • Hypotension • Mediastinal widening on chest X-ray accompanied with sudden reduction of chest tube drainage • End-organ malperfusion • Decreased cardiac output • Evidence of undrained pericardial effusions with or without compression

The operative steps required to reopen a recent sternotomy are fairly simple and include reopening of the skin and subcutaneous tissues, followed by removing the sternal wires and spreading the sternum gently with the surgeon's fingers. A retractor is then placed and clot burden removed. A thorough exploration for the source of bleeding should be undertaken, with the understanding that there may be no identifiable single source in many cases. All surgical sites and cannulation sites should be evaluated carefully. In more than half of the patients returning to operating room, the surgical team can locate an obvious bleeding site (Karthik et al. 2004). However, there are a considerable number of patients in whom just the act of removing the clot burden and associated fibrin split products, along with the additional administration of blood products and coagulation factors, may be enough to improve multifocal small bleeding areas. If other, more significant areas of bleeding are encountered, they must be addressed surgically. Following completion of the re-exploration, the chest may be closed or left open with a temporary dressing as the situation dictates.

7.7.3 Clinical Outcome

Patients who require reoperation for bleeding have a demonstrable increase in morbidity and mortality as compared to their peers, although there is obviously some degree of selection bias (patients who are sicker or required a more extensive operation will tend to have more bleeding issues in general). However, most studies demonstrate that there is a distinct chance for increased morbidity and mortality in patients with reoperation due to bleeding. The incidence of reoperation after adult cardiac surgery is 2–9% (Moulton et al. 1996; Charalambous et al. 2006; Vivacqua et al. 2011). In these patients, the main predictor of outcome is the time gap between surgery and resternotomy. If there is a time interval more than 12 hours before starting reoperation, there is increased risk of other unwanted complications including but not limited to:

- Noncardiac complications like sternal wound infections, renal failure postoperative CNS complications including stroke
- Increased need for transfusion
- Prolonged mechanical ventilation
- Increased chance of using assist devices such as intra-aortic balloon pump (Nalysnyk et al. 2003; Karthik et al. 2004; Pompilio et al. 2011; Vivacqua et al. 2011; Stone et al. 2012; Biancari et al. 2016; Kinnunen et al. 2017)

References

National Clinical Guideline Centre (UK). Blood transfusion. London: National Institute for Health and Care Excellence (UK); 2015a. NICE Guideline, No. 24. 16, Cryoprecipitate: thresholds and targets. https://www.ncbi.nlm.nih.gov/books/NBK338779/.

National Clinical Guideline Centre (UK). Blood transfusion. London: National Institute for Health and Care Excellence (UK); 2015b. NICE Guideline, No. 24. 17, Cryoprecipitate: doses. https://www.ncbi.nlm.nih.gov/books/NBK338787/.

Abrishami A, Chung F, Wong J. Topical application of antifibrinolytic drugs for on-pump cardiac surgery: a systematic review and meta-analysis. Can J Anaesth. 2009;56:202–12.

Alfredsson J, Neely B, Neely ML, Bhatt DL, Goodman SG, Tricoci P, Mahaffey KW, Cornel JH, White HD, Fox KA, Prabhakaran D, Winters KJ, Armstrong PW, Ohman EM, Roe MT. Predicting the risk of bleeding during dual antiplatelet therapy after acute coronary syndromes. Heart. 2017;103:1168–76.

Bakchoul T, Zollner H, Greinacher A. Current insights into the laboratory diagnosis of HIT. Int J Lab Hematol. 2014;36:296–305.

Balsam LB, Timek TA, Pelletier MP. Factor eight inhibitor bypassing activity (FEIBA) for refractory bleeding in cardiac surgery: review of clinical outcomes. J Card Surg. 2008;23:614–21.

Biancari F, Tauriainen T, Perrotti A, Dalen M, Faggian G, Franzese I, Chocron S, Ruggieri VG, Bounader K, Gulbins H, Reichart D, Svenarud P, Santarpino G, Fischlein T, Puski T, Maselli D, Dominici C, Nardella S, Mariscalco G, Gherli R, Musumeci F, Rubino AS, Mignosa C, De Feo M, Bancone C, Gatti G, Maschietto L, Santini F, Salsano A, Nicolini F, Gherli T, Zanobini M, Saccocci M, D'Errigo P, Kinnunen EM, Onorati F. Bleeding, transfusion and the risk of stroke after coronary surgery: a prospective cohort study of 2357 patients. Int J Surg. 2016;32:50–7.

Bignami E, Cattaneo M, Crescenzi G, Ranucci M, Guarracino F, Cariello C, Baldassarri R, Isgro G, Baryshnikova E, Fano G, Franco A, Gerli C, Crivellari M, Zangrillo A, Landoni G. Desmopressin after cardiac surgery in bleeding patients. A multicenter randomized trial. Acta Anaesthesiol Scand. 2016;60:892–900.

Bojko B, Vuckovic D, Mirnaghi F, Cudjoe E, Wasowicz M, Jerath A, Pawliszyn J. Therapeutic monitoring of tranexamic acid concentration: high-throughput analysis with solid-phase microextraction. Ther Drug Monit. 2012;34:31–7.

Brascia D, Reichart D, Onorati F, Perrotti A, Ruggieri VG, Bounader K, Verhoye JP, Santarpino G, Fischlein T, Maselli D, Dominici C, Mariscalco G, Gherli R, Rubino AS, De Feo M, Bancone C, Gatti G, Santini F, Dalen M, Saccocci M, Faggian G, Tauriainen T, Kinnunen EM, Nicolini F, Gherli T, Rosato S, Biancari F. Validation of bleeding classifications in coronary artery bypass grafting. Am J Cardiol. 2017;119:727–33.

Cappabianca G, Mariscalco G, Biancari F, Maselli D, Papesso F, Cottini M, Crosta S, Banescu S, Ahmed AB, Beghi C. Safety and efficacy of prothrombin complex concentrate as first-line treatment in bleeding after cardiac surgery. Crit Care. 2016;20:5.

Carvalho M, Rodrigues A, Gomes M, Carrilho A, Nunes AR, Orfao R, Alves A, Aguiar J, Campos M. Interventional algorithms for the control of coagulopathic bleeding in surgical, trauma, and postpartum settings: recommendations from the share network group. Clin Appl Thromb Hemost. 2016;22:121–37.

Charalambous CP, Zipitis CS, Keenan DJ. Chest reexploration in the intensive care unit after cardiac surgery: a safe alternative to returning to the operating theater. Ann Thorac Surg. 2006;81:191–4.

Colson PH, Gaudard P, Fellahi JL, Bertet H, Faucanie M, Amour J, Blanloeil Y, Lanquetot H, Ouattara A, Picot MC. Active bleeding after cardiac surgery: a prospective observational multicenter study. PLoS One. 2016;11:e0162396.

Cooper JD, Ritchey AK. Response to treatment and adverse events associated with use of recombinant activated factor VII in children: a retrospective cohort study. Ther Adv Drug Saf. 2017;8:51–9.

Crowther M, Cook D, Guyatt G, Zytaruk N, McDonald E, Williamson D, Albert M, Dodek P, Finfer S, Vallance S, Heels-Ansdell D, McIntyre L, Mehta S, Lamontagne F, Muscedere J, Jacka M, Lesur O, Kutsiogiannis J, Friedrich J, Klinger JR, Qushmaq I, Burry L, Khwaja K, Sheppard JA, Warkentin TE. Heparin-induced thrombocytopenia in the critically ill: interpreting the 4Ts test in a randomized trial. J Crit Care. 2014;29:470.e477–15.e477.

Cuker A, Gimotty PA, Crowther MA, Warkentin TE. Predictive value of the 4Ts scoring system for heparin-induced thrombocytopenia: a systematic review and meta-analysis. Blood. 2012;120:4160–7.

Curley GF, Shehata N, Mazer CD, Hare GM, Friedrich JO. Transfusion triggers for guiding RBC transfusion for cardiovascular surgery: a systematic review and meta-analysis*. Crit Care Med. 2014;42:2611–24.

Dacey LJ, Munoz JJ, Johnson ER, Leavitt BJ, Maloney CT, Morton JR, Olmstead EM, Birkmeyer JD, O'Connor GT. Effect of preoperative aspirin use on mortality in coronary artery bypass grafting patients. Ann Thorac Surg. 2000;70:1986–90.

Desborough MJ, Oakland K, Brierley C, Bennett S, Doree C, Trivella M, Hopewell S, Stanworth SJ, Estcourt LJ. Desmopressin use for minimising perioperative blood transfusion. Cochrane Database Syst Rev. 2017a;7:Cd001884.

Desborough MJ, Oakland KA, Landoni G, Crivellari M, Doree C, Estcourt LJ, Stanworth SJ. Desmopressin for treatment of platelet dysfunction and reversal of antiplatelet agents: a systematic review and meta-analysis of randomized controlled trials. J Thromb Haemost. 2017b;15:263–72.

Dietrich W, Faraoni D, von Heymann C, Bolliger D, Ranucci M, Sander M, Rosseel P. ESA guidelines on the management of severe perioperative bleeding: comments on behalf of the subcommittee on transfusion and Haemostasis of the European Association of Cardiothoracic Anaesthesiologists. Eur J Anaesthesiol. 2014;31:239–41.

Dotsch TM, Dirkmann D, Bezinover D, Hartmann M, Treckmann JW, Paul A, Saner FH. Assessment of standard laboratory tests and rotational thromboelastometry for the prediction of postoperative bleeding in liver transplantation. Br J Anaesth. 2017;119:402–10.

Durandy Y. Use of blood products in pediatric cardiac surgery. Artif Organs. 2015;39:21–7.

Eaton MP. Antifibrinolytic therapy in surgery for congenital heart disease. Anesth Analg. 2008;106:1087–100.

Eerenberg ES, Kamphuisen PW, Sijpkens MK, Meijers JC, Buller HR, Levi M. Reversal of rivaroxaban and dabigatran by prothrombin complex concentrate: a randomized, placebo-controlled, crossover study in healthy subjects. Circulation. 2011;124:1573–9.

Engoren MC, Habib RH, Zacharias A, Schwann TA, Riordan CJ, Durham SJ. Effect of blood transfusion on long-term survival after cardiac operation. Ann Thorac Surg. 2002;74:1180–6.

Faraoni D, Goobie SM. The efficacy of antifibrinolytic drugs in children undergoing noncardiac surgery: a systematic review of the literature. Anesth Analg. 2014;118:628–36.

Farm M, Bakchoul T, Frisk T, Althaus K, Odenrick A, Norberg EM, Berndtsson M, Antovic JP. Evaluation of a diagnostic algorithm for heparin-induced thrombocytopenia. Thromb Res. 2017;152:77–81.

Favaloro EJ, McCaughan G, Pasalic L. Clinical and laboratory diagnosis of heparin induced thrombocytopenia: an update. Pathology. 2017;49:346–55.

Ferraris VA, Brown JR, Despotis GJ, Hammon JW, Reece TB, Saha SP, Song HK, Clough ER, Shore-Lesserson LJ, Goodnough LT, Mazer CD, Shander A, Stafford-Smith M, Waters J, Baker RA, Dickinson TA, Fitz Gerald DJ, Likosky DS, Shann KG. 2011 update to the Society of Thoracic Surgeons and the Society of Cardiovascular Anesthesiologists blood conservation clinical practice guidelines. Ann Thorac Surg. 2011;91:944–82.

Ferraris VA, Ferraris SP, Saha SP, Hessel EA 2nd, Haan CK, Royston BD, Bridges CR, Higgins RS, Despotis G, Brown JR, Spiess BD, Shore-Lesserson L, Stafford-Smith M, Mazer CD, Bennett-Guerrero E, Hill SE, Body S. Perioperative blood transfusion and blood conservation in cardiac surgery: the Society of Thoracic Surgeons and the Society of Cardiovascular Anesthesiologists clinical practice guideline. Ann Thorac Surg. 2007;83:S27–86.

Ghadimi K, Levy JH, Welsby IJ. Prothrombin complex concentrates for bleeding in the perioperative setting. Anesth Analg. 2016;122:1287–300.

Greinacher A. Clinical practice. Heparin-induced thrombocytopenia. N Engl J Med. 2015;373:252–61.

Groom RC, Akl BF, Albus R, Lefrak EA. Pediatric cardiopulmonary bypass: a review of current practice. Int Anesthesiol Clin. 1996;34:141–63.

Guzzetta NA, Russell IA, Williams GD. Review of the off-label use of recombinant activated factor VII in pediatric cardiac surgery patients. Anesth Analg. 2012;115:364–78.

Jobes DR, Sesok-Pizzini D, Friedman D. Reduced transfusion requirement with use of fresh whole blood in pediatric cardiac surgical procedures. Ann Thorac Surg. 2015;99:1706–11.

Karthik S, Grayson AD, McCarron EE, Pullan DM, Desmond MJ. Reexploration for bleeding after coronary artery bypass surgery: risk factors, outcomes, and the effect of time delay. Ann Thorac Surg. 2004;78:527–34; discussion 534.

Kincaid EH, Monroe ML, Saliba DL, Kon ND, Byerly WG, Reichert MG. Effects of preoperative enoxaparin versus unfractionated heparin on bleeding indices in patients undergoing coronary artery bypass grafting. Ann Thorac Surg. 2003;76:124–8; discussion 128.

Kinnunen EM, De Feo M, Reichart D, Tauriainen T, Gatti G, Onorati F, Maschietto L, Bancone C, Fiorentino F, Chocron S, Bounader K, Dalen M, Svenarud P, Faggian G, Franzese I, Santarpino G, Fischlein T, Maselli D, Dominici C, Nardella S, Gherli R, Musumeci F, Rubino AS, Mignosa C, Mariscalco G, Serraino FG, Santini F, Salsano A, Nicolini F, Gherli T, Zanobini M, Saccocci M, Ruggieri VG, Philippe Verhoye J, Perrotti A, Biancari F. Incidence and prognostic impact of bleeding and transfusion after coronary surgery in low-risk patients. Transfusion. 2017;57:178–86.

Koch A, Pernow M, Barthuber C, Mersmann J, Zacharowski K, Grotemeyer D. Systemic inflammation after aortic cross clamping is influenced by toll-like receptor 2 preconditioning and deficiency. J Surg Res. 2012;178(2). https://doi.org/10.1016/j.jss.2012.04.052.

Koch CG, Li L, Sessler DI, Figueroa P, Hoeltge GA, Mihaljevic T, Blackstone EH. Duration of red-cell storage and complications after cardiac surgery. N Engl J Med. 2008;358:1229–39.

Koster A, Faraoni D, Levy JH. Antifibrinolytic therapy for cardiac surgery: an update. Anesthesiology. 2015;123:214–21.

Lee GC, Kicza AM, Liu KY, Nyman CB, Kaufman RM, Body SC. Does rotational thromboelastometry (ROTEM) improve prediction of bleeding after cardiac surgery? Anesth Analg. 2012;115:499–506.

Lee GM, Arepally GM. Diagnosis and management of heparin-induced thrombocytopenia. Hematol Oncol Clin North Am. 2013;27:541–63.

Lei C, Xiong LZ. Perioperative red blood cell transfusion: what we do not know. Chin Med J. 2015;128:2383–6.

Levy JH, Welsby I, Goodnough LT. Fibrinogen as a therapeutic target for bleeding: a review of critical levels and replacement therapy. Transfusion. 2014;54:1389–405; quiz 1388.

Lo GK, Juhl D, Warkentin TE, Sigouin CS, Eichler P, Greinacher A. Evaluation of pretest clinical score (4 T's) for the diagnosis of heparin-induced thrombocytopenia in two clinical settings. J Thromb Haemost. 2006;4:759–65.

McQuilten ZK, Crighton G, Brunskill S, Morison JK, Richter TH, Waters N, Murphy MF, Wood EM. Optimal dose, timing and ratio of blood products in massive transfusion: results from a systematic review. Transfus Med Rev. 2018;32(1):6–15.

Mehta RH, Sheng S, O'Brien SM, Grover FL, Gammie JS, Ferguson TB, Peterson ED. Reoperation for bleeding in patients undergoing coronary artery bypass surgery: incidence, risk factors, time trends, and outcomes. Circ Cardiovasc Qual Outcomes. 2009;2:583–90.

Mirmansoori A, Farzi F, Sedighinejad A, Imantalab V, Mohammadzadeh A, Atrkar Roushan Z, Ghazanfar Tehran S, Nemati M, Dehghan A. The effect of desmopressin on the amount of bleeding in patients undergoing coronary artery bypass graft surgery with a cardiopulmonary bypass pump after taking anti-platelet medicine. Anesth Pain Med. 2016;6:e39226.

Momeni M, Carlier C, Baele P, Watremez C, Van Dyck M, Matta A, Kahn D, Rennotte MT, Glineur D, de Kerchove L, Jacquet LM, Thiry D, Gregoire A, Eeckhoudt S, Hermans C. Fibrinogen concentration significantly decreases after on-pump versus off-pump coronary artery bypass surgery: a systematic point-of-care ROTEM analysis. J Cardiothorac Vasc Anesth. 2013;27:5–11.

Moulton MJ, Creswell LL, Mackey ME, Cox JL, Rosenbloom M. Reexploration for bleeding is a risk factor for adverse outcomes after cardiac operations. J Thorac Cardiovasc Surg. 1996;111:1037–46.

Murphy GJ, Pike K, Rogers CA, Wordsworth S, Stokes EA, Angelini GD, Reeves BC. Liberal or restrictive transfusion after cardiac surgery. N Engl J Med. 2015;372:997–1008.

Nalysnyk L, Fahrbach K, Reynolds MW, Zhao SZ, Ross S. Adverse events in coronary artery bypass graft (CABG) trials: a systematic review and analysis. Heart. 2003;89:767–72.

Ng W, Jerath A, Wasowicz M. Tranexamic acid: a clinical review. Anaesthesiol Intensive Ther. 2015;47:339–50.

Omar HR, Enten G, Karlnoski R, Ching YH, Mangar D, Camporesi EM. Recombinant activated factor VII significantly reduces transfusion requirements in cardiothoracic surgery. Drug R&D. 2015;15:187–94.

Orsini S, Noris P, Bury L, Heller PG, Santoro C, Kadir RA, Butta NC, Falcinelli E, Cid AR, Fabris F, Fouassier M, Miyazaki K, Lozano ML, Zuniga P, Flaujac C, Podda GM, Bermejo N, Favier R, Henskens Y, De Maistre E, De Candia E, Mumford AD, Ozdemir GN, Eker I, Nurden P, Bayart S, Lambert MP, Bussel J, Zieger B, Tosetto A, Melazzini F, Glembotsky AC, Pecci A, Cattaneo M, Schlegel N, Gresele P. Bleeding risk of surgery and its prevention in patients with inherited platelet disorders. Haematologica. 2017;102:1192–203.

Patrono C, Bachmann F, Baigent C, Bode C, De Caterina R, Charbonnier B, Fitzgerald D, Hirsh J, Husted S, Kvasnicka J, Montalescot G, Garcia Rodriguez LA, Verheugt F, Vermylen J, Wallentin L, Priori SG, Alonso Garcia MA, Blanc JJ, Budaj A, Cowie M, Dean V, Deckers J, Fernandez Burgos E, Lekakis J, Lindahl B, Mazzotta G, Morais J, Oto A, Smiseth OA, Morais J, Deckers J, Ferreira R, Mazzotta G, Steg PG, Teixeira F, Wilcox R. Expert consensus document on the use of antiplatelet agents. The task force on the use of antiplatelet agents in patients with atherosclerotic cardiovascular disease of the European society of cardiology. Eur Heart J. 2004;25:166–81.

Payani N, Foroughi M, Bagheri A, Rajaei S, Dabbagh A. Effect of local fibrinogen administration on postoperative bleeding in coronary artery bypass graft patients. J Cell Mol Anesth. 2016;1:23–7.

Payani N, Foroughi M, Dabbagh A. The effect of intravenous administration of active recombinant factor VII on postoperative bleeding in cardiac valve reoperations; a randomized clinical trial. Anesth Pain Med. 2015;5:e22846.

Pifarre R, Babka R, Sullivan HJ, Montoya A, Bakhos M, El-Etr A. Management of postoperative heparin rebound following cardiopulmonary bypass. J Thorac Cardiovasc Surg. 1981;81:378–81.

Pompilio G, Filippini S, Agrifoglio M, Merati E, Lauri G, Salis S, Alamanni F, Parolari A. Determinants of pericardial drainage for cardiac tamponade following cardiac surgery. Eur J Cardiothorac Surg. 2011;39:e107–13.

Pouplard C, Gueret P, Fouassier M, Ternisien C, Trossaert M, Regina S, Gruel Y. Prospective evaluation of the '4Ts' score and particle gel immunoassay specific to heparin/PF4 for the diagnosis of heparin-induced thrombocytopenia. J Thromb Haemost. 2007;5:1373–9.

Prat NJ, Meyer AD, Ingalls NK, Trichereau J, DuBose JJ, Cap AP. Rotational thromboelastometry significantly optimizes transfusion practices for damage control resuscitation in combat casualties. J Trauma Acute Care Surg. 2017a;83:373–80.

Prat NJ, Meyer AD, Ingalls NK, Trichereau J, DuBose JJ, Cap AP. ROTEM significantly optimizes transfusion practices for damage control resuscitation in combat casualties. J Trauma Acute Care Surg. 2017b. https://doi.org/10.1097/TA.0000000000001568.

Prechel MM, Walenga JM. Complexes of platelet factor 4 and heparin activate toll-like receptor 4. J Thromb Haemost. 2015;13:665–70.

Ranucci M, Isgro G, Soro G, Conti D, De Toffol B. Efficacy and safety of recombinant activated factor vii in major surgical procedures: systematic review and meta-analysis of randomized clinical trials. Arch Surg. 2008;143:296–304; discussion 304.

Rao VK, Lobato RL, Bartlett B, Klanjac M, Mora-Mangano CT, Soran PD, Oakes DA, Hill CC, van der Starre PJ. Factor VIII inhibitor bypass activity and recombinant activated factor VII in cardiac surgery. J Cardiothorac Vasc Anesth. 2014;28:1221–6.

Remy KE, Natanson C, Klein HG. The influence of the storage lesion(s) on pediatric red cell transfusion. Curr Opin Pediatr. 2015;27:277–85.

Salter BS, Weiner MM, Trinh MA, Heller J, Evans AS, Adams DH, Fischer GW. Heparin-induced thrombocytopenia: a comprehensive clinical review. J Am Coll Cardiol. 2016;67:2519–32.

Sandset PM. CXCL4-platelet factor 4, heparin-induced thrombocytopenia and cancer. Thromb Res. 2012;129(Suppl 1):S97–100.

Schmidt DE, Halmin M, Wikman A, Ostlund A, Agren A. Relative effects of plasma, fibrinogen concentrate, and factor XIII on ROTEM coagulation profiles in an in vitro model of massive transfusion in trauma. Scand J Clin Lab Invest. 2017;77:397–405.

Schouten ES, van de Pol AC, Schouten AN, Turner NM, Jansen NJ, Bollen CW. The effect of aprotinin, tranexamic acid, and aminocaproic acid on blood loss and use of blood products in major pediatric surgery: a meta-analysis. Pediatr Crit Care Med. 2009;10:182–90.

Sharma V, Fan J, Jerath A, Pang KS, Bojko B, Pawliszyn J, Karski JM, Yau T, McCluskey S, Wasowicz M. Pharmacokinetics of tranexamic acid in patients undergoing cardiac surgery with use of cardiopulmonary bypass*. Anaesthesia. 2012;67:1242–50.

Solomon C, Pichlmaier U, Schoechl H, Hagl C, Raymondos K, Scheinichen D, Koppert W, Rahe-Meyer N. Recovery of fibrinogen after administration of fibrinogen concentrate to patients with severe bleeding after cardiopulmonary bypass surgery. Br J Anaesth. 2010;104:555–62.

Song HK, Tibayan FA, Kahl EA, Sera VA, Slater MS, Deloughery TG, Scanlan MM. Safety and efficacy of prothrombin complex concentrates for the treatment of coagulopathy after cardiac surgery. J Thorac Cardiovasc Surg. 2014;147:1036–40.

Sorensen B, Bevan D. A critical evaluation of cryoprecipitate for replacement of fibrinogen. Br J Haematol. 2010;149:834–43.

Stone GW, Clayton TC, Mehran R, Dangas G, Parise H, Fahy M, Pocock SJ. Impact of major bleeding and blood transfusions after cardiac surgery: analysis from the acute catheterization and urgent intervention triage strategY (ACUITY) trial. Am Heart J. 2012;163:522–9.

Tanaka KA, Mazzeffi M, Durila M. Role of prothrombin complex concentrate in perioperative coagulation therapy. J Intensive Care. 2014;2:60.

Teoh KH, Young E, Blackall MH, Roberts RS, Hirsh J. Can extra protamine eliminate heparin rebound following cardiopulmonary bypass surgery? J Thorac Cardiovasc Surg. 2004;128:211–9.

Tettey M, Aniteye E, Sereboe L, Edwin F, Kotei D, Tamatey M, Entsuamensah K, Amuzu V, Frimpong-Boateng K. Predictors of post operative bleeding and blood transfusion in cardiac surgery. Ghana Med J. 2009;43:71–6.

Theusinger OM, Baulig W, Seifert B, Emmert MY, Spahn DR, Asmis LM. Relative concentrations of haemostatic factors and cytokines in solvent/detergent-treated and fresh-frozen plasma. Br J Anaesth. 2011;106:505–11.

Tokushige A, Shiomi H, Morimoto T, Ono K, Furukawa Y, Nakagawa Y, Kadota K, Ando K, Shizuta S, Tada T, Tazaki J, Kato Y, Hayano M, Abe M, Hamasaki S, Ohishi M, Nakashima H, Mitsudo K, Nobuyoshi M, Kita T, Imoto Y, Sakata R, Okabayashi H, Hanyu M, Shimamoto M, Nishiwaki N, Komiya T, Kimura T. Incidence and outcome of surgical procedures after coronary artery bypass grafting compared with those after percutaneous coronary intervention: a report from the coronary revascularization demonstrating outcome study in Kyoto PCI/CABG registry Cohort-2. Circ Cardiovasc Interv. 2014;7:482–91.

Turecek PL, Varadi K, Gritsch H, Schwarz HP. FEIBA: mode of action. Haemophilia. 2004;10(Suppl 2):3–9.

Vivacqua A, Koch CG, Yousuf AM, Nowicki ER, Houghtaling PL, Blackstone EH, Sabik JF 3rd. Morbidity of bleeding after cardiac surgery: is it blood transfusion, reoperation for bleeding, or both? Ann Thorac Surg. 2011;91:1780–90.

Wademan BH, Galvin SD. Desmopressin for reducing postoperative blood loss and transfusion requirements following cardiac surgery in adults. Interact Cardiovasc Thorac Surg. 2014;18:360–70.

Warmuth M, Mad P, Wild C. Systematic review of the efficacy and safety of fibrinogen concentrate substitution in adults. Acta Anaesthesiol Scand. 2012;56:539–48.

Wikkelso A, Wetterslev J, Moller AM, Afshari A. Thromboelastography (TEG) or thromboelastometry (ROTEM) to monitor haemostatic treatment versus usual care in adults or children with bleeding. Cochrane Database Syst Rev. 2016;8:Cd007871.

Wikkelso A, Wetterslev J, Moller AM, Afshari A. Thromboelastography (TEG) or rotational thromboelastometry (ROTEM) to monitor haemostatic treatment in bleeding patients: a systematic review with meta-analysis and trial sequential analysis. Anaesthesia. 2017;72:519–31.

Yang L, Stanworth S, Baglin T. Cryoprecipitate: an outmoded treatment? Transfus Med. 2012;22:315–20.

Yank V, Tuohy CV, Logan AC, Bravata DM, Staudenmayer K, Eisenhut R, Sundaram V, McMahon D, Olkin I, McDonald KM, Owens DK, Stafford RS. Systematic review: benefits and harms of in-hospital use of recombinant factor VIIa for off-label indications. Ann Intern Med. 2011;154:529–40.

Zhu JF, Cai L, Zhang XW, Wen YS, Su XD, Rong TH, Zhang LJ. High plasma fibrinogen concentration and platelet count unfavorably impact survival in non-small cell lung cancer patients with brain metastases. Chin J Cancer. 2014;33:96–104.

Cardiovascular Complications and Management After Adult Cardiac Surgery

8

Antonio Hernandez Conte and Andrew G. Rudikoff

Abstract

Over the last several decades, the risk profile and severity index of patients undergoing cardiac surgery have increased as cardiac surgery has become more sophisticated. Cardiac surgical patients in the twenty-first century are older, have greater disease burden, and possess diminished physiologic reserve, including decreased ventricular function. Many of these patients have already undergone prior cardiac interventions and need additional, more complex surgical procedures. Consequently, these patients are at risk for developing major postoperative complications. Recognition and management of these complications are paramount to the cardiac anesthesiologist and intensivist.

Preoperatively, cardiac centers worldwide are developing risk calculators to stratify cardiac surgery patients. Large databases (i.e., Society of Thoracic Surgeons) and the use of risk tools (i.e., EuroSCORE, STS score) have focused on predicting complications post-cardiac surgery. The EuroSCORE model (standard and logistic) has been used to predict in-hospital mortality, 3-month mortality, prolonged length of stay (≫12 days), and major postoperative complications (intraoperative stroke, stroke over 24 h, postoperative myocardial infarction,

A. H. Conte, M.D., M.B.A. (✉)
University of California, Irvine School of Medicine, Orange, CA, USA

Kaiser Permanente Los Angeles Medical Center, Los Angeles, CA, USA
e-mail: Antonio.Conte@kp.org

A. G. Rudikoff, M.D.
Kaiser Permanente Los Angeles Medical Center, Los Angeles, CA, USA
e-mail: Andrew.G.Rudikoff@kp.org

A. Dabbagh et al. (eds.), *Postoperative Critical Care for Adult Cardiac Surgical Patients*, https://doi.org/10.1007/978-3-319-75747-6_8

deep sternal wound infection, re-exploration for bleeding, sepsis and/or endocarditis, gastrointestinal complications, postoperative renal failure, and respiratory failure).

Recognition of complications postoperatively is done through continuous invasive and noninvasive monitoring. This is accomplished via continuous electrocardiogram (ECG), arterial blood pressure measurement via arterial catheter, frequent arterial blood gas sampling, central venous pressure (CVP) measurement via central venous catheter, pulse oximetry, and evaluation of chest tube drainage. Additionally, the use of a pulmonary artery (PA) catheter and mixed venous oxygen saturation may be indicated. Chest X-rays are used to assess pleural effusions; transthoracic and transesophageal echocardiography can diagnose cardiac tamponade, illuminate postoperative structural abnormalities, and assess right and left ventricular function postoperatively.

The main insult usually sustained by the patient requiring cardiac surgery is related to inadequate myocardial contraction accompanied by low cardiac output with potentially compromised central and peripheral systemic indices. Poor diastolic function is linked to the inability to wean from cardiopulmonary bypass. Patients who cannot be weaned from CPB may require alternative means of extracorporeal support after separation from CPB. Innovative techniques for circulatory support devices have been developed, and newer more advanced and portable devices continue to enter the mainstay of modern-day cardiac practice. Initially, intra-aortic balloon pumps (IABPs) and centrifugal pumps were developed, whereas now rapidly evolving technical changes have led to new and improved pneumatic and electrically driven internal assist devices that are smaller and provide a less invasive means of insertion. These devices are being increasingly utilized in an effort to provide supportive assistance to one or both ventricle with increased safety and durability. Additionally, for patients who sustain permanent myocardial damage during cardiac surgery or with end-stage heart disease, multiple devices for extracorporeal support may be utilized as bridges to transplantation or as destination therapy.

Despite the utmost diligence and care in managing the patient undergoing cardiac surgery, multiple complications may ensue in the immediate postoperative period. This chapter will discuss the major complications that can arise and various treatment measures that may be employed by the cardiac anesthesiologist, cardiac surgeon, and critical care intensivist.

Keywords

Cardiovascular effects of common inotropic agents · Cardiac complications · Postoperative myocardial infarction · Postoperative hemodynamic instability · Low cardiac output · Cardiogenic shock · Arrhythmias · Vasoplegic syndrome · Postoperative cardiac tamponade · Cardiopulmonary resuscitation (CPR) after cardiac surgery · Circulatory assist devices

8.1 Background

Over the last several decades, the risk profile and severity index of patients undergoing cardiac surgery have increased as cardiac surgery has become more sophisticated. Cardiac surgical patients in the twenty-first century are older, have greater disease burden, and possess diminished physiologic reserve, including decreased ventricular function. Many of these patients have already undergone prior cardiac interventions and need additional, more complex surgical procedures. Consequently, these patients are at risk for developing major postoperative complications. Recognition and management of these complications are paramount to the cardiac anesthesiologist and intensivist.

Preoperatively, cardiac centers worldwide are developing risk calculators to stratify cardiac surgery patients. Large databases (i.e., Society of Thoracic Surgeons) and the use of risk tools (i.e., EuroSCORE, STS score) have focused on predicting complications post-cardiac surgery. The EuroSCORE model (standard and logistic) has been used to predict in-hospital mortality, 3-month mortality, prolonged length of stay (≫12 days), and major postoperative complications (intraoperative stroke, stroke over 24 h, postoperative myocardial infarction, deep sternal wound infection, re-exploration for bleeding, sepsis and/or endocarditis, gastrointestinal complications, postoperative renal failure, and respiratory failure). In a recent study, data on 5051 consecutive patients (isolated [74.4%] or combined coronary artery bypass grafting [11.1%], valve surgery [12.0%], and thoracic aortic surgery [2.5%]) were prospectively collected. In-hospital mortality was 3.9% and 16.1% of patients who had one or more major complications, respectively. Standard EuroSCORE also showed very good discriminatory ability and good calibration in predicting postoperative renal failure, sepsis, 3-month mortality, prolonged length of stay, and respiratory failure. These outcomes can be predicted accurately using the standard EuroSCORE which is very simple and easy in its calculation. The 2nd chapter of this book, titled "Risk and Outcome Assessments" provides a full discussion on the latter topics.

Recognition of complications postoperatively is done through continuous invasive and noninvasive monitoring. This is accomplished via continuous electrocardiogram (ECG), arterial blood pressure measurement via arterial catheter, frequent arterial blood gas sampling, central venous pressure (CVP) measurement via central venous catheter, pulse oximetry, and evaluation of chest tube drainage. Additionally, the use of a pulmonary artery (PA) catheter and mixed venous oxygen saturation may be indicated. Chest X-rays are used to assess pleural effusions; transthoracic and transesophageal echocardiography can diagnose cardiac tamponade, illuminate postoperative structural abnormalities, and assess right and left ventricular function postoperatively.

The main insult usually sustained by the patient requiring cardiac surgery is related to inadequate myocardial contraction accompanied by low cardiac output with potentially compromised central and peripheral systemic indices. Poor diastolic function is linked to the inability to wean from cardiopulmonary bypass. Patients who cannot be weaned from CPB may require alternative means of extracorporeal support after separation from CPB. Innovative techniques for circulatory support devices have been developed, and newer more advanced and portable devices continue to enter the mainstay of modern-day cardiac practice. Initially, intra-aortic balloon pumps (IABPs) and centrifugal pumps were developed, whereas now rapidly evolving technical changes have led to new and improved pneumatic and electrically driven internal assist devices that are smaller and provide a less invasive means of insertion. These devices are being increasingly utilized in an effort to provide supportive assistance to one or both ventricle with increased safety and durability. Additionally, for patients who sustain permanent myocardial damage during cardiac surgery or with end-stage heart disease, multiple devices for extracorporeal support may be utilized as bridges to transplantation or as destination therapy.

Despite the utmost diligence and care in managing the patient undergoing cardiac surgery, multiple complications may ensue in the immediate postoperative period. This chapter will discuss the major complications that can arise and various treatment measures that may be employed by the cardiac anesthesiologist, cardiac surgeon, and critical care intensivist.

8.2 Cardiac Monitoring

Upon arrival to the ICU, the postoperative cardiac surgical patient requires diligent and continuous hemodynamic monitoring; this is accomplished via continuous electrocardiogram (ECG), arterial blood pressure measurement via arterial catheter, frequent arterial blood gas sampling, central venous pressure (CVP) measurement via central venous catheter, pulse oximetry, and evaluation of chest tube drainage. Additionally, the use of a pulmonary artery (PA) catheter may be indicated, and its use has validated in patients who manifest pulmonary hypertension, severe low cardiac output, and partition of right and left ventricular failure. However, PA catheter use is associated with multiple risks and higher morbidity and mortality when indiscriminately utilized.

The main aim post-cardiac surgery is to maintain optimal hemodynamics and end-organ perfusion. The postoperative cardiac surgical patient commonly demonstrates persistent hypovolemia. After CBP, the inflammatory system is upregulated, resulting in increased capillary permeability and rapid distribution of fluid to extravascular compartment. One way to assess hypovolemia is through CVP, which is considered an approximation of preload. Though CVP can be an unreliable surrogate of preload, it is recommended to keep CVP > 10 mmHg by volume repletion; by the same respect, a CVP > 20 mmHg may warrant diuresis. Before volume administration, hemodynamic response to increasing preload can be assessed by passive leg raising.

After cardiac surgery, reduced myocardial function may be due to a wide variety of causes including inadequate valve repair, newly arising transient valvular dysfunction, insufficient revascularization, ischemic reperfusion injury, myocardial edema, reduced preload, and increased afterload. The adequacy of cardiac performance during the postoperative period in the intensive care unit (ICU) is assessed by cardiac index, arterial blood pressure, pedal pulses, skin temperature, mixed venous oxygen saturation level, urinary volume, and metabolic acidosis. Possible indicators of insufficient cardiac performance are:

Mean arterial pressure < 60 mmHg
Serum lactate > 2 mmol/L
Urinary output < 0.5 mL/h
Svo_2 < 60% with Sao_2 > 95%

Central mixed venous oxygen saturation (SVO_2) is a very accurate indicator of tissue perfusion, as it demonstrates the relationship between oxygen supply (determined by cardiac output) and demand (metabolic state). However, SVO_2 can only be obtained via use of a PA catheter.

Causes of low cardiac output after cardiac surgery may be evaluated by electrocardiogram, chest X-ray, hemodynamic data, cardiac indices obtained via PA catheter, and/or transesophageal/transthoracic echocardiography (TEE/TTE). ECG changes may be suggestive of myocardial ischemia or infarction, significant chest tube drainage, and blood collection, or signs of tamponade may be noted through chest X-ray, and echocardiography can delineate new ventricular wall motion abnormalities, decreased ejection fraction (EF), and new or residual valvular pathology.

8.2.1 Cardiovascular Effects of Common Inotropic Agents

The primary treatment for low cardiac output states is to utilize pharmacologic therapy. Specific classes of pharmacologic agents are instituted based upon the cause of low cardiac output state. Catecholamines are typically utilized as first-line therapeutic agents and exert their cardiovascular effects through α, β_1, β_2, and dopaminergic receptors. α receptor activation causes arterial vascular smooth muscle contraction and an increase in systemic vascular resistance (SVR). β_1 receptor stimulation in the myocardium causes increased contractility and conduction velocity. β_2 receptor activation causes vascular smooth muscle relaxation and reduction in SVR. Dopaminergic receptor activation in the kidney and splanchnic circulation causes organ vasodilation. Epinephrine in low doses acts at β_1 receptors and in high dose acts at α receptors. Norepinephrine is a potent α receptor agonist and enhances SVR via vasoconstriction. Phenylephrine is an α receptor agonist used in bolus setting to correct hypotension.

Pharmacologic support in patients with low cardiac output may be obligatory in the postoperative period. However, prior to instituting inotropic/pressor therapy, optimization of preload status, afterload status, and SVR must be considered as cardiac output is a function of myocardial contractility and hemodynamic conditions (afterload and preload). Additionally, inotropic and pressor therapy may yield additional adverse effects which may undermine the optimization of the post-cardiac surgery patient.

8.3 Cardiac Complications

8.3.1 Postoperative Myocardial Ischemia

While a large majority of cardiothoracic surgery is performed to optimize vascular supply to the heart via coronary artery bypass grafting, postoperative myocardial ischemia (PMI) and associated perioperative myocardial infarction (MI) remain significant complications in the postoperative setting.

The Society of Thoracic Surgeons (STS) National (United States) Database was established in 1989 as an initiative for quality improvement and patient safety among cardiothoracic surgeons. The STS maintains a clinical database for every cardiothoracic surgical procedure performed. The STS database has defined perioperative ischemia as the occurrence of at least one of the following markers: (1) electrocardiographic changes consistent with ischemia, (2) elevation of serum markers (i.e., troponin), and (3) reduced systolic ejection fraction. According to the most recent review of the STS database, the incidence of PMI is 1%.

8.3.1.1 Diagnosis of Postoperative Myocardial Ischemia (PMI)

The diagnosis of PMI is based upon STS guidelines. The most common laboratory tool for assessment of PMI is measurement of troponin I or cardiac troponin. Patients who manifested elevated preoperative levels of troponin may *not* necessarily imply PMI in the postoperative period. In addition, patients who underwent coronary artery bypass grafting (CABG) with the use of cardiopulmonary bypass (CPB) were more likely to have elevated levels of troponin compared to patients who were "off-pump." Additionally, troponin levels were more apt to remain within normal limits if CPB during CABG was not utilized. Elevation of the MB fraction of creatine kinase may also be measured and may be indicative of PMI. Since the majority of PMI may occur while a postoperative cardiac surgical patient is still intubated, symptoms associated with angina may not be elicited; therefore, electrocardiographic detection with follow-up laboratory assessment is paramount and critical to detection of PMI in the immediate postoperative period.

The type of cardiac surgery performed may allow the clinician to more accurately assess the etiology for PMI. In CABG cases, patients may be prone to closure of newly created vascular coronary conduits, as well as residual myocardial injury secondary to poor myocardial protection or low-flow cardiac states. Patients having undergone valve repair or replacement, especially aortic valve replacement with or without aortic root surgery, may be prone to anatomic disturbances in coronary blood flow originating at the coronary ostia. Diagnosis may require echocardiographic evaluation of left and right main coronary ostia or definitive invasive cardiac catheterization to rule out reocclusion or new occlusion of coronary ostia or their tributaries.

8.3.1.2 Management

Treatment of coronary myocardial ischemia and PMI is targeted at maneuvers to improve or restore coronary perfusion. In the absence of arterial hypotension, the initiation of intravenous venodilators (i.e., nitroglycerin), arterial vasodilators (i.e., sodium nitroprusside), and calcium channel blockers (i.e., nifedipine, nicardipine) may yield significant improvement in coronary perfusion. In addition, the administration of calcium channel blockers (i.e., nifedipine, nicardipine, clevidipine) may ameliorate vasospasm in cardiac arterial blood vessels.

The need to augment oxygen-carrying capacity may also require the administration of red blood cells. Patients not responding to restoration of arterial diastolic pressure concomitant with the use of preferential pressors and/or vasodilators may necessitate further evaluation with cardiac catheterization or invasive cardiac assessment with a pulmonary artery catheter. Efforts should be made to initiate the appropriate treatment intervention as soon as possible to rapidly institute definitive therapy.

8.3.2 Postoperative Hemodynamic Instability

Patients undergoing cardiac surgery undergo significant alterations in temperature, circulating blood volume, initiation of cardiopulmonary bypass, myocardial protection with plegic solutions, and total circulatory arrest render this patient population extremely susceptible to residual hemodynamic lability upon arrival in the intensive care unit.

8.3.2.1 Low Cardiac Output

Afterload, preload, and myocardial contractility are the main determinants of heart performance. Cardiac contraction cannot be considered independent from the vascular system, and manipulation of both afterload and preload is necessary for optimal cardiac function. Review of the Starling curve is important in understanding this physiologic relationship, and it is important for the clinician to develop an estimation a particular patient's Starling curve status.

Low cardiac output is the most critical complication after cardiac surgery. It is defined as the need for inotropic infusion support (for longer than 30 min), use of IAPB, or inotropic support to achieve cardiac output >2.2 L/m^2/min and preserve systolic blood pressure > 90 mmHg despite afterload reduction, optimization of preload, and correction of electrolytes and blood gases. Low cardiac output plays an important role in morbidity and mortality after cardiac surgery.

Some causes of low cardiac output syndrome include incomplete myocardial revascularization, insufficient myocardial protection during aortic cross-clamp, reperfusion injury, and systemic inflammatory response. During aortic cross-clamp, myocardial perfusion is interrupted; a bloodless field is provided at the expense of potential myocardial ischemia. A cardioplegic solution is used to arrest the heart and decrease the ischemic damage of myocardium during these intervals. Although there is no consensus about type, time, temperature, route of administration, and volume of cardioplegic solution, many studies had shown that inadequate myocardial preservation during surgery leads to postoperative low cardiac output. Therefore, improved ways of cardiac protection can minimize myocardial injury.

Low cardiac output (i.e., left ventricular ejection fraction <40%) in the postoperative period is associated with prolonged length of stay and further complicated by higher morbidity and mortality. Additionally, there is an increased utilization of healthcare resources to manage this subset of patients. Studies have shown that there are multiple independent predictors of low cardiac output after aortic valve and mitral valve replacement. These include:

Preoperative renal disease
Increasing age and frailty
Female sex
Redo-surgery and small aortic valve size
Urgency of the operation and CPB time

The most important predictor of low cardiac output after CABG is preoperative left ventricular dysfunction (EF < 20%). Management of low cardiac output due to left heart failure consists of increasing contractility, afterload reduction, and preload limitation. For right heart failure, in addition to inotropic agents, adequate preload status and reduction in pulmonary vascular resistance are recommended. In low cardiac output states that do not respond to inotropic support and IABP, the use of a temporary percutaneous ventricular assist device (i.e., Impella, Tandem Heart) as a bridge to recovery or transplantation may be advised.

8.3.2.2 Diagnosis

The critical care team should accurately and efficiently review the patient's preoperative hemodynamic and intraoperative hemodynamic history as well as noting significant events which may have deviated from the usual and customary management of a cardiothoracic surgical patient.

Diagnosis should include assessment of systolic and diastolic blood pressure trends as well as calculation of perfusion pressure and total peripheral resistance and estimation of cardiac output and/or cardiac index. Changes in the patient's cardiac rhythm and rate should also be assessed to determine if deviations from the intraoperative status have occurred. Loss of circulating blood volume should also be determined by assessing chest tube drainage or reductions in urinary output.

8.3.2.3 Management

The implementation of vasopressors, vasodilators, and/or inotropic agents may be necessary based upon the specific hemodynamic disturbance or etiology of ventricular dysfunction. However, definitive therapy should be aimed at determining the underlying etiology for the respective change (i.e., hypovolemia causing hypotension). Persistent hypotension despite pressor therapy may warrant further support such as administration of colloids or blood products. Hypertension may denote inadequate pain relief or lack of adequate sedation; therefore, opioids or sedatives may be warranted. Transesophageal echocardiography (TEE) may be of assistance in delineating cardiac specific pathology contributing to hemodynamic compromise.

Implementation of inotropic support should be based upon more specific findings delineated by use of a pulmonary artery catheter or echocardiography. Low cardiac output states secondary to diminution of stroke volume can be augmented by the use of fluids or pharmacologic therapy (i.e., epinephrine, norepinephrine, dobutamine, dopamine, or milrinone). The implementation of temporary pacing may ameliorate deficient cardiac rate contributing to low cardiac output. Therefore, pacing should be considered as an additional intervention. The insertion of an IABP should be reserved only for instances of refractory hemodynamic compromise unresponsive to pharmacologic support and pacing support.

8.3.3 Arrhythmias

Numerous rhythm disturbances may manifest themselves in patients having undergone cardiac surgery. Electrophysiologic cardiac abnormalities may be secondary to manual manipulation of the heart, arrest with plegic solutions, anatomic/mechanical disruption of electrical pathways, and/or impaired cardiac perfusion resulting in ischemia.

8.3.3.1 Diagnosis

The diagnosis of rhythm disturbances can be accurately assessed with a minimum of two-lead electrocardiographic monitoring; however, more occult arrhythmias may necessitate twelve-lead electrocardiographic evaluation. Arrhythmias may include but are not limited to bradyarrhythmias, tachyarrhythmias, malignant tachyarrhythmias, and multiple degrees of heart block.

The most common arrhythmia occurring in both the acute and later phases of postoperative recovery is the appearance of atrial fibrillation. A recent study of the STS database revealed that atrial fibrillation occurs with an annual incidence of 20% with the mean occurrence on postoperative day 3,, but the range was from 0 to 21 days after surgery. A review of multiple studies indicates that atrial fibrillation occurs in 10–40% of patients' post-cardiac surgery. Although prophylactic therapy with beta-adrenergic blockers reduces the incidence of postoperative atrial fibrillation, this arrhythmia remains an important cause of increased hospital stays and expenses after heart surgery.

Predictors of atrial fibrillation during hospitalization include age greater than 65, history of intermittent atrial fibrillation, atrial pacing, and chronic obstructive pulmonary disease. Additionally, atrial fibrillation is common after coronary artery bypass surgery (CABG) and results in prolonged hospitalization. Predictors *after* discharge were atrial fibrillation during hospitalization, valve surgery, and pulmonary hypertension. Patients with atrial fibrillation had almost twice the hospital mortality of patients without atrial fibrillation.

8.3.3.2 Management

Sinus rhythm is the rhythm of choice with respect to optimizing cardiac performance and ventricular filling. Electrical cardioversion or pharmacologic intervention with pacing may be necessary to establish and maintain normal sinus rhythm. Bradycardia can be treated with external or internal pacing and/or the administration of anticholinergics and/or catecholamines. Although atropine (10–40 mcg/kg) and glycopyrrolate (10–20 mcg/kg) are two useful anticholinergics, they are usually not effective in the postoperative setting. Catecholamines such as epinephrine, norepinephrine, isoproterenol, and ephedrine may also be used to treat symptomatic bradycardia. Sinus bradycardia with an adequate stroke volume may respond to anticholinergics; however, bradycardic patients with depressed ventricular performance should likely receive a more potent catecholamine such as epinephrine. More serious bradycardias (e.g., ventricular escape or idioventricular rhythms) will require more aggressive therapy.

Perioperative tachycardia responds well to electrical cardioversion and/or pharmacologic therapy. In the absence of electrolyte disturbances, new onset atrial flutter and atrial fibrillation are receptive to synchronized cardioversion. Post-electrocardioversion pacing can also help to control dysrhythmias. Bi-atrial pacing has been shown to be effective in preventing post-CABG atrial fibrillation than single-site atrial pacing. Beta-blockers (e.g., metoprolol, propranolol), calcium channel blockers (e.g., verapamil, diltiazem), and digoxin can also be used to help control the rate. Ventricular tachycardias can be treated with magnesium, lidocaine, bretylium, procainamide, and direct-current cardioversion. The treatment of ventricular fibrillation is immediate asynchronous electrical cardioversion.

After initial rhythm correction maneuvers, intravenous medications such as lidocaine (1–3 mg/kg), procainamide (250–500 mg load then 15–60 mcg/kg/min), bretylium (5–10 mg/kg), and amiodarone (1–5 mg/kg) may be instituted to help suppress further rhythm disturbance, and continuous infusions of these medications are often necessary. The onset of atrial fibrillation may be mitigated by the use of beta-blockers, angiotensin-converting enzyme (ACE) inhibitor, supplemental potassium, amiodarone, or nonsteroidal anti-inflammatory drugs when initiated in the preoperative period and continued through the operative phase. However, implementation of any of these agents is not completely effective; however, they do contribute to diminished rates of atrial fibrillation.

8.4 Vasoplegic Syndrome

Vasoplegia is one form of vasodilatory shock and common complications during or after cardiac surgery. The incidence of perioperative vasoplegia or vasoplegic syndrome may develop during or after cardiopulmonary pulmonary bypass (CPB) and ranges from 5 to 25%. Vasoplegic syndrome is characterized by significant hypotension, high or normal cardiac outputs and low systemic vascular resistance (SVR), and increased requirements for fluids and vasopressors during or after CPB.

The cause of reduced vascular tone is a matter of controversy, but it is postulated that endothelial dysregulation during CPB leading to an inflammatory response may play an important role. Vasoplegic syndrome is multifactorial, resulting on the one hand from pathologic activation of several vasodilator mechanisms and on the other from resistance to vasopressors; these pathways are dynamic and an interaction between the two is commonly seen. Activation of adenosine triphosphate-sensitive potassium channels (K_{ATP} channels) in the plasma membrane of vascular smooth muscle, activation of the inducible form of nitric oxide (NO) synthase, and deficiency of the hormone vasopressin are the prime culprits responsible for derailment of vascular tone. Known risk factors for developing vasoplegia include preoperative use of certain drugs (β-blockers, angiotensin-converting enzyme inhibitors, calcium channel blockers, and amiodarone), pre-CPB arterial hemodynamic instability, length of CPB, need for pre-CPB vasopressors, core temperature on CPB, and the intraoperative use of aprotinin.

A patient independent risk factor was the type of surgery being performed. Compared with coronary artery bypass grafting, valve procedures and surgery specifically intended for the treatment of heart failure were associated with an increased risk; however, aortic surgery and reoperations were protective against the development of vasoplegic syndrome. The mechanism of protection for these two groups remains speculative. Additionally, higher additive EuroSCORE was also associated with a higher incidence of vasoplegic syndrome.

Vasoplegic syndrome carries a poor prognosis. Specifically, norepinephrine-refractory vasoplegia is associated with an increase in morbidity and mortality. Catecholamine-refractory vasoplegic syndrome lasting for more than 36–48 h may have a mortality rate as high as 25%. Among patients who developed post-CPB vasoplegia, 57.4% had a bad outcome (defined as either death or a hospital length of stay >10 days) versus only 22.9% of non-vasoplegic patients.

8.4.1 Vasoplegic Syndrome Treatment

Vasoplegia does not usually respond to volume expansion. Norepinephrine, phenylephrine, high-dose dopamine, and vasopressin can increase systemic vascular resistance and maintain perfusion pressure after CPB. If there is no physiologic response to vasoconstrictor agents, methylene blue is recommended; see Table 8.1 for drugs, dosages, and site of action. Greater dosages of vasopressin, >0.04 U/min have not been shown to be beneficial when compared with norepinephrine alone, most likely because of poor microcirculatory perfusion. To date most literature has been published describing the post-CPB use of methylene blue as a therapeutic intervention of last resort to reverse vasoplegia.

Table 8.1 Summary of pressors and inotropes

Drug	Mechanism of action	Dose	Physiologic effects
Phenylephrine	α1 agonist	• 40–100 μg bolus • 0.5–10 μg/min infusion	Peripheral vasoconstriction, no inotropic action
Norepinephrine	α1, α2, and β1 agonist	• 4–10 μg bolus • 10–300 ng/kg/min	Potent vasoconstrictor with potential gut ischemia; increases pulmonary vascular resistance; arrhythmias
Vasopressin	V1 (independent of adrenergic receptors)	• 1–6 U/h infusion	Mesenteric ischemia at doses >6 U/h
Methylene blue	Inhibition of guanylate cyclase	• 2 mg/kg bolus	• Hemolytic anemia in patients with G6PD deficiency
		• 0.5 mg/kg/h for 6 h	• Greenish-blue coloration of urine and skin

8.5 Postoperative Cardiac Tamponade (POCT)

POCT is a specific type of circulatory failure due to compression of right heart (and sometimes left heart) chambers by blood or fluid accumulation in the pericardial sac after cardiac surgery; POCT may be seen from 1 to 8% of cardiac surgeries. This accumulation of fluid leads to increased pressure in the pericardial cavity and a decreased systemic venous return; this accumulation of fluid results in a pericardial effusion and may worsen to create tamponade physiology. However, clinically insignificant pericardial effusions are very common after open heart surgery. POCT is typically secondary to either surgical bleeding (i.e., suture lines, cannulation site, and branches of internal mammary artery) or secondary to CPB-related coagulation abnormalities. Characteristics and outcomes of patients who develop POCT are poorly defined.

The diagnosis of cardiac tamponade is based on clinical presentation, central venous pressure monitoring, and chest X-ray; transthoracic and/or transesophageal echocardiography yield the most accurate diagnostic information. It should be suspected in any patients with clinical hemodynamic instability (elevated central venous pressure, decreased systemic blood pressure, and urine output) in association with increased need for inotropic agents in the setting of significant chest tube drainage. Echocardiographic findings may demonstrate diastolic collapse of right atrium (and right ventricle) and lack of inferior vena cava collapse during inspiration. Diastolic collapse of left heart chambers may occur in the presence of discrete localized fluid accumulation.

Independent risk factors for POCT are type of surgery: aortic aneurysm, heart transplant, and valve surgery in comparison with CABG alone. Additionally POCT is associated with female gender, increased PTT preoperatively, renal failure, prolonged CPB time, pulmonary thromboembolism, and elevated BSA. POCT is especially common after valve surgery where oral chronic anticoagulant agents were usually utilized preoperatively. Postoperative anticoagulation is also considered to be a major contributing factor to the development of pericardial effusions and POCT *after* open heart surgery. The site and size of pericardial effusions after open heart surgery may be related specifically to the type of surgery; however, pericardial effusions causing POCT tend to be located posteriorly or circumferentially and are usually classified as moderate or large.

Some studies have shown that posterior pericardiotomy during cardiac surgery prevents blood accumulation in the posterior of left ventricular wall. Redo-sternotomy and mediastinal re-exploration, clot removal, and search for the probable site(s) of bleeding are the only efficient treatments of POCT after cardiac surgery. Late pericardial effusion and delayed tamponade may occur after cardiac surgery; diagnosis may be difficult. In this specific instance of POCT, it may occur due to pericardial adhesion, and the pericardial effusion is typically localized in the posterior portion of the heart. Transesophageal echocardiography is the most sensitive and specific diagnostic modality and can demonstrate the presence, size, and site of localized effusion and guide the approach to drainage.

8.6 Cardiac Arrest and Cardiopulmonary Resuscitation (CPR) After Cardiac Surgery

The incidence of cardiac arrest after cardiac surgery is less than 3%. The outcome is better than other causes of cardiac arrest due to a wide array of reversible etiologies and is also typically a witnessed arrest. The most common causes of postoperative cardiac arrest are ventricular fibrillation, major bleeding, and tamponade; all of them are usually treated immediately as they are recognized promptly in the ICU. As multiple hemodynamic indices (i.e., arterial pressure, pulse oximetry, ECG monitoring, and central venous pressure line) are observed continuously in the ICU, this allows for rapid identification of a critical event ensued by a rapid response. It has been shown that prompt management of cardiac arrest leads to improved outcomes and survival in these patients; ICU staff must be trained to manage this situation effectively and rapidly.

Among the predisposing factors leading to cardiac arrest, myocardial infarction has the worst prognosis. Hence it is rational that the CPR guidelines after cardiac surgery differ from cardiac arrest in other settings. The last guideline protocol for resuscitation after cardiac surgery was in 2009, and it was recommended for use in ICU for all patients post-sternotomy. The following is a summary of the guidelines:

(a) *Diagnosis of cardiac arrest*
- Because of full monitoring of intubated patients in ICU, verification of any "flat line" in monitors must be checked by central pulse palpation (i.e., femoral, carotid) for 10 s.
- As a clinical point, ECG lead displacement will not imitate ventricular fibrillation (VF) or asystole pattern; it causes "flat line" with preserved pressure lines.

(b) *Defibrillation attempts*
- A precordial thumb is recommended within 10 s of VT/VF onset but does not replace defibrillation. When VF is recognized, three consecutive biphasic defibrillation shocks (between 150 and 360 J) are recommended to restore cardiac output. It must be done consecutively without intervening CPR. Its time sequence is emphasized before starting external cardiac massage.
- If defibrillation fails, a bolus of intravenous amiodarone (300 mg) is recommended. If amiodarone is not available, 1 mg/kg of lidocaine may be given.
- If the patient had severe bradycardia or asystole and cannot be treated by cardioversion, a single dose of 3 mg of atropine is recommended. Epicardial pacing should be instituted at 90 beats/min.
- If adequate cardiac output is not achieved, CPR should be started. In pulseless electrical activity, the pacemaker must be set to "off" to rule out VF.

(c) *Timing of external cardiac massage*
- With VF or VT, if either defibrillation was not accessible or was unsuccessful (after three failed attempts), external cardiac massage must be started. Techniques should apply pressure in the middle of sternum, 100 beats/min, and press down 4–5 cm in depth. The efficacy of cardiac massage can be assessed by arterial trace on monitor; systolic impulse must be over 60 mmHg.
- In the presence of a balloon-expandable valve stent (i.e., TAVR), there is the risk of valve damage during external cardiac massage.

(d) *Airway control*
- The second person in attendance during a cardiac arrest is responsible for respiratory state. In intubated patients, oxygen on ventilator is increased to 100%, and PEEP is omitted. If the patient is not intubated, 100% oxygen with a bag valve and mask should be initiated with 2 breathes for every 30 chest compression. Bilateral and equal lung expansion must be checked.
- Capnography confirms position of endotracheal tube and quality of CPR. A rough way to assess lung compliance is disconnection from the ventilator and continuation with bag/valve ventilation; if there is adequate ventilation, reconnection to the ventilator occurs.
- Occlusion or malposition of endotracheal tube must be ruled out whenever lung inflation is not easy; in this condition the endotracheal tube should be removed, and bag/valve ventilation with airway is continued.
- If tension pneumothorax is suspected, a large bore Angiocath catheter is placed in second intercostal space at anterior midclavicular line with immediate insertion of a chest tube.

(e) *Emergent sternotomy*
- After failed defibrillation or pacemaker activation, there is proven benefit for resternotomy in the ICU. If the pressure generated by compression is not enough, the cause of arrest may be massive bleeding, tamponade, or tension pneumothorax, and emergent resternotomy should be accelerated. It is a common belief among cardiac surgeons that if initial resuscitation is not successful, resternotomy should be performed.

- Location of internal mammary artery and other grafts should be considered before internal massage.
- Re-exploration sternotomy should be considered if tension pneumothorax or cardiac tamponade is suspected. Additionally, an open chest allows for internal cardiac massage; this can improve coronary and cerebral perfusion pressure more than doubling of external massage. Return of spontaneous circulation may be increased as well.

(f) *Administration of drugs*

- During CPR, all medication infusions must be stopped. Although concern about severe hypertension and major bleeding after adrenaline (epinephrine) use is justifiable, epinephrine is nonetheless recommended when reversible causes of cardiac arrest are excluded; 1 mg of epinephrine should be administered for asystole/pulseless electrical activity and after the second failed cardioversion in VT/VF is used.
- All drugs should be administered via a central venous catheter when available.

(g) *Cardiac arrest in the setting of IABP*

- When pacemaker is activated, cardiac arrest may be identified by changes in pressure trace of CVP and pulse oximetry on monitor. Pressure trigger of IABP is turned on during cardiac massage with maximum augmentation with 1:1 counter pulsation to increase cardiac massage effect. Internal trigger must be set up whenever there is a period without cardiac massage.

(h) *Mechanical circulatory support after cardiac arrest*

- Mechanical circulatory support (CPB, extracorporeal membrane oxygenation) may be effective when spontaneous circulation has not been started by internal massage.

8.7 Circulatory Assist Devices

8.7.1 Intra-aortic Balloon Pump (IABP)

The intra-aortic balloon pump (IABP) is the most commonly utilized mechanical circulatory assist device in cardiac surgery and has been used since the late 1960s. It is used after cardiac surgery, coronary angioplasty, myocardial infarction, and other low output conditions, as the first step in the treatment of cardiogenic shock. IABP increases coronary artery perfusion pressure (and thus improves oxygen supply) during diastole by inflation and decreases the metabolic demand of myocardium (afterload reduction) in systole by deflating. The drive mechanism is pneumatic (helium). This volume replacement during cardiac cycles may increase cardiac output by 20%, but it cannot provide complete mechanical support.

IABP is used to facilitate CPB weaning intraoperatively when hemodynamic stabilization is not adequate despite adequate preload and afterload and use of inotropic agents. It provides a protective method against hemodynamic deterioration during the early postoperative period in the ICU. It is believed that use of preoperative IABP has better outcomes compared to later insertion in the intraoperative or postoperative period. Studies had suggested that prophylactic IABP (instead of rescue therapy for cardiovascular instability) may decrease mortality and morbidity and improve outcome in high-risk cardiac surgery patients, who have at least two of following conditions: unstable angina at the time of surgery, redo operations, congestive heart failure in spite of full-dose medical treatment, EF < 30%, and left main artery stenosis>75%.

The use of levosimendan in lieu of IABP is controversial, and it is disputed that it can be as effective as IABP in high-risk cardiac surgery patients. Levosimendan is the only inotropic agent that increases the sensitivity of myocardial contractile protein to calcium (others act by raising intracellular calcium). It decreases myocardial demand and afterload and increases cardiac index.

The insertion technique for IABP is either percutaneously or insertion under direct visualization by surgical exposure of the femoral artery (retrograde approach). When there is no access through femoral artery (due to aortic occlusion or previous surgery), transthoracic arch and axillary, subclavian, and iliac arteries are suggested (antegrade approach). The complication rate for IABP is low; however, distal embolic events and/or limb ischemia is the most common complication with frequent need for vascular intervention (i.e., arterial embolectomy). The size of balloon pump catheter, female sex, presence of peripheral arterial diseases, and duration of IABP use are predictors of IABP-related complications. Limitations of IABP are small body size, right ventricular failure, profound heart failure, and tachyarrhythmia.

8.7.2 Ventricular Assist Device (VAD)

While the intra-aortic balloon pump (IABP) is very helpful for hemodynamic instability, it only increases cardiac output by 10–20%. Therefore, the definitive treatment for severe cardiac decompensation relies on the use of a ventricular assist device (VAD). Circulatory assist devices have been designed and utilized to support the heart by providing forward flow, bridge to recovery, heart transplant, or destination therapy; they have been shown to improve quality of life and outcome. VADs may be used for short- and long-term support, without removal of the native heart. VADs are commonly labeled as LVAD (left), RVAD (right), BiVAD (biventricular), and TAH (total artificial heart). VADs may be implantable via an intracardiac approach or externally (abdominal wall or intraperitoneal); a midsternotomy and use of CPB are necessary for insertion of inlet tube from the heart to device and outlet tube from device to the aorta. The device power source may be electrical or pneumatic; forward flow may be pulsatile or continuous. VADs require long-term anticoagulation; however, patients have nearly unlimited mobility. Newer generation of assist devices are smaller, require less complex surgical implantation, have less blood-surface contact, and provide longer durability.

VADs are of great benefit in cases of reversible ventricular dysfunction. It was shown that patients who underwent elective VAD placement had better outcomes than when inserted in emergent or urgent situations. VADs are not recommended in patients with terminal severe comorbidities (i.e., severe hepatic or pulmonary dysfunction, chronic dialysis, sepsis, and metastatic cancer). The most common complications are bleeding, infection, and thromboembolic events.

8.7.3 Extracorporeal Membrane Oxygenation (ECMO)

Extracorporeal membrane oxygenation (ECMO) is used instead of conventional cardiopulmonary bypass for reversible respiratory or cardiac failure and/or whenever there is no response to usual therapies (optimized preload state, use of inotropic agents, and ventilator support). The sole advantage of ECMO is its application in emergency situation (at the bedside and operating room) and as a satisfactory partial cardiopulmonary support for both the heart (left and right) and lung for severe, acute, and reversible dysfunction.

In less than 1% of patients after routine cardiac surgery operations, there is failure to wean off CPB in spite of high-dose inotropic agents, pressors, and placement of IABP. Emergency surgery, repeat surgeries, severe LV dysfunction, renal failure, and younger age are predictors of postcardiotomy pump failure and need for ECMO support. The cause of low cardiac output syndrome in the aforementioned scenarios may be related to systemic inflammatory response during CPB, myocardial ischemia, and/or reperfusion injury. Other indications for implementing ECMO include cardiogenic shock with correctable pathology, bridge to transplantation, myocarditis, postpartum cardiomyopathy, and cardiac arrest. ECMO is not suggested in the presence of sepsis, multi-organ failure, and severe neurologic deficit and absolutely contraindicated in active bleeding and whenever recovery of cardiac function due to severe underlying disease is not expected.

The ECMO circuit is composed of a blood-pumping device (roller/centrifugal pump), inflow and outflow cannula, membrane oxygenator, hemofilter, heparin-coated circuit, and heat exchanger. There are two methods of cannula insertion: peripheral and central (transthoracic). Peripheral arterial and venous cannulation are performed percutaneously by Seldinger technique, cutdown, or both. Central cannulation can be accomplished by sternotomy or thoracotomy. Whenever there is lung dysfunction with normal circulatory state, venovenous type of ECMO is applied. Venoarterial ECMO is recommended for acute heart failure or if both heart failure and respiratory insufficiency/failure is present. The adequacy of perfusion is determined by serum lactate level, mixed venous oxygen saturation, and arterial base deficit.

Activated clotting time must be kept around 180–200 s during use of ECMO in order to prevent thrombosis and hemorrhagic events. Other described complications and causes of in- hospital death with ECMO include ischemia of lower limbs, organ system dysfunction (lung, renal, and neurologic), sepsis, DIC, myocardial failure, and oxygenation failure. Vascular complications with venovenous cannulation are less than arterial cannulation. Open vascular exposure, use of antegrade catheter to increase limb perfusion, rapid clinical diagnosis, and intervention to remove cannula and replace vascular access reduce ischemic events. Chapter 20 of this book deals with ECMO as a separate chapter with more details for interested audiences.

Bibliography

Afilalo J, Mottillo S, Eisenberg MJ, Alexander KP, Noiseux N, Perrault LP, Morin J-F, Langlois Y, Ohayon SM, Monette J. Addition of frailty and disability to cardiac surgery risk scores identifies elderly patients at high risk of mortality or major morbidity. Circ Cardiovasc Qual Outcomes. 2012;5:222–8.

Atoui R, Ma F, Langlois Y, Morin JF. Risk factors for prolonged stay in the intensive care unit and on the ward after cardiac surgery. J Card Surg. 2008;23:99–106.

Camm AJ, Kirchhof P, Lip GY, Schotten U, Savelieva I, Ernst S, Van Gelder IC, Al-Attar N, Hindricks G, Prendergast B. Guidelines for the management of atrial fibrillation: the Task Force for the Management of Atrial Fibrillation of the European Society of Cardiology (ESC). Eur Heart J. 2010;31:2369–429.

Fischer GW, Levin MA. Vasoplegia during cardiac surgery: current concepts and management. Semin Thorac Cardiovasc Surg. 2010;22:140–4.

Kuvin JT, Harati NA, Pandian NG, Bojar RM, Khabbaz KR. Postoperative cardiac tamponade in the modern surgical era. Ann Thorac Surg. 2002;74:1148–53.

Mathew JP, Fontes ML, Tudor IC, James Ramsay J, Duke P, Mazer CD, Barash PG, Hsu PH, Mangano DT, Investigators of the Ischemia Research and Education Foundation; Multicenter Study of Perioperative Ischemia Research Group. A multicenter risk index for atrial fibrillation after cardiac surgery. JAMA. 2004;291:1720–9.

O'Neill WW, Kleiman NS, Moses J, Henriques JP, Dixon S, Massaro J, Palacios I, Maini B, Mulukutla S, Džavík V. A prospective randomized clinical trial of hemodynamic support with Impella 2.5 TM versus intra-aortic balloon pump in patients undergoing high-risk percutaneous coronary intervention: the PROTECT II study. Circulation. 2012;126(14):1717–27.

Parolari A, Pesce LL, Trezzi M, Cavallotti L, Kassem S, Loardi C, Pacini D, Tremoli E, Alamanni F. EuroSCORE performance in valve surgery: a meta-analysis. Ann Thorac Surg. 2010;89:787–93, 793.e1–2.

Toumpoulis IK, Anagnostopoulos CE, Swistel DG, DeRose JJ Jr. Does EuroSCORE predict length of stay and specific postoperative complications after cardiac surgery? Eur J Cardiothorac Surg. 2005;27:128–33.

Winkelmayer WC, Levin R, Avorn J. Chronic kidney disease as a risk factor for bleeding complications after coronary artery bypass surgery. Am J Kidney Dis. 2003;41:84–9.

9 Gastrointestinal Complications and Their Management After Adult Cardiac Surgery

Jamel Ortoleva and Edward A. Bittner

Abstract

Gastrointestinal complications (GICs) following cardiac surgery are often severe and contribute to substantial morbidity and mortality. The diagnosis of GICs remains difficult because symptoms and signs are often subtle, or nonspecific, and this commonly leads to delay in definitive diagnosis and treatment. Preventive strategies, coupled with early recognition and aggressive management, provide the foundation of the general clinical approach to addressing these complications. Overall, a high index of clinical suspicion and a low threshold for investigation and definitive management are recommended in patients with nonroutine clinical progress after cardiac surgery. It is imperative that all clinicians who care for postoperative cardiac surgical patients be familiar with the full spectrum of potential GICs in this patient population, as well as the general therapeutic approaches to these complications.

J. Ortoleva, M.D.
Adult Cardiothoracic Anesthesiology Program, Yale-New Haven Hospital, New Haven, CT, USA
e-mail: Ortoleva@partners.org

E. A. Bittner, M.D., Ph.D., M.S.Ed. (✉)
Critical Care-Anesthesiology Fellowship, Massachusetts General Hospital, Harvard Medical School, Boston, MA, USA

Surgical Intensive Care Unit, Massachusetts General Hospital, Harvard Medical School, Boston, MA, USA

Department of Anesthesia, Critical Care and Pain Medicine, Massachusetts General Hospital, Harvard Medical School, Boston, MA, USA
e-mail: ebittner@partners.org

A. Dabbagh et al. (eds.), *Postoperative Critical Care for Adult Cardiac Surgical Patients*, https://doi.org/10.1007/978-3-319-75747-6_9

Keywords
Gastrointestinal complications · Risk factors · Pathophysiology · Epidemiology · Ileus · Colonic pseudo-obstruction · Dysphagia · Gastritis · Esophagitis · Gastrointestinal bleeding · Acute cholecystitis · Acute mesenteric ischemia · Liver dysfunction · Pancreatitis · Gastrointestinal complications related to mechanical assist devices

9.1 Introduction

Gastrointestinal complications (GIC) after cardiac surgery encompass a heterogeneous group of pathologies, ranging from a simple, temporary paralytic ileus to more serious, life-threatening conditions, such as gastrointestinal hemorrhage, cholecystitis, acute pancreatitis, liver failure, and mesenteric ischemia. Although relatively infrequent, these complications are often severe, resulting in a prolonged hospitalization and increased cost and high mortality. Despite the advances in perioperative care of cardiac surgery patients, the incidence of postoperative GICs and associated mortality has not changed substantially since the earliest reports (Diaz-Gomez et al. 2010). Recent improvements in surgical technique and perioperative care to reduce GICs may have been offset by the increasing complexity of cardiac surgery with older and sicker patients undergoing operations.

The clinical diagnosis of GICs is often difficult as a result of multiple factors, including differences in typical clinical signs and symptoms compared with noncardiac surgery patients, the impact of medications affecting assessment (e.g., sedatives, neuromuscular-blocking agents and analgesics), and underlying patient comorbidities. Diagnosis may further be impaired by the tendency to underestimate potentially lethal consequences of GICs because of their relative infrequency and the fact that they lack a "visible connection" to the primary target organ of cardiac surgery (Karangelis et al. 2011).

The pathogenesis of GICs is complex, not fully understood, and often multifactorial. Risk factors for GICs have been identified and may enable the use of preventive strategies, prompt early investigation, and allow early identification of complications in the perioperative period. Delayed recognition of these complications leads to a high incidence of morbidity and mortality; therefore prompt diagnosis and treatment are essential. This chapter reviews the epidemiology, clinical features, and treatment of patients developing GICs after cardiac surgery.

9.2 Epidemiology

9.2.1 Incidence

The incidence of gastrointestinal complications following cardiothoracic surgery ranges widely from <1% to 5.5% of patients and is associated with mortality rates between 14 and 61% (Vassiliou et al. 2008; Zhang et al. 2009).The most common GICs include ileus, gastrointestinal (GI) bleeding, bowel ischemia, and pancreatitis. Perforation of a duodenal ulcer, hepatic failure, and cholecystitis occur less frequently. The wide variation in incidence of GICs may be accounted for by differences in patients studied, surgical technique, and reporting. Previous reports on the incidence and risk factors for these complications have largely focused on patients undergoing coronary artery bypass grafting (CABG) rather than the larger population of cardiac surgical procedures. With the broader application of percutaneous transluminal coronary angioplasty, the population of patients referred for cardiac surgery has significantly changed with a majority of patients in tertiary centers undergoing more complex procedures including combined valve/CABG, multiple valve, and aortic procedures. In addition the current population of cardiac surgical patients are often older and present with significant preoperative comorbidities including atherosclerotic diseases. These factors potentially increase the risk of abdominal organ hypoperfusion and thromboembolic events, which represent two major pathophysiologic mechanisms of ischemic complications. The high mortality in cardiac surgical patients that develop GICs has been attributed to delayed diagnosis and treatment, which often precipitates multisystem organ failure. However, these patients frequently have serious associated medical problems and limited physiologic reserved, which diminishes their ability to survive a major ischemic, septic, or hemorrhagic insult. During the last decade, significant advances have also been made in the perioperative management of patients undergoing cardiac surgery, which might favorably impact the incidence of GICs. These changes in the cardiac surgical population and advances in management have raised the question of the validity of previously reported incidence and risk factors for the occurrence of GICs.

Variation in the incidence of GICs might also be explained by an inconsistency in definitions in different studies. For example, a retrospective study by Mangi et al. analyzed 8709 patients undergoing cardiac surgery and reported an incidence of GICs of 0.5% (Mangi et al. 2005). These authors only reported patients with GICs which required a general surgical consult. Using this definition, only the "sickest" patients were included, particularly those with ischemic bowel disease. Patients with GICs managed with medical or endoscopic treatment without surgical consult were not reported in their series. In contrast in a national multicenter investigation that included more than 2.5 million CABG procedures, the reported GIC rate was 4.1% (Rodriguez et al. 2007). In this analysis rare GICs such as intraabdominal abscess, *Clostridium difficile* infection, esophageal ulceration, and diverticulitis were included which likely explains the higher incidence of GICs in their analysis. Some literature suggests a reduction in the incidence of both ischemic and, more markedly, of hemorrhagic GICs (Filsoufi et al. 2007; Ashfaq et al. 2015).While the precise explanation for this finding has not been elucidated, it has been suggested that the lower incidence of GICs might lie in systematic application of preventive measures and new advances in the intraoperative management of patients undergoing cardiac surgery.

9.2.2 Risk Factors

Numerous risk factors have been reported for GICs after cardiac surgery (Vassiliou et al. 2008; Gulkarov et al. 2014). In general, patients with comorbidities and those with a prolonged or complicated postoperative course are most likely to develop GICs. Although for each complication there may be individual risk factors, as a

Table 9.1 Risk factors for GI complications after cardiac surgery

Preoperative	Intraoperative	Postoperative
Advanced age	Valvular or combined CABG/valve surgery	Prolonged mechanical ventilation
Decreased left ventricular ejection fraction (<40%)	Emergency surgery	Need for reoperation (re-sternotomy or re-thoracotomy)
Peripheral vascular disease	Prolonged CPB time	Stroke
Peptic ulcer disease	Increased blood transfusion	Postoperative infection or sepsis (including sternal wound infection)
Chronic kidney disease	Presence of arrhythmias	Acute kidney injury
Diabetes mellitus		Need for vasopressors or IABP after surgery
COPD		
Use of preoperative inotropic support or IABP		

general principle, those factors that lead to reduced peripheral blood delivery and tissue oxygenation increase the incidence significantly. Some of the identified factors seem to be universally present across different studies; some others are likely unique to specific study populations. Many patients with GICs present with more than one complication (Filsoufi et al. 2007). Risk factors for GICs may be classified as pre-, intra-, or postoperative (Table 9.1). Commonly cited preoperative risk factors include advanced age, chronic renal failure, hepatic insufficiency, peripheral vascular disease, diabetes mellitus, chronic obstructive respiratory disease, preexisting gastrointestinal disease, congestive heart failure, prior myocardial infarction, low cardiac output state, and use of inotropic support or an intra-aortic balloon pump (IABP). Intraoperative risk factors include prolonged cardiopulmonary bypass (CPB) duration, valvular surgery, emergency surgery, increased blood transfusion, use of IABP, and the presence of arrhythmias. Postoperative risk factors for GICs include prolonged mechanical ventilation, an acute kidney injury, a deep sternal wound infection, and a low cardiac output state.

Based on identified risk factors, risk stratification scores have been developed to estimate the probability for the patient to develop a GIC after cardiac surgery (Díaz-Gómez et al. 2010; Karangelis et al. 2011; Vassiliou et al. 2008; Zhang et al. 2009; Mangi et al. 2005; Rodriguez et al. 2007; Filsoufi et al. 2007; Ashfaq et al. 2015; Gulkarov et al. 2014). Risk stratification based on identification of such scores may influence operative strategy or heighten the index of suspicion of the treating clinician when confronted with a postoperative course which deviates from the expected norm. Finally, risk stratification scores for GICs may provide clinically relevant information indicating subsets of patients most likely to benefit from invasive procedures such as laparotomy and may provide a framework for providing patients and their families with realistic expectations should such complications occur.

9.3 Pathophysiology

Under normal conditions, the splanchnic circulation receives 20% of cardiac output and accounts for 20% of total body oxygen consumption (Allen 2014). Blood is supplied to the liver, stomach, pancreas, and duodenum by the celiac artery, the superior mesenteric artery supplies the pancreas, duodenum, jejunum and ileum, ascending and transverse colon, and the descending and sigmoid colon are supplied by the inferior mesenteric artery, with each major artery branching from the abdominal aorta. The splanchnic circulation acts not only as perfusion to the abdominal organs but also as a blood reservoir, enabling compensatory autotransfusion into the central circulation (of approximately 800 mL blood) in response to hypovolemia, catecholamines, or low cardiac output (Hessel 2004). The splanchnic supply is usually autoregulated by resistance arterioles, which dilate in response to a decrease in mean arterial pressure (MAP) or accumulation of metabolites. However, the splanchnic circulation is unable to autoregulate perfusion at extremes of pressure or flow and therefore is vulnerable to alterations in these parameters during cardiopulmonary bypass (CPB), hemorrhage, hypovolemia, or arrhythmias.

Splanchnic hypoperfusion and impaired oxygen-induced ischemia are thought to be the primary cause of most GICs after cardiac surgery (Moneta et al. 1985; Ohri and Velissaris 2006). Hypoperfusion may be caused by reduced or suboptimal cardiac output, impaired regional blood flow, or inadequate systemic MAP. Additional injury likely occurs through systemic inflammation and systemic inflammatory response syndrome (SIRS), release of inflammatory mediators, nonpulsatile blood flow, hypothermia, drug therapy, and mechanical factors.

The SIRS response occurs as a result of surgical stress, contact with the CPB circuit, mechanical ventilation, and ischemia itself which may exacerbate SIRS together with reperfusion injury. The inflammatory and complement cascades release mediators which have vasoconstrictor actions and cytokine activation have been implicated in vascular endothelial dysfunction and damage (Ohri and Velissaris 2006). All these factors contribute to a maldistribution of blood flow and impaired mucosal oxygen delivery.

CPB causes renin release and activation of the renin-angiotensin-aldosterone axis with secretion of angiotensin II, a potent vasoconstrictor. Vasoactive drugs commonly used in the perioperative period such as norepinephrine and vasopressin are also associated with splanchnic hypoperfusion. In addition hypothermia used with CPB is associated with vasoconstriction and altered regional blood flow and distribution (Slater et al. 2001).

Mechanical factors that may contribute to GI ischemia include micro- and macro-emboli resulting from air, atheroma, thrombus, or debris and hepatic and GI congestion related to venous cannula placement. Mechanical ventilation especially requiring high positive end-expiratory pressure (PEEP) can result in hypotension and impaired cardiac output, leading to splanchnic vasoconstriction and hypoperfusion. In combination these factors result in the shunting of blood away from the GI system, leading to organ ischemia and damage.

Nonischemic mechanisms may also contribute to the development of GICs after cardiac surgery including bacterial translocation (resulting from altered mucosal barriers and blood flow), adverse drug reactions (e.g., over-anticoagulation, amiodarone-induced hepatotoxicity), and iatrogenic organ injury (e.g., malpositioned surgical drains).

9.4 Diagnostic Considerations

Early diagnosis of GICs in cardiac surgery patients is often challenging. Clinical presentation varies with pathology, no single diagnostic test will reliably diagnose or exclude all intra-abdominal pathology, and investigation should be directed by patient history and presentation. A patient's complaint of abdominal pain in the appropriate clinical setting is often the most sensitive indicator of significant GI pathology. Other clinical indices that should prompt efforts for early recognition of GICs include abdominal bloating, persistent ileus, sepsis, or GI bleeding. Multi-organ failure, metabolic derangement, and cardiovascular instability are nonspecific and often late signs of complications. Overall, a low threshold for investigation in those patients with nonroutine postoperative courses is recommended. In addition to a review of risk factors and physical exam, initial laboratory testing should include serum lactate, glucose, a hepatic panel (transaminases, bilirubin, alkaline phosphatase, and gamma-glutamyl transpeptidase), coagulation parameters, and complete blood count including white blood cell count and differential. These may be followed by abdominal radiography, ultrasound or computed tomography scanning, upper and lower endoscopy, and diagnostic laparoscopy or laparotomy as indicated.

9.5 Treatment Considerations

Since early diagnosis of GICs after cardiac surgery is difficult and patients are often critically ill at the time complications are recognized, management of these serious, often life-threatening, problems is challenging. Initial treatment is often conservative, but when it fails, prompt surgical intervention is necessary. Timely operation or intervention may be lifesaving in patients who are unable to compensate from the severe hemodynamic disturbances of a refractory abdominal complication, such as major bleeding or sepsis. Hesitation to intervene because the patient "had recent cardiovascular surgery" should not be a barrier. Special considerations are necessary for postcardiac surgical patients undergoing abdominal surgery (Dong et al. 2012). The lower end of the sternal wound should be protected from contact with the abdominal incision to prevent contamination and reduce the risk of sternal infection and mediastinitis. Prophylaxis against bacterial endocarditis should be instituted, especially in patients with a prosthetic vessel or valve(s). Finally patients who are anticoagulated require judicious reversal and re-institution of anticoagulation after abdominal surgery.

9.6 Specific Conditions

The clinical presentation, suggested diagnostic tests, and management considerations for specific conditions are described in the following sections and summarized in Table 9.2.

Table 9.2 Summary of gastrointestinal complications, common clinical presentations, and suggested investigations (adapted from Allen 2014)

Complication	Clinical presentation	Diagnosis	Management
Ileus	Abdominal distension and pain Nausea/vomiting	Abdominal radiograph	Suppositories, enemas, prokinetic agents Mobilization Minimizing opioids Correction of electrolyte abnormalities Nasogastric tube decompression
Colonic pseudo-obstruction	Abdominal distension and pain	Colonic dilation and fluid levels on abdominal radiograph	Neostigmine and colonoscopic decompression
Dysphagia	Odynophagia, hoarseness Coughing or gagging when swallowing	Videofluoroscopic swallow study or fiber-optic endoscopic evaluation of swallowing	Modification of eating and swallowing Nasoenteral tube or parenteral feeding
Gastritis and esophagitis	Gnawing or burning ache or abdominal pain Nausea or vomiting	Tests for ***H. pylori*** Endoscopy	Initiate enteral feeding H2 receptor blockers or proton pump inhibitors
GI bleeding Upper: duodenal or gastric ulceration Lower GIT: diverticulitis, AV malformations	Blood/melena per rectum Hematochezia Hemodynamic instability	Hemoglobin Lactate dehydrogenase Endoscopy (evidence or site of bleeding identified and potentially treated)	Intravenous fluid resuscitation Correction of coagulopathy Proton pump inhibitors Endoscopy for clipping or sclerotherapy to bleeding vessels Angiography, surgery (if lower gastrointestinal tract bleeding with arteriovenous malformation or diverticulitis)
Mesenteric ischemia Occlusive: emboli or thrombus Nonocclusive mesenteric ischemia (NOMI): hypoperfusion	Shock Abdominal pain and distension Intolerant of enteral nutrition GI bleeding	Complete blood count (leukocytosis) Lactate Abdominal radiograph (distended bowel, thickened bowel, evidence of ileus) Computed tomography Mesenteric angiography (global impairment of perfusion) Colonoscopy (ischemic bowel) Laparotomy (ischemic bowel)	Intravenous fluid resuscitation Circulatory support (inotropes or vasopressors) Antibiotic therapy Embolectomy, thrombectomy, and endarterectomy, as well as endovascular techniques such as balloon angioplasty, percutaneous stenting, and thrombolysis Laparotomy and bowel resection if perforation

(continued)

Table 9.2 (continued)

Complication	Clinical presentation	Diagnosis	Management
Peptic ulcer perforation	Abdominal pain, distension peritonitis	Abdominal radiograph (peritoneal air) Computed tomography scan abdomen (peritoneal air, collection)	Intravenous fluid resuscitation Proton pump inhibitor high dose Laparotomy-vagotomy and oversew of ulcer or resection Enteral rest and nasogastric drainage
Pancreatitis	Shock Epigastric and back pain Nausea and vomiting Abdominal distension	Amylase Lipase Computed tomography scan abdomen (pancreatic inflammation, free fluid, necrosis)	Intravenous fluid resuscitation Postpyloric feeding or intravenous nutrition Supportive therapy Analgesia Percutaneous drainage or surgical treatment
Cholecystitis Calculous or acalculous	Often 10–15 days postsurgery Right upper quadrant pain Fever Leukocytosis SIRS/shock	Liver function tests (elevated) Ultrasound (thickened gallbladder and common bile duct, ±gallstones) CT scan of abdomen Laparoscopy	Surgery (calculous) with cholecystectomy Antibiotics ± percutaneous drainage (acalculous)
Hepatic dysfunction	May be asymptomatic Jaundice	Elevated liver function tests (most commonly hyperbilirubinemia, transaminitis) Abdominal ultrasound (exclude obstruction, thrombosis, collections) Hepatitis serology screen (exclude as cause)	Stop potential hepatotoxins Supportive

9.7 Ileus

Ileus is a common GIC which in its simplest form affects almost every patient undergoing cardiac surgery (Karangelis et al. 2011). Perioperative fasting, effects of anesthetic agents, opioids, and decreased patient mobility all contribute to the intestinal dysfunction, which in the vast majority of cases resolves spontaneously in the early postoperative period. In a small proportion of patients, the ileus persists after the fourth postoperative day and requires the use of suppositories, enemas, and promotility agents (i.e., metoclopramide, erythromycin) or methylnaltrexone to facilitate clinical resolution. Close clinical monitoring, patient mobilization, minimizing the use of postoperative opioids, and correction of serum electrolyte abnormalities are usually successful in restoring or improving intestinal function. Cases that remain unresponsive are often managed with nasogastric suction, which should be continued until the return of bowel function. It is important to recognize that the appearance of clinically significant new ileus, especially when accompanied by severe abdominal pain, may indicate a more serious underlying problem such as mesenteric ischemia or pancreatitis.

9.8 Colonic Pseudo-obstruction

Colonic pseudo-obstruction (Ogilvie's syndrome) is an acute dilatation of the colon without any mechanical obstruction which occurs in up to 3.5% of patients undergoing cardiac or thoracic surgery (Guler et al. 2011). It may also develop after noncardiac surgery or systemic illness. It is characterized by massive colonic dilatation and the presence of fluid levels on abdominal radiograph. While the pathophysiology has not been fully elucidated, this condition seems to be associated with a disturbance of the autonomic innervation of the colon. Untreated, colonic pseudo-obstruction can lead to cecal overdistention and subsequent perforation. Perforation is more likely to occur if the cecal diameter exceeds 10–12 cm (De Giorgio and Knowles 2009). Two common management modalities for colonic pseudo-obstruction, used alone or in combination, are neostigmine administration and colonoscopic decompression. Surgical options for more refractory disease include cecal decompression (i.e., cecostomy) and colonic resection with ostomy creation.

9.9 Dysphagia

Dysphagia is a common complaint following cardiac surgery. The etiology of postoperative dysphagia is often multifactorial, including contributions from gastroesophageal reflux, local tissue trauma and inflammation from surgery, endotracheal intubation, intraoperative transesophageal echocardiography, and other potential factors such as recurrent/superior laryngeal nerve injury (Grimm et al. 2015). Affected patients are at increased risk for complications such as aspiration and pneumonia. Risk factors for dysphagia after cardiac surgery include male gender, low body mass index, chronic lung disease, cerebrovascular disease, placement of ventricular assist device or heart transplantation, hypothermic circulatory arrest, and prolonged postoperative mechanical ventilation. Early consultation with a speech language pathologist is vital to accurately diagnose patients with dysphagia in the immediate postoperative period. Therapy consists of modification of eating behavior and swallowing technique and in some more severe cases enteral tube or parenteral feeding.

9.10 Gastritis and Esophagitis

Gastritis and esophagitis are among the more common GICs in the cardiac surgery patient population. The etiology is multifactorial, with contributing factors including mucosal hypoperfusion, preexisting history of gastric or esophageal mucosal disorders, and the use of nonsteroidal anti-inflammatory drugs. Esophagitis is often associated with gastro-esophageal reflux, a particular concern for postsurgical patients due to the potential for pulmonary aspiration. Management of esophagitis and gastritis during the perioperative period includes avoidance of hypotension, avoiding delay in enteral feeding, and aggressive management with H2 receptor blockers or proton pump inhibitors. Diagnosis of esophagitis and gastritis is typically based on history and clinical symptoms with endoscopy as the most commonly utilized diagnostic modality. Maintaining head-of-bed elevation is an important preventive measure for postoperative patients with gastro-esophageal reflux and high pulmonary aspiration risk.

9.11 GI Hemorrhage

Gastrointestinal bleeding (GIB) is among the most common GICs following cardiac surgical procedures. In general, upper GIB occurs more frequently than lower GIB, with most hemorrhages (>90%) occurring proximal to the ligament of Treitz (Yilmaz et al. 1996). The two most common etiologies of upper GIB in cardiac surgical patients are duodenal ulceration and gastric erosion. Gastric and duodenal ulceration following cardiac surgery are likely secondary to systemic hypoperfusion with subsequent development of mucosal ischemia and erosion. Contributing factors include preoperative fasting, coagulation disorders, history of gastric or duodenal ulcer disease, and prolonged mechanical ventilation.

The initial step in diagnosis of GIB is the insertion of a nasogastric tube and lavage of gastric contents which aids in determining if the GI hemorrhage is proximal to the ligament of Treitz. Medical therapy is attempted first and includes the administration of proton pump inhibitors, red blood cell transfusion, and correction of coagulopathy. If medical management fails, upper endoscopy is the next step in evaluation and treatment of potential bleeding source(s). Endoscopic interventions are aimed at stopping the bleeding by cauterization, vasoconstrictive agent injection, or both. Endovascular embolization is now considered the first-line therapy for massive UGI bleeding that is refractory to endoscopic management (Loffroy et al. 2015). Surgical intervention is indicated if the patient fails medical endoscopic and endovascular treatment. In general, the presence of continued hemodynamic instability and a predetermined transfusion threshold (e.g., >4–6 units of packed red blood cells) are utilized as "triggers" for surgery.

As with upper GI bleeding, management of lower GI hemorrhage following cardiac surgical procedures begins with hemodynamic resuscitation and normalization of coagulation parameters. If the bleeding does not stop, the next step is the identification of the source of hemorrhage, either endoscopically or by imaging (e.g., angiography). In many cases, the bleeding can be controlled endoscopically or with endovascular embolization. Surgery is reserved for the failure of non-operative therapies.

Of note, gastrointestinal hemorrhage has been reported with increased frequency in cardiac patients with ventricular assist devices, with higher bleeding rates seen among recipients of nonpulsatile devices as compared to pulsatile devices (Cheng et al. 2014). Nonpulsatile ventricular assist devices far outnumber pulsatile devices, and thus GI hemorrhage will continue to be an important issue in this patient population for the foreseeable future.

9.12 Acute Cholecystitis

Acute cholecystitis after cardiac surgery is rare but carries a high mortality (Passage et al. 2007). Many cases of acute cholecystitis are "acalculous" and result from a variety of factors including systemic hypoperfusion, the SIRS, prolonged fasting, and the use of opioid medications. Typical symptoms of acute cholecystitis include right upper quadrant pain and tenderness on examination. However, diagnosis is often delayed in postcardiac surgical patients due to the presence of mechanical ventilation and sedation. For patients with acute cholecystitis, diagnosis is most often confirmed with right upper quadrant ultrasound or CT scan. Initial conservative treatment with transition to surgery in cases with lack of clinical improvement after 48 h is often recommended. The definitive treatment of acute cholecystitis is cholecystectomy for patients who are able to tolerate surgery. For poor surgical candidates, percutaneous cholecystostomy can serve as "bridging" therapy until the patient is ready to undergo cholecystectomy. Mortality rates associated with acalculous cholecystitis are significant which may reflect the overall poor general health status of patients at risk for this complication.

9.13 Acute Mesenteric Ischemia

Acute mesenteric ischemia (AMI) is a potentially life-threatening complication of cardiac surgery that can occur within hours to several days after surgery. AMI can affect any part of the small or large intestine and lead to devastating complications including mucosal sloughing, gangrenous changes of the bowel wall, and perforation. Mortality rates for patients with AMI exceed 40% in recent series (Eris et al. 2013; Viana et al. 2013). Common causes of AMI include embolism to the superior mesenteric artery, acute thrombosis of an atherosclerotic plaque with previous partial occlusion, splanchnic vasoconstriction leading to low flow and regional ischemia (referred to as nonocclusive mesenteric ischemia, NOMI), and mesenteric venous thrombosis. AMI after cardiac surgery most often is due to a NOMI and is related to a reduction in the splanchnic blood flow, which can be due to low cardiac output, and aggravated by cardiovascular support, such as vasopressors, and by preexisting atherosclerotic disease. The classic sign of AMI is abdominal pain out of proportion to physical examination findings; however many patients with intestinal ischemia after cardiac surgery have vague and nonspecific symptoms. Other symptoms are also present inconsistently and may include nausea, vomiting, and diarrhea. Physical examination is often unremarkable unless peritonitis has developed. During the late stages of AMI, abdominal distension and guarding, as well as systemic complications, may develop.

The most common laboratory abnormalities in patients with AMI are an unexplained lactic acidosis, hemoconcentration, and leukocytosis. However, even at the time when mesenteric ischemia is confirmed at laparotomy, an elevation of serum lactate may not be present (Acosta et al. 2009). Abdominal radiographs are of little help in the diagnosis of mesenteric ischemia. The presence of dilated loops of bowel is nonspecific, and thickened bowel loops or "thumbprinting" caused by submucosal edema or hemorrhage is inconsistently seen. Doppler sonography is useful in diagnosing chronic mesenteric arterial occlusive disease but has limited role in AMI. In the setting of high clinical suspicion, sigmoidoscopy or colonoscopy can aid in diagnosis of colonic ischemia. Computed tomography angiography provides direct visualization of the mesenteric vasculature, intestines, and mesentery allowing fast and accurate diagnosis of AMI. Angiography is the gold standard diagnostic test in acute mesenteric artery occlusion, providing both anatomical visualization of the vessels and therapeutic options (e.g., intravascular administration of vasodilators and thrombolytics).

Treatment of AMI consists of volume resuscitation, broad-spectrum antibiotics, vasodilators, and intravenous heparin at therapeutic doses which should be initiated without delay. Although surgical revascularization has been the standard management for restoring visceral blood flow, embolectomy, thrombectomy, and endarterectomy as well as endovascular techniques such as balloon angioplasty, percutaneous stenting, thrombolysis, and thrombus extraction have all been used with favorable outcomes. Angiographically proven NOMI can be treated with intra-arterial infusion of tolazoline, papaverine, or prostaglandin E2, after the selective intra-arterial catheterization of the SMA. If the patient develops signs of bowel infarction such as peritonitis, worsening sepsis, or metabolic acidosis during treatment, laparotomy is indicated.

9.14 Liver Dysfunction

Liver dysfunction can affect up to 10% of patients after cardiac surgery and can range in severity from mild liver enzyme elevation to fulminant failure (Sabzi and Faraji 2015). Consequences of severe liver failure include impaired clearance of hepatically metabolized drugs, coagulopathy, and encephalopathy. Risk factors for postoperative liver dysfunction include preexisting liver disease, prolonged CPB time, low cardiac output states necessitating administration of inotropic agents and/or IABP, volume of blood transfusion, and combined CABG and valve operations. Side effects of anesthetic drugs, as well as mechanical pressure from a low-placed inferior vena cava cannula, can also contribute to postoperative hepatic dysfunction. Treatment is supportive with control of fluids and electrolytes and replenishment of nutrient and coagulation factors. Worsening encephalopathy, jaundice, and ascites are important clinical markers of decompensation of liver function. Monitoring of coagulation and also maintaining vigilance for signs of postoperative bleeding should be continued beyond the usual postoperative monitoring period. Intravascular catheters should be removed as soon as they are no longer needed because of the increased risk of catheter-related sepsis in patients with liver impairment.

9.15 Pancreatitis

Acute pancreatitis is a relatively uncommon complication following cardiac surgery ranging in severity from subclinical amylase and lipase elevations to severe hemorrhagic, necrotic pancreatitis. Hypoperfusion from CPB, perioperative bleeding, SIRS, micro-embolization, and a history of preexisting pancreatic or gallstone disease are factors that increase the risk of acute pancreatitis. Clinically significant pancreatitis usually occurs slightly later following cardiac surgery than other GICs, such as bleeding or mesenteric ischemia. Patients typically complain of upper abdominal and left upper quadrant pain, nausea, vomiting, and/or abdominal distension. Laboratory values including elevated amylase and lipase are usually present. However, due to the high incidence of hyperamylasemia in cardiac surgery patients (exceeding 33%), clinical correlation is required before definitive diagnosis of pancreatitis is made (Fernandez-del Castillo et al. 1991). Management of acute pancreatitis postcardiac surgery follows that for noncardiac surgery patients.

9.16 GICs Related to Mechanical Assist Devices

The expanding use of mechanical cardiac assist technologies, i.e., ventricular assist devices (VADs), intra-aortic balloon pumps (IABPs), and extracorporeal membrane oxygenation devices (ECMO), is associated with clinically significant GICs.

- Patients who undergo VAD placement are at risk for a number of potential GICs, including abdominal infection, bowel injury, acalculous cholecystitis, pancreatitis, various hernias, gastric outlet obstruction, peritoneal fluid leaks, and mesenteric ischemia.
- IABPs have long been used for perioperative circulatory support in patients with low cardiac output. Despite improving coronary perfusion and reducing left ventricular afterload, IABP use is a known risk factor for gastrointestinal complications including gastrointestinal bleeding, bowel ischemia, and pancreatitis. In addition, malposition of the IABP balloon has been established as a primary factor leading to compromised visceral blood flow (Rastan et al. 2010).
- ECMO has been associated with embolic phenomena of the systemic circulation, end-organ ischemia, gastrointestinal hemorrhage, and abdominal compartment syndrome.

9.17 Prevention

A number of strategies have been suggested for prevention of GICs after cardiac surgery:

Preoperative preparation

- Use of preoperative risk stratification models may allow preventive strategies to be used pre- and intraoperatively as well as prompt earlier investigation, diagnosis, and management of complications postoperatively.
- Prophylactic gastric acid suppression using H2 blockers or proton pump inhibitors has been recommended to reduce the risk of peptic and duodenal ulcers and GI bleeding (Patel and Som 2013). Prophylactic acid-suppressive therapy has been associated with an increased incidence of pneumonia and other complications in hospitalized patients; therefore a practical approach is to initiate treatment during perioperative period and discontinue the therapy once normal oral intake is re-established.
- Preoperative hemodynamic optimization with correction of hypovolemia and anemia and support of cardiac output (e.g., inotrope therapy or IABP if required) may be beneficial for maintaining perfusion of the organs of the GI tract, thereby reducing GICs. However there are no large clinical trials to validate this approach. At present there remains considerable debate around the use of preoperative transfusion, and to date, no minimal preoperative hemoglobin target or threshold has been established.

Intraoperative prevention

- Intraoperative maintenance of adequate cardiac output and oxygenation is important; however, the exact hemodynamic parameters for adequate cardiac output and oxygen delivery are unknown and likely vary between patients.
- Several methods for monitoring GI perfusion, including measurement of gastric pH, ultrasound of blood flow in hepatic or mesenteric vessels, and measurement of intestinal transport functions, have been described but are not presently used clinically.
- Aspirin treatment within 48 h postoperatively has been associated with a reduction in both the incidence and mortality of GICs in CABG surgery (Mangano 2002).
- Milrinone infusion in patients undergoing CABG resulted in reduced gastric mucosal acidosis and lower inflammatory marker and endotoxin levels in a small RCT (Mollhoff et al. 1999). However other inotropic and vasoactive therapies such as epinephrine, dopamine, dobutamine, and vasopressin have been associated with reduced blood flow to the splanchnic circulation despite increases in MAP and systemic blood flow. It is likely that these detrimental effects are attributable at least in part to the mesenteric arteriolar constriction which is marked in response to systemic vasoconstrictors and overrides normal autoregulation. Minimizing the use of pure vasoconstrictors has been suggested through the use of inotropes if support for MAP targets is required.
- Modification of CPB as a preventive strategy to reduce GICs has been proposed and investigated with few strategies shown to be clearly effective in reducing the incidence or severity of GICs (Table 9.3).

Table 9.3 Modifications of CPB have been proposed to reduce GI complications investigations (adapted from Allen 2014)

• Minimize gaseous microemboli and atheroemboli (through the use of epiaortic scanning for cannula site selection, avoidance of excess aortic manipulation, meticulous de-airing)
• Transfusion to avoid severe anemia
• Use of CPB circuits with biocompatible surfaces
• Reduction of blood-air interfaces
• Minimize surface area and volume of the CPB circuit
• Use of pulsatile CPB flow
• Off-pump CABG surgery
• Use of internal mammary-based pedicled grafts
• Use of proximal anastomotic devices to avoid clamping the aorta in such patients
• Screening for heparin-induced thrombocytopenia (HIT) and active prophylaxis against HIT
• Fast-track extubation pathways and/or minimizing sedation to enable earlier recognition of a GICs

Conclusion

GICs following cardiac surgical procedures continue to significantly contribute to morbidity and mortality. The diagnosis of GICs remains difficult because symptoms and signs are often subtle, or nonspecific, and this commonly leads to delay in definitive diagnosis and treatment. Preventive strategies, coupled with early recognition and aggressive management, provide the foundation of the general clinical approach to addressing these complications. Overall, a high index of clinical suspicion and a low threshold for investigation and definitive management are recommended in patients with nonroutine clinical progress after cardiac surgery. Therefore, it is imperative that all clinicians who care for postoperative cardiac surgical patients be familiar with the full spectrum of potential GICs in this patient population, as well as the general therapeutic approaches to these complications.

References

Acosta S, Sonesson B, Resch T. Endovascular therapeutic approaches for acute superior mesenteric artery occlusion. Cardiovasc Intervent Radiol. 2009;32(5):896–905.

Allen SJ. Gastrointestinal complications and cardiac surgery. J Extra Corpor Technol. 2014;46:142–9.

Ashfaq A, Johnson DJ, Chapital AB, Lanza LA, DeValeria PA, Arabia FA. Changing trends in abdominal surgical complications following cardiac surgery in an era of advanced procedures. A retrospective cohort study. Int J Surg. 2015;15:124–8.

Cheng A, Williamitis CA, Slaughter MS. Comparison of continuous-flow and pulsatile-flow left ventricular assist devices: is there an advantage to pulsatility? Ann Cardiothorac Surg. 2014;3:573–81.

De Giorgio R, Knowles CH. Acute colonic pseudo-obstruction. Br J Surg. 2009;96:229–39.

Díaz-Gómez JL, Nutter B, Xu M, Sessler DI, Koch CG, Sabik J, Bashour CA. The effect of postoperative gastrointestinal complications in patients undergoing coronary artery bypass surgery. Ann Thorac Surg. 2010;90:109–15.

Dong G, Liu C, Xu B, Jing H, Li D, Wu H. Postoperative abdominal complications after cardiopulmonary bypass. J Cardiothorac Surg. 2012;7:108.

Eris C, Yavuz S, Yalcinkaya S, Gucu A, Toktas F, Yumun G, Erdolu B, Ozyazicioglu A. Acute mesenteric ischemia after cardiac surgery: an analysis of 52 patients. ScientificWorldJournal. 2013;2013:631534.

Fernandez-del Castillo C, Harringer W, Warshaw AL, Vlahakes GJ, Koski G, Zaslavsky AM, Rattner DW. Risk factors for pancreatic cellular injury after cardiopulmonary bypass. N Engl J Med. 1991;325:382–7.

Filsoufi F, Rahmanian PB, Castillo JG, Scurlock C, Legnani PE, Adams DH. Predictors and outcome of gastrointestinal complications in patients undergoing cardiac surgery. Ann Surg. 2007;246(2):323–9.

Grimm JC, Magruder JT, Ohkuma R, Dungan SP, Hayes A, Vose AK, Orlando M, Sussman MS, Cameron DE, Whitman GJ. A novel risk score to predict dysphagia after cardiac surgery procedures. Ann Thorac Surg. 2015;100:568–74.

Gulkarov I, Trocciola SM, Yokoyama CC, Girardi LN, Krieger KK, Isom OW, Salemi A. Gastrointestinal complications after mitral valve surgery. Ann Thorac Cardiovasc Surg. 2014;20(4):292–8.

Guler A, Sahin MA, Atilgan K, Kurkluoglu M, Demirkilic U. A rare complication after coronary artery bypass graft surgery: Ogilvie's syndrome. Cardiovasc J Afr. 2011;22:335–7.

Hessel EA 2nd. Abdominal organ injury after cardiac surgery. Semin Cardiothorac Vasc Anesth. 2004;8:243–63.

Karangelis D, Oikonomou K, Koufakis T, Tagarakis GI. Gastrointestinal complications following heart surgery: an updated review. Eur J Cardiovasc Med. 2011;1:34–7.

Loffroy R, Favelier S, Pottecher P, Estivalet L, Genson PY, Gehin S, Cercueil JP, Krause D. Transcatheter arterial embolization for acute nonvariceal upper gastrointestinal bleeding: indications, techniques and outcomes. Diagn Interv Imaging. 2015;96:731–44.

Mangano DT. Aspirin and mortality from coronary bypass surgery. N Engl J Med. 2002;347: 1309–17.

Mangi AA, Christison-Lagay ER, Torchiana DF, Warshaw AL, Berger DL. Gastrointestinal complications in patients undergoing heart operation: an analysis of 8709 consecutive cardiac surgical patients. Ann Surg. 2005;241:895–901; discussion 901–894.

Mollhoff T, Loick HM, Van Aken H, Schmidt C, Rolf N, Tjan TD, Asfour B, Berendes E. Milrinone modulates endotoxemia, systemic inflammation, and subsequent acute phase response after cardiopulmonary bypass (CPB). Anesthesiology. 1999;90:72–80.

Moneta GL, Misbach GA, Ivey TD. Hypoperfusion as a possible factor in the development of gastrointestinal complications after cardiac surgery. Am J Surg. 1985;149:648–50.

Ohri SK, Velissaris T. Gastrointestinal dysfunction following cardiac surgery. Perfusion. 2006;21:215–23.

Passage J, Joshi P, Mullany DV. Acute cholecystitis complicating cardiac surgery: case series involving more than 16,000 patients. Ann Thorac Surg. 2007;83:1096–101.

Patel AJ, Som R. What is the optimum prophylaxis against gastrointestinal haemorrhage for patients undergoing adult cardiac surgery: histamine receptor antagonists, or proton-pump inhibitors? Interact Cardiovasc Thorac Surg. 2013;16:356–60.

Rastan AJ, Tillmann E, Subramanian S, Lehmkuhl L, Funkat AK, Leontyev S, Doenst T, Walther T, Gutberlet M, Mohr FW. Visceral arterial compromise during intra-aortic balloon counterpulsation therapy. Circulation. 2010;122:S92–9.

Rodriguez F, Nguyen TC, Galanko JA, Morton J. Gastrointestinal complications after coronary artery bypass grafting: a national study of morbidity and mortality predictors. J Am Coll Surg. 2007;205:741–7.

Sabzi F, Faraji R. Liver function tests following open cardiac surgery. J Cardiovasc Thorac Res. 2015;7:49–54.

Slater JM, Orszulak TA, Cook DJ. Distribution and hierarchy of regional blood flow during hypothermic cardiopulmonary bypass. Ann Thorac Surg. 2001;72:542–7.

Vassiliou I, Papadakis E, Arkadopoulos N, Theodoraki K, Marinis A, Theodosopoulos T, Palatianos G, Smyrniotis V. Gastrointestinal emergencies in cardiac surgery. A retrospective analysis of 3,724 consecutive patients from a single center. Cardiology. 2008;111(2):94–101.

Viana FF, Chen Y, Almeida AA, Baxter HD, Cochrane AD, Smith JA. Gastrointestinal complications after cardiac surgery: 10-year experience of a single Australian centre. ANZ J Surg. 2013;83:651–6.

Yilmaz AT, Arslan M, Demirkilc U, Ozal E, Kuralay E, Bingol H, Oz BS, Tatar H, Ozturk OY. Gastrointestinal complications after cardiac surgery. Eur J Cardiothorac Surg. 1996;10:763–7.

Zhang G, Wu N, Liu H, Lv H, Yao Z, Li J. Case control study of gastrointestinal complications after cardiopulmonary bypass heart surgery. Perfusion. 2009;24:173–8.

Renal Complications and Their Management After Adult Cardiac Surgery 10

Juan M. Perrone and Gaston Cudemus

Abstract

Acute kidney injury (AKI) is a serious postoperative complication following cardiac surgery. Despite the incidence of AKI requiring temporary renal replacement therapy being low, it is nonetheless associated with high morbidity and mortality. Therefore, preventing AKI associated with cardiac surgery can dramatically improve outcomes in these patients. The pathogenesis of AKI is multifactorial, and many attempts to prevent or treat renal injury have been met with limited success. This chapter will discuss the incidence and risk factors for cardiac surgery-associated AKI, including the pathophysiology, potential biomarkers of injury, and treatment modalities.

Keywords

Epidemiology · Definition and staging · Pathophysiology · Nephrotoxins · Ischemia and ischemia-reperfusion injury · Atheroembolism · Exposure to CPB · Risk factors and biomarkers · Strategies for renal protection and management of CSA-AKI · Strategies for renal protection · Cardiopulmonary bypass management of CSA-AKI · General principles · Postoperative management · Renal replacement therapy

J. M. Perrone, M.D. (✉)
Department of Anesthesiology, Critical Care and Pain Medicine, Massachusetts General Hospital, Harvard Medical School, Boston, MA, USA
e-mail: jperrone@partners.org

G. Cudemus, M.D.
Cardiothoracic Anesthesiology and Critical Care, Department of Anesthesia, Critical Care and Pain Medicine, Corrigan Minehan Heart Center, Boston, MA, USA

Division of Cardiac Surgery, Massachusetts General Hospital, Harvard Medical School, Boston, MA, USA
e-mail: gcudemus@mgh.harvard.edu

A. Dabbagh et al. (eds.), *Postoperative Critical Care for Adult Cardiac Surgical Patients*, https://doi.org/10.1007/978-3-319-75747-6_10

10.1 Epidemiology

Acute kidney injury following cardiac surgery is among the top causes of AKI (Hoste et al. 2015). Depending on the underlying baseline characteristics and the type of surgery, the incidence reaches up to 39% with 1–6.5% of the patients affected requiring renal replacement therapy (RRT). AKI is independently associated with higher mortality (up to 60% when severe enough) and an almost eightfold increased risk for the development of chronic kidney disease (CKD) (Mangano et al. 2009). Although the varying definitions of kidney dysfunction have made it difficult to compare epidemiologic and outcomes studies, there is clear evidence in large cohort studies that the risk of mortality is proportional to the degree of severity of kidney injury. With advances in cardiopulmonary bypass (CPB) techniques and ICU care, there has been a decrease in mortality despite the increased incidence of AKI (Cooper et al. 2006). The identification of patients at risk of AKI and early prevention may offer a reduction in morbidity and mortality of cardiac surgery patients.

10.2 Definition and Staging

In 2008, the Acute Dialysis Quality Initiative (ADQI) defined CSA-AKI as "an abrupt deterioration in kidney function following cardiac surgery as evidenced by a reduction in glomerular filtration rate (GFR)." This group recommended to use the Acute Kidney Injury Network (AKIN) definition for AKI, which was at that time an updated revision of the risk, injury, failure, loss, and end-stage kidney disease (RIFLE) definition for AKI. In 2012, the Kidney Disease: Improving Global Outcomes (KDIGO) consensus group published the newest version of these definitions (Kidney disease: Improving Global Outcomes (KDIGO) Acute Kidney Injury Work Group 2012). This definition and grading system is based on the functional biomarkers serum creatinine (SCr) and urine output and defines three severity grades of AKI (Table 10.1). The KDIGO guidelines define AKI as an increase in SCr ≥0.3 mg/dL within 48 h or an increase in SCr ≥1.5 times baseline that is known or presumed to have occurred within the prior 7 days or urine volume < 0.5 mL/kg/h for 6 h. Although a majority of CSA-AKI is directly related to cardiac surgery and will occur immediately following cardiac surgery, there may still be a large variation in cause, timing, and duration of CSA-AKI. Therefore, the implementation of the KDIGO guidelines in perioperative cardiac surgical patients requires attention to the following points. First, increase of SCr must be greater than 1.5 times baseline SCr. This baseline SCr must reflect the kidney function of the patient in steady-state condition, within 7 days before occurrence of AKI. For elective cardiac surgery patients, this will be the preoperative value. However, when this is not the case and the patient is unstable, this preoperative value cannot be used as a baseline. In these patients, a representative value from the preceding 3 months may serve as a baseline value. This requires clinical judgment as sometimes several SCr values are available. Second, a patient may also qualify when there is an absolute increase of SCr of 0.3 mg/dL or greater within a 48-h time window. One should notice that for every new sample, the reference value also moves forward in time, since the 48-h time

Table 10.1 The kidney disease: improving global outcomes, diagnosis, and grading system for acute kidney injury

(a) AKI is defined by either an increase of serum creatinine or an episode of oliguria		
Increase of serum creatinine ≥0.3 mg/dL within 48 h		
Increase of serum creatinine ≥1.5-fold above baseline, known or assumed to have occurred within 7 days		
Urine volume < 0.5 mL/kg/h for 6 h		
(b) AKI severity is staged by the worst of either SCr changes or oliguria		
Stage	Serum creatinine	Urine output
1	≥1.5–1.9 times baseline or >0.3 mg/dL increase	<0.5 mL/kg/h for 6–12 h
2	≥2.0–2.9 times baseline	<0.5 mL/kg/h for ≥12 h
3	≥3.0 times baseline or Increase of serum creatinine to ≥4.0 mg/dL or RRT or In patients <18 year, decrease of eGFR to <35 mL/min per 1.73 m^2	<0.3 mL/kg/h for ≥24 h or Anuria for ≥12 h

AKI acute kidney injury, *eGFR* estimated glomerular filtration rate, *SCr* serum creatinine

window must be met. Third, a patient may classify when urine output is less than 0.5 mL/kg/h for a period of 6 h. This implicates that every hour during a 6-h time period, the oliguria criterion should be met. This requires strict timing of urine output measurements.

10.3 Pathophysiology

The pathogenesis of AKI in cardiac surgery is complex and not completely understood. It is thought to be due to a combination of nephrotoxins, ischemia, and inflammatory and atheroembolic mechanisms (Stafford-Smith 2005).

10.3.1 Nephrotoxins

Nephrotoxin exposure frequently occurs prior to and following cardiac surgery. Antibiotics such as beta-lactams, vancomycin, or aminoglycosides can cause acute interstitial nephritis or direct injury. Commonly, patients are taking angiotensin-converting enzyme inhibitors (ACEi) prior to surgery, which inhibit renal efferent arteriolar vasoconstriction. Postoperatively, patients may be exposed to potentially nephrotoxic medications, such as diuretics and antibiotics. Free hemoglobin (Hb) is another potential nephrotoxin thought to contribute to AKI in patients after cardiac surgery. Longer time on CPB and lower CPB flows are associated with the development of AKI. This association may be because of hemolysis and the release of free-Hb (Fischer et al. 2002).

10.3.2 Ischemia and Ischemia-Reperfusion Injury

Renal perfusion during the perioperative period is critical for prevention of AKI in the cardiac surgery patient. Even if the patient does not suffer kidney dysfunction in the preoperative period, the effects of anesthesia and exposure to CPB can lead to loss of autoregulation and are a proposed mechanism for perioperative ischemia-reperfusion injury. Renal hypoperfusion is often the initial insult in cardiac surgery-associated AKI, which leads to a reduction in blood flow to the highly metabolic renal medulla. Patients who have had a recent acute coronary event or have severe valvular heart disease with compromised ventricular function may have decreased cardiac output and impaired renal perfusion. In a recent observational study, Lannemyr et al. evaluated the renal effects of normothermic CPB in 18 patients undergoing open cardiac surgery. Their major finding was that despite a 33% increase in systemic perfusion flow rate during CPB, a renal oxygen supply/demand mismatch developed. This was most likely caused by renal vasoconstriction, which in combination with hemodilution decreased renal oxygen delivery by 20% during CPB. This impairment in renal oxygenation was accompanied by a release of a tubular injury marker (NAG) and was further aggravated after weaning from CPB (Lannemyr et al. 2017).

10.3.3 Atheroembolism

Renal atheroembolism from the ascending aorta during operative aortic manipulation is also believed to contribute to postoperative AKI. Macroscopic and microscopic emboli may be freed during aortic cannulation and clamping and released during CPB. This is supported by studies that demonstrate that the number of Doppler-detected emboli during CABG surgery is associated with risk of postoperative kidney dysfunction. Strategies to avoid aortic cross-clamping and the usage of devices that limit aortic manipulation have been used, but none have so far been demonstrated to be effective at preventing postoperative AKI (Nakamoto et al. 2001).

10.3.4 Exposure to Cardiopulmonary Bypass and Activation of Inflammatory Pathways

The use of the CPB pump is known to cause a systemic inflammatory response syndrome (SIRS) and has been associated with elevations in levels of pro-inflammatory cytokines compared with operations done off-pump, suggesting that the CPB pump is the culprit in the activation of inflammation during cardiac surgery. Initial studies conducted prior to consensus definitions of AKI encountered difficulties with outcomes due to varying experience of surgical teams. Despite numerous randomized and nonrandomized trials, this issue remained controversial. In 2012, the CORONARY trial randomized 4752 patients to compare short- and long-term outcomes of patients undergoing off-pump versus on-pump CABG with surgeons experienced with OPCAB (Lamy et al. 2012). At 30 days, the investigators demonstrated no difference in the primary outcomes (death, stroke, myocardial infarction, or AKI requiring RRT) between the two groups. However, off-pump CABG was associated with less transfusion and reoperation for bleeding, less AKI, less respiratory infections or failure, and more early revascularizations. Further follow-up and analyses at 5 years are being performed to detect if these benefits are maintained in the long term. Despite equivocal support for OPCAB, there is some evidence that a subgroup of patients with preexisting kidney dysfunction has a lower risk for AKI during OPCAB.

10.4 Risk Factors and Biomarkers

In order to prevent perioperative kidney injury, it is important to identify those patients who are at risk of developing AKI. Evidence from epidemiological studies has established major risk factors for developing CSA-AKI (Table 10.2). These

Table 10.2 Risk factors for developing acute kidney injury in cardiac surgery (from Hoste et al. 2015)

Preoperative
• Female gender
• Reduced LV function or congestive cardiac failure
• Previous cardiac surgery
• Recent preoperative coronary angiogram
• Emergent surgery
• Preoperative IABP insertion
• Comorbidities (diabetes mellitus, chronic obstructive pulmonary disease)
• Use of ACE inhibitors, angiotensin receptor blockers
• Nephrotoxic medications: aminoglycosides, vancomycin, NSAIDs
Intraoperative
• Duration of CPB
• Cross-clamp time
• Type of cardiac surgery (i.e. valve surgery as opposed to pure CABG)
• Perioperative red cell transfusion
• Nephrotoxins
• Hemodilution: hematocrit <25%
• Low MAP
Postoperative
• Postoperative blood loss
• Postoperative transfusion requirement
• Myocardial infarction
• Nephrotoxic drugs
• Need for emergent reoperation
• Urinary tract obstruction
• Sepsis/SIRS

ACE angiotensin-converting enzyme, *CABG* coronary artery bypass graft, *CPB* cardiopulmonary bypass, *IABP* intra-aortic balloon pump, *LV* left ventricular, *MAP* mean arterial pressure, *NSAIDs* nonsteroidal anti-inflammatory drugs, *SIRS* systemic inflammatory response syndrome studies have shown that of all the identified risk factors for AKI, the severity of preexisting chronic kidney disease is the best predictor of postoperative requirement for dialysis. Approximately 10–20% of patients with an elevated baseline preoperative SCr of between 2 and 4 mg/dL will require RRT in the postoperative period. In patients with a preoperative SCr >4.0 mg/dL, 25–28% will need RRT (Chertow et al. 2012).

Despite significant advances in our understanding of the pathophysiology of CSA-AKI, there is a paucity of options for prevention and treatment. One reason that is frequently cited is the inherent delay from injury to diagnosis due to the common reliance on SCr as the principal diagnostic marker for AKI. Serum creatinine provides a good estimate of the GFR in patients with stable chronic kidney disease. However, creatinine is a poor measure of kidney injury during acute stages of kidney dysfunction. Rises in SCr concentration often lag behind the kidney injury by 48–72 h. The relationship between creatinine and GFR is not linear and thus GFR declines by more than 50% before a significant change occurs in SCr. Furthermore, SCr concentration is influenced by numerous factors independent of the kidney, including gender, age, race, muscle mass, diurnal variation, metabolism, volume of distribution, medications, and protein intake (Kellum et al. 2015).

Interventions to prevent AKI or treat early AKI would ideally be guided by a biomarker or panel of biomarkers that diagnose AKI shortly after the time of actual injury, in the same way as troponin elevation and ST changes signal myocardial injury. More than 50 candidate biomarkers have been investigated as indicators of kidney injury (McIlroy et al. 2010). Two of these, insulin-like growth factor-binding protein 7 (IGFBP7) and tissue inhibitor of metalloproteinases-2 (TIMP-2) have demonstrated excellent performance in predicting CSA-AKI and were used to identify high-risk patients in a recent randomized controlled clinical trial (Meersch et al. 2014).

10.5 Strategies for Renal Protection and Management of CSA-AKI

10.5.1 General Principles

Cardiac surgery-associated AKI shares the same management principles common to all forms of AKI, and these have considerable overlap with preventive interventions set forward by the "KDIGO bundle" described below. CSA-AKI does not have a specific therapy, but meticulous clinical attention is needed to support the patient until (if) AKI resolves. The kidney possesses remarkable capacity to repair itself even after severe, dialysis-requiring AKI. The key to managing AKI in the cardiac intensive care unit is based on the recognition of the contributing factors to kidney injury and dysfunction. Following the KDIGO guidelines, the management of AKI stage 1 focuses primarily on (1) assessing and treating the etiology, (2) removing and avoiding insults, (3) optimizing hemodynamics, and (4) managing complications. If AKI stage 2–3 develops, (5) check for renal dosing of medications and (6) assess for renal replacement therapy.

10.5.2 KDIGO Bundle

The 2012 KDIGO guidelines proposed strategies for the prevention of AKI that included the discontinuation of all nephrotoxic agents and consideration of alternatives to radiocontrast agents, the assurance of volume status and perfusion pressure, functional hemodynamic monitoring, close monitoring of serum creatinine levels and urinary output, and avoidance of hyperglycemia (Cooper et al. 2006). In a recent randomized controlled trial, Meersch and colleagues studied the effect of the "KDIGO bundle" in patients at high risk of AKI who had undergone cardiac surgery (Meersch et al. 2017). Patients at high risk were identified by assessing postoperative urine levels of IGFBP7 and TIMP-2. The investigators found that rates of AKI were significantly lower in patients who received the bundled intervention than in patients who received standard care, including the specification to keep mean arterial pressure > 65 mmHg and central venous pressure 8–10 mmHg (55.1% vs. 71.7%; absolute risk reduction of 16.6%; 95% CI 5.5%–27.9%; $P = 0.004$). Furthermore, implementation of the bundle resulted in significantly improved hemodynamics, less hyperglycemia, and lower use of ACEi or angiotensin II-receptor blockers (ARBs) compared with control patients. This study is the first to demonstrate the effectiveness of an intervention to prevent AKI in susceptible patients (Kellum 2017).

10.5.3 Volume and Fluid Management

In general, crystalloid-based resuscitation with balanced salt solutions is the first choice. Hypervolemia in oliguric or anuric AKI may be life-threatening due to acute pulmonary edema, especially in the cardiac surgical population. The initial approach should be to maintain euvolemia and avoid venous congestion and fluid overload. This is particularly important in patients who have recently received intravenous radiocontrast. Colloids have traditionally been an attractive option because of their potential capacity to expand the plasma volume more efficiently than crystalloid solutions. Nonetheless, colloids have not been demonstrated to be superior to crystalloids, and although theoretically they may improve maintenance of intravascular volume longer than crystalloids, this has not been proven to be advantageous in the cardiac surgical population (Romagnoli et al. 2016). In addition, a recent retrospective study has shown an association between albumin administration and increased rates of AKI in patients undergoing on-pump cardiac surgery (Frenette et al. 2014). Based on available literature, caution should be paid on using colloids in cardiac surgery patients, and balanced crystalloid solutions should be used preferentially.

10.5.4 Functional Hemodynamic Monitoring and Management

Once fluid status has been optimized, efforts should concentrate on maintaining renal blood flow, oxygenation, and renal perfusion pressure. In low cardiac output states, inotropes may be used to improve renal perfusion, and vasopressors may be used in vasodilated states. There have been concerns with using norepinephrine in hypotension; however, there is no evidence that it compromises renal blood flow in patients who are adequately fluid resuscitated. It has been demonstrated that norepinephrine significantly increases renal blood flow with an improvement in urine output and creatinine clearance in vasodilated patients (Redfors et al. 2011). Vasopressin may also be used in cases of catecholamine-resistant vasodilatory shock. The goal in clinical practice is maintenance of a systemic mean arterial pressure of between 65 and 75 mmHg. These goals should be individualized according to the usual baseline blood pressure, particularly in patients with preexisting hypertension or kidney impairment.

A second component of hemodynamic management is the presence of ventricular dysfunction and valvular diseases; these may cause renal dysfunction and can be simultaneously worsened by AKI. Venous congestion, as evidenced by increases in CVP, will cause an increase in renal subcapsular pressure reducing GFR (Damman et al. 2009). Identifying patients who will respond to fluids by increasing left ventricular stroke volume is important in order to optimize cardiac output and minimize fluid overload. This should be accomplished with the use of dynamic measures of fluid responsiveness based on ultrasound and heart-lung interaction in mechanically ventilated patients, such as pulse pressure variation, stroke volume variation, and passive leg raise. Accurate prediction and assessment of fluid responsiveness is a crucial skill necessary to optimize forward flow and avoid fluid overload, venous hypertension, and renal congestion (Marik 2016). This is particularly important in the postoperative cardiac surgical patient with compromised right ventricular function. Prompt identification of RV dysfunction is of major importance as fluid management becomes challenging, and severe venous congestion is very likely, whereas rapid treatment of right heart dysfunction becomes a priority to reduce congestive kidney failure and favor recovery of renal function.

Management of acute RV dysfunction is challenging as LV preload may also be compromised due to interventricular interdependence. On the contrary, in the case of fluid overload and insufficient response to diuretics, slow and controlled volume unloading through continuous renal replacement therapy might be necessary.

A detailed understanding of the management of vasoactive and inotropic infusions is necessary, and it is beyond the scope of this chapter. Catecholamines (norepinephrine, epinephrine, and dobutamine) may improve RV function with direct inotropic effect but also by increasing systolic aortic pressure, thus improving RV myocardial perfusion. Phosphodiesterase inhibitors and pulmonary vasodilators are used to reduce RV afterload and improve its interaction with the pulmonary circulation. Importantly, these drugs may cause systemic hypotension and decreased coronary perfusion, compromising myocardial performance. Given this scenario, the combination of norepinephrine and milrinone is a common effective combination (Aya et al. 2013).

10.6 Pharmacologic Interventions

Despite extensive research into pharmacologic interventions to prevent or treat established AKI, there have been no drugs that clearly demonstrate improved clinical outcomes.

10.6.1 Diuretics

Diuretics increase urine output by decreasing tubular reabsorption through several different mechanisms. While diuretics may increase urine output in some patients, there is no conclusive evidence that loop diuretics prevent AKI or improve clinical outcomes. Furthermore, diuretics may be detrimental to the kidney, as studies have shown that furosemide increases perioperative serum creatinine concentration in cardiac patients, potentially by decreasing intravascular volume. A meta-analysis of RCTs demonstrated that loop diuretics were associated with a shorter duration of RRT and increased urine output. However, this did not translate into improvements in mortality or rate of independence from RRT. Currently, guidelines suggest only using them in the management of volume overload to promote diuresis, thereby facilitating fluid, acid-base and electrolyte control (Bagshaw et al. 2007).

10.6.2 Dopamine

Dopamine acts on several receptors that increase renal blood flow and perfusion pressure. Dopaminergic receptor-mediated renal vasodilation increases renal blood flow, beta-adrenoreceptor activation increases cardiac output, and alpha-adrenoreceptor stimulation increases renal perfusion. Low-dose dopamine (1–3 μg/kg/min) and its effect on AKI have been extensively studied. Although dopamine has been demonstrated to increase postoperative urine output, multiple studies and large RCTs have demonstrated that it does not prevent AKI or the need for RRT, increases the incidence of atrial fibrillation, and does not reduce mortality in critically ill patients with early acute kidney dysfunction in the ICU (Friedrich et al. 2005).

10.6.3 Fenoldopam

Fenoldopam is a selective dopamine-1 receptor agonist capable of increasing urine output in patients with AKI. Initial studies suggested some renoprotective properties of fenoldopam in contrast-induced nephropathy. Gillies et al. conducted a systematic review and meta-analysis of randomized controlled trials comparing fenoldopam with placebo to prevent AKI after major surgery (Gillies et al. 2015). In this analysis, perioperative treatment with fenoldopam was associated with a significant reduction in postoperative AKI, but it had no impact on renal replacement therapy or hospital mortality.

10.6.4 N-acetylcysteine

N-acetylcysteine is an antioxidant that enhances the endogenous glutathione scavenging system and has shown promise as a renoprotective agent by attenuating intravenous contrast-induced nephropathy. Current evidence does not support the use of NAC to prevent AKI in cardiac surgery. Trials in the perioperative and ICU settings have shown a lack of renal protection of NAC in high-risk cardiac surgery patients. Several meta-analyses assessing NAC in cardiac surgery have been performed to assess its renoprotective properties. None have demonstrated an improvement in the postoperative increase in creatinine or kidney injury requiring RRT (Naughton et al. 2008).

10.7 Renal Replacement Therapy

The initiation of RRT is indicated to treat volume overload unresponsive to diuretics, uremic signs and symptoms, severe metabolic acidosis, and hyperkalemia. RRT removes solutes, alters electrolyte concentration in the extracellular fluid, and removes extracellular fluid. Multiple modalities of RRT are currently available, and these include intermittent hemodialysis, continuous renal replacement therapies, and hybrid therapies, such as sustained low-efficiency dialysis (SLED). Importantly, KDIGO guidelines suggest using continuous RRT for hemodynamically unstable patients rather than standard intermittent RRT. Although the goal in cardiac surgery and ICU is to prevent AKI from developing, RRT remains the mainstay supportive therapy in managing AKI meeting the abovementioned criteria (Gaudry et al. 2016).

The role of RRT during CPB is unclear. Initial pilot studies have demonstrated a reduction in inflammatory markers with hemofiltration; however, this did not result in an improvement in morbidity or mortality. Despite this, hemofiltration may be effective in patients with AKI or chronic disease by blood volume control, blood conservation, and the management of the effects of kidney dysfunction.

Similarly, the optimal timing for initiation of RRT for patients who develop AKI is not known. Early initiation of RRT (i.e., in the absence of life-threatening complications) has been suggested as a means to better control acid-base status, electrolyte imbalances, extracellular volume status, and systemic inflammation. A small single-centered study assessed 44 patients undergoing CABG surgery with preoperative SCr concentration greater than 2.5 mg/dL but not requiring dialysis. The group that had preoperative dialysis demonstrated a decrease in mortality and incidence of AKI requiring dialysis (Durmaz et al. 2003). Despite this, there is not enough evidence to support the routine use of prophylactic RRT in high-risk patients undergoing cardiac surgery.

However, earlier RRT may also expose patients who might otherwise recover from the unnecessary risks of vascular access and expense and complications of this therapy. While earlier initiation of RRT is done in some centers, the evidence for it is predominantly derived from observational studies (Mehta 2016).

Conclusions

CSA-AKI is associated with significant morbidity and mortality. Although intense and promising research is ongoing, no specific pharmacologic strategy for CSA-AKI resolution can be recommended yet. A better understanding of the pathophysiology of AKI in cardiac surgery may allow optimization of the perioperative and postoperative care of these patients. Biomarkers and the early identification of patients at risk of AKI may lead to improved outcomes. Patient selection, risk stratification, meticulous attention to prevention, and aggressive early intervention with targeted hemodynamic management remain the best available tools.

References

Hoste EA, Bagshaw SM, Bellomo R, Cely CM, Colman R, Cruz DN, et al. Epidemiology of acute kidney injury in critically ill patients: the multinational AKI-EPI study. Intensive Care Med. 2015;41:1411–23.

Mangano CM, Diamondstone LS, Ramsay JG, Aggarwal A, Herskowitz A, Mangano DT. Renal dysfunction after myocardial revascularization: risk factors, adverse outcomes, and hospital resource utilization. The Multicenter Study of Perioperative Ischemia Research Group. Ann Intern Med. 2009;128:194–203.

Cooper WA, O'Brien SM, Thourani VH, et al. Impact of renal dysfunction on outcomes of coronary artery bypass surgery: results from the Society of Thoracic Surgeons National Adult Cardiac Database. Circulation. 2006;113:1063–70.

Kidney disease: Improving Global Outcomes (KDIGO) Acute Kidney Injury Work Group. KDIGO clinical practice guideline for acute kidney injury. Kidney Int. 2012;2:1–138.

Stafford-Smith M. Evidence-based renal protection in cardiac surgery. Semin Cardiothorac Vasc Anesth. 2005;9:65–76.

Fischer UM, Weissenberger WK, Warters RD, et al. Impact of cardiopulmonary bypass management on postcardiac surgery renal function. Perfusion. 2002;17:401–6.

Lannemyr L, Bragadottir G, Krumbholz V, Redfors B, Sellgren J, Ricksten S-E. Effects of cardiopulmonary bypass on renal perfusion, filtration, and oxygenation in patients undergoing cardiac surgery. Anesthesiology. 2017;126:205–13.

Nakamoto S, Kaneda T, Inoue T, et al. Disseminated cholesterol embolism after coronary artery bypass grafting. J Card Surg. 2001;16:410–3.

Lamy A, Devereaux PJ, Prabhakaran D, et al. Off-pump or on-pump coronary-artery bypass grafting at 30 days. NEJM. 2012;366:1489–97.

Chertow GM, Lazarus JM, Christiansen CL, et al. Preoperative renal risk stratification. Circulation. 2012;95:878–84.

Kellum JA, Sileanu FE, Murugan R, et al. Classifying AKI by urine output versus serum creatinine level. J Am Soc Nephrol. 2015;26:2231–8.

McIlroy DR, Wagener G, Lee HT. Biomarkers of acute kidney injury: an evolving domain. Anesthesiology. 2010;112:998–1004.

Meersch M, Schmidt C, Van Aken H, Martens S, Rossaint J, et al. Urinary TIMP-2 and IGFBP7 as early biomarkers of acute kidney injury and renal recovery following cardiac surgery. PLoS One. 2014;9(3):e93460. https://doi.org/10.1371/journal.pone.0093460.

Meersch M, Schmidt C, Hoffmeier A, Van Aken H, Wempe C, Gerss J, Zarbock A. Prevention of cardiac surgery-associated AKI by implementing the KDIGO guidelines in high risk patients identified by biomarkers: the PrevAKI randomized controlled trial. Intensive Care Med. 2017;43(11):1551–61. https://doi.org/10.1007/s00134-016-4670-3.

Kellum JA. AKI: the myth of inevitability is finally shattered. Nat Rev Nephrol. 2017 Mar;13(3):140–1.

Romagnoli S, Rizza A, Ricci Z. Fluid status assessment and management during the perioperative phase in adult cardiac surgery patients. J Cardiothorac Vasc Anesth. 2016;30:1076–84.

Frenette AJ, Bouchard J, Bernier P, et al. Albumin administration is associated with acute kidney injury in cardiac surgery: a propensity score analysis. Crit Care. 2014;18:602.

Redfors B, Bragadottir G, Sellgren J, Sward K, Ricksten SE. Effects of norepinephrine on renal perfusion, filtration and oxygenation in vasodilatory shock and acute kidney injury. Instensive Care Med. 2011;37:60–7.

Damman K, van Deursen VM, Navis G, et al. Increased central venous pressure is associated with impaired renal function and mortality in a broad spectrum of patients with cardiovascular disease. J Am Coll Cardiol. 2009;53:582–8.

Marik PE. Fluid responsiveness and the six guiding principles of fluid resuscitation. Crit Care Med. 2016;44:1920–2.

Aya HD, Cecconi M, Hamilton M, et al. Goal-directed therapy in cardiac surgery: a systematic review and meta-analysis. Br J Anaesth. 2013;110:510–5.

Bagshaw SM, Delaney A, Haase M, Ghali WA, Bellomo R. Loop diuretics in the management of acute renal failure: a systematic review and meta-analysis. Crit Care Resusc. 2007;9:60–8.

Friedrich JO, Adhikari N, herridge MS, Beyene J. Meta-analysis: low-dose dopamine increases urine output but does not prevent renal dysfunction or death. Ann Intern Med. 2005;142:510–24.

Gillies MA, Kakar V, Parker RJ, Honore PM, Ostermann M. Fenoldopam to prevent acute kidney injury after major surgery: a systematic review and meta-analysis. Crit Care. 2015;19:449.

Naughton F, Wijeysundera D, Karkouti K, Tait G, Beattie WS. N-acetylcysteine to reduce renal failure after cardiac surgery: a systematic review and meta-analysis. Can J Anaesth. 2008;55:827–35.

Gaudry S, Hajage D, Schortgen F, et al. Initiation strategies for renal-replacement therapy in the intensive care unit. NEJM. 2016;375:122–33.

Durmaz I, Yagdi T, Calkavur T, et al. Prophylactic dialysis in patients with renal dysfunction undergoing on-pump coronary artery bypass surgery. Ann Thorac Surg. 2003;75:859–64.

Mehta RL. Renal-replacement therapy in the critically ill: does timing matter? NEJM. 2016;375:175–6.

Respiratory Complications and Management After Adult Cardiac Surgery

11

Michael Nurok, Oren Friedman, and Erik R. Dong

Abstract

The respiratory system's primary function is to exchange oxygen and carbon dioxide as part of metabolism. This is accomplished by moving blood and air into approximation in the alveoli through mass action driven by the heart and lung. The physical properties of the heart and lung dictate how the respiratory system functions and can dysfunction in pathologic states. These principles inform evidence-based strategies for mechanical ventilation and the rationale for treating frequently encountered respiratory complications following cardiac surgery.

Keywords

Respiratory physiology and pathophysiology · Respiratory mechanics · Gas exchange · Ventilation and perfusion · Cardiopulmonary interactions · Pulmonary response to general anesthesia and cardiac surgery · Risk factors for postoperative respiratory failure · Mechanical ventilation · Indications for mechanical ventilation · Complications of mechanical ventilation · Direct consequences · Indirect consequences · Complications of mechanical ventilation · Reducing postoperative respiratory failure · Preoperative risk stratification · Intraoperative management to reduce respiratory failure · Postoperative strategies to reduce respiratory failure · Ventilation modes · Volume control ventilation · Pressure control

M. Nurok, M.D. (✉)
Cardiac Surgery Intensive Care Unit, Cedars-Sinai Medical Center, Los Angeles, CA, USA
e-mail: Michael.Nurok@cshs.org

O. Friedman, M.D.
Critical Care Medicine, Pulmonary Medicine, Cardiothoracic Surgery and Transplant Team, Cedars-Sinai Medical Center, Los Angeles, CA, USA

E. R. Dong, D.O., M.D.
Critical Care Cardiology, Heart Institute, Cedars-Sinai Medical Center, Los Angeles, CA, USA

A. Dabbagh et al. (eds.), *Postoperative Critical Care for Adult Cardiac Surgical Patients*, https://doi.org/10.1007/978-3-319-75747-6_11

ventilation · Pressure support · Alternative modes · Noninvasive ventilation · Positive end-expiratory pressure · Auto-i-PEEP · Oxygen and ventilation goals · Work of breathing on mechanical ventilation · Discontinuation of mechanical ventilation · Readiness for spontaneous breathing trial (SBT) · Performing spontaneous breathing trials · High-flow oxygen · Mechanical ventilation in specific scenarios · ARDS · Mechanical ventilation during VV ECMO for ARDS · Strategies for managing specific perioperative disease states · Pleural effusion · Acute respiratory distress syndrome · Pneumothorax/hemothorax · Pulmonary edema · Obstructive airway disease · Pneumonia and ventilator-associated events · Pulmonary hypertension

11.1 Respiratory Physiology and Pathophysiology

11.1.1 Respiratory Mechanics

The respiratory system is made of two components, the lung and chest wall. The chest wall includes the rib cage, abdomen, and diaphragm. The physical properties of the lung and chest wall contribute to how breathing occurs. Inspiration is an active process principally involving the diaphragm. Inspiration can be augmented by the external intercostal muscles as "bucket handles," pulling the ribs upward and forward, thereby expanding the thorax in the lateral and anteroposterior direction. Accessory muscles including the scalene and sternocleidomastoid muscles also contribute to respiration during periods of exertion.

Expiration during normal tidal breathing is predominantly a passive process governed by the elastic properties of the chest wall and lung that oppose active expansion during inspiration. Under some circumstances including exercise, expiration can become an active process with contribution of the abdominal muscles increasing abdominal pressure and elevating the diaphragm as well as the internal intercostals pulling the ribs down and inward. Accessory muscles, including the sternocleidomastoids, pectoralis, and trapezius, may contribute ventilation under conditions of high demand.

Under normal conditions the visceral and parietal pleura are tightly opposed, and the pressure in the potential space between these two layers is slightly negative (Jaeger and Blank 2011). Normally the two layers move in unison; however disruption of the layers by either air or fluid has a significant negative effect on respiratory mechanics.

To understand respiratory physiology, it is important to understand pressure changes across the lung and chest wall. Transpulmonary (also called transmural) pressure is the difference in pressure between inside the lung (alveoli) and outside the lung (intrapleural space). When transpulmonary pressure is increased by either expansion of the chest wall in spontaneous respiration or introduction of positive pressure in mechanical ventilation, airflow occurs and the respiratory system increases its volume. It is important to understand that elevated transpulmonary pressure is thought to drive lung injury and that without knowing transpulmonary

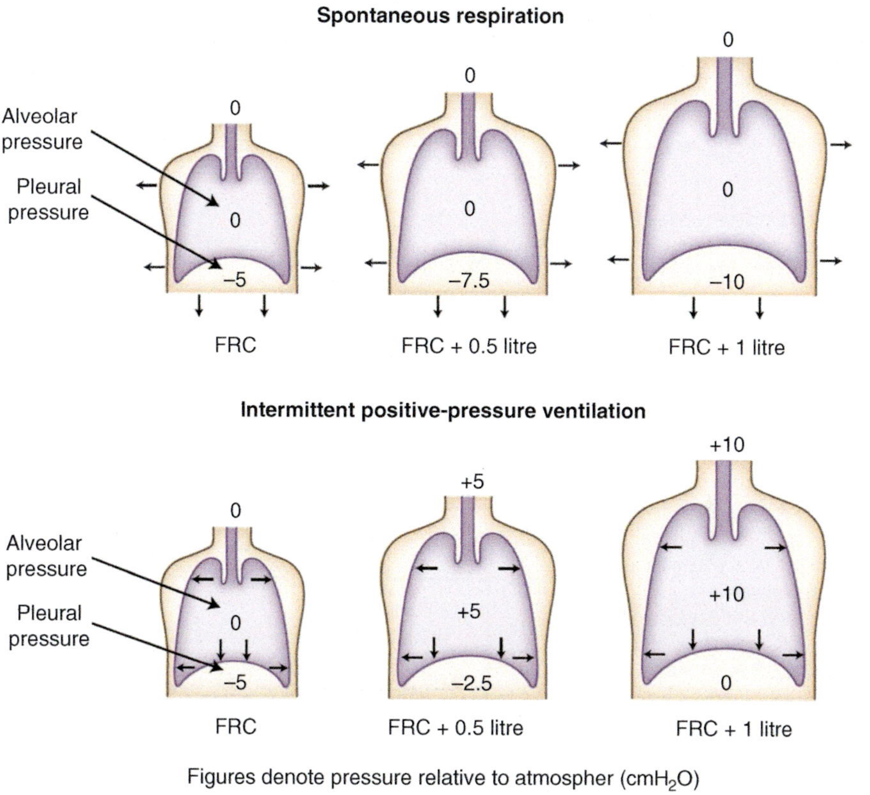

Fig. 11.1 Demonstrates the variable relationship between airway and alveolar pressures and transpulmonary pressure (alveolar minus pleural pressure) in health with spontaneous and intermittent positive pressure ventilation. With permission of Springer (Nurok M and Topulos GP 2012a)

pressure, the clinician will need to rely on imprecise surrogates (Vt/kg, driving pressure, plateau pressure) to infer whether ventilator settings may be harmful. Figures 11.1 and 11.2 demonstrate the variable relationship between airway pressures and transpulmonary pressure.

The lung and chest wall both have unique elastic properties; however their equilibrium positions are different as demonstrated in Fig. 11.3. The isolated chest wall contains approximately ¾ of total lung capacity in the relaxed position, whereas the isolated lung contains under ¼ of total lung capacity in the relaxed position. The relaxation of the total respiratory system (lung and chest wall combined as a functional unit) is volume of gas in the system with a transmural pressure of zero and is often used synonymously with functional residual capacity. Strictly speaking, the definition of FRC is the volume of gas in the lung at end expiration. Under some conditions the relaxation volume of the respiratory system and FRC may be different. FRC is clinically significant in that retaining gas in the lung at the end of expiration is important to prevent alveolar collapse.

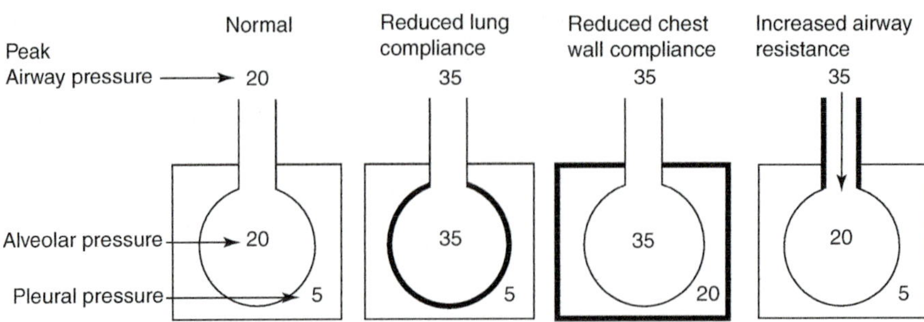

Fig. 11.2 Transpulmonary pressure gradients in different pathologic states with mechanical ventilation. Although peak airway pressures may be similarly elevated in these disease states, the transpulmonary pressures can be markedly different. With permission (Buckley and Gillham 2007)

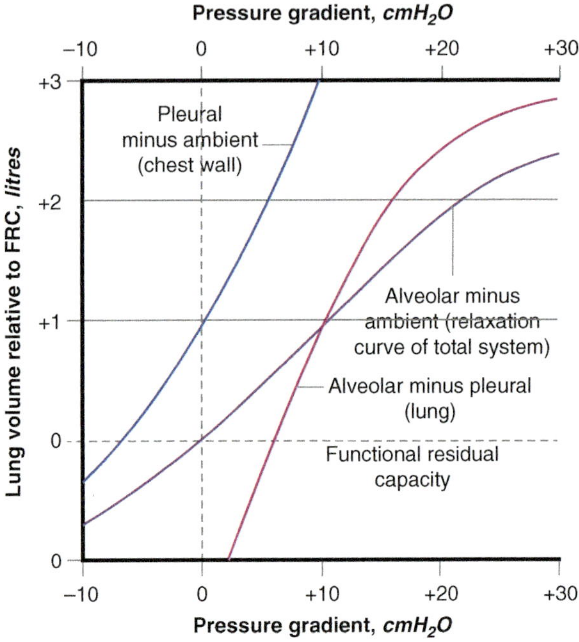

Fig. 11.3 Diagram showing different pleural pressures with mechanical and spontaneous ventilation and diagram of lung volume vs. transmural pressure. With permission of Springer (Nurok M and Topulos GP 2012a)

The change in volume per unit change in pressure is called compliance. Compliance is generally expressed as the slope of the pressure-volume curve. While the isolated normal lung is easily distensible with a compliance of approximately 200 mL/cm H_2O, the compliance of the system as a whole is in the range of 50–80 mL/cm H_2O due to the contribution of the significantly stiffer (i.e., relatively noncompliant) chest wall (Jaeger and Blank 2011; West 2012a, b). Decreases in compliance can be caused by pathologic processes that make the chest wall more stiff (e.g., obesity or scleroderma), or lung more stiff (e.g., pulmonary edema, acute respiratory distress syndrome), or both. Differentiating the etiology of decreased compliance (chest wall vs. lung) requires the measurement of intrapleural pressure. Esophageal pressure is commonly used as a surrogate for intrapleural pressure (Akoumianaki et al. 2014).

11.1.2 Gas Exchange

The lung achieves gas exchange at the alveolar-blood interface through passive diffusion. Key variables governing diffusion are the area of alveoli available, the partial pressure of gas on both sides of the interface, and the thickness of the interface (West 2012a, b). Because CO_2 is more soluble than O_2, its diffusion rate is 20 times higher. For this reason, diffusion limitation of CO_2 is much more common for O_2 than CO_2.

Oxygen and carbon dioxide transfer in the normal lung are largely *perfusion limited*. In disease states where the alveolar membrane is thickened (e.g., pulmonary edema) and decreased in area (e.g., COPD) or the diffusion characteristics of the capillary/alveolar membrane are otherwise abnormal (e.g., pulmonary hypertension), *diffusion limitation* can also be introduced.

11.1.3 Ventilation and Perfusion

The respiratory system accomplishes gas exchange by placing blood and air in close proximity. In general, most alveolar units are in close relationship to pulmonary capillaries; however a range of possible relationships exist including states of pure shunt where pulmonary capillaries perfuse regions with nonfunctional or nonexistent alveoli and regions of pure dead space where functional alveoli exist but are not in proximity to pulmonary capillaries or these capillaries are nonfunctional. See Fig. 11.4. Shunt predominantly influences oxygenation and widens the A-a gradient, whereas dead space widens the alveolar to end-tidal PCO2 gradient.

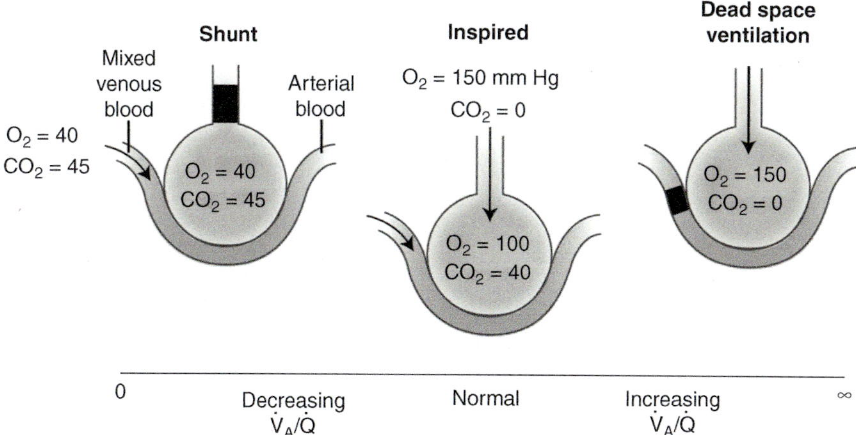

Fig. 11.4 Effects of different V/Q ratios. With permission of Springer (Nurok M and Topulos GP 2012b)

Both ventilation and perfusion are greatest in the dependent region of the lung because of gravity and the fact that dependent alveoli sit on a more compliant portion of the pressure-volume curve in spontaneously breathing subjects. Because of the greater density of blood compared to the lung, the ratio of V to Q is highest in the nondependent regions of the lung and lowest in dependent regions. In addition to this vertical heterogeneity of V/Q relationships, there is also more ventilation and perfusion in the center of the thorax and less toward the periphery following arborization of the pulmonary vascular tree (Hakim et al. 1987; Glenny et al. 2000).

11.1.4 Cardiopulmonary Interactions

The pressures to which the visceral and parietal pleura are exposed are also transmitted to the pericardium and great vessels and therefore affect cardiac and vascular physiology. These anatomical relationships mean that changes in respiratory physiology have highly relevant effects on cardiac performance that must be considered in critically ill patients, in particular, those receiving mechanical ventilation. These effects of cardiopulmonary interactions are often exaggerated in patients with impaired cardiac function.

Increases in intrathoracic pressure as seen with positive pressure ventilation lead to decrease venous return to the right atrium (Henderson et al. 2010). Spontaneous ventilation has the opposite effect. Right ventricular afterload is increased at low lung volumes due to decrease in size and therefore increase in resistance of extraalveolar vessels at low lung volumes and compression of alveolar vessels at high lung volumes (see Fig. 11.5).

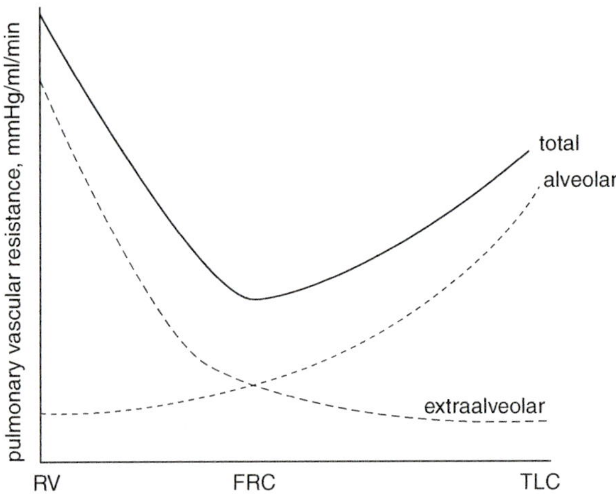

Fig. 11.5 The relationship between lung volumes and pulmonary vascular resistance with contributions from the alveolar and extraalveolar vasculature. With permission of Springer (Bronicki R and Anas N 2009)

Left heart preload is decreased as a result of decreased right heart preload from positive pressure ventilation and the effects of increased pulmonary vascular resistance. If PVR is significantly elevated, then transseptal ventricular pressure gradient may reverse, and the right ventricle may bow toward the left ventricle further decreasing its filling.

Increased intrathoracic pressure decreases left ventricular afterload. This is thought to happen because the increase in intrathoracic pressure is transmitted to the intrathoracic aorta but not the extrathoracic aorta thereby increasing forward flow from the intrathoracic aorta to the extrathoracic portion. This permits the left ventricle to discharge against a relatively volume depleted intrathoraic aorta.

11.1.5 Pulmonary Response to General Anesthesia and Cardiac Surgery

The provision of general anesthesia has negative effects on the respiratory system, some of which may endure for up to 24 h. These include impaired ventilator response to hypercarbia and hypoxia, reduced tidal volume with spontaneous ventilation, decrease in functional residual capacity, dependent atelectasis, decreased compliance, increased work of breathing, increased shunt and dead space, impaired V/Q matching, inhibition of hypoxic pulmonary vasoconstriction, predisposition to obstruction, and altered surfactant function (Friedrich 2012).

Surgery causes an inflammatory response as a result of tissue trauma, blood loss, transfusion, and hypothermia. The inflammatory response to cardiopulmonary bypass (CPB) is additive and has important effects on the respiratory system. CPB increases capillary permeability, complement activation, leukocyte activation, and cytokine release. These effects are thought to occur when the blood components of the immune system are exposed to the foreign materials of the CPB circuit. In addition, following removal of an aortic cross clamp, there are elements of ischemia-reperfusion injury to several major organs including the heart, lungs, kidneys, liver, and brain with subsequent immune system activation. Finally, the presence of endotoxemia post-CPB is also thought to play a role in the inflammatory cascade, although the etiology of these elevated endotoxin levels is still a matter of investigation (Laffey et al. 2002).

The robust inflammatory response to cardiac surgery may create a systemic inflammatory response syndrome (SIRS) that can be associated with organ dysfunction including myocardial depression, renal failure, acute lung injury, and multiple organ dysfunction syndrome (MODS). MODS develops with an incidence of 11% after CPB and has a mortality rate of 41% (Laffey et al. 2002).

Respiratory dysfunction is common after cardiac surgery occurring in anywhere between 5 and 25% of patients (Canver and Chanda 2003; Filsoufi et al. 2008). Studies have also suggested an elevated mortality, up to 25% in patients who develop respiratory failure (Canver and Chanda 2003). A contemporary study of approximately 6000 patients from 2008 found an overall incidence of 9% but up to 17% in multiple valve surgeries and 22% in aortic surgeries

(Filsoufi et al. 2008). The modern era of cardiac surgery is marked by more heterogenous and complex procedures which may expose patients to greater risk of respiratory complications.

The lungs are exposed to a significant inflammatory response post-cardiac surgery. Although general anesthesia will cause atelectasis in most patients, there is additional insult to the lungs in cardiac surgery as compared with other major surgeries that is attributed to the cardiopulmonary bypass (CPB) circuit (Taggart et al. 1993). Inflammation may be a result of contact with foreign material in the CPB circuit, ischemia-reperfusion injury as circulation changes from CPB to pulsatile native flow, and collapse and re-expansion of lungs. Despite recognition of reduced systemic inflammation in patients undergoing off-pump CABG compared to on pump, there has been no demonstrable difference in post-op gas exchange or incidence of respiratory failure (Ng et al. 2002). Clearly, there are additional sources of inflammation in cardiac surgery contributing to respiratory failure that are not well understood. In addition to the inflammation from CPB, patients undergoing cardiac surgery are at high risk for acute lung injury (ALI) given collapse and re-expansion of the lung, possible breach of the pleural space, reperfusion injury, and potential for blood transfusions.

There are also mechanical effects on respiration when the chest is entered. Altered chest wall compliance occurs with thoracotomy and sternotomy. Thoracic surgery is associated with reduction in lung volumes in a restrictive pattern (both FEV1 and FVC will decrease proportionally); vital capacity can remain reduced up to 1 week. Functional residual capacity is also reduced 30% (Braun et al. 1978; Berrizbeitia et al. 1989). The effects are likely a combination of changes to interposition of rib cage and sternum, postoperative pain/splinting, and effects on diaphragm function (Ford et al. 1983). Atelectasis occurs in up to 70% of patients after cardiac surgery (Jain et al. 1991). Atelectasis is more severe with a larger number of grafts, longer operative and bypass time, and violation of pleural space (Wilcox et al. 1985). When lungs are re-expanded after surgery, some alveoli units may be filled with fluid and may not be functional until the fluid is redistributed There is also decrease in tidal volume and loss of sighing (due to pain) which can exacerbate atelectasis. Large pleural chest tubes also contribute to pain. Thoracotomy incisions such as those used for minimally invasive direct CABG may have worse pain. Pleural effusions, usually left sided and exudative, are common after surgery and may contribute to respiratory impairment if large enough.

11.1.6 Risk Factors for Postoperative Respiratory Failure

Risk factors associated with respiratory failure include advanced age, decreased EF, and renal failure (Filsoufi et al. 2008). Additional factors contributing to the risk include CPB time, sepsis from endocarditis, GI bleeding, renal failure, sternal wound infection, new stroke, and bleeding requiring reoperation (Canver and Chanda 2003) (Table 11.1).

Table 11.1 Common risk factors for postoperative respiratory failure

Preoperative risk factors (Arozullah et al. 2000; Filsoufi et al. 2008)	Intraoperative characteristics	Postoperative characteristics (Canver and Chanda 2003)
Smoking (Warner et al. 1989)	Reoperation, CPB time greater than 4–6 h (Canver and Chanda 2003; Rajakaruna et al. 2005; Bailey et al. 2011)	Mediastinal bleeding and need for re-exploration (Karthik et al. 2004; Ranucci et al. 2008)
Age > 70	Significant volume administration during surgery	New neurologic events
COPD, especially with more severe disease (Kroenke et al. 1993)	Need for inotropes and/or mechanical circulatory support to wean off bypass	Worsening hemodynamic instability
Neuromuscular disease affecting respiratory muscles	Aortic cases and/or need for circulatory arrest	*Gastrointestinal bleeding*
Diabetes	Emergent surgery	*Renal failure*
Inability to climb one flight of stairs		*Sternal wound infection*
Renal failure		*Sepsis and endocarditis*
Cardiogenic shock prior to surgery		
Low ejection fraction		

11.2 Mechanical Ventilation

11.2.1 Indications for Mechanical Ventilation

Intubation and institution of mechanical ventilation in the perioperative period can be thought of as planned and unplanned events. The institution of mechanical ventilation as a component of general anesthesia is obviously necessary for the surgery itself. Cardiac surgery distinguishes itself from other major surgeries by the practice of leaving patients intubated at the end of the procedure. Mechanical ventilation (MV) is necessary in the immediate postoperative period in the vast majority of patients. Due to its routine use to facilitate care, MV management can be expected to follow a common path. As opposed to unplanned mechanical ventilation, the majority of patients will not have superimposed respiratory failure, and the duration of MV will be brief.

Prolonged ventilation and unplanned reintubation in the cardiac surgery intensive care unit (CSICU) may be necessary as a result of non-pulmonary organ failure, perioperative complications, frank respiratory failure, or need for airway protection. Examples of non-pulmonary organ failure requiring prolonged ventilation include severe cardiogenic shock, renal failure and subsequent right ventricular volume overload, and sepsis from endocarditis or other sources. Perioperative complications such as mediastinal bleeding, graft failure requiring cardiac catheterization, severe vasoplegia requiring high-dose vasopressors, and phrenic nerve injury can also extend mechanical ventilation. Airway protection may be necessary for patients who have an acute neurologic event (such as stroke or seizure), airway trauma (such as severe epistaxis from NG placement), and need for diagnostic studies (such as TEE, endoscopy).

Unplanned reintubation for respiratory failure is sometimes necessary. Although often divided into hypoxemic (oxygenation failure) and hypercapnic (ventilatory failure), respiratory failure is commonly a mixture of both. The ventilator management for prolonged intubation or unplanned reintubation is by nature more complex. As opposed to following a typical protocol, it necessitates diagnosing the etiology of respiratory failure, proper ventilator management specific to that etiology, need for resolution of the inciting event before weaning, and application of appropriate weaning strategies. Refer to the section on ventilator management for specifics.

11.2.2 Complications of Mechanical Ventilation

11.2.2.1 Direct Consequences

1. Ventilator-associated pneumonia: The risk for developing VAP increases every day as patient remains intubated.
2. Oropharyngeal and tracheal trauma: Mouth and pharyngeal mucosal damage, glottic edema, vocal cord trauma, ischemic injury to tracheal mucosa from endotracheal tube cuff, and loss of glottic reflexes (swallowing, secretion clearance, airway protection) with prolonged intubation.
3. Ventilator-induced diaphragm dysfunction: Prolonged mechanical ventilation especially with minimal patient effort (minimal diaphragm contraction either from prolonged sedatives or over support without patient-triggered breaths) can lead to diaphragm atrophy (Sassoon et al. 2002; Vassilakopoulos and Petrof 2004).

11.2.2.2 Indirect Consequences

Critical illness neuromuscular disorders: Both neuropathy and myopathy can lead to profound weakness and are related to decreased mobility from prolonged bed rest and neuromuscular blockade.

Delirium: ICU delirium can be caused or exacerbated by the use of benzodiazepines for sedation, prolonged immobilization, sleep deprivation, and inability to communicate (due to intubation) (Inouye et al. 1999) (Table 11.2).

11.2.3 Reducing Postoperative Respiratory Failure

Preoperative risk stratification: In a national surgical quality improvement program database with over 450 k patients, the odds for postoperative pulmonary complications attributable to COPD were 2.36. COPD was an independent predictor of postoperative pneumonia, failure to wean from mechanical ventilation, and reintubation (Gupta et al. 2013).

Table 11.2 Ventilator related complications

Complications of mechanical ventilation	Description	Manifestations
Barotrauma	High mean airway pressures and high transpulmonary pressure	Pneumothorax Pneumomediastinum
Volutrauma	High tidal volumes Cyclical opening/closing of alveoli	Worsens ALI Secondary organ injury
Oxygen toxicity	High inspired oxygen	Worsens/causes ALI
Ventilator dyssynchrony	Mismatch between patient's demands and machine settings	Increased work of breathing Worse gas exchange Can lead to low SVO2
Intrinsic i-PEEP	Dynamic hyperinflation	Hemodynamic compromise

Preoperative pulmonary function tests remain controversial, but may be helpful in identifying patients so high risk that the surgery should be cancelled or delayed. That being said there is no clearly definable PFT threshold that can be deemed too high risk, and many patients with poor PFTs would be identified high risk on clinical grounds alone. If PFTs are available, it is generally accepted that a FEV1 and FVC less than 70% predicted and a ratio < 65% predicts an increased risk of complications (Gass and Olsen 1986). It is logical to assume the worse the FEV1, the less effective cough the patient can generate and the higher risk of developing atelectasis, pneumonia, and respiratory failure in general. Studies that have examined PFTs with clinical features often show that clinical features are more predictive than PFTs (Williams-Russo et al. 1992).

Although a routine preoperative arterial blood gas is not necessary, it can be very helpful in severe COPD patients. Knowledge of pre-existing CO_2 retention and the patient's baseline $PaCO_2$ is helpful and should be used to titrate ventilator settings. The patient's baseline $PaCO_2$ should be targeted, as their slightly acidic pH baseline is usually low to mid 7.3s. A normal CO_2 should not be targeted as this will lead to bicarbonate excretion, subsequent worsening acidosis on weaning, and prolonged mechanical ventilation (Gladwin and Pierson 1998).

Patients with underlying lung disease should be as optimized as possible before surgery. A preoperative course of bronchodilators, antibiotics, and steroids may be necessary in a patient with an acute exacerbation of chronic bronchitis. Certainly, one should delay elective cardiac surgery if the patient is in the throngs of an asthma or COPD exacerbation or interstitial lung disease flare.

Intraoperative management to reduce respiratory failure: As noted above, CPB and cardiac surgery place patients at risk for acute lung injury. Lung protective ventilation (LPV), marked by tidal volumes less than or equal to 6 cm^3/kg and use of i-PEEP, is essential in the management of established lung injury. But LPV has also been studied as a preventative strategy. Higher intraoperative tidal volume (TV) during pneumonectomy has been found to correlate with the likelihood of developing postoperative respiratory failure (Fernandez-Perez et al. 2006). Intraoperative LPV has been shown to decrease post-op respiratory failure in major abdominal surgery (Futier et al. 2013). In two small trials of patients undergoing CABG, high

TVs and low i-PEEP were associated with higher levels of bronchoscopically sampled inflammatory markers than patients who received low TV and high i-PEEP strategy (Wrigge et al. 2005; Zupancich et al. 2005). A single-center trial of 150 cardiac surgery patients randomized to 6 vs. 10 cm^3/kg tidal volume intraoperatively found a higher percentage of patients extubated at 6 h post-op and less reintubations in the lower TV group (Sundar et al. 2011). Another trial found that tidal volumes 10 cm^3/kg or greater in mechanically ventilated patients after cardiac surgery were a significant risk factor for single and multiple organ failure and a prolonged stay in the ICU (Lellouche et al. 2012). We recommend 6–8 cm^3/kg tidal volume intraoperative and immediately postoperative, with the use of i-PEEP for lung recruitment if there is evidence of lung injury.

In addition, intraoperative strategies to reduce the amount of neuromuscular blockade, avoidance of total muscle suppression, and judicious use of reversal agents may help reduce postoperative respiratory muscle weakness. Residual effects of neuromuscular blockade can reduce respiratory muscle strength, impair glottic reflexes, and prolong the need for ventilation (Bevan 2000; Murphy et al. 2005). Clinicians should be mindful that the lingering effects of NMB may be difficult to detect but clinically relevant, (Kopman et al. 1997) especially in patients with marginal respiratory function at baseline.

11.2.3.1 Postoperative Strategies to Reduce Respiratory Failure

Fast-track extubation: There has been widespread acceptance of early extubation after cardiac surgery. Earlier extubation has putative benefits including a reduction in respiratory complications and improvements in early mobilization. So-called "fast-track" protocols generally refer to extubation within 6 h of surgery. Fast track is facilitated by favoring short-acting sedatives postoperatively and limiting opiate and benzodiazepine use during surgery (Myles and McIlroy 2005). Early extubation after CABG reduces costs (Cheng et al. 1996a, b) and resources and does not lead to any increase in perioperative morbidity (Cheng et al. 1996a, b). Early extubation is associated with less atelectasis and better spirometry (Johnson et al. 1997). In a cohort study, fast-track patients were less likely to develop pneumonia (London et al. 1997). Early physical therapy and occupational therapy is an important goal; it has been associated with faster discharge and decreased delirium (Schweickert et al. 2009). There is consensus that patients should be extubated once euthermic, hemostatic, and hemodynamically stable. The need for vasopressors and inotropes is ok as long as there is not a clear trend of worsening hemodynamics or signs of hypoperfusion. Once these practical criteria are met, sedation is stopped, the patient is woken, and then a SBT is performed.

Limiting sedation during mechanical ventilation: Cardiac surgery patients who require extended ventilation or reintubation for respiratory failure should be approached with an aggressive strategy to limit sedation and liberate from the ventilator. Mechanically ventilated patients are prone to ventilator-associated pneumonia, upper GI hemorrhage, bacteremia, baraotrauma, venous thromboembolism, sinusitis, and cholestasis. Ventilator-associated pneumonia is arguably one of the worse complications of long-term ventilation, its cumulative risk increases over time (Cook et al. 1998), and the associated mortality is very high (Chastre and Fagon 2002). These complications can be decreased by ensuring patients are not intubated any longer than absolutely necessary. Daily sedative interruption (Schweickert et al. 2004) can reduce intubation time and limit the related complications listed above. A landmark trial showed that once daily awakening, i.e., discontinuation of sedation in ICU patients, leads to earlier extubation and decreased length of stay (Kress et al. 2000). Daily interruptions of sedation do not appear to have any adverse mental health effects and in fact may reduce symptoms of PTSD (Kress et al. 2003; Treggiari et al. 2009; Strom et al. 2010). The Awake and Breathe trial randomized 336 patients to daily awakening trials combined with spontaneous breathing trials or usual care sedation plus daily SBT and found that patients spend less time intubated, had shorter ICU and hospital stays, and improved survival. In fact, for every seven patients treated with this intervention, one life was saved (Girard et al. 2008). A protocol of no sedation (pain control with opiates only) led to more days without mechanical ventilation and a shorter ICU stay (Strom et al. 2010). In summary, there is tremendous evidence in support of limiting or even eliminating sedative infusions in critical care with the goal of reducing duration of mechanical ventilation and its many associated complications.

11.2.4 Ventilation Modes

Contrary to popular opinion, there is no evidence that any one particular ventilator mode is superior to or offers any outcome advantage over others. However, there are characteristics of particular modes that are useful for managing specific conditions. All modes require setting Fio2, i-PEEP, and triggering (either pressure or flow).

Volume control ventilation: In AC/VC breaths are mandatory, and the ventilator delivers a set tidal volume with each breath delivered. The ventilator cycles to exhalation when that volume is finished. It is the preferred mode in most clinical settings. Breaths can be triggered by the ventilator or the patient. Tidal volume is set and is constant whether there are mandated breaths or assisted (patient-triggered breaths). Once the tidal volume is delivered, the ventilator "cycles" to exhalation. Airway pressures are dependent on the volume set and the patient's lung compliance (but are not directly manipulated). Flow (the speed of the delivered tidal volume) can be adjusted. Critically ill patients tend to favor a fast flow rate. A high flow allows a large tidal volume to be delivered in a shorter time, leaving more time for exhalation and avoidance of hyperinflation. A consequence of increased flow is higher peak airway pressure, but this will often be preferable to ventilator dyssynchrony or air trapping.

The patient can be completely sedated and even paralyzed on AC/VC and be assured a certain minute ventilation. Tidal volumes can of course be strictly controlled which offers an advantage when lung protective ventilation (such as with ARDS) is necessary.

Pressure control ventilation: In AC/PC, pressure is set and tidal volume varies based on lung compliance, patient effort, and timing of cycling. As opposed to AC in which flow is adjusted, in PC the inspiratory time or inspiratory/expiration (I/E) ratio is adjusted. Time therefore determines cycling from inspiration to exhalation and will affect the volume delivered. Some critically ill patients may be more synchronous on pressure control mode, but because this is hard to predict, it will require making changes at the bedside and observing. There is an obvious advantage if maintaining strict airway pressures is desired. There is a practical advantage in using AC/PC mode during ventilation on VV ECMO, as it allows control of driving pressure, and it can act as a barometer for patient improvement. As lung compliance improves, tidal volumes will climb.

Pressure support: Similar to AC/PC, PS is a pressure-targeted mode. However, neither volume nor cycling nor respiratory rate is determined by the clinician, but instead relates to the patient's interaction with the ventilator. The patient has the ability to take large or small breaths and set their own respiratory rate. The ventilator cycles to exhalation based on a decrement in flow. When the patient nears the end of their breath, flow drops and the ventilator cycles to exhalation. The setup has a natural advantage in maximizing ventilator synchrony. Awake patients and patients with vigorous spontaneous respiratory efforts commonly respond well to this mode. It is a misnomer that patients are "less supported" on PS, as one can achieve just as high level of support by dialing up the inspiratory pressure as with any other mode. Pressure support at low levels is also a commonly used mode for ventilator weaning.

SIMV remains popular in many surgical ICUs and can be understood as a mixture of controlled mode and pressure support. Typically, a tidal volume and respiratory rate are set similarly to volume control, but for breaths taken above the set respiratory rate, the ventilator delivers a pressure support breath. The mode can lead to dyssynchrony and/or under supported patients if either the respiratory rate is too low or the pressure support is too minimal. SIMV leads to delayed weaning, despite the popular belief that it facilitates earlier separation from the ventilator (Esteban et al. 1995).

Alternative modes: Some centers prefer using airway pressure release ventilation for patients with ARDS. It is similar in concept to pressure control ventilation but with a long inspiratory interval held at a high airway pressure and short "release" breaths to facilitate ventilation. There are various proprietary modifications to APRV, but they share in common maintenance of sustained high airway pressure to improve oxygenation and maintain airway recruitment. Although some clinical trials have demonstrated improved oxygenation in ARDS with the use of APRV (Varpula et al. 2003; Varpula et al. 2004), none have shown meaningful improvement in outcomes. High-frequency oscillation ventilation has also been used in ARDS and relies on sustained high airway pressure. Ventilation is achieved through high-frequency pulsations. Although theoretically advantageous in terms of oxygenation with minimal atelectrauma, a large randomized control trial in ARDS found no advantage over standard ventilation (Ferguson et al. 2013).

Noninvasive ventilation: NIVV can be extremely helpful and beneficial for respiratory failure secondary to two common situations in cardiac surgery care, COPD exacerbation (Ram et al. 2004), and acute pulmonary edema (Lightowler et al. 2003; Vital et al. 2008). NIVV can reduce work of breathing during COPD, improve minute ventilation, improve oxygenation, and decrease dynamic airway collapse. The beneficial physiology of positive pressure ventilation in the setting of acute pulmonary edema involves reduction of cardiac preload, reduction of afterload, and redistribution of pulmonary volume away from the lung. NIVV is best applied to patients with readily reversible respiratory failure. The patient who is acutely hypertensive with pulmonary edema who can be reversed with vasodilators and diuretics would be an appropriate candidate. On the other hand, a patient with postoperative cardiogenic shock and pulmonary edema who may need VA ECMO would be a poor candidate for NIVV.

Two important randomized controlled trials examined NIVV as a rescue ventilation in patients who fail extubation and found no differences in reintubation rates, delayed reintubation in the NIVV arm, and worse outcomes in patients who received NIVV (Keenan et al. 2002; Esteban et al. 2004). After failing an extubation trial, NIVV not only delays the inevitable reintubation but exposes patients to potentially harmful period of under support. A declining patient on NIVV will require progressively higher levels of support. The higher the FIO_2 and pressure settings on NIVV, the riskier the intubation.

Positive end-expiratory pressure: All modes will require setting positive end-expiratory pressure (PEEP). PEEP represents the lowest airway pressure that the lung will be allowed to fall to on end exhalation. It is commonly misunderstood as pushing air back into the lung on exhalation, when in fact it is more akin to providing a bottom limit to the decline in airway pressure. PEEP allows more alveoli to remain open at the end of a breath. Over time the application of PEEP will lead to cyclical recruitment of alveoli and an improvement in oxygenation. PEEP improves oxygenation best in pathologic states that involve shunt from collapsed or filled alveoli such as pneumonia, ARDS, pulmonary edema, and atelectasis. Although increasing peak airway pressure and tidal volume can recruit lung on inspiration, the lung will derecruit again on exhalation. The cyclical opening and closing of alveoli is thought to be a key mechanism for ventilator-induced lung injury. PEEP on the other hand maintains alveolar recruitment and is a less injurious method of lung recruitment. Even patients with healthy lungs will benefit from a small amount of i-PEEP to prevent derecruitment during intubation. Five of PEEP is applied nearly universally. PEEP can have adverse consequences especially at overly high levels. It can lead to hemodynamic impairment by decreasing RV preload. High alveolar pressures can lead to west zone 1 conditions (alveolar pressure exceeds capillary pressure), a regional fall in blood flow, and increase in dead space ventilation. High PEEP can lead to a global rise in pulmonary vascular resistance through this same mechanism and exacerbation of right heart dysfunction. PEEP can also cause overdistension and damage of normal alveolar segments especially when there is normal lung adjacent to un-recruitable consolidation.

Auto PEEP/intrinsic PEEP(i-PEEP): It is also crucially important for the critical care clinician to recognize that PEEP set on a ventilator may be less than the total PEEP the patient experiences. Measured "extrinsic" PEEP does not take into account "intrinsic" also known as auto-PEEP. i-PEEP relates to residual volume in the alveoli due to incomplete emptying before the subsequent breath is delivered.

Patients with obstructive airway disease and air trapping and those who are tachypneic with large tidal volumes are at risk of developing i-PEEP. Metabolic acidosis and large dead space fraction (common in patients with shock) can also lead to i-PEEP (Rossi et al. 1995). The best diagnostic tool for identifying i-PEEP is the expiratory flow curve on the ventilator graphics. Ventilator graphics typically display inhalation as a positive deflection and exhalation as a negative deflection. The X-axis denotes zero flow state. If expiratory flow does not return to the X-axis before the subsequent breath, i-PEEP is suggested. The hemodynamic consequences can be severe. i-PEEP will increase the juxta-cardiac right atrial pressure and reduce venous return. Consequences on venous return are amplified by hypovolemic states (Berlin 2014). The hemodynamic consequences of pericardial tamponade, right ventricular failure, pulmonary hypertension, and hemorrhage will all be exacerbated by the presence of i-PEEP. Temporarily disconnecting the patient from the ventilator to allow decompression can demonstrate an immediate and startling improvement in blood pressure in these situations.

Oxygen and ventilation goals: The goals of mechanical ventilation are to achieve acceptable oxygenation and ventilation to support the patient's physiology. "Normal" PO_2 and $PaCO_2$ are less important than adequate PO_2 and $PaCO_2$. Hyperoxia has been shown to be deleterious in a number of different critical illnesses (Martin and Grocott 2013). Hyperoxia can lead to resorption atelectasis as well as oxidative injury. Hyperoxia post-cardiac arrest has been linked to worse survival and worse neurologic outcomes (Kilgannon et al. 2010; Kilgannon et al. 2011) presumably due to the exacerbation of reperfusion injury. Part of the strategy of applying i-PEEP in ARDS is to allow the downward titration of harmful FiO_2. VV ECMO is also believed to offer the avoidance of toxic FiO_2 to the injured alveolar space. Experience has shown safety allowing SaO_2 to fall to 88% during ARDS and permissive hypercapnia (to allow for low tidal volumes) down to pH in the 7.2 range. For most routine post-cardiac surgery patients, a SaO_2 goal of 92% or above should suffice. Since hypoxia/hypercapnia and acidosis can increase PVR, patients with severe pulmonary hypertension and/or RV failure may benefit from maintaining gas exchange in the normal range. Patients with intracranial hypertension are also sensitive to CO_2 clearance and will require stricter titration.

Work of breathing on mechanical ventilation: One major goal of MV is to decrease work of breathing, an important concept to be mindful of in mechanical ventilation. It is easier for clinicians to recognize if MV is successfully improving gas exchange. But there is a common misconception that the action of placing someone on the ventilator alone will decrease work of breathing. With the exception of deep sedation or paralysis, the diaphragm will continue to contract while on mechanical ventilation. Workload is shared between the patient's muscles and the machine. Care must be taken to make sure that the ventilator is set appropriately, or else the patient may experience a higher work of breathing. Factors influencing the work of breathing include lung and chest compliance, airway resistance, i-PEEP, endotracheal tube diameter (Shapiro et al. 1986), and minute ventilation (Marini et al. 1985; Polese et al. 1999).

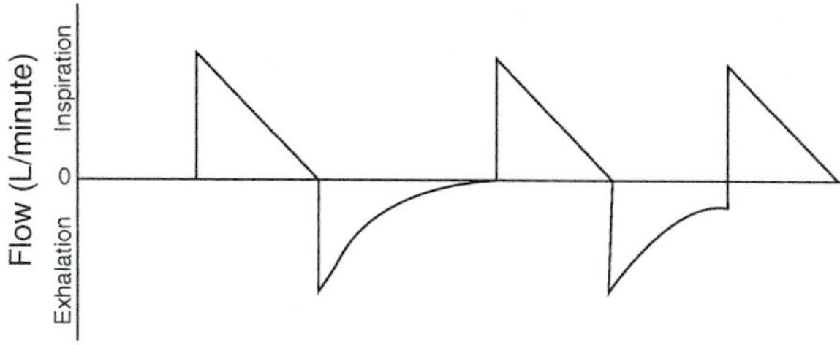

Fig. 11.6 This is a flow time curve which is available on all modern mechanical ventilators. In the first breath the expiratory flow returns to zero and there is no I-i-PEEP. There is incomplete exhalation on the second breath, and expiratory flow is still present before the third breath. This can occur in a cyclical fashion resulting in dynamic hyperinflation and possible hemodynamic compromise

Examples of ventilator dyssynchrony:

1. Ineffective triggering (patient attempts to take a breath but the effort does not trigger the ventilator).
2. Patient makes an expiratory effort before the ventilator cycles from inhalation to exhalation.
3. Patient desires a larger breath and has persistent inspiratory efforts even as the ventilator has cycled to exhalation.

Ventilator dyssynchrony can lead to increased work of breathing (Leung et al. 1997) and should be addressed first by adjusting the ventilator rather than resorting to deeper sedation (Fig. 11.6).

11.2.5 Discontinuation of Mechanical Ventilation

The term "weaning" is often applied to discontinuation of MV but it is misleading. It suggests a false belief that liberation from MV is best accomplished by slowly reducing the level of support. In fact, the most efficient method for determining whether a patient still needs the ventilator is to perform a daily test of withdrawal of ventilator support (spontaneous breathing trials, SBT) while monitoring to see if the patient can function without it.

Readiness for spontaneous breathing trial (SBT): Clinicians have long strived to develop reliable criteria to assess a patient's readiness to undergo a SBT. Considerable investigations of various readiness criteria (including negative inspiratory force, oxygenation and i-PEEP levels, minute ventilation) have been studied. Most criteria do not aide care perhaps because SBTs even if failed are not dangerous, and many more patients than recognized will pass a SBT if performed. Consensus conferences have concluded that the application of weaning predictors prior to performing a SBT is not necessary (MacIntyre et al. 2001; Boles et al. 2007). Patients should undergo a SBT when there has been clinical improvement, reversal of the underlying cause of respiratory failure, adequate oxygenation, and the presence of spontaneous breathing efforts (Epstein 2009).

Routine postoperative patients should undergo a SBT when they are rewarmed and achieve hemostasis and stabilization of hemodynamics and awake enough to participate in the SBT.

Performing spontaneous breathing trials: In a landmark trial, 546 patients were randomized to four methods of ventilator weaning, pressure support with progressive withdrawal of the inspiratory pressure, SIMV with gradual reduction of respiratory rate, or once or intermittent (at least two times a day) trials of unassisted breathing via T-piece circuit. Neither once daily nor multiple daily trials of spontaneous breathing led to the fastest weaning. SIMV led to the slowest weaning (Esteban et al. 1995).

SBTs are best accomplished by either using a low level of pressure support or T piece (which involves application of oxygen only with no mechanical support). Although randomized control trials of T-piece versus pressure support trials have not proven a superiority to either approach (Jones et al. 1991; Farias et al. 2001), there is rationale for using T piece in certain scenarios. T-piece trial offers the best representation of the patient's post-extubation physiology. Positive pressure as previously mentioned can reduce preload and afterload and can keep pulmonary edema at bay. For patients with severe LV or RV dysfunction, pulmonary edema and hypertension strongly consider a T-piece trial prior to extubation to be sure that the patient is ready. Pressure support trials offer the theoretical advantage of mildly assisting the patient so as to overcome the resistance in the endotracheal tube. There is also the advantage of being able to monitor tidal volumes and respiratory rate on the ventilator console, as opposed to T-piece trials in which there is more reliance on the subjective physical appearance of the patient. The clinician must be careful not to over support the patient during a pressure support SBT by applying to high a level of inspiratory pressure and thereby not subjecting the patient to a stringent enough test. We recommend no higher than 5/5 for a true SBT. Readiness for extubation should be demonstrated by RR under 30, adequate oxygenation with an applied FiO_2 of 40% or less, i-PEEP of 5 or less, and the absence of visible respiratory distress or worsening hemodynamics during the trial. A low rapid shallow breathing index (RSBI) (tidal volume in liters divided by the respiratory rate) is desired. A number greater than 105 during a T-piece readiness trial has been associated with subsequent successful SBT (Meade et al. 2001; Yang and Tobin 1991). Many extrapolate that metric to SBTs in general, including PS trials. A strong cough, ability to follow commands, and minimal secretions are desired but not absolutely necessary.

11.2.6 High-Flow Oxygen

High-flow oxygen plays an important role in the care of patients with severe hypoxic respiratory failure. The device delivers very high flow rates and allows much higher effective oxygen delivery than other noninvasive methods, humidification, and a small amount of i-PEEP. A recent important randomized controlled trial of patients in respiratory failure found a survival benefit with nasal high-flow oxygen therapy when compared with 100% NRB mask and noninvasive ventilation; however patients with cardiogenic pulmonary edema and hemodynamic instability were excluded (Frat et al. 2015). High-flow O_2 may have the benefit of allowing cough and secretion clearance, humidification of inspired gas, and less ventilator-induced lung injury than NIVV, and it may be an important tool for addressing hypoxic respiratory failure in the post-op patient absence of pulmonary edema or shock.

11.2.7 Mechanical Ventilation in Specific Scenarios

ARDS The presence of bilateral pulmonary infiltrates in combination with a P/F ratio < 200 meets criteria for ARDS. An older study from 1996 examined 3848 patients after cardiac surgery and found an incidence of 1% of ARDS with a mortality rate of 68% (Christenson et al. 1996). Since then improvements in CPB technique and management of ARDS have likely brought both the incidence and mortality down.

It is vitally important to pay strict attention to ventilator settings as ventilator-induced lung injury is a major factor contributing to the mortality in this condition. The landmark ARMA trial solidified the practice of a lung protective ventilation (LPV) strategy targeting a tidal volume of 6 cm^3/kg of ideal body weight. It is important that ideal body weight is used as opposed to actual body weight which can lead to erroneously high tidal volume targets. In the ARMA trial, a plateau pressure < 30 was also targeted. An important recent trial found that the driving pressure (difference between the plateau pressure and i-PEEP) independently and strongly correlated with survival in ARDS. When Vt was reduced or i-PEEP was increased, they were only beneficial if associated with decreases in driving pressure (Amato et al. 2015). Although, more trials are needed to understand the role of driving pressure further, this important finding may turn out to be the key variable we should target in ARDS.

Experience has shown the safety of permissive hypercapnia as well as acceptance of O_2 saturations as low as 88% and PaO_2 in the 55–60 range in order to apply low tidal volumes and limit oxygen toxicity.

Application of i-PEEP is particularly beneficial in ARDS as it can improve oxygenation, allow reduction of FiO_2, and limit VILI. There is no one universally accepted way for appropriately adjusting i-PEEP in ARDS. In the ARMA trial demonstrating mortality benefit to low tidal volume ventilation in ARDS, i-PEEP level was chosen based on a prespecified scale at each FiO_2 level. A separate study of high versus low i-PEEP applied indiscriminately in ARDS did not lead to an improvement in outcomes (Briel et al. 2010). A trial of i-PEEP individually titrated to a positive transpulmonary pressure measured by esophageal balloon did show an improvement in gas exchange (Talmor et al. 2008). i-PEEP should be set on an individual basis, but there are no studies that identify an optimal method.

The following methods have been used to optimize i-PEEP:

1. Titrate to maximal lung compliance
2. Titrate to best end-tidal CO_2 (reflecting maximal ventilation and avoidance of overdistension/dead space ventilation)
3. Titrate to the optimal hemodynamic protocol (either using PA catheter or echo)
4. Titrate to lung recruitment visualized on bedside ultrasound
5. Titrate to transpulmonary pressure

In summary, trials have not identified a superior method to adjust i-PEEP. i-PEEP should be individualized to each patient. There is agreement that too low will lead to atelectrauma/impaired gas exchange/lung derecruitment and too high can lead to barotrauma/adverse hemodynamics/impaired gas exchange.

Prone positioning in severe ARDS (P/F ratio < 150) improves mortality (Guerin et al. 2013). Early neuromuscular blockade has been shown in one trial to improve mortality and can certainly be helpful in guaranteeing lung protective ventilation (Papazian et al. 2010). Nitric oxide, although commonly used to improve oxygenation in severe ARDS, has not been shown to improve mortality (Adhikari et al. 2007).

Veno-venous (VV) ECMO is increasingly used to treat patients with severe ARDS who have refractory gas exchange abnormalities despite LPV and i-PEEP or whom are unable to achieve LPV. A trial showed improved mortality in patients who were transferred to an ECMO center although only 75% of those patients ultimately received ECMO (Peek et al. 2009). A large RCT for ECMO in severe ARDS (EOLIA) is underway.

Mechanical ventilation during VV ECMO for ARDS: One of the major propertied benefits of VV ECMO is the allowance of consistent lung protective ventilation. All patients should be treated with tidal volumes of 6 cm^3/kg or less, and a large survey of current practice showed majority of centers target a TV 4–6 cm^3/kg (Marhong et al. 2014). There has been vast interest in ventilating patients with ultra-lung protective ventilation (decreasing tidal volumes below 6 cm^3/kg) to theoretically offer even more lung protection. In a recent review of 49 studies of patients on VV ECMO, and approximately 2000 patients, a plateau <25 and TV < 4 cm^3/kg (as opposed to 4–6 cm^3/kg) were associated with improved mortality (Marhong et al. 2015). An analysis of patients on VV ECMO for H1N1 found that low driving pressure and a plateau pressure < 25 correlated with mortality in ARDS (Pham et al. 2013). An additional trial showed that driving pressure under 10 was a major determinant of survival during VV ECMO (Neto et al. 2016). We recommend aiming for a tidal volume between 4 and 6 cm^3/kg and a driving pressure of 10 or less. Limit ventilator FIO_2 as much as possible ideally down to 21%. Set i-PEEP at 10 and increase only if it leads to a reduction in driving pressure.

11.3 Strategies for Managing Specific Perioperative Disease States

11.3.1 Pleural Effusion

Nearly half of patients undergoing cardiac surgery will develop pleural effusions (Light 2002). Generally speaking these occur as a direct result of surgical trauma and do not need aggressive treatment or drainage. However, a small subset of individuals may require further workup and treatment. Variables that may help determine the clinical course include timing of onset, size/volume of effusion, progression of accumulation, and associated cardiopulmonary symptoms.

Non-specific pleural effusions are especially common following coronary artery bypass grafting and cardiac transplantation and less so after valvular surgery (Heidecker and Sahn 2006). Non-specific effusions may be considered early (less than 30 days from surgery) or late (greater than 30 days from surgery). Common causes of these effusions include interruption of the mediastinal lymphatic system, pleurotomy, topical cardiac cooling, postpericardiotomy syndrome (PPCS), and pericarditis.

Symptomatic effusions may necessitate further evaluation including chest x-ray, chest CT, echocardiography, or ultrasound and ultimately drainage with or without drain placement. These latter, more complex cases may be caused by chylothorax, infectious mediastinitis, heart failure, pulmonary embolus, empyema, pneumonia, and catheter erosion into the pleural space.

11.3.2 Acute Respiratory Distress Syndrome

Acute respiratory distress syndrome (ARDS) is a highly morbid condition comprised of a continuum of acute hypoxemic respiratory failure with diffuse pulmonary infiltrates (Ware and Matthay 2000). In 2012, the Berlin Definition of ARDS categorized the syndrome into mild, moderate, and severe with the inclusion criteria of bilateral infiltrates not attributed to heart failure/fluid overload, pleural effusions, nodes, or atelectasis and onset within 1 week of clinical insult. The spectrum of severity is classified by the ratios of partial pressure of oxygen (PaO_2) to fraction of inspired oxygen (FiO_2): mild (200 mmHg < PaO_2/FiO_2 < or equal to 300), moderate (100 mmHg < PaO_2/FiO_2 < or equal to 200), and severe (PaO_2/FiO_2 < or equal to 100) with i-PEEP of at least 5 cmH_2O (Force et al. 2012).

Up to 20% of patients undergoing cardiac surgery may develop ARDS, with a mortality rate as high as 80% which is nearly double that of the general population (Stephens et al. 2013). ARDS is associated with prolonged hospital/ICU stay and long-term physical and psychosocial morbidity (Mikkelsen et al. 2012). Variables leading to increased risk include but are not limited to cardiopulmonary bypass, transfusion of allogenic blood products, aspiration pneumonia, ventilator-induced lung injury (VILI), hypothermic circulatory arrest, pulmonary contusion, ischemia reperfusion, and drug toxicity (Stephens et al. 2013).

Identification and minimization of risk factors are the mainstays in decreasing the incidence of ARDS post-cardiac surgery. However, when the diagnosis is made, focus of treatment remains supportive with the goal of minimizing further trauma to the damaged lung. This includes low-volume ventilation strategies, meticulous fluid administration, avoidance of blood product transfusion, paralysis, prone ventilation, and extracorporeal membrane oxygenation (ECMO) in the most severe cases (Amato et al. 1998; Gattinoni et al. 2001; Papazian et al. 2010).

11.3.3 Pneumothorax/Hemothorax

Air in the pleural space, or pneumothorax, can be attributed to the mechanisms of:

- Communication between the pleural space and the atmosphere
- Communication between the pleural space and alveolar ventilation
- Presence of an organism capable of producing gas (Noppen and De Keukeleire 2008)

In patients without diagnosed lung disease, these can be considered primary spontaneous pneumothoraces. In those with pre-existing conditions such as emphysema, ARDS, and cystic fibrosis, they are considered secondary spontaneous pneumothoraces (Haynes and Baumann 2010). Iatrogenic pneumothoraces are those caused by surgical/procedural violations of the pleural space during cardiac/lung surgery, thoracentesis, central line placement, or positive pressure ventilation (Yarmus and Feller-Kopman 2012). In patients who are spontaneously breathing, clinical signs and symptoms may include acute respiratory distress, hypoxemia, hypercapnia, pleuritic chest pain, unilateral breath sounds, hypotension, and tachycardia. Intubated patients may develop increased airway pressures, hemodynamic compromise, and tracheal deviation if transformation to a tension pneumothorax occurs.

Along with clinical suspicion, the mainstay in the diagnosis of pneumothorax is radiographic imaging. Chest radiography will demonstrate the absence of distal lung markings in pneumothorax, and CT remains the gold standard in obtaining precise information regarding size and location (Kelly et al. 2006). Additionally, ultrasound has recently become a preferred diagnostic modality due to high sensitivity, accessibility, and low cost (Yarmus and Feller-Kopman 2012).

Post-cardiac surgery patients often present with mediastinal bleeding that can traverse the open pleural space and create a hemothorax. Signs and symptoms may be similar to those found in pneumothorax however may additionally be accompanied by anemia and hemodynamic instability associated with hypovolemic shock. The treatment for both pneumothorax and hemothorax involves drainage of air/blood via tube thoracostomy to facilitate re-expansion of the lung and closure of the space between the parietal and visceral pleura. However, when faced with the emergent nature of a tension pneumothorax, immediate tube or needle decompression may be necessary and precede any diagnostic imaging.

11.3.4 Pulmonary Edema

Postoperative pulmonary edema is a common complication among patients in the cardiac surgical intensive care unit, the etiology of which can be either cardiac or non-cardiac in origin. Cardiac-induced pulmonary edema is a result of elevation in pulmonary blood flow leading to pulmonary venous hypertension, and an increase in pulmonary capillary wedge pressure (PCWP) (Meyer and Krishnamani 2010) demonstrated that extravasation of intravascular fluid occurs as PCWP exceeds plasma colloid osmotic pressure (typically at 28 mmHg) (Jeremias and Brown 2010). With continuation of this process, the interstitial space can no longer tolerate fluid accumulation, and it begins to collect in the alveoli. Clinically, this presents as respiratory distress, hypercapnia, hypoxia, crackles, wheezes, and rales in addition to an elevated jugular venous pressure, new murmurs, and S3/S4 heart sounds. Further diagnostic evidence can be found with chest radiography, troponin, B-type natriuretic peptide, and electrocardiogram. Echocardiogram and PCWP measurements (with a pulmonary artery catheter) can assess the left ventricle and confirm depressed function. In cardiogenic edema, the goal is to address the underlying pathology by decreasing intrapulmonary fluid with the use of diuretics along with simultaneous optimization of left ventricular function using inotropes and/or vasodilators (decrease pre/afterload).

Non-cardiac pulmonary edema can occur with systemic inflammation in response to cardiopulmonary bypass, blood transfusion, sepsis, neurogenic insult, post-pneumonectomy, and re-expansion following thoracentesis or with lung transplantation. In these cases, management is focused on treating the underlying etiology and supporting the patient. Independent of cause, severe edema may require positive pressure ventilation, which can reduce the work of breathing, reduce the shunt fraction, and improve oxygenation.

11.3.5 Obstructive Airway Disease

The preoperative workup of the cardiac surgical patient focuses on the diagnosis and optimization of obstructive airway disease. Asthma and chronic obstructive pulmonary disease (COPD) are the most commonly diagnosed illness in this population. In both conditions the underlying mechanism involves airflow resistance and inflammation; however only in asthma is this acutely reversible. COPD can be broken down into emphysema, chronic bronchitis, or a combination of the two. Furthermore, patients may suffer from both asthma and COPD simultaneously and have a significantly higher risk of bronchospasm in the postoperative setting.

Clinically, bronchospasm presents as increased work of breathing, accessory/intercostal muscle use, pulsus paradoxus, and wheezing. Mechanically ventilated patients may have an acute elevation in peak inspiratory pressures, alterations in expiratory capnography waveforms, and auto-i-PEEP. Treatment is centered on the administration of inhaled beta2-agonists and noninvasive positive pressure ventilation (NPPV) (Brochard et al. 1990). NPPV has been shown by Brouchard et al. to improve gas exchange by increasing tidal volumes with reduction of respiratory rate and symptoms.

Despite the nonreversible airflow obstruction in COPD, symptomatic relief can be achieved with the use of inhaled bronchodilators. Beta-2 adrenergic agonists (increased smooth muscle relaxation via increased intracellular CAMP) and inhaled cholinergic antagonist (decreased intracellular cGMP) can both be used. Longer-acting B2-agonists (salmeterol) and phosphodiesterase inhibitors (aminophylline), however, have failed to exhibit any benefit during both acute exacerbations and bronchospasm (van Noord et al. 2000). In circumstances refractory to traditional therapy, racemic epinephrine can be used as a rescue agent. Similar approaches can be employed in severe asthma exacerbations as bronchodilators, supplemental oxygen, and systemic epinephrine have all been shown to improved airflow. Additionally, intravenous steroids can be considered, with the understanding that onset will not be immediate. When conventional therapy fails to improve oxygenation, intubation, and mechanical ventilation, paralysis may be required.

In any patient with obstructive airway disease, the respiratory therapist and bedside nurse must be aggressive in facilitating the clearance of secretions with frequent suctioning, ensuring adequate hydration, administering mucolytics, providing aerosolized gas flow, and performing chest physiotherapy. When mechanical ventilation is necessary, the underlying obstruction increases the risk of "dynamic hyperinflation" or auto-i-PEEP that can severely compromise hemodynamics and lead to cardiac arrest. Clinicians should identify and avoid auto-i-PEEP early. Ventilation strategies should include reduction of respiratory rate and/or tidal volumes in addition to increasing flow rates to prolong time for exhalation. In circumstances of extreme bronchospasm and air trapping (severe asthma), paralysis may be necessary to avoid auto-i-PEEP. The resultant hypercapnia is often more tolerable than the detrimental hemodynamic effects of auto-i-PEEP.

11.3.6 Pneumonia and Ventilator-Associated Events

The incidence of pneumonia after cardiac surgery can be as high as 2–10%, with a risk of mortality of 20–30% (Hortal et al. 2009). Allou and colleagues demonstrated independent risk factors including duration of cardiopulmonary bypass, age, COPD, intraoperative blood transfusion, and left ventricular ejection fraction (Allou et al. 2014). The main culprits of infection are *Haemophilus influenzae* and *Streptococcus* with rare but complicated cases caused by methicillin-resistant *S. Aureus* (MRSA), *Serratia*, *Klebsiella pneumoniae*, and *Enterobacter*. Mechanisms of infection can be attributed to pre-procedure colonization of bacteria, impaired host defense from medications/critical illness, and aspiration of contaminated fluids, which can all be influenced by presurgical hospitalization (Kollef 1999). If pneumonia is diagnosed in patients 48 h post intubation and mechanical ventilation, it is defined as ventilator-associated pneumonia (VAP). VAP is associated with high morbidity and mortality—up to 50% in one series (Heyland et al. 1999)—however it is hard to know whether VAP alone is responsible for the high mortality or if the incidence is higher in sicker patients.

The diagnosis of pneumonia can be a challenge in the postoperative patient. Many of the classic signs of infection including tachycardia, leukocytosis, and fever are also present in the postsurgical patient experiencing cytokine release and inflammation. Common abnormal findings on a postoperative chest x-ray, including asymmetrical pulmonary edema, pleural effusions, lung contusion, and regional atelectasis, can be difficult to differentiate from pneumonia. Clinicians do a very poor job diagnosing VAP on clinical grounds alone, with high rates of missed diagnoses and over diagnosis (Fagon et al. 1993; Torres et al. 1994). Given the diagnostic challenge, we recommend bronchoscopically derived invasive quantitative cultures (Chastre and Fagon 2002). Although studies in broad ICU populations have not conclusively found a benefit to invasive versus clinical diagnosis (Sole Violan et al. 2000; Shorr et al. 2005), many have found an invasive approach leads to improved diagnostic accuracy, a reduction in inappropriate antimicrobial therapy, (Bonten et al. 1997), and, in some instances, improved outcomes (Sanchez-Nieto et al. 1998; Fagon et al. 2000).

The treatment of pneumonia should include broad-spectrum antibiotics that provide antimicrobial activity against organisms that have a high incidence of infection at the institution. Once cultures result and the species of pathogen can be identified, coverage should be narrowed. Patients susceptible to multidrug-resistant infections should be empirically started on combination therapy including antipseudomonal cephalosporins (cefepime, ceftazidime) or a carbapenem (imipenem, meropenem) or piperacillin-tazobactam in addition to therapy covering for MRSA (vancomycin, linezolid). Antifungal agents should be considered in the immunosuppressed population.

In response to the lack of sufficient epidemiological data regarding VAP, the CDC coined the term "ventilator-associated event (VAE)," in 2014. This terminology captured a broader group of patients including those with worsening oxygenation after initial stability, with a 20% increase in FiO_2 and/or an increase of i-PEEP by 3 cm H_2O (Raoof et al. 2014). To further differentiate VAEs (infectious and noninfectious), the CDC proposes the following tiers:

Tier 1: Ventilator-associated condition (VAC)—sustained hypoxemia >2 days, etiology non-specific.

Tier 2: Infection-related ventilator-associated complication (IVAC)—sustained hypoxemia, signs/symptoms of infection (temp>38 C or WBC > 12,000 cells/mm or <4000 cells/mm), and new antimicrobial therapy >4 days.

Tier 3: Probable or possible ventilator-associated pneumonia (VAP)—additional culture positivity of endotracheal tube aspirate, sputum, BAL, lung tissue or protected brushing, and/or purulent secretions (>25 neutrophils and <10 squamous epithelial per low-power field). Excluded are the pathogens not commonly seen in VAP: *Enterococcus*, coagulase-negative *Staphylococcus*, and *Candida*.

11.3.7 Pulmonary Hypertension

The diagnosis of pulmonary hypertension (PH) has been associated with an increased risk of postoperative morbidity and mortality in both non-cardiac and cardiac surgery (Roques et al. 1999; Ramakrishna et al. 2005). By consensus, PH is considered when mean pulmonary artery pressures (PAP) are greater than or equal to 25 mmHg at rest or greater than or equal to 30 mmHg with exercise.

PH is a condition further stratified based on location of causation: precapillary, capillary, postcapillary, and by plausible etiology. In 2013, the World Health Organization classified PH into five groups (Hill and Farber 2008):

1. Pulmonary arterial hypertension (inheritable PH, idiopathic PH, PH resulting from connective tissue disorders, and HIV), caused by proliferation of smooth muscle/endothelial cells leading to obstruction of the pulmonary vasculature
2. PH secondary to left heart disease (elevated left heart pressures) consisting of both systolic/diastolic heart failure and valvular pathology (regurgitation/stenosis) of the mitral/aortic valves or both
3. PH secondary to lung disease and/or persistent hypoxemia (interstitial lung disease, COPD, obstructive sleep apnea) resulting in hypertrophy of the arterial smooth muscle
4. PH resulting from embolic/thrombotic obstruction of blood flow through the pulmonary vasculature
5. PH due to unclear etiology and usually multifactorial mechanisms (glycogen storage diseases, sarcoidosis, hemolytic anemia)

In patients undergoing cardiac surgery, the origin of PH is typically postcapillary, group 2 (Hill et al. 2009). The increased risk of postoperative complications arises from the potential for right ventricular (RV) ischemia and cor pulmonale (Haddad et al. 2009). From a physiological standpoint, there are multiple mechanisms behind this phenomenon:

- PH increases RV afterload and therefore oxygen demand.
- Compensatory right ventricular hypertrophy (PH increases afterload) increases the amount of myocardial tissue requiring oxygenation.
- As PAP (right ventricular systolic pressures) nears systemic blood pressures, the myocardium is no longer perfused in systole and diastole.
- Decreased RV compliance with RVH combined with increased RV end-diastolic pressures worsens RV ischemia.
- RV failure and dilation alter LV structure resulting in decreased cardiac output.

Additionally, there are numerous perioperative variables that can lead to exacerbations in PH (Ortega et al. 2013). Clinicians managing patients on chronic medical therapy for PH must emphasize the importance of medication adherence in the preoperative setting. Administration of preoperative analgesic and anxiolytic medications (opioids/benzodiazepines) can result in reduced respiratory function leading to hypoxia, hypercapnia, and respiratory acidosis which can increase PAP. Finally, the introduction of noxious stimuli including surgical stimulation and pain can elevate PAP. Variables associated with specific operations include embolization of bone/cement to the pulmonary artery during orthopedic procedures, removal of pulmonary vasculature during lung resections, systemic inflammatory response syndrome with cardiopulmonary bypass in cardiac surgery, pneumoperitoneum with carbon dioxide insufflation during laparoscopic surgery, and large fluid shifts often encountered in major surgeries.

When managing postoperative patients with PH and right ventricular failure, clinicians must be extraordinarily vigilant and familiar with the complex and vast array of etiologies. The mainstay of treatment is accurate diagnosis and reversal of the underlying culprit. Depending on the type of PH being managed and with careful consideration of all hemodynamic parameters, there are pharmacologic therapies that can be used in this population. Although often affecting systemic blood pressure inhaled prostaglandins, nitric oxide can be delivered through endotracheal tubes for rapid improvement in hemodynamics. Intravenous vasodilators such as calcium channel blockers, nitroglycerin, and sodium nitroprusside can be beneficial along with the PDE-3 antagonist milrinone. For longer-term management, PDE-5 inhibitors (tadalafil, sildenafil) have been shown to improve hemodynamics.

To successfully treat and manage PH in the postoperative patient, clinicians must have a full understanding of the complex physiology behind all groups of PH. With this knowledge and manipulation of hemodynamics, patients can have safe and successful recoveries from all types of surgical procedures.

Additional Reading Section

Physiology and Pathophysiology

Henderson WR, Griesdale DE, Walley KR, Sheel AW. Clinical review: Guyton—the role of mean circulatory filling pressure and right atrial pressure in controlling cardiac output. Crit Care. 2010b;14(6):243. https://doi.org/10.1186/cc9247.

Jaeger JM, Blank RS. Essential anatomy and physiology of the respiratory system and the pulmonary circulation. In: Slinger PD, editor. Principles and practice of anesthesia for thoracic surgery. New York: Springer; 2011b. p. 51–69.

Laffey JG, Boylan JF, Cheng DC. The systemic inflammatory response to cardiac surgery: implications for the anesthesiologist. Anesthesiology. 2002b;97(1):215–52.

Lumb AB, Nunn JF. Nunn's applied respiratory physiology. 6th ed. Edinburgh, Philadelphia: Elsevier Butterworth Heinemann; 2005.

Martin DS, Grocott MP. Oxygen therapy in critical illness: precise control of arterial oxygenation and permissive hypoxemia. Crit Care Med. 2013b;41(2):423–32. https://doi.org/10.1097/CCM.0b013e31826a44f6

West JB. Respiratory physiology: the essentials. 9th ed. Philadelphia: Wolters Kluwer Health/Lippincott Williams & Wilkins; 2012.

Mechanical Ventilation

Akoumianaki E, Maggiore SM, Valenza F, Bellani G, Jubran A, Loring SH, Loring SH, Pelosi P, Talmor D, Grasso S, Chiumello D, Guérin C, Patroniti N, Ranieri VM, Gattinoni L, Nava S, Terragni PP, Pesenti A, Tobin M, Mancebo J, Brochard L, PLUG Working Group (Acute Respiratory Failure Section of the European Society of Intensive Care Medicine). The application of esophageal pressure measurement in patients with respiratory failure. Am J Respir Crit Care Med. 2014b;189(5):520–31. https://doi.org/10.1164/rccm.201312-2193CI.

Barr J, Fraser GL, Puntillo K, Ely EW, Gelinas C, Dasta JF, Davidson JE, Devlin JW, Kress JP, Joffe AM, Coursin DB, Herr DL, Tung A, Robinson BR, Fontaine DK, Ramsay MA, Riker RR, Sessler CN, Pun B, Skrobik Y, Jaeschke R, American College of Critical Care Medicine. Clinical practice guidelines for the management of pain, agitation, and delirium in adult patients in the intensive care unit. Crit Care Med. 2013;41(1):263–306. https://doi.org/10.1097/CCM.0b013e3182783b72.

Bojar RM. Respiratory management. In: Bojar RM, editor. Manual of perioperative care in adult cardiac surgery. 5th ed. Wiley-Blackwell: Hoboken; 2011.

Buckley D, Gillham M. Invasive respiratory support. In: Sidebotham D, McKee A, Gillham M, Levy JH, editors. Cardiothoracic critical care. Philadelphia: Butterworth Heinemann Elsevier; 2007b.

Gilstrap D, MacIntyre N. Patient-ventilator interactions. Implications for clinical management. Am J Respir Crit Care Med. 2013;188(9):1058–68. https://doi.org/10.1164/rccm.201212-2214CI.

Hasan A. Understanding mechanical ventilation: a practical handbook. 2nd ed. Dordrecht: Springer; 2010.

Hess DR, Fessler HE. Respiratory controversies in the critical care setting. Should noninvasive positive-pressure ventilation be used in all forms of acute respiratory failure? Respir Care. 2007;52(5):568–78; discussion 578–581

Hill N. Noninvasive positive-pressure ventilation. In: Tobin MJ, editor. Principles and practice of mechanical ventilation. 3rd ed. New York: McGraw-Hill Medical; 2013.

Slutsky AS, Ranieri VM. Ventilator-induced lung injury. N Engl J Med. 2013;369(22):2126–36. https://doi.org/10.1056/NEJMra1208707.

Fast- Track Considerations

Myles PS, McIlroy D. Fast-track cardiac anesthesia: choice of anesthetic agents and techniques. Semin Cardiothorac Vasc Anesth. 2005b;9(1):5–16.

Zhu F, Lee A, Chee YE. Fast-track cardiac care for adult cardiac surgical patients. Cochrane Database Syst Rev. 2012;10:Cd003587. https://doi.org/10.1002/14651858.CD003587.pub2.

Pulmonary Hypertension

Minai OA, Yared JP, Kaw R, Subramaniam K, Hill NS. Perioperative risk and management in patients with pulmonary hypertension. Chest. 2013;144(1):329–40. https://doi.org/10.1378/chest.12-1752.

Simonneau G, Gatzoulis MA, Adatia I, Celermajer D, Denton C, Ghofrani A, Gomez Sanchez MA, Krishna Kumar R, Landzberg M, Machado RF, Olschewski

H, Robbins IM, Souza R, Souza R. Updated clinical classification of pulmonary hypertension. J Am Coll Cardiol. 2013;62(25 Suppl):D34–41. https://doi.org/10.1016/j.jacc.2013.10.029.

ARDS

The Acute Respiratory Distress Syndrome Network. Ventilation with lower tidal volumes as compared with traditional tidal volumes for acute lung injury and the acute respiratory distress syndrome. The Acute Respiratory Distress Syndrome Network. N Engl J Med. 2000;342(18):1301–8. https://doi.org/10.1056/NEJM200005043421801.

The ARDS Definition Task Force, Ranieri VM, Rubenfeld GD, Thompson BT, Ferguson ND, Caldwell E, Fan E, Camporota L, Slutsky AS. Acute respiratory distress syndrome: the Berlin Definition. JAMA. 2012;307(23):2526–33. https://doi.org/10.1001/jama.2012.5669.

Guerin C, Reignier J, Richard JC, Beuret P, Gacouin A, Boulain T, Mercier E, Badet M, Mercat A, Baudin O, Clavel M, Chatellier D, Jaber S, Rosselli S, Mancebo J, Sirodot M, Hilbert G, Bengler C, Richecoeur J, Gainnier M, Bayle F, Bourdin G, Leray V, Girard R, Baboi L, Ayzac L, PROSEVA Study Group. Prone positioning in severe acute respiratory distress syndrome. N Engl J Med. 2013b;368(23):2159–68. https://doi.org/10.1056/NEJMoa1214103.

Kutlu CA, Williams EA, Evans TW, Pastorino U, Goldstraw P. Acute lung injury and acute respiratory distress syndrome after pulmonary resection. Ann Thorac Surg. 2000;69(2):376–80.

Wagnetz D, De Perrot M. Postthoracotomy surgical management and complications. In: Slinger PD, editor. Principles and practice of anesthesia for thoracic surgery. New York: Springer; 2011. p. 661–73.

Pulmonary Edema

Meyer T, Krishnamani R. Acute heart failure and pulmonary edema. In: Jeremias A, Brown DL, editors. Cardiac intensive care. Philadelphia: Saunders; 2010b. p. 291–308.

Key Terms and Definitions

Acute respiratory failure: The acute inability to maintain normal blood gas partial pressures of oxygen and/or carbon dioxide. Acute respiratory failure is caused by ventilatory failure (failure to maintain normal alveolar gas partial pressure) or venous admixture due to a spectrum of ventilation and perfusion mismatch.

Acute respiratory distress syndrome (ARDS): A syndrome of lung injury from multiple etiologies characterized by hypoxemia of varying degrees quantified by the PaO2/FiO2 ratio. This syndrome develops within 1 week of a known clinical insult with new or worsening respiratory symptoms not explained by fluid overload or cardiac failure. The current definition requires bilateral opacities that are not fully explained by effusions, lobar collapse, or nodules.

Compliance: A quantification of the change in volume caused by a given change in pressure. In mechanically ventilated patients, "dynamic compliance" is measured while airflow is present and is calculated as Cdyn = Vt/(Ppeak-i-PEEP). Static compliance (Cstat = Vt/(Pplateau-i-PEEP)) is measured after inspiration has ended and when airflow has terminated. Dynamic compliance is decreased with increased airflow resistance, whereas static compliance is not affected.

Dead space: Variously refers to lung regions of pure dead space (V/Q = infinity, i.e., ventilation without perfusion), areas with high V/Q ratios, and the solution to the dead space equation.

Positive end-expiratory pressure (i-PEEP): The pressure in alveoli above atmospheric pressure at end expiration. Extrinsic i-PEEP is delivered by a mechanical ventilator and by convention is referred to as continuous positive airway pressure (CPAP) in non-intubated patients. Intrinsic or "auto"-i-PEEP occurs because of incomplete expiration due to obstructive lung pathology and "air trapping."

Pulmonary vascular resistance (PVR): The resistance that must be overcome by the right ventricle to create forward flow in the pulmonary vasculature. Calculated as the difference between mean PA pressure and LAP divided by the cardiac output.

Shunt: Variously refers to lung regions of pure shunt where $V/Q = 0$ (i.e., perfusion without ventilation), to areas of very low V/Q ratios, and to the solution to the shunt equation for venous admixture.

Spontaneous awakening trial (SAT): The first step in ventilator liberation where sedatives are stopped but active analgesics are maintained. The goal of the SAT is to determine the patient's appropriateness for a spontaneous breathing trial and usually requires that the patient opens their eyes to verbal stimulus and tolerates the interruption of sedation for a sustained period without exhibiting signs of sustained agitation, tachypnea, desaturation, dysrhythmia, or respiratory distress.

Spontaneous breathing trial (SBT): A trial of spontaneous ventilation following a successful spontaneous awakening trial to evaluate the patient's appropriateness for ventilator liberation. The intensivist should assess for the adequacy of gas exchange, respiratory mechanics, and hemodynamic stability. In addition, prior to extubation, consideration should be given to the degree of patient comfort, the predicted ability for the patient to protect their airway after extubation, and the difficulty of resecuring the airway should the patient require reintubation. An SBT should be conducted daily in intubated patients.

Transpulmonary pressure: The pressure across the lung parenchyma (also referred to as transmural pressure) and defined as alveolar pressure, the pressure inside the lung, minus pleural pressure. During mechanical ventilation the change in pleural pressure required for a given volume change is dominated by chest wall mechanics and is positive during lung inflation. Unlike pleural pressure, the change in transpulmonary pressure across the lung required for a given volume change is the same during both spontaneous and mechanical ventilation.

References

Adhikari NK, Burns KE, Friedrich JO, Granton JT, Cook DJ, Meade MO. Effect of nitric oxide on oxygenation and mortality in acute lung injury: systematic review and meta-analysis. BMJ. 2007;334:779.

Akoumianaki E, Maggiore SM, Valenza F, Bellani G, Jubran A, Loring SH, Pelosi P, Talmor D, Grasso S, Chiumello D, Guerin C, Patroniti N, Ranieri VM, Gattinoni L, Nava S, Terragni PP, Pesenti A, Tobin M, Mancebo J, Brochard L, PLUG Working Group (Acute Respiratory

Failure Section of the European Society of Intensive Care Medicine). The application of esophageal pressure measurement in patients with respiratory failure. Am J Respir Crit Care Med. 2014;189:520–31.

Allou N, Bronchard R, Guglielminotti J, Dilly MP, Provenchere S, Lucet JC, Laouenan C, Montravers P. Risk factors for postoperative pneumonia after cardiac surgery and development of a preoperative risk score*. Crit Care Med. 2014;42:1150–6.

Amato MB, Barbas CS, Medeiros DM, Magaldi RB, Schettino GP, Lorenzi-Filho G, Kairalla RA, Deheinzelin D, Munoz C, Oliveira R, Takagaki TY, Carvalho CR. Effect of a protective-ventilation strategy on mortality in the acute respiratory distress syndrome. N Engl J Med. 1998;338:347–54.

Amato MB, Meade MO, Slutsky AS, Brochard L, Costa EL, Schoenfeld DA, Stewart TE, Briel M, Talmor D, Mercat A, Richard JC, Carvalho CR, Brower RG. Driving pressure and survival in the acute respiratory distress syndrome. N Engl J Med. 2015;372:747–55.

Arozullah AM, Daley J, Henderson WG, Khuri SF. Multifactorial risk index for predicting postoperative respiratory failure in men after major noncardiac surgery. The National Veterans Administration Surgical Quality Improvement Program. Ann Surg. 2000;232:242–53.

Bailey ML, Richter SM, Mullany DV, Tesar PJ, Fraser JF. Risk factors and survival in patients with respiratory failure after cardiac operations. Ann Thorac Surg. 2011;92:1573–9.

Berlin D. Hemodynamic consequences of auto-PEEP. J Intensive Care Med. 2014;29:81–6.

Berrizbeitia LD, Tessler S, Jacobowitz IJ, Kaplan P, Budzilowicz L, Cunningham JN. Effect of sternotomy and coronary bypass surgery on postoperative pulmonary mechanics. Comparison of internal mammary and saphenous vein bypass grafts. Chest. 1989;96:873–6.

Bevan DR. Recovery from neuromuscular block and its assessment. Anesth Analg. 2000;90:S7–13.

Boles JM, Bion J, Connors A, Herridge M, Marsh B, Melot C, Pearl R, Silverman H, Stanchina M, Vieillard-Baron A, Welte T. Weaning from mechanical ventilation. Eur Respir J. 2007;29:1033–56.

Bonten MJ, Bergmans DC, Stobberingh EE, van der Geest S, De Leeuw PW, van Tiel FH, Gaillard CA. Implementation of bronchoscopic techniques in the diagnosis of ventilator-associated pneumonia to reduce antibiotic use. Am J Respir Crit Care Med. 1997;156:1820–4.

Braun SR, Birnbaum ML, Chopra PS. Pre- and postoperative pulmonary function abnormalities in coronary artery revascularization surgery. Chest. 1978;73:316–20.

Briel M, Meade M, Mercat A, Brower RG, Talmor D, Walter SD, Slutsky AS, Pullenayegum E, Zhou Q, Cook D, Brochard L, Richard JC, Lamontagne F, Bhatnagar N, Stewart TE, Guyatt G. Higher vs lower positive end-expiratory pressure in patients with acute lung injury and acute respiratory distress syndrome: systematic review and meta-analysis. JAMA. 2010;303:865–73.

Brochard L, Isabey D, Piquet J, Amaro P, Mancebo J, Messadi AA, Brun-Buisson C, Rauss A, Lemaire F, Harf A. Reversal of acute exacerbations of chronic obstructive lung disease by inspiratory assistance with a face mask. N Engl J Med. 1990;323:1523–30.

Bronicki RA, Anas NG. Cardiopulmonary interaction. Pediatr Crit Care Med. 2009;10(3):p316. https://journals.lww.com/pccmjournal/Abstract/2009/05000/Cardiopulmonary_interaction.6.aspx.

Buckley D, Gillham M. Invasive respiratory support. In: Cardiothoracic critical care. Philadelphia: Butterworth Heinemann Elsevier; 2007, p. 420.

Canver CC, Chanda J. Intraoperative and postoperative risk factors for respiratory failure after coronary bypass. Ann Thorac Surg. 2003;75:853–7; discussion 857–858.

Chastre J, Fagon JY. Ventilator-associated pneumonia. Am J Respir Crit Care Med. 2002;165:867–903.

Cheng DC, Karski J, Peniston C, Asokumar B, Raveendran G, Carroll J, Nierenberg H, Roger S, Mickle D, Tong J, Zelovitsky J, David T, Sandler A. Morbidity outcome in early versus conventional tracheal extubation after coronary artery bypass grafting: a prospective randomized controlled trial. J Thorac Cardiovasc Surg. 1996a;112:755–64.

Cheng DC, Karski J, Peniston C, Raveendran G, Asokumar B, Carroll J, David T, Sandler A. Early tracheal extubation after coronary artery bypass graft surgery reduces costs and improves resource use. A prospective, randomized, controlled trial. Anesthesiology. 1996b;85:1300–10.

Christenson JT, Aeberhard JM, Badel P, Pepcak F, Maurice J, Simonet F, Velebit V, Schmuziger M. Adult respiratory distress syndrome after cardiac surgery. Cardiovasc Surg. 1996;4:15–21.

Cook DJ, Walter SD, Cook RJ, Griffith LE, Guyatt GH, Leasa D, Jaeschke RZ, Brun-Buisson C. Incidence of and risk factors for ventilator-associated pneumonia in critically ill patients. Ann Intern Med. 1998;129:433–40.

Epstein SK. Weaning from ventilatory support. Curr Opin Crit Care. 2009;15:36–43.

Esteban A, Frutos-Vivar F, Ferguson ND, Arabi Y, Apezteguia C, Gonzalez M, Epstein SK, Hill NS, Nava S, Soares MA, D'Empaire G, Alia I, Anzueto A. Noninvasive positive-pressure ventilation for respiratory failure after extubation. N Engl J Med. 2004;350:2452–60.

Esteban A, Frutos F, Tobin MJ, Alia I, Solsona JF, Valverdu I, Fernandez R, de la Cal MA, Benito S, Tomas R, et al. A comparison of four methods of weaning patients from mechanical ventilation. Spanish Lung Failure Collaborative Group. N Engl J Med. 1995;332:345–50.

Fagon JY, Chastre J, Hance AJ, Domart Y, Trouillet JL, Gibert C. Evaluation of clinical judgment in the identification and treatment of nosocomial pneumonia in ventilated patients. Chest. 1993;103:547–53.

Fagon JY, Chastre J, Wolff M, Gervais C, Parer-Aubas S, Stephan F, Similowski T, Mercat A, Diehl JL, Sollet JP, Tenaillon A. Invasive and noninvasive strategies for management of suspected ventilator-associated pneumonia. A randomized trial. Ann Intern Med. 2000;132:621–30.

Farias JA, Retta A, Alia I, Olazarri F, Esteban A, Golubicki A, Allende D, Maliarchuk O, Peltzer C, Ratto ME, Zalazar R, Garea M, Moreno EG. A comparison of two methods to perform a breathing trial before extubation in pediatric intensive care patients. Intensive Care Med. 2001;27:1649–54.

Ferguson ND, Slutsky AS, Meade MO. High-frequency oscillation for ARDS. N Engl J Med. 2013;368:2233–4.

Fernandez-Perez ER, Keegan MT, Brown DR, Hubmayr RD, Gajic O. Intraoperative tidal volume as a risk factor for respiratory failure after pneumonectomy. Anesthesiology. 2006;105:14–8.

Filsoufi F, Rahmanian PB, Castillo JG, Chikwe J, Adams DH. Predictors and early and late outcomes of respiratory failure in contemporary cardiac surgery. Chest. 2008;133:713–21.

Force ADT, Ranieri VM, Rubenfeld GD, Thompson BT, Ferguson ND, Caldwell E, Fan E, Camporota L, Slutsky AS. Acute respiratory distress syndrome: the Berlin Definition. JAMA. 2012;307:2526–33.

Ford GT, Whitelaw WA, Rosenal TW, Cruse PJ, Guenter CA. Diaphragm function after upper abdominal surgery in humans. Am Rev Respir Dis. 1983;127:431–6.

Frat JP, Thille AW, Mercat A, Girault C, Ragot S, Perbet S, Prat G, Boulain T, Morawiec E, Cottereau A, Devaquet J, Nseir S, Razazi K, Mira JP, Argaud L, Chakarian JC, Ricard JD, Wittebole X, Chevalier S, Herbland A, Fartoukh M, Constantin JM, Tonnelier JM, Pierrot M, Mathonnet A, Beduneau G, Deletage-Metreau C, Richard JC, Brochard L, Robert R, for the FLORALI Study Group and the REVA Network. High-flow oxygen through nasal cannula in acute hypoxemic respiratory failure. N Engl J Med. 2015;372:2185–96.

Friedrich A. Management of common complications following thoracic surgery. In: Hartigan PM, editor. Practical handbook of thoracic anesthesia. New York: Springer; 2012. p. 291–310.

Futier E, Constantin JM, Paugam-Burtz C, Pascal J, Eurin M, Neuschwander A, Marret E, Beaussier M, Gutton C, Lefrant JY, Allaouchiche B, Verzilli D, Leone M, De Jong A, Bazin JE, Pereira B, Jaber S, IMPROVE Study Group. A trial of intraoperative low-tidal-volume ventilation in abdominal surgery. N Engl J Med. 2013;369:428–37.

Gass GD, Olsen GN. Preoperative pulmonary function testing to predict postoperative morbidity and mortality. Chest. 1986;89:127–35.

Gattinoni L, Tognoni G, Pesenti A, Taccone P, Mascheroni D, Labarta V, Malacrida R, Di Giulio P, Fumagalli R, Pelosi P, Brazzi L, Latini R, Prone-Supine Study Group. Effect of prone positioning on the survival of patients with acute respiratory failure. N Engl J Med. 2001;345:568–73.

Girard TD, Kress JP, Fuchs BD, Thomason JW, Schweickert WD, Pun BT, Taichman DB, Dunn JG, Pohlman AS, Kinniry PA, Jackson JC, Canonico AE, Light RW, Shintani AK, Thompson JL, Gordon SM, Hall JB, Dittus RS, Bernard GR, Ely EW. Efficacy and safety of a paired sedation and ventilator weaning protocol for mechanically ventilated patients in intensive care (Awakening and Breathing Controlled trial): a randomised controlled trial. Lancet. 2008;371:126–34.

Gladwin MT, Pierson DJ. Mechanical ventilation of the patient with severe chronic obstructive pulmonary disease. Intensive Care Med. 1998;24:898–910.

Glenny RW, Lamm WJ, Bernard SL, An D, Chornuk M, Pool SL, Wagner WW Jr, Hlastala MP, Robertson HT. Selected contribution: redistribution of pulmonary perfusion during weightlessness and increased gravity. J Appl Physiol (1985). 2000;89:1239–48.

Guerin C, Reignier J, Richard JC, Beuret P, Gacouin A, Boulain T, Mercier E, Badet M, Mercat A, Baudin O, Clavel M, Chatellier D, Jaber S, Rosselli S, Mancebo J, Sirodot M, Hilbert G, Bengler C, Richecoeur J, Gainnier M, Bayle F, Bourdin G, Leray V, Girard R, Baboi L, Ayzac L, PROSEVA Study Group. Prone positioning in severe acute respiratory distress syndrome. N Engl J Med. 2013;368:2159–68.

Gupta H, Ramanan B, Gupta PK, Fang X, Polich A, Modrykamien A, Schuller D, Morrow LE. Impact of COPD on postoperative outcomes: results from a national database. Chest. 2013;143:1599–606.

Haddad F, Couture P, Tousignant C, Denault AY. The right ventricle in cardiac surgery, a perioperative perspective: II. Pathophysiology, clinical importance, and management. Anesth Analg. 2009;108:422–33.

Hakim TS, Lisbona R, Dean GW. Gravity-independent inequality in pulmonary blood flow in humans. J Appl Physiol (1985). 1987;63:1114–21.

Haynes D, Baumann MH. Management of pneumothorax. Semin Respir Crit Care Med. 2010;31:769–80.

Heidecker J, Sahn SA. The spectrum of pleural effusions after coronary artery bypass grafting surgery. Clin Chest Med. 2006;27:267–83.

Henderson WR, Griesdale DE, Walley KR, Sheel AW. Clinical review: Guyton—the role of mean circulatory filling pressure and right atrial pressure in controlling cardiac output. Crit Care. 2010;14:243.

Heyland DK, Cook DJ, Griffith L, Keenan SP, Brun-Buisson C. The attributable morbidity and mortality of ventilator-associated pneumonia in the critically ill patient. The Canadian Critical Trials Group. Am J Respir Crit Care Med. 1999;159:1249–56.

Hill NS, Farber HW. 2008. Pulmonary hypertension. In: Hargett CW TV, editor. Contemporary cardiology. Totowa, NJ: Humana Press. p 1 online resource (xv, 444 p.).

Hill NS, Roberts KR, Preston IR. Postoperative pulmonary hypertension: etiology and treatment of a dangerous complication. Respir Care. 2009;54:958–68.

Hortal J, Giannella M, Perez MJ, Barrio JM, Desco M, Bouza E, Munoz P. Incidence and risk factors for ventilator-associated pneumonia after major heart surgery. Intensive Care Med. 2009;35:1518–25.

Inouye SK, Bogardus ST Jr, Charpentier PA, Leo-Summers L, Acampora D, Holford TR, Cooney LM Jr. A multicomponent intervention to prevent delirium in hospitalized older patients. N Engl J Med. 1999;340:669–76.

Jaeger JM, Blank RS. Essential anatomy and physiology of the respiratory system and the pulmonary circulation. In: Slinger PD, editor. Principles and practice of anesthesia for thoracic surgery. New York: Springer; 2011. p. 51–69.

Jain U, Rao TL, Kumar P, Kleinman BS, Belusko RJ, Kanuri DP, Blakeman BM, Bakhos M, Wallis DE. Radiographic pulmonary abnormalities after different types of cardiac surgery. J Cardiothorac Vasc Anesth. 1991;5:592–5.

Jeremias A, Brown DL. Cardiac intensive care. 2nd ed. Philadelphia, PA: Saunders/Elsevier; 2010.

Johnson D, Thomson D, Mycyk T, Burbridge B, Mayers I. Respiratory outcomes with early extubation after coronary artery bypass surgery. J Cardiothorac Vasc Anesth. 1997;11:474–80.

Jones DP, Byrne P, Morgan C, Fraser I, Hyland R. Positive end-expiratory pressure vs T-piece. Extubation after mechanical ventilation. Chest. 1991;100:1655–9.

Karthik S, Grayson AD, McCarron EE, Pullan DM, Desmond MJ. Reexploration for bleeding after coronary artery bypass surgery: risk factors, outcomes, and the effect of time delay. Ann Thorac Surg. 2004;78:527–34; discussion 534

Keenan SP, Powers C, McCormack DG, Block G. Noninvasive positive-pressure ventilation for postextubation respiratory distress: a randomized controlled trial. JAMA. 2002;287:3238–44.

Kelly AM, Weldon D, Tsang AY, Graham CA. Comparison between two methods for estimating pneumothorax size from chest X-rays. Respir Med. 2006;100:1356–9.

Kilgannon JH, Jones AE, Parrillo JE, Dellinger RP, Milcarek B, Hunter K, Shapiro NI, Trzeciak S, Emergency Medicine Shock Research Network (EMShockNet) Investigators. Relationship between supranormal oxygen tension and outcome after resuscitation from cardiac arrest. Circulation. 2011;123:2717–22.

Kilgannon JH, Jones AE, Shapiro NI, Angelos MG, Milcarek B, Hunter K, Parrillo JE, Trzeciak S, Emergency Medicine Shock Research Network (EMShockNet) Investigators. Association between arterial hyperoxia following resuscitation from cardiac arrest and in-hospital mortality. JAMA. 2010;303:2165–71.

Kollef MH. The prevention of ventilator-associated pneumonia. N Engl J Med. 1999;340:627–34.

Kopman AF, Yee PS, Neuman GG. Relationship of the train-of-four fade ratio to clinical signs and symptoms of residual paralysis in awake volunteers. Anesthesiology. 1997;86:765–71.

Kress JP, Gehlbach B, Lacy M, Pliskin N, Pohlman AS, Hall JB. The long-term psychological effects of daily sedative interruption on critically ill patients. Am J Respir Crit Care Med. 2003;168:1457–61.

Kress JP, Pohlman AS, O'Connor MF, Hall JB. Daily interruption of sedative infusions in critically ill patients undergoing mechanical ventilation. N Engl J Med. 2000;342:1471–7.

Kroenke K, Lawrence VA, Theroux JF, Tuley MR, Hilsenbeck S. Postoperative complications after thoracic and major abdominal surgery in patients with and without obstructive lung disease. Chest. 1993;104:1445–51.

Laffey JG, Boylan JF, Cheng DC. The systemic inflammatory response to cardiac surgery: implications for the anesthesiologist. Anesthesiology. 2002;97:215–52.

Lellouche F, Dionne S, Simard S, Bussieres J, Dagenais F. High tidal volumes in mechanically ventilated patients increase organ dysfunction after cardiac surgery. Anesthesiology. 2012;116:1072–82.

Leung P, Jubran A, Tobin MJ. Comparison of assisted ventilator modes on triggering, patient effort, and dyspnea. Am J Respir Crit Care Med. 1997;155:1940–8.

Light RW. Clinical practice. Pleural effusion. N Engl J Med. 2002;346:1971–7.

Lightowler JV, Wedzicha JA, Elliott MW, Ram FS. Non-invasive positive pressure ventilation to treat respiratory failure resulting from exacerbations of chronic obstructive pulmonary disease: cochrane systematic review and meta-analysis. BMJ. 2003;326:185.

London MJ, Shroyer AL, Jernigan V, Fullerton DA, Wilcox D, Baltz J, Brown JM, MaWhinney S, Hammermeister KE, Grover FL. Fast-track cardiac surgery in a Department of Veterans Affairs patient population. Ann Thorac Surg. 1997;64:134–41.

MacIntyre NR, Cook DJ, Ely EW Jr, Epstein SK, Fink JB, Heffner JE, Hess D, Hubmayer RD, Scheinhorn DJ, American College of Chest Physicians; American Association for Respiratory Care; American College of Critical Care Medicine. Evidence-based guidelines for weaning and discontinuing ventilatory support: a collective task force facilitated by the American College of Chest Physicians; the American Association for Respiratory Care; and the American College of Critical Care Medicine. Chest. 2001;120:375S–95S.

Marhong JD, Munshi L, Detsky M, Telesnicki T, Fan E. Mechanical ventilation during extracorporeal life support (ECLS): a systematic review. Intensive Care Med. 2015;41:994–1003.

Marhong JD, Telesnicki T, Munshi L, Del Sorbo L, Detsky M, Fan E. Mechanical ventilation during extracorporeal membrane oxygenation. An international survey. Ann Am Thorac Soc. 2014;11:956–61.

Marini JJ, Capps JS, Culver BH. The inspiratory work of breathing during assisted mechanical ventilation. Chest. 1985;87:612–8.

Martin DS, Grocott MP. Oxygen therapy in critical illness: precise control of arterial oxygenation and permissive hypoxemia. Crit Care Med. 2013;41:423–32.

Meade M, Guyatt G, Cook D, Griffith L, Sinuff T, Kergl C, Mancebo J, Esteban A, Epstein S. Predicting success in weaning from mechanical ventilation. Chest. 2001;120:400S–24S.

Meyer T, Krishnamani R. "Acute heart failure and pulmonary edema" in cardiac intensive care. 2nd ed. Philadelphia, PA: Saunders/Elsevier; 2010.

Mikkelsen ME, Christie JD, Lanken PN, Biester RC, Thompson BT, Bellamy SL, Localio AR, Demissie E, Hopkins RO, Angus DC. The adult respiratory distress syndrome cognitive outcomes study: long-term neuropsychological function in survivors of acute lung injury. Am J Respir Crit Care Med. 2012;185:1307–15.

Murphy GS, Szokol JW, Marymont JH, Franklin M, Avram MJ, Vender JS. Residual paralysis at the time of tracheal extubation. Anesth Analg. 2005;100:1840–5.

Myles PS, McIlroy D. Fast-track cardiac anesthesia: choice of anesthetic agents and techniques. Semin Cardiothorac Vasc Anesth. 2005;9:5–16.

Neto AS, Schmidt M, Azevedo L, Bein T, Brochard L, Beutel G, Combes A, Costa E, Hodgson C, Lindskov C, Lubnow M, Lueck C, Michaels A, Paiva JA, Park M, Pesenti A, Pham T, Quintel M, Marco Ranieri V, Ried M, Roncon-Albuquerque R, Slutsky A, Takeda S, Terragni P, Vejen M, Weber-Carstens S, Welte T, Gama de Abreu M, Pelosi P, Schultz M, Network RR, Investigators PN. Associations between ventilator settings during extracorporeal membrane oxygenation for refractory hypoxemia and outcome in patients with acute respiratory distress syndrome: a pooled individual patient data analysis. Intensive Care Med. 2016;42:1672–84.

Ng CS, Wan S, Yim AP, Arifi AA. Pulmonary dysfunction after cardiac surgery. Chest. 2002;121:1269–77.

Noppen M, De Keukeleire T. Pneumothorax. Respiration. 2008;76:121–7.

Nurok M, Topulos GP. Practical Handbook of Thoracic Anesthesia by Philip M. Hartigan (ed). Respiratory Physiology. 2012a. p. 20.

Nurok M, Topulos GP. Practical Handbook of Thoracic Anesthesia by Philip M. Hartigan (ed). Respiratory Physiology. 2012b. p. 33.

Ortega RC, et al. Intraoperative management of patients with pulmonary hypertension advances in pulmonary hypertension. Adv Pulm Hypertens. 2013;12:18–23.

Papazian L, Forel JM, Gacouin A, Penot-Ragon C, Perrin G, Loundou A, Jaber S, Arnal JM, Perez D, Seghboyan JM, Constantin JM, Courant P, Lefrant JY, Guerin C, Prat G, Morange S, Roch A, Investigators AS. Neuromuscular blockers in early acute respiratory distress syndrome. N Engl J Med. 2010;363:1107–16.

Peek GJ, Mugford M, Tiruvoipati R, Wilson A, Allen E, Thalanany MM, Hibbert CL, Truesdale A, Clemens F, Cooper N, Firmin RK, Elbourne D, CESAR trial collaboration. Efficacy and economic assessment of conventional ventilatory support versus extracorporeal membrane oxygenation for severe adult respiratory failure (CESAR): a multicentre randomised controlled trial. Lancet. 2009;374:1351–63.

Pham T, Combes A, Roze H, Chevret S, Mercat A, Roch A, Mourvillier B, Ara-Somohano C, Bastien O, Zogheib E, Clavel M, Constan A, Marie Richard JC, Brun-Buisson C, Brochard L, Network RR. Extracorporeal membrane oxygenation for pandemic influenza A(H1N1)-induced acute respiratory distress syndrome: a cohort study and propensity-matched analysis. Am J Respir Crit Care Med. 2013;187:276–85.

Polese G, Lubli P, Mazzucco A, Luzzani A, Rossi A. Effects of open heart surgery on respiratory mechanics. Intensive Care Med. 1999;25:1092–9.

Rajakaruna C, Rogers CA, Angelini GD, Ascione R. Risk factors for and economic implications of prolonged ventilation after cardiac surgery. J Thorac Cardiovasc Surg. 2005;130:1270–7.

Ram FS, Picot J, Lightowler J, Wedzicha JA. Non-invasive positive pressure ventilation for treatment of respiratory failure due to exacerbations of chronic obstructive pulmonary disease. Cochrane Database Syst Rev. 2004;1:CD004104.

Ramakrishna G, Sprung J, Ravi BS, Chandrasekaran K, McGoon MD. Impact of pulmonary hypertension on the outcomes of noncardiac surgery: predictors of perioperative morbidity and mortality. J Am Coll Cardiol. 2005;45:1691–9.

Ranucci M, Bozzetti G, Ditta A, Cotza M, Carboni G, Ballotta A. Surgical reexploration after cardiac operations: why a worse outcome? Ann Thorac Surg. 2008;86:1557–62.

Raoof S, Baumann MH, Critical Care Societies C. An official multi-society statement: ventilator-associated events: the new definition. Crit Care Med. 2014;42:228–9.

Roques F, Nashef SA, Michel P, Gauducheau E, de Vincentiis C, Baudet E, Cortina J, David M, Faichney A, Gabrielle F, Gams E, Harjula A, Jones MT, Pintor PP, Salamon R, Thulin L. Risk factors and outcome in European cardiac surgery: analysis of the EuroSCORE multinational database of 19030 patients. Eur J Cardiothorac Surg. 1999;15:816–22; discussion 822–813

Rossi A, Polese G, Brandi G, Conti G. Intrinsic positive end-expiratory pressure (PEEPi). Intensive Care Med. 1995;21:522–36.

Sanchez-Nieto JM, Torres A, Garcia-Cordoba F, El-Ebiary M, Carrillo A, Ruiz J, Nunez ML, Niederman M. Impact of invasive and noninvasive quantitative culture sampling on outcome of ventilator-associated pneumonia: a pilot study. Am J Respir Crit Care Med. 1998;157:371–6.

Sassoon CS, Caiozzo VJ, Manka A, Sieck GC. Altered diaphragm contractile properties with controlled mechanical ventilation. J Appl Physiol (1985). 2002;92:2585–95.

Schweickert WD, Gehlbach BK, Pohlman AS, Hall JB, Kress JP. Daily interruption of sedative infusions and complications of critical illness in mechanically ventilated patients. Crit Care Med. 2004;32:1272–6.

Schweickert WD, Pohlman MC, Pohlman AS, Nigos C, Pawlik AJ, Esbrook CL, Spears L, Miller M, Franczyk M, Deprizio D, Schmidt GA, Bowman A, Barr R, McCallister KE, Hall JB, Kress JP. Early physical and occupational therapy in mechanically ventilated, critically ill patients: a randomised controlled trial. Lancet. 2009;373:1874–82.

Shapiro M, Wilson RK, Casar G, Bloom K, Teague RB. Work of breathing through different sized endotracheal tubes. Crit Care Med. 1986;14:1028–31.

Shorr AF, Sherner JH, Jackson WL, Kollef MH. Invasive approaches to the diagnosis of ventilator-associated pneumonia: a meta-analysis. Crit Care Med. 2005;33:46–53.

Sole Violan J, Fernandez JA, Benitez AB, Cardenosa Cendrero JA, Rodriguez de Castro F. Impact of quantitative invasive diagnostic techniques in the management and outcome of mechanically ventilated patients with suspected pneumonia. Crit Care Med. 2000;28:2737–41.

Stephens RS, Shah AS, Whitman GJR. Lung injury and acute respiratory distress syndrome after cardiac surgery. Ann Thorac Surg. 2013;95:1122–9.

Strom T, Martinussen T, Toft P. A protocol of no sedation for critically ill patients receiving mechanical ventilation: a randomised trial. Lancet. 2010;375:475–80.

Sundar S, Novack V, Jervis K, Bender SP, Lerner A, Panzica P, Mahmood F, Malhotra A, Talmor D. Influence of low tidal volume ventilation on time to extubation in cardiac surgical patients. Anesthesiology. 2011;114:1102–10.

Taggart DP, el-Fiky M, Carter R, Bowman A, Wheatley DJ. Respiratory dysfunction after uncomplicated cardiopulmonary bypass. Ann Thorac Surg. 1993;56:1123–8.

Talmor D, Sarge T, Malhotra A, O'Donnell CR, Ritz R, Lisbon A, Novack V, Loring SH. Mechanical ventilation guided by esophageal pressure in acute lung injury. N Engl J Med. 2008;359:2095–104.

Torres A, el-Ebiary M, Padro L, Gonzalez J, de la Bellacasa JP, Ramirez J, Xaubet A, Ferrer M, Rodriguez-Roisin R. Validation of different techniques for the diagnosis of ventilator-associated pneumonia. Comparison with immediate postmortem pulmonary biopsy. Am J Respir Crit Care Med. 1994;149:324–31.

Treggiari MM, Romand JA, Yanez ND, Deem SA, Goldberg J, Hudson L, Heidegger CP, Weiss NS. Randomized trial of light versus deep sedation on mental health after critical illness. Crit Care Med. 2009;37:2527–34.

van Noord JA, de Munck DR, Bantje TA, Hop WC, Akveld ML, Bommer AM. Long-term treatment of chronic obstructive pulmonary disease with salmeterol and the additive effect of ipratropium. Eur Respir J. 2000;15:878–85.

Varpula T, Jousela I, Niemi R, Takkunen O, Pettila V. Combined effects of prone positioning and airway pressure release ventilation on gas exchange in patients with acute lung injury. Acta Anaesthesiol Scand. 2003;47:516–24.

Varpula T, Valta P, Niemi R, Takkunen O, Hynynen M, Pettila VV. Airway pressure release ventilation as a primary ventilatory mode in acute respiratory distress syndrome. Acta Anaesthesiol Scand. 2004;48:722–31.

Vassilakopoulos T, Petrof BJ. Ventilator-induced diaphragmatic dysfunction. Am J Respir Crit Care Med. 2004;169:336–41.
Vital FM, Saconato H, Ladeira MT, Sen A, Hawkes CA, Soares B, Burns KE, Atallah AN. Non-invasive positive pressure ventilation (CPAP or bilevel NPPV) for cardiogenic pulmonary edema. Cochrane Database Syst Rev. 2008;1:CD005351.
Ware LB, Matthay MA. The acute respiratory distress syndrome. N Engl J Med. 2000;342:1334–49.
Warner MA, Offord KP, Warner ME, Lennon RL, Conover MA, Jansson-Schumacher U. Role of preoperative cessation of smoking and other factors in postoperative pulmonary complications: a blinded prospective study of coronary artery bypass patients. Mayo Clin Proc. 1989;64:609–16.
West JB. Respiratory physiology: the essentials. 9th ed. Philadelphia: Wolters Kluwer Health/Lippincott Williams & Wilkins; 2012a.
West JB. Respiratory physiology—the essentials. 6th ed. Philadelphia: Lippincott Williams & Wilkins; 2012b.
Wilcox P, Baile EM, Hards J, et al. Phrenic nerve function and its relationship to atelectasis after coronary artery bypass grafting. Thorax. 1985;40:293–9.
Williams-Russo P, Charlson ME, MacKenzie CR, Gold JP, Shires GT. Predicting postoperative pulmonary complications. Is it a real problem? Arch Intern Med. 1992;152:1209–13.
Wrigge H, Uhlig U, Baumgarten G, Menzenbach J, Zinserling J, Ernst M, Dromann D, Welz A, Uhlig S, Putensen C. Mechanical ventilation strategies and inflammatory responses to cardiac surgery: a prospective randomized clinical trial. Intensive Care Med. 2005;31:1379–87.
Yang KL, Tobin MJ. A prospective study of indexes predicting the outcome of trials of weaning from mechanical ventilation. N Engl J Med. 1991;324:1445–50.
Yarmus L, Feller-Kopman D. Pneumothorax in the critically ill patient. Chest. 2012;141:1098–105.
Zupancich E, Paparella D, Turani F, Munch C, Rossi A, Massaccesi S, Ranieri VM. Mechanical ventilation affects inflammatory mediators in patients undergoing cardiopulmonary bypass for cardiac surgery: a randomized clinical trial. J Thorac Cardiovasc Surg. 2005;130:378–83.

Central Nervous System Care in Postoperative Adult Cardiac Surgery

12

Ali Dabbagh

Abstract

CNS dysfunction after cardiac surgery is considered among the most important etiologies for morbidities and mortalities after cardiac surgery and patients undergoing cardiac surgery might be affected by unwanted CNS complications; this is a well-established finding in many studies.

Although postoperative period-related factors constitute only about one-fifth (20%) of etiologies of postoperative CNS complications of cardiac surgery, the CNS complications are not usually seen intraoperatively; those CNS complications seen first during the hospitalization period are usually encountered in ICU.

Two main classifications are used for categorizing postoperative CNS injuries in cardiac surgery patients. The first is mainly a clinical classification (including type I and type II disorders), while the second is a time-based classification (including early and late diseases).

Advanced age, high preoperative creatinine level, prior neurological event, prolonged cardiopulmonary bypass time, and female gender are considered as early risk factors, while prior neurologic event, diabetes mellitus, unstable angina, previous cerebral vascular disease, need for inotropic support, and postoperative atrial fibrillation are considered as delayed risk factors. Aortic atherosclerosis is considered as both an acute and a chronic risk factor. The underlying mechanisms are classified into five main classes: patient-related etiologies, intraoperative surgical etiologies, intraoperative anesthetic etiologies, intraoperative extracorporeal circulation (ECC) etiologies, and postoperative period-related etiologies; a number of potential etiologies have been proposed in each class. Prevention strategies include pharmacologic neuroprotection and CPB-related techniques. Novel and older technologies are used to improve the CNS outcome.

A. Dabbagh, M.D.
Cardiac Anesthesiology Department, Anesthesiology Research Center, Faculty of Medicine, Shahid Beheshti University of Medical Sciences, Tehran, Iran
e-mail: alidabagh@sbmu.ac.ir

A. Dabbagh et al. (eds.), *Postoperative Critical Care for Adult Cardiac Surgical Patients*, https://doi.org/10.1007/978-3-319-75747-6_12

Keywords
Classification and mechanisms of CNS dysfunction after cardiac surgery General considerations of CNS dysfunction after cardiac surgery · Classification of CNS injuries · Type I and type II injuries · Time-based classification of postoperative CNS injuries · Risk factors of CNS injuries · Mechanisms and potential etiologies of CNS injuries · Prevention strategies · Pharmacologic neuroprotection · CPB-related equipment · Neurologic monitoring

12.1 Classification and Mechanisms of CNS Dysfunction After Cardiac Surgery

12.1.1 General Considerations of CNS Dysfunction After Cardiac Surgery

CNS dysfunction after cardiac surgery is considered among the most important etiologies for morbidities and mortalities after cardiac surgery and patients undergoing cardiac surgery might be affected by unwanted CNS complications; this is a well-established finding in many studies. Postoperative cerebral dysfunction after cardiac surgery is one of the most devastating complications and the least desired morbidity after cardiac surgery; it would affect not only the short-term clinical outcome adversely, but also the long-term quality of life; in such a way that "*neurocognitive decline after cardiac surgery might be seen in up to three quarters of patients at hospital discharge and persist in a third of patients up to 6 months after surgery ... and also, are associated with decreased quality of life.*" As the population of elderly undergoing cardiac surgery increases, these complications are seen more frequently. Although postoperative period-related factors constitute only about one-fifth (20%) of etiologies of postoperative CNS complications of cardiac surgery, the CNS complications are not usually seen intraoperatively; instead, unpredicted CNS complications during hospitalization are often experienced in ICU (Roach et al. 1996; Hogue et al. 1999; Newman et al. 2001; Sato et al. 2002; Hogue et al. 2008a, b, c; Mathew et al. 2009; Lombard and Mathew 2010; Hedberg et al. 2011; Bartels et al. 2013; Mashour et al. 2013; Fink et al. 2015; Biancari et al. 2016; Brascia et al. 2017a, b; Karhausen et al. 2017; Kinnunen et al. 2017; Dabbagh 2014a, b; Dabbagh and Ramsay 2017a, b).

12.1.2 Classification of CNS Injuries After Cardiac Surgery

Two main classifications are used for categorizing postoperative CNS injuries in cardiac surgery patients. The first is mainly a clinical classification, while the second is a time-based classification.

12.1.2.1 Type I and Type II Injuries

Cerebral complications after cardiac surgery have been categorized into type I and type II injuries (Roach et al. 1996; Newman et al. 2001; Carrascal et al. 2005; Smith 2006; Marasco et al. 2008; Liu et al. 2009; Lombard and Mathew 2010; Fink et al. 2015).

Type I injuries: These usually comprise neurologic deficits. Though they do not have a high incidence, the severity and poor outcome could never be neglected. Frank stroke has the most serious outcome; its incidence is about 1% following CABG. Type I injuries include the following:

- Fatal and nonfatal stroke (motor, sensory, or language deficit or a combination of them)
- Hypoxic encephalopathy
- Focal neurologic injury
- TIA (transient ischemic attack)
- Coma at discharge
- Stupor at discharge

Type I injury could happen in 1–4% of closed-chamber and 8–9% of open-chamber cardiac surgeries.

Type II injuries: Neurologic disorders other than type I which are also more common than the previous class of disorders include the following:

- New deterioration of intellectual function
- Confusion
- Agitation
- Memory deficit
- Seizures without evidence of focal injury
- Disorientation
- Problem-solving ability deficit
- Attention and concentration impairment
- Language problems
- Psychomotor performance problems
- Learning and memory problems
- Mental processing speed deficit
- Intelligence deficit
- Usually, delirium is among the most common acute presentations of CNS disorders (more discussion about postoperative delirium and its management is presented in the next paragraphs of this chapter)

Type II injury could happen in over 50% of the patients at the time of discharge from hospital and about 30% of the patients six times after operation.

12.1.2.2 Time-Based Classification of Postoperative CNS Injuries

Another classification involves the time interval after surgery, based on the fact that "early and delayed stroke differ in their related risk factors." Based on Karhausen et al. definition, early stroke occurs during 0–1 postoperative days of surgery; however, stroke during ≥2 postoperative days is categorized under delayed stroke; having relatively different etiologic factors, early strokes are primarily due to one of the following items (Karhausen et al. 2017):

- Particulate and gaseous embolism during surgery
- Intraoperative hemodynamic perturbations
- Both of the above

However, late strokes are mainly the ultimate outcome of "prothrombotic postoperative state" which are promoted by the following etiologies during and after cardiac surgery:

- Humoral and cellular inflammatory responses
- Platelet activation

The risk factors for early and late CNS disorders are discussed in the next section. Early postoperative cognitive dysfunction is an important predictor of "late postoperative cognitive dysfunction" 5 years later after surgery. It has been mentioned that early stroke has right cerebral hemisphere predominance rather than the left hemisphere, while delayed stroke involves a uniform distribution. About one-fifth (20%) of postoperative CNS complications of cardiac surgery occur due to postoperative events, while 80% are directly related to intraoperative events (Hogue et al. 1999; Nathan et al. 2007; Hogue et al. 2008a, b, c; Hedberg et al. 2011; Hedberg and Engstrom 2012; Bartels et al. 2013; Mashour et al. 2013).

12.1.3 Risk Factors of CNS Injuries

Usually, a time-based classification is considered for classification of the risk factors, having the following two categories for classifications of risk factors for postoperative cerebral disorders after cardiac surgery (Hogue et al. 1999; Hedberg et al. 2011).

Early *stroke risk factors are:*

- Advanced age
- High preoperative creatinine level
- Prior neurological event
- Aortic atherosclerosis area of involvement
- Longer duration of cardiopulmonary bypass
- Female gender with a 7-fold increased risk of early stroke and a 1.7-fold increased risk of delayed stroke

Delayed *stroke risk factors are*

- Prior neurological event
- Diabetes
- Aortic atherosclerosis
- Unstable angina
- Previous cerebral vascular disease
- Need for inotropic support
- Atrial fibrillation in postoperative period (combined end points of low cardiac output and atrial fibrillation)
- Low cardiac output (combined end points of low cardiac output and atrial fibrillation)
- Moderate-to-severe postoperative thrombocytopenia which is as an independent risk factor (Karhausen et al. 2017)

12.1.4 Mechanisms and Potential Etiologies of CNS Injuries

One of the most prominent features in "post-cardiac surgery cerebral disorders" is that their etiologies are not distinct; but a number of interrelated factors are responsible for the occurrence of these clinical disorders; however, a general classification could be as follows:

- Patient-related factors
- Intraoperative surgical factors
- Intraoperative anesthetic factors
- Intraoperative extracorporeal circulation (ECC) factors
- Postoperative period-related factors: about one-fifth (20%) of postoperative CNS complications of cardiac surgery occur due to postoperative events, while 80% are directly related to intraoperative events

There are a relatively great bulk of studies discussing the main potential mechanisms and risk factors for postoperative CNS disorders. Such studies have led us to consider potential CNS disorders in these patients more deeply and assess a number of risk factors considered as highly probable or possible etiologic or promoting factors. So, when dealing with cardiac surgery patients in the perioperative period, especially the postoperative period, we need to consider these probable mechanisms and potential risk factors in order to manage the patients appropriately; here a brief discussion of these mechanisms and risk factors is presented based on previous studies (Bucerius et al. 2004; Carrascal et al. 2005; Karkouti et al. 2005; McKhann et al. 2005; Selnes et al. 2005; Selnes and McKhann 2005; McKhann et al. 2006; Heckman et al. 2007; van Dijk et al. 2007; Hogue et al. 2008a, b, c; Marasco et al. 2008; Nelson et al. 2008; Fahy et al. 2009; Funder et al. 2009; Grigore et al. 2009; Grocott 2009; Lazar et al. 2009; Liu et al. 2009; Sheehy et al. 2009; Coburn et al. 2010; Lombard and Mathew 2010; Rudolph et al. 2010;

Hedberg et al. 2011; Messerotti Benvenuti et al. 2012a, b; Moller et al. 2012; Sun et al. 2012; Bartels et al. 2013; Bruggemans 2013; Knipp et al. 2013; Mashour et al. 2013; Reinsfelt et al. 2013; Dvir et al. 2014; Fink et al. 2015; Flaherty et al. 2015; Biancari et al. 2016; Brascia et al. 2017a, b; Karhausen et al. 2017; Kinnunen et al. 2017):

- First of all, postoperative CNS complications after cardiac surgery are usually **ischemic** type; less than 5% of them have a hemorrhagic origin. However, "*CPB-related inflammation, microemboli, and hypoperfusion*" are related mainly to acute (short term) neurocognitive disorders and "*underlying cerebrovascular disease in CABG candidates*" is mainly responsible for the late neurocognitive impairments (occurring 1–5 years postoperatively).
- There is a direct relationship between aortic atherosclerosis and postoperative CNS problems: "***aortic atherosclerosis and cerebral atherosclerosis are concomitant pathologies***." Till now, the main possible etiology for postoperative CNS complications is the underlying atherosclerotic process of the patient involving all the arterial system including the coronary arteries and the cerebral vascular system. Aortic atheroma (even when it is not as a plaque) is disrupted during thoracic aortic manipulations, including aortic cannulation, aortic cross clamping, and proximal anastomosis of grafts. Also, perfusion through the arterial cannula of CPB has a "sandblasting effect" which increases the risk of CNS injury; epi-aortic scanning is the most sensitive method for detecting aortic atherosclerosis to find appropriate place for cannulation, while palpation of the aorta by surgeon's finger is not as effective.
- **Microemboli** are originated both from *fatty nature* of embolic particles and the presence of aluminum and silicone in the aspirates of the cardiotomy suction; both types could occlude CNS end arteries. Lipid microemboli cause small capillary and arteriolar dilatations (SCADs), generally in the range of 10–70 μm; most of lipid microemboli are shed into brain end arteries through cardiotomy suction.
- **CABG approaches vs. endovascular carotid catheterization**: Using or avoiding **CPB** has been considered as a potential mechanism of injury with extensive studies assessing its effects. From one aspect, **off-pump surgery** has less aortic manipulations and potentially prevents CPB-related microemboli and inflammation; on the other hand, "*aortic manipulations by the surgeon during proximal grafting*" and "*hypotension episodes at the time of cardiac maneuvering for distal grafting*" are two possible mechanisms which could cause CNS injury in off-pump patients. Possibly this is why no significant difference (regarding postoperative CNS events) has been demonstrated between on-pump and off-pump groups. Finally, "**CPB alone does not cause enough neuro-inflammatory changes leading to increased long term cognitive dysfunction**." However, the cognitive outcome of adult patients between two methods (i.e., surgical vs. endovascular revascularization of coronary arteries) seems similar (Fink et al. 2015)

- Against the discussions related to on-pump and off-pump procedures, **the time interval for using extracorporeal circulation** and CPB is considered as a real risk factor for postoperative CNS dysfunction, since it boosts the inflammatory response, though a number of studies have failed to find a strong relationship in between.
- **CNS hypoperfusion** during CPB is an important risk factor. MAP between 50 and 80 mmHg is a target blood pressure for maintaining cerebral autoregulation functioning; the role of MAP is especially important in maintaining both cortical end arteries and cerebral collateral arteries. However, patients undergoing cardiac surgery usually have comorbidities; so, their cerebral autoregulation would function in higher pressures and upper limit of blood pressure for MAP during CPB is considered more appropriate for these patients. Even in patients undergoing off-pump cardiac surgery, any blood pressure derangement might have a great impact on CNS outcome. It seems that cerebral oximetry could help us control cerebral perfusion with much more exactness.
- **Hypothermia** during cardiac surgery has been used as an organ protective strategy; however, its effect on CNS outcome is yet to be defined since it has not been demonstrated to be effective in protecting CNS. On the other side, **hyperthermia** is a potent CNS risk factor usually occurring if slow rewarming strategies are not used for CPB weaning: 2 °C difference of CPB perfusate temperature and nasopharyngeal temperature improve outcome compared with 6 °C.
- As mentioned earlier, **time interval after surgery** is another factor since the risk factors of "early and delayed stroke" are different.
- The main CNS insult happens during the operation; however, about 20% of the strokes are the result of **postoperative events**, which mandates enough vigilance during postoperative period.
- **Particle emboli**: Both *macroemboli* (atherosclerotic debris originating from the thoracic aorta) and *microemboli* (fatty particles or gaseous emboli) are considered as important etiologies for cerebral injuries.
- **Gender**: Female gender is associated with a 5- to 7-fold increased risk of early stroke and a 1.5- to 2-fold increased risk of delayed stroke.
- **Previous history** of cerebrovascular events has a strong impact on chance of stroke after CABG or other cardiac surgeries; previous neurocognitive disorders have a non-negligible impact on the chance of postoperative occurrence of neurocognitive disorders.
- **Bleeding** after cardiac surgery, especially there is severe bleeding, mandating **transfusion** independently increases the risk of stroke after CABG (Biancari et al. 2016; Brascia et al. 2017a, b; Kinnunen et al. 2017).
- **Moderate-to-severe postoperative thrombocytopenia**: After on-pump CABG surgery, an independent association has been demonstrated between "*moderate-to-severe postoperative thrombocytopenia* and postoperative stroke"; also, postoperative moderate-to-severe postoperative thrombocytopenia has predictive value in timing of stroke (Karhausen et al. 2017). In other studies on patients

undergoing transcatheter aortic valve replacement (TAVR), the severity of thrombocytopenia after procedure has been demonstrated as "*an excellent and easily obtainable marker demonstrating worse short- and long-term outcomes*" after the procedure (Dvir et al. 2014; Flaherty et al. 2015).

- **Tight glycemic control** in diabetic and nondiabetic adult patients undergoing cardiac surgery was considered as a neuroprotective strategy; however, during recent years, evidence demonstrated "tight glycemic control" as an equivocal strategy regarding *patient outcome* and *mortality rate*, compared with conventional glucose management; a possible mechanism is the relatively high resistance against insulin during cardiopulmonary bypass with latent hypoglycemia after CPB, especially kin postoperative period which could induce cerebral hazards.
- **Anemia** is another major potential risk factor for postoperative CNS injury, especially if the hematocrit level during CPB is below 22% in patients at risk of CNS injury, in such a way that for each 1% fall in the level of hematocrit, a 10% increase in CNS injury chance has been shown; the possible mechanism for this finding is decreased cerebral oxygen delivery accompanied with increased embolic load due to compensatory cerebral arterial dilatation; however, it is not still proved that packed cell transfusion in order to compensate for anemia could prevent CNS injury, so we have to weigh the risk and benefit of transfusion in such cases.
- **Genetic predisposition** is another potential mechanism, explained in a number of studies, including genetic variants of CRP and interleukin 6 and also apolipoprotein E (APOE) genotype.
- **Atrial fibrillation** is the most common arrhythmia in postoperative period of cardiac surgery, occurring in >30% of the patients, and has a clear and direct relationship with postoperative CNS injury.
- **Advanced age** is "the main predictive factor which could foresee the occurrence of permanent postoperative neuropsychological defects" (mainly type II injury).
- Impaired **left ventricular function**: Heart failure is associated with impaired cognitive function (primarily presented as delirium in hospitalized patients).
- **Valvular surgery** is an important risk factor for increased prevalence of postoperative cognitive decline than other cardiac procedures; it is possible that microembolic events are the major reason for this fact.
- Postoperative neurocognitive disorders would affect the **cortical white matter of the brain** mainly due to inflammatory mechanisms with a number of markers like "Alzheimer-associated amyloid β."
- In a retrospective observational study in more than 6000 CABG patients, peripheral vascular disease, critical preoperative state, and intraoperative insertion of intra-aortic balloon pump had relationship with postoperative stroke (Karhausen et al. 2017) (Table 12.1).

Table 12.1 Proposed risk factors for post-cardiac surgery cerebral dysfunction

Patient-related factors:
1. Risk factors related to *patient pathophysiologic status*
• CPB-related inflammatory response
• Intraoperative hypoperfusion and hemodynamic perturbations
• Intraoperative cerebral oxygenation status
• Intraoperative anesthetics used during operation
2. Risk factors related to *underlying patient status*
• Perioperative comorbid states (diabetes mellitus, hypertension, atherosclerosis especially in ascending aorta, previous cerebrovascular pathologies, peripheral vascular disease, critical preoperative state)
• Preoperative cerebral blood flow (CBF) velocity, which demonstrates cerebral perfusion status (even preoperative left-sided hypoperfusion could be a risk factor)
• Old age
• Perioperative sleep status (risk of sleep apnea)
• Perioperative administration of medications
3. Risk factors related to *patient social status*
• Underlying social class and social status
• Postoperative administration of rehabilitation care
• Underlying level of education
• Gender
• Ethnic differences
Procedure-related factors (intraoperative and postoperative surgical factors, anesthetic factors, and extracorporeal circulation "ECC" factors):
• Using cardiotomy suction (time of using suction during surgery, using cell saver and arterial filter)
• Duration of aortic cross clamp
• Using hypothermia, optimal rewarming, severity, and duration of hypothermia (especially if using DHCA)
• Hyperthermia after CPB
• Deairing management during surgery
• Type of surgery (especially valve surgery or involving the aortic root)
• Intraoperative use of epi-aortic scanning by the surgeon for aortic cannulation
• Unstable hemodynamic status before, during, or after CPB
• Location of the possible side of hypoperfusion during operation (left vs. right carotid system)
• Using or avoiding CPB (on pump vs. off pump)
• Duration of CPB
• Amount of bleeding and volume of transfused blood
• Readmission to the operating theatre for control of acute postoperative bleeding
• Intraoperative insertion of intra-aortic balloon pump
Only one-fifth (20%) of postoperative CNS complications of cardiac surgery occur due to ***postoperative events***
• Hyperthermia after CPB
• Hypotension
• Amount of bleeding and volume of transfused blood
• Moderate-to-severe postoperative thrombocytopenia
• Readmission to the operating theatre for control of acute postoperative bleeding

12.2 Prevention Strategies

12.2.1 Pharmacologic Neuroprotection

Though a number of pharmaceutical agents have been proposed as neuroprotective agents, none has been fully proved yet; however, the following agents have been demonstrated to be effective in suppressing the ischemic penumbra in some studies (Hogue et al. 2007; Nelson et al. 2008; Mitchell et al. 2009; Lombard and Mathew 2010; Benggon et al. 2012; Dabbagh and Rajaei 2012; Zhang et al. 2012; Bruggemans 2013):

- Intraoperative lidocaine might have neuroprotective effects through suppressing the inflammatory response in cardiac surgery patients.
- Thiopental mainly decreases the embolic load (possibly due to cerebral vasoconstriction).
- Propofol might decrease the oxygen consumption during ischemic period.
- Postoperative donepezil might have therapeutic (rather than preventive) effects for postoperative cognitive dysfunction.
- 17β-Estradiol might limit ischemic injury of the neuronal tissue in women undergoing cardiac surgery.
- In some studies, antagonists of N-methyl-D-aspartate have been demonstrated as neuroprotective agents; among them, anesthetics could be mentioned as the prototype of these drugs used for cardiac surgery patients. Usually, these pharmaceuticals are blamed for their neuroapoptotic effects; however, some agents like ***xenon*** and ***dexmedetomidine*** may have neuroprotective effects; on the other hand, although ***ketamine*** might have adverse neurodevelopmental effects in neonatal animal brain studies, it might be effective in decreasing postoperative neurocognitive dysfunction after cardiac surgery. Magnesium is another agent with potential anti-inflammatory effects, being an antagonist of NMDA.
- Dextromethorphan, nimodipine, aprotinin, remacemide, beta-blockers, pexelizumab, and a number of other agents have been proposed; however none have been conclusive yet.

12.2.2 CPB-Related Equipment

A full description of the CPB-related factors affecting the CNS is discussed in detail in this book in a separate chapter titled "*Chap. 18: Cardiopulmonary bypass: postoperative effects*."

12.3 ICU Delirium in Adult Cardiac Surgery

Delirium is "*a common, complex and multifactorial syndrome resulting from global organic cerebral dysfunction*" and based on DSM-5 (Diagnostic and Statistical Manual of Mental Disorders, Fifth Edition) or ICD-10 (10th revision of the

International Statistical Classification of Diseases and Related Health Problems) classifications it is defined as "*a neurocognitive disorder or a neuropsychiatric syndrome with its hallmark as disturbed attention and awareness developing over a short period of time*" (Aldecoa et al. 2017; Bush et al. 2017a, b).

Postoperative delirium may even start in the recovery room and be continued as long as the fifth postoperative day or even afterwards. In the elderly, postoperative delirium is even a more dynamic and much more complex process; meanwhile, the frequency of postoperative delirium is really high; in some studies, 25–88% of patients admitted to ICU have been challenging with delirium; diagnosis of delirium: due to the fluctuating nature of delirium symptoms and signs and also due to deficient routine tests for screening cognitive functions, delirium is often misdiagnosed or underdiagnosed (McNicoll et al. 2003; Ouimet et al. 2007; Hosie et al. 2013; El Hussein et al. 2015; Aldecoa et al. 2017; Bush et al. 2017a, b; Zheng et al. 2017).

Risk factors for delirium: In the "Clinical practice guidelines for the management of pain, agitation, and delirium in adult patients in the intensive care unit" published by The American College of Critical Care Medicine (ACCM) in 2013, among all potential risk factors, the following four baseline risk factors are considered as having positive and significant association with ICU delirium development:

- Preexisting dementia
- History of hypertension
- History of alcoholism
- High severity of illness at admission

Also, the above guideline has stated that "coma is an independent risk factor for the development of delirium in ICU patients" (Barr et al. 2013). However, when considering non-pharmacologic interventions for treatment of delirium in the next paragraphs, the following classification of potential delirium risk factors is considered (Van Rompaey et al. 2009; Bruno and Warren 2010; Shehabi et al. 2010):

- Acute illness
- Host factors including age or chronic health problems
- Iatrogenic or environmental factors

The impact of delirium on healthcare outcome: The most common unwanted consequences of delirium are the following (Breitbart et al. 2002; Neufeld et al. 2016; Aldecoa et al. 2017; Bush et al. 2017a, b):

- Risk of mortality is increased.
- There is significant chance of functional impairment, leading to some catastrophic events like patient falls which are increased due to delirium.
- Healthcare costs are increased.

- Length of mechanical ventilation, ICU admission, and hospital stay are all prolonged.
- Preexisting dementia would aggravate; at the same time, the potential risk for de novo dementia is increased; dementia is considered as a remarkable risk factor for delirium development during and after the ICU admission.
- For patients and their relatives and also for caregivers and healthcare providers, delirium imposes "significant psychological distress" (Breitbart et al. 2002).

Patient monitoring: A number of well-known scales have been proposed for detection and monitoring of delirium, both for level of consciousness and monitoring of delirium, in the "Clinical practice guidelines for the management of pain, agitation, and delirium in adult patients in the intensive care unit" published by The American College of Critical Care Medicine (ACCM) in 2013; the two following screening scales are recommended as the most valid and reliable tools for delirium monitoring in adult ICU, suggesting their use as routine monitoring tools feasible in clinical practice at least once per shift (Barr et al. 2013):

- Confusion Assessment Method for the ICU (CAM-ICU)
- Intensive Care Delirium Screening Checklist (ICDSC)

Some studies suggest routine using of the above two tools at least once per shift. For neurologic monitoring, detailed discussion is presented in another chapter of the book titled "*Chap. 12: CNS Complications & Management after adult Cardiac Surgery*".

Treatment of delirium: Currently, the cornerstone for prophylaxis and treatment of delirium is multicomponent non-pharmacological interventions and supportive care, though pharmacological options have been proposed for many years (Bruno and Warren 2010; NICE 2010; Barr et al. 2013; Abraha et al. 2015; Martinez et al. 2015; Bannon et al. 2016).

Non-pharmacologic interventions for prevention and treatment of ICU delirium

Non-pharmacologic interventions are based on the classification of delirium risk factors which could be divided as:

1. Acute illness
2. Host factors including age or chronic health problems
3. Iatrogenic or environmental factors

Under each of the above three risk factors, a number of related items are categorized (Van Rompaey et al. 2009; Bruno and Warren 2010). For modification and compensation of these above three risk factors, a number of non-pharmacologic interventions have been proposed by studies, including but not limited to those presented in Table 12.2.

Pharmacologic options for the prevention and treatment of ICU delirium:

Routine use of antipsychotics for prevention or treatment of perioperative delirium in adults is not proved as an evidence-based approach (Neufeld et al. 2016).

Table 12.2 Non-pharmacologic interventions for prevention and treatment of delirium in ICU patients (Needham 2008; Schweickert et al. 2009; Bruno and Warren 2010; Shehabi et al. 2010; Barr et al. 2013; NICE 2014; Abraha et al. 2015; Hu et al. 2015; Knauert et al. 2015; Martinez et al. 2015; Bannon et al. 2016; Pulak and Jensen 2016; Aldecoa et al. 2017; Bush et al. 2017a, b)

Interventions for compensation or prevention of sleep deprivation
• Restoration of normal pattern of sleep (i.e., increasing night sleep, decreasing daytime sleep, and restoration of circadian sleep pattern; also increasing REM sleep fractions and decreasing nighttime arousal)
• Providing appropriate pattern of light (simulating or using natural light and/or using bright light with designed sleep/wakefulness pattern); ICU night light levels may be between 5 and 1400 lux, while melatonin secretion is affected with light levels between 100 and 500 lux; avoiding light variation; instead using continuous indirect low-grade light
• Using eye masks
• Reducing or minimizing background noise (noise levels not exceeding 35 dB) especially when there is high-level noise due to patient care activities or other environmental noises which may even peak to 85 dB
• Using earplugs, or other noise control strategies
• Increasing patient comfort during patient care for improvement of sleep
• Holding as much therapeutic procedures and interventions as possible during the time of sleep; i.e., holding nonurgent blood sampling, temporarily removing catheters, holding respiratory treatments temporarily, timely removal of physical restraints
Interventions for improved patient comfort
• Modification of pain
• Modification of stress and anxiety
• Making unpleasant effects of mechanical ventilation tolerable
• Meanwhile rational use of analgesics and sedatives and prevention of heavy sedation as much as possible
• Ensuring adequate fluid intake
• Increasing patient autonomy (for example setting the time of nonurgent procedures with the patient)
• Massage therapy: effleurage massage or even using a simple 3-min backrub
Interventions for improving exercise and physical therapy
• Application of passive or active exercises for improving range of motion
• Encouraging the patient for doing active exercises by himself/herself
• Avoidance of prolonged bed rest as soon as possible
• Early active mobilization
Interventions for avoidance of social isolation and/or stimulating cognitive activities
• Removing language, cultural, and sensory barriers
• Music therapy
• Using media like television
• Frequent reorientation of the patient to place, person, and time (at least once per shift)
• Presence of the family members in patient bedside (needs them to be oriented and trained about the importance of their presence)
• Bringing items of significance by family members from home to bedside
Interventions for pharmacologic prevention of delirium
• Modification of potential deliriogenic drugs or avoiding them (e.g., benzodiazepines)
• Using potential prophylactic drugs for premedication, anesthesia, or sedation (e.g., clonidine, dexmedetomidine)

Even, in the elderly, the net impact of antipsychotics may be towards increasing mortality, especially when the dose is increased (Maust et al. 2015). None of the currently available medications used for delirium are FDA approved; this is why the following antipsychotics are not considered in the format of “formal recommendations” for treatment of delirium; most of them are considered as “off-label” drugs for delirium. The use of antipsychotics for treatment of delirium has historically been considered despite the above limitations and potential concerns regarding the adverse effects, leading to the following results in brief (Maglione et al. 2011; Teslyar et al. 2013; Inouye et al. 2014; Fok et al. 2015; Mu et al. 2015; Santos et al. 2015; Serafim et al. 2015; Schrijver et al. 2016; Siddiqi et al. 2016; Mo and Yam 2017):

- *Haloperidol (Haldol®)*: For prevention and treatment of delirium, haloperidol is the most quoted antipsychotic; however, the last word about its dosing regimen and even the net harm-benefit profile of the drug for ICU delirium is yet to be said; some studies have questioned its benefits over the harms.
- *Atypical antipsychotics*: The evidence in support of these drugs in ICU delirium is even fewer compared to that of haloperidol; however, future studies would possibly determine whether to use these drugs as the therapeutic or preventive pharmacologic agents for ICU delirium, if their proposed “lower incidence of QTc prolongation and neurologic adverse effects” compared with haloperidol are proved (Table 12.3).

Table 12.3 Drugs for ICU delirium (Maglione et al. 2011; Mo and Yam 2017; Dabbagh et al. 2017)

Drug	Peak of effect	Dosing	Adverse effects/comments
Haloperidol (Haldol®)	Very rapid (especially IV route)	IV: 5 mg per day divided into 2–4 doses	• QT interval abnormalities: Torsades de pointes, ventricular fibrillation and ventricular tachycardia
		Oral: 0.5–5 mg for 2–3 times a day; based on symptoms	• Risk of extrapyramidal side effects or other CNS problems like neuroleptic malignant syndrome (rare)
		Discontinue in patients with QTc > 500 ms	
Risperidone (Risperdal®)	Oral: 1 h	Oral tablets: 0.25, 0.5, 1, 2, 3, and 4 mg	• **Has oral and solution forms**
		Dose: 0.5–8 mg/day orally	• Risk of extrapyramidal side effects or other CNS adverse effects including seizure and sleep abnormalities and also gastrointestinal problems
			• Needs hepatic and renal adjustment

Table 12.3 (continued)

Drug	Peak of effect	Dosing	Adverse effects/comments
Olanzapine * **(off-label use)**	Oral: 6 h IM: 30 min	2.5–20 mg/day oral 5–10 mg/day IM	• **Has oral and IM forms** • Needs to monitor for QT interval prolongation • Needs to monitor for potential arrhythmias • CNS side effects like seizure and extrapyramidal adverse effects • No need for hepatic or renal adjustment
Quetiapine * **(seroquel) (off-label use)**	Oral: 90 min	100–400 mg/day divided by 2 daily doses	• **Has oral form** • Needs to monitor for QT interval prolongation • Needs to monitor for potential arrhythmias • CNS side effects like seizure and extrapyramidal adverse effects • Less Parkinson-like effects than the other second-generation antipsychotics • Needs hepatic adjustment
Ziprasidone * **(off-label use)**	Oral: 6 h	Oral: 20–80 mg/2 times/day	• **Has oral and IM forms**
	IM: 1 h	IM: 40 mg/day; divided by 6–12 doses	• No need for hepatic or renal adjustment

*Olanzapine, quetiapine, and ziprasidone are not among the commonly used drugs for postoperative delirium; their use should be with extreme cautions

12.4 Neurologic Monitoring

Novel and older technologies are used to improve the CNS outcome. This monitoring is used more commonly nowadays. A full description of the neurologic monitoring in cardiac surgery is discussed in detail in this book in a separate chapter titled "*Central nervous system monitoring*". However, a brief discussion is presented here. The main currently available CNS monitoring are the following:

- Clinical assessment of CNS status and of sedation in postoperative period (intensive care unit)
- Classic electroencephalogram (EEG) including multichannel or unichannel EEG
- Monitoring depth of anesthesia
- Evoked potentials (including motor evoked potential, somatosensory evoked potential, and auditory evoked potential)
- Regional cerebral oximetry (rSO_2) by near-infrared spectroscopy technique (NIRS)

- Jugular vein oxygen saturation ($SjvO_2$)
- Transcranial Doppler (TCD)
- Other modes for assessment of cerebral blood flow

A full description of these devices is found in this book in the chapter discussing Chap. 12: CNS Complications & Management after adult Cardiac Surgery.

References

Abraha I, Trotta F, Rimland JM, Cruz-Jentoft A, Lozano-Montoya I, Soiza RL, Pierini V, Dessi Fulgheri P, Lattanzio F, O'Mahony D, Cherubini A. Efficacy of non-pharmacological interventions to prevent and treat delirium in older patients: a systematic overview. The SENATOR project ONTOP Series. PLoS One. 2015;10:e0123090.

Aldecoa C, Bettelli G, Bilotta F, Sanders RD, Audisio R, Borozdina A, Cherubini A, Jones C, Kehlet H, MacLullich A, Radtke F, Riese F, Slooter AJ, Veyckemans F, Kramer S, Neuner B, Weiss B, Spies CD. European Society of Anaesthesiology evidence-based and consensus-based guideline on postoperative delirium. Eur J Anaesthesiol. 2017;34:192–214.

Bannon L, McGaughey J, Clarke M, McAuley DF, Blackwood B. Impact of non-pharmacological interventions on prevention and treatment of delirium in critically ill patients: protocol for a systematic review of quantitative and qualitative research. Syst Rev. 2016;5:75.

Barr J, Fraser GL, Puntillo K, Ely EW, Gelinas C, Dasta JF, Davidson JE, Devlin JW, Kress JP, Joffe AM, Coursin DB, Herr DL, Tung A, Robinson BR, Fontaine DK, Ramsay MA, Riker RR, Sessler CN, Pun B, Skrobik Y, Jaeschke R. Clinical practice guidelines for the management of pain, agitation, and delirium in adult patients in the intensive care unit. Crit Care Med. 2013;41:263–306.

Bartels K, McDonagh DL, Newman MF, Mathew JP. Neurocognitive outcomes after cardiac surgery. Curr Opin Anaesthesiol. 2013;26:91–7.

Benggon M, Chen H, Applegate R, Martin R, Zhang JH. Effect of dexmedetomidine on brain edema and neurological outcomes in surgical brain injury in rats. Anesth Analg. 2012;115:154–9.

Biancari F, Tauriainen T, Perrotti A, Dalen M, Faggian G, Franzese I, Chocron S, Ruggieri VG, Bounader K, Gulbins H, Reichart D, Svenarud P, Santarpino G, Fischlein T, Puski T, Maselli D, Dominici C, Nardella S, Mariscalco G, Gherli R, Musumeci F, Rubino AS, Mignosa C, De Feo M, Bancone C, Gatti G, Maschietto L, Santini F, Salsano A, Nicolini F, Gherli T, Zanobini M, Saccocci M, D'Errigo P, Kinnunen EM, Onorati F. Bleeding, transfusion and the risk of stroke after coronary surgery: a prospective cohort study of 2357 patients. Int J Surg. 2016;32:50–7.

Brascia D, Garcia-Medina N, Kinnunen EM, Tauriainen T, Airaksinen J, Biancari F. Impact of transfusion on stroke after cardiovascular interventions: meta-analysis of comparative studies. J Crit Care. 2017a;38:157–63.

Brascia D, Reichart D, Onorati F, Perrotti A, Ruggieri VG, Bounader K, Verhoye JP, Santarpino G, Fischlein T, Maselli D, Dominici C, Mariscalco G, Gherli R, Rubino AS, De Feo M, Bancone C, Gatti G, Santini F, Dalen M, Saccocci M, Faggian G, Tauriainen T, Kinnunen EM, Nicolini F, Gherli T, Rosato S, Biancari F. Validation of bleeding classifications in coronary artery bypass grafting. Am J Cardiol. 2017b;119:727–33.

Breitbart W, Gibson C, Tremblay A. The delirium experience: delirium recall and delirium-related distress in hospitalized patients with cancer, their spouses/caregivers, and their nurses. Psychosomatics. 2002;43:183–94.

Bruggemans EF. Cognitive dysfunction after cardiac surgery: pathophysiological mechanisms and preventive strategies. Neth Heart J. 2013;21:70–3.

Bruno JJ, Warren ML. Intensive care unit delirium. Crit Care Nurs Clin North Am. 2010;22:161–78.

Bucerius J, Gummert JF, Borger MA, Walther T, Doll N, Falk V, Schmitt DV, Mohr FW. Predictors of delirium after cardiac surgery delirium: effect of beating-heart (off-pump) surgery. J Thorac Cardiovasc Surg. 2004;127:57–64.

Bush SH, Marchington KL, Agar M, Davis DH, Sikora L, Tsang TW. Quality of clinical practice guidelines in delirium: a systematic appraisal. BMJ Open. 2017a;7:e013809.

Bush SH, Tierney S, Lawlor PG. Clinical assessment and management of delirium in the palliative care setting. Drugs. 2017b;77(15):1623–43.

Carrascal Y, Casquero E, Gualis J, Di Stefano S, Florez S, Fulquet E, Echevarria JR, Fiz L. Cognitive decline after cardiac surgery: proposal for easy measurement with a new test. Interact Cardiovasc Thorac Surg. 2005;4:216–21.

Coburn M, Fahlenkamp A, Zoremba N, Schaelte G. Postoperative cognitive dysfunction: incidence and prophylaxis. Anaesthesist. 2010;59:177–84; quiz 185

Dabbagh A. Postoperative CNS care. In: Dabbagh A, Esmailian F, Aranki S, editors. Postoperative critical care for cardiac surgical patients. 1st ed. New York: Springer; 2014a. p. 245–56.

Dabbagh A. Postoperative central nervous system monitoring. In: Dabbagh A, Esmailian F, Aranki S, editors. Postoperative critical care for cardiac surgical patients. 1st ed. New York: Springer; 2014b. p. 129–59.

Dabbagh A, Rajaei S. Xenon: a solution for anesthesia in liver disease? Hepat Mon. 2012;12:e8437.

Dabbagh A, Ramsay MAE. Postoperative central nervous system management in patients with congenital heart disease. In: Dabbagh A, Conte AH, Lubin L, editors. Congenital heart disease in pediatric and adult patients: anesthetic and perioperative management. 1st ed. New York: Springer; 2017a. p. 829–50.

Dabbagh A, Ramsay MAE. Central nervous system monitoring in pediatric cardiac surgery. In: Dabbagh A, Conte AH, Lubin L, editors. Congenital heart disease in pediatric and adult patients: anesthetic and perioperative management. 1st ed. New York: Springer; 2017b. p. 279–316.

Dabbagh A, Talebi Z, Rajaei S. Cardiovascular pharmacology in pediatric patients with congenital heart disease. In: Dabbagh A, Conte AH, Lubin L, editors. Congenital heart disease in pediatric and adult patients: anesthetic and perioperative management. 1st ed. New York: Springer; 2017. p. 117–95.

Dvir D, Genereux P, Barbash IM, Kodali S, Ben-Dor I, Williams M, Torguson R, Kirtane AJ, Minha S, Badr S, Pendyala LK, Loh JP, Okubagzi PG, Fields JN, Xu K, Chen F, Hahn RT, Satler LF, Smith C, Pichard AD, Leon MB, Waksman R. Acquired thrombocytopenia after transcatheter aortic valve replacement: clinical correlates and association with outcomes. Eur Heart J. 2014;35:2663–71.

El Hussein M, Hirst S, Salyers V. Factors that contribute to underrecognition of delirium by registered nurses in acute care settings: a scoping review of the literature to explain this phenomenon. J Clin Nurs. 2015;24:906–15.

Fahy BG, Sheehy AM, Coursin DB. Glucose control in the intensive care unit. Crit Care Med. 2009;37:1769–76.

Fink HA, Hemmy LS, MacDonald R, Carlyle MH, Olson CM, Dysken MW, McCarten JR, Kane RL, Garcia SA, Rutks IR, Ouellette J, Wilt TJ. Intermediate- and long-term cognitive outcomes after cardiovascular procedures in older adults: a systematic review. Ann Intern Med. 2015;163:107–17.

Flaherty MP, Mohsen A, Moore JB, Bartoli CR, Schneibel E, Rawasia W, Williams ML, Grubb KJ, Hirsch GA. Predictors and clinical impact of pre-existing and acquired thrombocytopenia following transcatheter aortic valve replacement. Catheter Cardiovasc Interv. 2015;85:118–29.

Fok MC, Sepehry AA, Frisch L, Sztramko R, Borger van der Burg BL, Vochteloo AJ, Chan P. Do antipsychotics prevent postoperative delirium? A systematic review and meta-analysis. Int J Geriatr Psychiatry. 2015;30:333–44.

Funder KS, Steinmetz J, Rasmussen LS. Cognitive dysfunction after cardiovascular surgery. Minerva Anestesiol. 2009;75:329–32.

Grigore AM, Murray CF, Ramakrishna H, Djaiani G. A core review of temperature regimens and neuroprotection during cardiopulmonary bypass: does rewarming rate matter? Anesth Analg. 2009;109:1741–51.

Grocott HP. PRO: temperature regimens and neuroprotection during cardiopulmonary bypass: does rewarming rate matter? Anesth Analg. 2009;109:1738–40.

Heckman GA, Patterson CJ, Demers C, St Onge J, Turpie ID, McKelvie RS. Heart failure and cognitive impairment: challenges and opportunities. Clin Interv Aging. 2007;2:209–18.

Hedberg M, Boivie P, Engstrom KG. Early and delayed stroke after coronary surgery—an analysis of risk factors and the impact on short- and long-term survival. Eur J Cardiothorac Surg. 2011;40:379–87.

Hedberg M, Engstrom KG. Stroke after cardiac surgery—hemispheric distribution and survival. Scand Cardiovasc J. 2012;47(3):136–44.

Hogue CW, Fucetola R, Hershey T, Freedland K, Davila-Roman VG, Goate AM, Thompson RE. Risk factors for neurocognitive dysfunction after cardiac surgery in postmenopausal women. Ann Thorac Surg. 2008a;86:511–6.

Hogue CW, Gottesman RF, Stearns J. Mechanisms of cerebral injury from cardiac surgery. Crit Care Clin. 2008b;24:83–98, viii–ix.

Hogue CW Jr, Freedland K, Hershey T, Fucetola R, Nassief A, Barzilai B, Thomas B, Birge S, Dixon D, Schechtman KB, Davila-Roman VG. Neurocognitive outcomes are not improved by 17beta-estradiol in postmenopausal women undergoing cardiac surgery. Stroke. 2007;38:2048–54.

Hogue CW Jr, Fucetola R, Hershey T, Nassief A, Birge S, Davila-Roman VG, Barzilai B, Thomas B, Schechtman KB, Freedland K. The role of postoperative neurocognitive dysfunction on quality of life for postmenopausal women 6 months after cardiac surgery. Anesth Analg. 2008;107:21–8.

Hogue CW Jr, Murphy SF, Schechtman KB, Davila-Roman VG. Risk factors for early or delayed stroke after cardiac surgery. Circulation. 1999;100:642–7.

Hosie A, Davidson PM, Agar M, Sanderson CR, Phillips J. Delirium prevalence, incidence, and implications for screening in specialist palliative care inpatient settings: a systematic review. Palliat Med. 2013;27:486–98.

Hu RF, Jiang XY, Chen J, Zeng Z, Chen XY, Li Y, Huining X, Evans DJ. Non-pharmacological interventions for sleep promotion in the intensive care unit. Cochrane Database Syst Rev. 2015;10:Cd008808.

Inouye SK, Marcantonio ER, Metzger ED. Doing damage in delirium: the hazards of antipsychotic treatment in elderly persons. Lancet Psychiatry. 2014;1:312–5.

Karhausen JA, Smeltz AM, Akushevich I, Cooter M, Podgoreanu MV, Stafford-Smith M, Martinelli SM, Fontes ML, Kertai MD. Platelet counts and postoperative stroke after coronary artery bypass grafting surgery. Anesth Analg. 2017;125:1129–39.

Karkouti K, Djaiani G, Borger MA, Beattie WS, Fedorko L, Wijeysundera D, Ivanov J, Karski J. Low hematocrit during cardiopulmonary bypass is associated with increased risk of perioperative stroke in cardiac surgery. Ann Thorac Surg. 2005;80:1381–7.

Kinnunen EM, De Feo M, Reichart D, Tauriainen T, Gatti G, Onorati F, Maschietto L, Bancone C, Fiorentino F, Chocron S, Bounader K, Dalen M, Svenarud P, Faggian G, Franzese I, Santarpino G, Fischlein T, Maselli D, Dominici C, Nardella S, Gherli R, Musumeci F, Rubino AS, Mignosa C, Mariscalco G, Serraino FG, Santini F, Salsano A, Nicolini F, Gherli T, Zanobini M, Saccocci M, Ruggieri VG, Philippe Verhoye J, Perrotti A, Biancari F. Incidence and prognostic impact of bleeding and transfusion after coronary surgery in low-risk patients. Transfusion. 2017;57:178–86.

Knauert MP, Haspel JA, Pisani MA. Sleep loss and circadian rhythm disruption in the intensive care unit. Clin Chest Med. 2015;36:419–29.

Knipp SC, Kahlert P, Jokisch D, Schlamann M, Wendt D, Weimar C, Jakob H, Thielmann M. Cognitive function after transapical aortic valve implantation: a single-centre study with 3-month follow-up. Interact Cardiovasc Thorac Surg. 2013;16:116–22.

Lazar HL, McDonnell M, Chipkin SR, Furnary AP, Engelman RM, Sadhu AR, Bridges CR, Haan CK, Svedjeholm R, Taegtmeyer H, Shemin RJ. The Society of Thoracic Surgeons practice guideline series: blood glucose management during adult cardiac surgery. Ann Thorac Surg. 2009;87:663–9.

Liu YH, Wang DX, Li LH, Wu XM, Shan GJ, Su Y, Li J, Yu QJ, Shi CX, Huang YN, Sun W. The effects of cardiopulmonary bypass on the number of cerebral microemboli and the incidence of cognitive dysfunction after coronary artery bypass graft surgery. Anesth Analg. 2009;109:1013–22.

Lombard FW, Mathew JP. Neurocognitive dysfunction following cardiac surgery. Semin Cardiothorac Vasc Anesth. 2010;14:102–10.

Maglione M, Maher AR, Hu J, Wang Z, Shanman R, Shekelle PG, Roth B, Hilton L, Suttorp MJ, Ewing BA, Motala A, Perry T. AHRQ comparative effectiveness reviews. In: Off-label use of atypical antipsychotics: an update. Rockville, MD: Agency for Healthcare Research and Quality (US); 2011.

Marasco SF, Sharwood LN, Abramson MJ. No improvement in neurocognitive outcomes after off-pump versus on-pump coronary revascularisation: a meta-analysis. Eur J Cardiothorac Surg. 2008;33:961–70.

Martinez F, Tobar C, Hill N. Preventing delirium: should non-pharmacological, multicomponent interventions be used? A systematic review and meta-analysis of the literature. Age Ageing. 2015;44:196–204.

Mashour GA, Avitsian R, Lauer KK, Soriano SG, Sharma D, Koht A, Crosby G. Neuroanesthesiology Fellowship Training: curricular guidelines from the Society for Neuroscience in Anesthesiology and Critical Care. J Neurosurg Anesthesiol. 2013;25:1–7.

Mathew JP, Mackensen GB, Phillips-Bute B, Grocott HP, Glower DD, Laskowitz DT, Blumenthal JA, Newman MF. Randomized, double-blinded, placebo controlled study of neuroprotection with lidocaine in cardiac surgery. Stroke. 2009;40:880–7.

Maust DT, Kim HM, Seyfried LS, Chiang C, Kavanagh J, Schneider LS, Kales HC. Antipsychotics, other psychotropics, and the risk of death in patients with dementia: number needed to harm. JAMA Psychiatry. 2015;72:438–45.

McKhann GM, Grega MA, Borowicz LM Jr, Bailey MM, Barry SJ, Zeger SL, Baumgartner WA, Selnes OA. Is there cognitive decline 1 year after CABG? Comparison with surgical and nonsurgical controls. Neurology. 2005;65:991–9.

McKhann GM, Grega MA, Borowicz LM Jr, Baumgartner WA, Selnes OA. Stroke and encephalopathy after cardiac surgery: an update. Stroke. 2006;37:562–71.

McNicoll L, Pisani MA, Zhang Y, Ely EW, Siegel MD, Inouye SK. Delirium in the intensive care unit: occurrence and clinical course in older patients. J Am Geriatr Soc. 2003;51:591–8.

Messerotti Benvenuti S, Zanatta P, Longo C, Mazzarolo AP, Palomba D. Preoperative cerebral hypoperfusion in the left, not in the right, hemisphere is associated with cognitive decline after cardiac surgery. Psychosom Med. 2012a;74:73–80.

Messerotti Benvenuti S, Zanatta P, Valfre C, Polesel E, Palomba D. Preliminary evidence for reduced preoperative cerebral blood flow velocity as a risk factor for cognitive decline three months after cardiac surgery: an extension study. Perfusion. 2012b;27:486–92.

Mitchell SJ, Merry AF, Frampton C, Davies E, Grieve D, Mills BP, Webster CS, Milsom FP, Willcox TW, Gorman DF. Cerebral protection by lidocaine during cardiac operations: a follow-up study. Ann Thorac Surg. 2009;87:820–5.

Mo Y, Yam FK. Rational use of second-generation antipsychotics for the treatment of ICU delirium. J Pharm Pract. 2017;30:121–9.

Moller CH, Penninga L, Wetterslev J, Steinbruchel DA, Gluud C. Off-pump versus on-pump coronary artery bypass grafting for ischaemic heart disease. Cochrane Database Syst Rev. 2012;3:CD007224.

Mu JL, Lee A, Joynt GM. Pharmacologic agents for the prevention and treatment of delirium in patients undergoing cardiac surgery: systematic review and metaanalysis. Crit Care Med. 2015;43:194–204.

Nathan HJ, Rodriguez R, Wozny D, Dupuis JY, Rubens FD, Bryson GL, Wells G. Neuroprotective effect of mild hypothermia in patients undergoing coronary artery surgery with cardiopulmonary bypass: five-year follow-up of a randomized trial. J Thorac Cardiovasc Surg. 2007;133:1206–11.

Needham DM. Mobilizing patients in the intensive care unit: improving neuromuscular weakness and physical function. JAMA. 2008;300:1685–90.

Nelson DP, Andropoulos DB, Fraser CD Jr. Perioperative neuroprotective strategies. Semin Thorac Cardiovasc Surg Pediatr Card Surg Annu. 2008:49–56. https://doi.org/10.1053/j.pcsu.2008.01.003.

Neufeld KJ, Yue J, Robinson TN, Inouye SK, Needham DM. Antipsychotic medication for prevention and treatment of delirium in hospitalized adults: a systematic review and meta-analysis. J Am Geriatr Soc. 2016;64:705–14.

Newman MF, Grocott HP, Mathew JP, White WD, Landolfo K, Reves JG, Laskowitz DT, Mark DB, Blumenthal JA. Report of the substudy assessing the impact of neurocognitive function on quality of life 5 years after cardiac surgery. Stroke. 2001;32:2874–81.

NICE. NCGCU. Delirium: diagnosis, prevention and management [Internet]. NICE Clinical Guidelines, No. 103. Treatment of delirium: non-pharmacological (hospital setting). 2010. https://www.ncbi.nlm.nih.gov/books/NBK65539/.

NICE. NIfHaCE. Delirium: quality statement two: interventions to prevent delirium, QS63. London: National Institute for Health and care Excellence. 2014. https://www.nice.org.uk/guidance/qs63.

Ouimet S, Kavanagh BP, Gottfried SB, Skrobik Y. Incidence, risk factors and consequences of ICU delirium. Intensive Care Med. 2007;33:66–73.

Pulak LM, Jensen L. Sleep in the intensive care unit: a review. J Intensive Care Med. 2016;31:14–23.

Reinsfelt B, Westerlind A, Blennow K, Zetterberg H, Ricksten SE. Open-heart surgery increases cerebrospinal fluid levels of Alzheimer-associated amyloid beta. Acta Anaesthesiol Scand. 2013;57:82–8.

Roach GW, Kanchuger M, Mangano CM, Newman M, Nussmeier N, Wolman R, Aggarwal A, Marschall K, Graham SH, Ley C. Adverse cerebral outcomes after coronary bypass surgery. Multicenter Study of Perioperative Ischemia Research Group and the Ischemia Research and Education Foundation Investigators. N Engl J Med. 1996;335:1857–63.

Rudolph JL, Schreiber KA, Culley DJ, McGlinchey RE, Crosby G, Levitsky S, Marcantonio ER. Measurement of post-operative cognitive dysfunction after cardiac surgery: a systematic review. Acta Anaesthesiol Scand. 2010;54:663–77.

Santos E, Cardoso D, Apostolo J, Neves H, Cunha M, Rodrigues M. Effectiveness of haloperidol prophylaxis in critically ill patients with a high risk for delirium: a systematic review of quantitative evidence protocol. JBI Database System Rev Implement Rep. 2015;13:83–92.

Sato Y, Laskowitz DT, Bennett ER, Newman MF, Warner DS, Grocott HP. Differential cerebral gene expression during cardiopulmonary bypass in the rat: evidence for apoptosis? Anesth Analg. 2002;94:1389–94.

Schrijver EJ, de Graaf K, de Vries OJ, Maier AB, Nanayakkara PW. Efficacy and safety of haloperidol for in-hospital delirium prevention and treatment: a systematic review of current evidence. Eur J Intern Med. 2016;27:14–23.

Schweickert WD, Pohlman MC, Pohlman AS, Nigos C, Pawlik AJ, Esbrook CL, Spears L, Miller M, Franczyk M, Deprizio D, Schmidt GA, Bowman A, Barr R, McCallister KE, Hall JB, Kress JP. Early physical and occupational therapy in mechanically ventilated, critically ill patients: a randomised controlled trial. Lancet. 2009;373:1874–82.

Selnes OA, Grega MA, Borowicz LM Jr, Barry S, Zeger S, Baumgartner WA, McKhann GM. Cognitive outcomes three years after coronary artery bypass surgery: a comparison of on-pump coronary artery bypass graft surgery and nonsurgical controls. Ann Thorac Surg. 2005;79:1201–9.

Selnes OA, McKhann GM. Neurocognitive complications after coronary artery bypass surgery. Ann Neurol. 2005;57:615–21.

Serafim RB, Bozza FA, Soares M, do Brasil PE, Tura BR, Ely EW, Salluh JI. Pharmacologic prevention and treatment of delirium in intensive care patients: a systematic review. J Crit Care. 2015;30:799–807.

Sheehy AM, Coursin DB, Keegan MT. Risks of tight glycemic control during adult cardiac surgery. Ann Thorac Surg. 2009;88:1384–5; author reply 1385–1386

Shehabi Y, Riker RR, Bokesch PM, Wisemandle W, Shintani A, Ely EW. Delirium duration and mortality in lightly sedated, mechanically ventilated intensive care patients. Crit Care Med. 2010;38:2311–8.

Siddiqi N, Harrison JK, Clegg A, Teale EA, Young J, Taylor J, Simpkins SA. Interventions for preventing delirium in hospitalised non-ICU patients. Cochrane Database Syst Rev. 2016;3:Cd005563.

Smith PK. Predicting and preventing adverse neurologic outcomes with cardiac surgery. J Card Surg. 2006;21(Suppl 1):S15–9.

Sun X, Lindsay J, Monsein LH, Hill PC, Corso PJ. Silent brain injury after cardiac surgery: a review: cognitive dysfunction and magnetic resonance imaging diffusion-weighted imaging findings. J Am Coll Cardiol. 2012;60:791–7.

Teslyar P, Stock VM, Wilk CM, Camsari U, Ehrenreich MJ, Himelhoch S. Prophylaxis with antipsychotic medication reduces the risk of post-operative delirium in elderly patients: a meta-analysis. Psychosomatics. 2013;54:124–31.

van Dijk D, Spoor M, Hijman R, Nathoe HM, Borst C, Jansen EW, Grobbee DE, de Jaegere PP, Kalkman CJ. Cognitive and cardiac outcomes 5 years after off-pump vs on-pump coronary artery bypass graft surgery. JAMA. 2007;297:701–8.

Van Rompaey B, Elseviers MM, Schuurmans MJ, Shortridge-Baggett LM, Truijen S, Bossaert L. Risk factors for delirium in intensive care patients: a prospective cohort study. Crit Care. 2009;13:R77.

Zhang XY, Liu ZM, Wen SH, Li YS, Li Y, Yao X, Huang WQ, Liu KX. Dexmedetomidine administration before, but not after, ischemia attenuates intestinal injury induced by intestinal ischemia-reperfusion in rats. Anesthesiology. 2012;116:1035–46.

Zheng HSA, Yahiaoui-Doktor M, Meissner W, Van Aken H, Zahn P, Pogatzki-Zahn E. Age and preoperative pain are major confounders for sex differences in postoperative pain outcome: a prospective database analysis. PLoS One. 2017;12:e0178659.

Infectious Diseases and Management After Cardiac Surgery

13

Antonio Hernandez Conte and Elizabeth Behringer

Abstract

The development of infectious diseases and/or inflammatory-related complications in postoperative cardiac surgical patient represents a diverse and complex array of clinical scenarios that may impact and complicate the hospital course of this patient population. Infectious diseases are different from other coexisting medical conditions in several respects. First, patients may have coexisting infectious diseases that may impact perioperative care when they come for surgery—these infections may be manifest or occult. Preexisting infectious diseases may be the reason for the surgery or may alter the risks associated with the surgery. Second, every patient undergoing surgery is at risk of acquiring an infectious disease during the perioperative period. Patients undergoing surgery are vulnerable to infection both at the surgical site and where natural defenses are breached, such as the respiratory tract, urinary tract, bloodstream, and sites of invasive monitoring. Acquired infectious diseases can be passed on to other patients and to health professionals in the perioperative period, and healthcare workers themselves may serve as active agents in transmitting infectious diseases to patients.

A. H. Conte, M.D., M.B.A. (✉)
University of California, Irvine, School of Medicine, Orange, CA, USA

Department of Anesthesiology, Kaiser Permanente Los Angeles Medical Center, Los Angeles, CA, USA
e-mail: Antonio.Conte@kp.org

E. Behringer, M.D.
Department of Cardiac Surgical Intensive Care Unit, Kaiser Permanente Los Angeles Medical Center, Los Angeles, CA, USA

A. Dabbagh et al. (eds.), *Postoperative Critical Care for Adult Cardiac Surgical Patients*, https://doi.org/10.1007/978-3-319-75747-6_13

Keywords
Surgical site infections · Sternal wound infections · Bloodstream infections · Deep sternal wound infections · Catheter-related infections · *Clostridium difficile* infection · Infectious diseases in post-cardiac transplant recipients · *Mycobacterium chimaera* infection

13.1 Background

The development of infectious diseases and/or inflammatory-related complications in postoperative cardiac surgical patient represents a diverse and complex array of clinical scenarios that may impact and complicate the hospital course of this patient population. Infectious diseases are different from other coexisting medical conditions in several respects. First, patients may have coexisting infectious diseases that may impact perioperative care when they come for surgery—these infections may be manifest or occult. Preexisting infectious diseases may be the reason for the surgery or may alter the risks associated with the surgery. Second, every patient undergoing surgery is at risk of acquiring an infectious disease during the perioperative period. Patients undergoing surgery are vulnerable to infection both at the surgical site and where natural defenses are breached, such as the respiratory tract, urinary tract, bloodstream, and sites of invasive monitoring. Acquired infectious diseases can be passed on to other patients and to health professionals in the perioperative period, and healthcare workers themselves may serve as active agents in transmitting infectious diseases to patients.

13.2 Surgical Site Infections

13.2.1 Background

Surgical site infections (SSIs) have been the focus of much attention during the past 30 years, and the major emphasis has been on completely preventing the occurrence of surgery-related infections and their associated morbidity and mortality. In 2002, the Centers for Medicare and Medicaid Services (CMS), in collaboration with the Centers for Disease Control (CDC), implemented the national Surgical Infection Prevention Project (SIPP). The key measures being monitored by this project are (1) the proportion of patients who receive parenterally administered antibiotics within 1 h prior to incision (within 2 h for vancomycin and fluoroquinolones), (2) the proportion of patients who receive prophylactic antimicrobial therapy consistent with published guidelines, and (3) the proportion of patients whose prophylactic antibiotic is discontinued within 24 h after surgery.

Despite the implementation of numerous sets of drug and policy guidelines, SSIs continue to occur at a rate of 2–5% for extra-abdominal surgery and up to 20% for intra-abdominal surgery, and affect approximately 500,000 patients annually. SSIs are among the most common causes of nosocomial infection, accounting for

14–16% of all nosocomial infections in hospitalized patients. SSIs are a major source of morbidity and mortality, rendering patients 60% more likely to spend time in the intensive care unit (ICU), five times more likely to require hospital readmission, and twice as likely to die. A recent resurgence in SSIs may be attributable to bacterial resistance, increased implantation of prosthetic and foreign materials, as well as poor immune status of many patients undergoing surgery. The universal adoption of simple measures, including frequent hand washing and appropriate administration of prophylactic antibiotics, has been emphasized as a method of decreasing the incidence of SSIs.

SSIs are divided into superficial infections (involving skin and subcutaneous tissues), deep infections (involving fascial and muscle layers), and infections of organs or tissue spaces (any area opened or manipulated during surgery). *S. aureus,* including methicillin-resistant *S. aureus,* is the predominant cause of SSIs. The increased proportion of SSIs caused by resistant pathogens and *Candida* species may reflect the increasing numbers of severely ill and immunocompromised surgical patients and the impact of widespread use of broad-spectrum antimicrobial drugs.

13.2.2 Risk Factors for Surgical Site Infections

The risk of developing an SSI is affected by patient-related, microbe-related, and wound-related factors. Patient-related factors include chronic illness, extremes of age, baseline immunocompetence or inherent/acquired immunocompromised, diabetes mellitus, and corticosteroid therapy. These factors are associated with an increased risk of developing an SSI.

Devitalized tissue, dead space, and hematomas are wound-related features associated with the development of SSIs. Historically, wounds have been described as *clean, contaminated,* and *dirty* according to the expected number of bacteria entering the surgical site. The presence of a foreign body (i.e., sutures or mesh) reduces the number of organisms required to induce an SSI. Interestingly, the implantation of major devices such as prosthetic joints and cardiac devices is not associated with a higher risk of SSIs. Risk factors for SSI are summarized in Table 13.1.

Table 13.1 Risk factors for surgical site infection (SSI)

Patient-related factors	Microbial factors	Wound-related factors
Extremes of age	Enzyme production	Devitalized tissue
Poor nutritional status	Polysaccharide capsule	Dead space
American Society of Anesthesiologists physical status score > 2	Ability to bind to fibronectin	Hematoma
Diabetes mellitus	Biofilm and slime formation	Contaminated surgery
Smoking		Presence of foreign material
Obesity		
Coexisting infections		
Colonization		
Immunocompromise		
Longer preoperative hospital stay		

Table 13.2 Criteria for diagnosis of a surgical site infection (SSI)

Type of SSI	Time course	Criteria (at least one must be present)
Superficial incisional SSI	Within 30 days of surgery	Superficial pus drainage
		Organisms cultured from superficial tissue or fluid
		Signs and symptoms (pain, redness, swelling, heat)
Deep incisional SSI	Within 30 days of surgery or within 1 year if prosthetic implant present	Deep pus drainage
		Dehiscence or wound opened by surgeon (for temperature > 38 ° C, pain, tenderness)
		Abscess (e.g., radiographically diagnosed)
Organ/space SSI	Within 30 days of surgery or within 1 year if prosthetic implant present	Pus from a drain in the organ/space
		Organisms cultured from aseptically obtained specimen of fluid or tissue in the organ/space
		Abscess involving the organ/space

13.2.3 Signs and Symptoms of SSIs

SSIs typically present within 30 days of surgery with localized inflammation of the surgical site and evidence of poor wound healing. Systemic features of infection, such as fever and malaise, may occur soon thereafter.

13.2.4 Diagnosis of SSIs

There may be nonspecific evidence of infection, such as an elevated white blood cell count, poor blood glucose control, and elevated levels of inflammatory markers, such as C-reactive protein. However, surgery is a great confounder, because surgery itself causes inflammation and thus renders surrogate markers of infection less reliable. Purulence at the wound sight is highly suggestive of infection. The gold standard in documenting a wound infection is growth of organisms in an aseptically obtained culture specimen. Approximately one-third of organisms cultured are staphylococci (*Staphylococcus aureus* and *Staphylococcus epidermidis*), *Enterococcus* species makes up more than 10%, and *Enterobacteriaceae* make up the bulk of the remaining culprits. Table 13.2 lists the criteria for diagnosing a SSI.

13.2.5 Preoperative Management

Active infections should be treated aggressively before surgery, and when possible surgery should be postponed until infection has resolved. If a localized area of infection is present at the intended surgical site, surgery should be postponed until the localized infection is treated and/or resolves spontaneously. If a patient has clinical evidence of infection, such as fever, chills, or malaise, efforts should be made to identify the source of the infectious process. Several studies have shown that smoking may increase not only the incidence of respiratory tract infection but also the incidence of wound infections. Preoperative cessation of smoking for 4–8 weeks before orthopedic surgery decreases the incidence of wound-related complications. Significant preoperative alcohol consumption may result in generalized immunocompromise. One month of preoperative alcohol abstinence reduces postoperative morbidity in alcohol users.

Diabetes mellitus is an independent risk factor for infection, and optimization of preoperative diabetes treatment may decrease perioperative infection. Malnutrition, whether manifesting as cachexia or obesity, is associated with an increased perioperative infection rate. Appropriate diet and/or weight loss may be beneficial before major surgery.

Staphylococcus aureus is the organism most commonly implicated in SSIs, and many individuals are carriers of *S. aureus* in the anterior nares. This carrier state has been identified as a risk factor for *S. aureus* wound infections. Topical mupirocin applied to the anterior nares has been successful in eliminating *S. aureus* and decreasing the risk of infection. However, there is concern that this practice may promote development of mupirocin-resistant *S. aureus.* Active surveillance programs to eliminate nasal colonization in hospital surgical personnel have controlled outbreaks of *S. aureus* SSIs and should be instituted as part of assertive infection control initiatives.

Hair clipping at the planned surgical site is acceptable, but shaving increases the risk of SSI, presumably due to microcuts serving as entry portals for microorganisms. Hair clipping should be performed with surgical razor devices (i.e., 3M™ Surgical Clippers). Preoperative skin cleansing with chlorhexidine has been shown to reduce the incidence of SSIs.

13.2.6 Intraoperative Management

It was recognized many years ago that prophylactic administration of antimicrobial agents prevents postoperative wound infections. This is particularly true when the procedure involves insertion of an artificial implant such as a heart valve or vascular graft. The organisms that are implicated in SSIs are usually those that are carried by the patient in the nose or on the skin. Unless the patient has been in the hospital for some time before surgery, these are usually community organisms that have not developed multiple drug resistance.

Timing of antibiotic prophylaxis (within 1 h prior to surgical incision) is important, since these organisms are introduced into the bloodstream at the time of incision. For cardiac surgery, the Joint Commission (formerly the Joint Commission on Accreditation of Healthcare Organizations) has recommended that the duration of prophylaxis be increased to 48 h, and dosing should occur every 4 h. A first-generation cephalosporin such as cefazolin is effective for many types of surgery. In general, the cephalosporins are effective against a wide spectrum of bacteria, possess a low incidence of side effects, and their tolerability makes them an ideal choice for surgical site infection prophylaxis. For high-risk patients and procedures, the selection of another appropriate antibiotic plays a critical role in decreasing the incidence of SSIs.

13.3 Deep Sternal Wound Infections

13.3.1 Etiology and Risk Factors

Deep sternal wound infection (DSWI) is a common complication after cardiac surgery with a reported incidence between 1 and 5% and is associated with a high mortality rate. DSWI is defined as one or more of the following: (1) deep sternal infection, which involves muscle and bone, with or without mediastinal involvement, as demonstrated by surgical exploration, with wound debridement and positive culture, or treatment with antibiotics, or (2) readmission within 30 days of surgery for DSWI. Despite the advances in detection and treatment with broad-spectrum antibiotic regimens, mortality remains high with a range of 10–20%. Microorganisms typically associated with DSWI include *Staphylococcus aureus, Staphylococcus epidermidis, Staphylococcus aureus, Acinetobacter, Pseudomonas, and Enterobacter.* The occurrence of DSWI is a reportable event and is tracked by state health regulatory agencies in the United States.

In a recent Australian study, there were 153 cases (1.3%) of DSWI reported from a total 11,848 cardiac surgical procedures. 78 cases (51%) required readmission for DSWI after the initial discharge, 70 of which had not been diagnosed during the first admission. The 30-day mortality rate from DSWI was 2.6%, and the overall mortality rate was 6.5%, which represented 2.2% of deaths. Significant preoperative risk factors associated with DSWI included diabetes, preoperative dialysis, respiratory disease, body mass index >25 kg/m^2, and angina CCS Class 3 or 4. The intraoperative factors were use of a ventricular assist device, cardiac transplantation, and a procedure involving the use of both internal thoracic arteries. In comparison to isolated CABG, valve procedures carried a higher risk of DSWI. Several studies have demonstrated that continuous intravenous insulin infusion decreases the risk of DSWI in diabetics.

Another study undertaken in Japan from 2004 to 2009 utilized the Japan Adult Cardiovascular Surgery Database. The authors found that the overall incidence of postoperative DSWI was 1.8%. The 30-day and operative mortality in patients with DSWI was higher after more complicated operative procedures. The incidence of re-exploration for bleeding in DSWI cases was 11.1%. Diabetes was a significant risk factor related to DSWI for all surgical groups.

Overall, 11 independent risk factors are associated with the development of DSWI. These risk factors could be divided into two groups: *patient related* (diabetes, obesity, prior myocardial infarction, chronic obstructive pulmonary disease, and aortic calcification) and *procedure related* (combined valve/CABG procedures, aortic surgery, CPB time, re-exploration for bleeding, respiratory failure, use of bilateral internal mammary artery). While hand hygiene by healthcare workers will continue to be an important step in preventing transmission of organisms, current data suggests that the patient's endogenous nasal and skin flora may pose a more significant risk for the development of DSWI. This is one potential target for a strategy to decrease the incidence of SSIs after cardiac surgery.

13.3.2 Prevention of Deep Sternal Wound Infections

Unfortunately, many of the associated risk factors associated with DSWI are not preventable. However, some factors are modifiable and their impact can be minimized. Strict glucose control in the perioperative period has been shown to decrease the incidence of surgical site infections, including DSWI. Insulin bolus and/or continuous infusions should attempt to achieve a glucose level between 80 and 120 mg/dL throughout the perioperative period.

In the United States and Europe, the primary pathogen in DSWIs is *S. aureus*. The anterior nares are the reservoir for Staphylococci which colonize the skin and lead to surgical site infections (SSIs). Given these facts, eradication of *S. aureus* from the nasal reservoir of patients would seem to be intuitively helpful. Mupirocin is a topical antibiotic structurally unlike any other antibiotic in clinical use. The nasal application of mupirocin is 91–100% effective in the short-term eradication of *S. aureus* and while *S. aureus* will repopulate the nasal flora this takes up to 22 weeks in 56% of patients. Additionally, mupirocin is also active against methicillin-resistant *S. aureus*. Reports from two institutions have now shown a benefit of mupirocin in preventing DSWIs.

Chlorhexidine can also be used to reduce staphylococcal colonization on the skin. Preoperative bathing or showering using 4% chlorhexidine gluconate has been shown to significantly reduce microbial counts on the skin. However, a meta-analysis comparing the efficacy of preoperative showering or bathing with chlorhexidine to other wash products in reducing surgical site infection in general surgery, vascular surgery, and urology patients failed to demonstrate a benefit. There has not been a randomized trial of this intervention in cardiac surgery patients. A theoretical advantage of using chlorhexidine is that in addition to reducing *Staphylococcus aureus* on the skin it also reduces coagulase-negative staphylococci and other microorganisms such as gram-negative bacteria. Studies have demonstrated that SSI rates after cardiac surgery have been successfully reduced through the use of chlorhexidine showers combined with nasal mupirocin compared to historical controls. Use of another skin cleanser 1% triclosan for whole-body washing preoperatively before cardiothoracic surgery in a patient population with a high methicillin-resistant *S. aureus* (MRSA) carriage rate (27%) significantly reduced MRSA SSIs. In an era of rising MRSA rates, this strategy merits further study.

Antibiotic prophylaxis to prevent SSIs has been discussed in the previous section; however, there are a few points particularly pertinent to cardiac surgery. As the most common pathogens isolated from sternal wound infections are the *Staphylococcus* species a first-generation cephalosporin (i.e., cefazolin) remains a clinically and cost-effective prophylactic antibiotic. Given the concern regarding methicillin-resistant *S. aureus* (MRSA), there has been discussion that vancomycin may be the prophylaxis of choice when a "cluster" of MRSA mediastinitis or incisional related SSI due to methicillin-resistant coagulase-negative staphylococci has been detected.

13.3.3 Treatment of Deep Sternal Wound Infections

DSWIs require immediate treatment upon detection. Established treatment includes institution of broad-spectrum antibiotics, sternal wound debridement, sternal wound drainage, open packing, and delayed closure of the sternal wound. Antibiotic treatment is targeted at cultured organisms and is instituted for an average of 6 weeks. A recent innovation in treatment involves the use of a vacuum-assisted closure (VAC) system in lieu of open packing.

A prospective study by Fuchs evaluated the effectiveness of utilizing vacuum-assisted closure system versus open packing for the treatment of DSWI. The authors found that baseline characteristics and a number of antibiotics did not differ between the two study groups; however, freedom from microbiological cultures was achieved earlier, C-reactive protein declined more rapidly, length of stay was shorter, sternal rewiring was performed earlier, and survival tended to be higher in the vacuum packing group compared to the open packing group.

13.4 Bloodstream Infections

Bloodstream infections (BSIs) are among the top three nosocomial infections. Anesthesiologists may play an important role in the prevention and often the treatment of BSIs. Central venous catheters are the major cause of nosocomial bacteremia and fungemia. Catheter-related bloodstream infections are common, costly, and potentially lethal. These infections are monitored by the National Nosocomial Infections Surveillance (NNIS) System of the CDC. A total of 80,000 cases of central venous catheter-associated BSI are estimated to occur annually in the United States, and the attributable mortality risk is estimated to be 12–25% for each infection. The NNIS System recommends that the rate of catheter-associated BSIs be expressed as the number of catheter-associated BSIs per 1000 days of central venous catheter exposure.

13.4.1 Signs and Symptoms

Patients typically have nonspecific signs of infection with no obvious source. There is no cloudy urine, purulent sputum, pus drainage, or wound inflammation. There is only an indwelling catheter. Inflammation at the catheter insertion site is suggestive. A sudden change in a patient's condition, such as mental status changes, hemodynamic instability, altered tolerance for nutrition, and generalized malaise, can indicate a BSI.

13.4.2 Diagnosis

Catheter-associated BSIs are defined as bacteremia or fungemia in a patient with an intravascular catheter with at least one blood culture positive for a recognized pathogen not related to another separate infection, clinical manifestations of infection, and no other apparent source for the BSI except the catheter. BSIs are considered to be associated with a central line if the line was in use during the 48-h period before the development of the BSI. If the time interval between the onset of infection and device use is longer than 48 h, then other sources of infection must be considered. The diagnosis is more compelling if, after catheter removal, the same organisms that grew in the blood culture grow from the catheter tip.

13.4.3 Prevention of Central Venous Catheter-Related Infections

Many central venous catheters are placed by anesthesiologists who may not be informed or aware about BSIs that develop days later. Preventing BSIs related to central venous catheters can be minimized by implementing a series of evidence-based steps shown to reduce catheter-related infection. A recent interventional study targeted *five* evidence-based procedures recommended by the CDC and identified as having the greatest effect in reducing the rate of catheter-related BSIs and the fewest barriers to implementation. The five interventions are (1) hand washing with soap and water or an alcohol cleanser before catheter insertion or maintenance, (2) using full-barrier precautions (hat, mask, and sterile gown, sterile area covering) during central venous catheter insertion, (3) cleaning the skin with chlorhexidine, (4) avoiding the femoral site and peripheral arms if possible, and (5) conducting routine daily inspection of catheters and removing them as soon as they are deemed unnecessary. In this study, use of these evidence-based interventions resulted in a large and sustained reduction (up to 66%) in rates of catheter-related BSIs that was maintained throughout the 18-month study period.

The subclavian and internal jugular venous routes carry less risk of infection than the femoral route, but the decision regarding anatomic location also has to consider the higher risk of pneumothorax with a subclavian catheter. During insertion, catheter contamination rates can be further reduced by rinsing gloved hands in a solution of chlorhexidine in alcohol before handling the catheter. Sterility must be maintained with frequent hand decontamination and cleaning of catheter ports with alcohol before accessing them. The same high standards of sterility should be applied with regional anesthetic catheters. Central venous catheters may be coated or impregnated with antimicrobial or antiseptic agents. These catheters have been associated with a lower incidence of BSIs. Concerns about widespread adoption of drug-impregnated catheters center on increased costs and promotion of antimicrobial resistance. However, use of such catheters may be indicated for the most vulnerable patients, such as those with severe immunocompromise.

13.4.4 Treatment and Postoperative Measures

The best "treatment" of central venous catheter-related BSIs is *prevention*. However, if infection is suspected, the source of the infection should be removed as soon as possible and broad-spectrum antimicrobial therapy should be initiated. Once culture results are available, antibiotic therapy can be targeted to the specific organism.

Because of antibiotic resistance patterns, it is difficult to strike a compromise between providing appropriate initial empirical coverage and not exhausting the last-line antimicrobial agents with the first salvo of antibiotic therapy. Treatment of patients with BSIs is similar to treatment of patients with sepsis.

Several postoperative management strategies can decrease the incidence of catheter-related BSI: (1) removal of central lines and pulmonary artery catheters as soon as possible, and (2) avoidance of unnecessary parenteral nutrition and even administration of dextrose-containing fluid, since these may be associated with an increased risk of BSI. Food and glucose can usually be withheld for a short period or delivered into the gut rather than into a vein.

13.5 *Clostridium difficile* Infection

13.5.1 Background

C. difficile is an anaerobic, gram-positive, spore-forming bacterium that is the major identifiable cause of antibiotic-associated diarrhea and pseudomembranous colitis. It is clear today that most antibiotics can alter bowel flora facilitating the growth of *C. difficile.* With the frequent use of broad-spectrum antibiotics, the incidence of *C. difficile* diarrhea has risen dramatically.

C. difficile infection is also the most common cause of diarrhea in healthcare settings, resulting in increased hospital stays and higher morbidity and mortality among patients. The prevalence of asymptomatic colonization in the hospital, especially in older people, is more than 20%. *C. difficile* is extremely hardy, can survive in the environment for prolonged periods of time, and is resistant to common disinfectants, which leads to transmission from contaminated surfaces and airborne spores. In approximately one-third of those colonized, *C. difficile* produces toxins that cause diarrhea. The two principal toxins are toxin A and toxin B. Toxin B is approximately 1000 times more cytotoxic than toxin A. Toxin A activates macrophages and mast cells. Activation of these cells causes the production of inflammatory mediators, which leads to fluid secretion and increased mucosal permeability. Toxin A is also an enterotoxin in that it loosens the tight junctions between the epithelial cells that line the colon, which helps toxin B enter into epithelial cells.

13.5.2 Risk Factors for C. *difficile* Infection

A number of risk factors for *C. difficile*-associated diarrhea have been identified: advanced age, severe underlying disease, gastrointestinal surgery, presence of a nasogastric tube, use of antiulcer medications, admission to an ICU, long duration of hospital stay, long duration of antibiotic administration (risk doubles after 3 days), use of multiple antibiotics, immunosuppressive therapy or general immunocompromise, recent surgery, and sharing of a hospital room with a *C. difficile*-infected patient.

13.5.3 Signs and Symptoms of *C. difficile* Infection

The most frequent symptoms of *C. difficile* infection are diarrhea and abdominal pain. Patients may be febrile with abdominal tenderness and distention. With perforation, patients may have an acute abdomen.

13.5.4 Diagnosis of *C. difficile* Infection

The gold standard for diagnosis of *C. difficile* infection is detection of *C. difficile* via enzyme-linked immunoassay for *C. difficile* toxins A and B in stool.

13.5.5 Treatment and Management of *C. difficile* Infection

Therapy for patients with *C. difficile*-associated diarrhea consists of fluid and electrolyte replacement, withdrawal of current antibiotic therapy if possible, and institution of targeted antibiotic treatment to eradicate *C. difficile.* Antibiotic treatment should be given orally, if possible. The first-line regimen is oral metronidazole 400 mg three times daily. An alternative is oral vancomycin 125 mg four times daily. Vancomycin has a theoretical advantage over metronidazole, since it is not well absorbed and may therefore reach the site of infection better. The major downside to vancomycin is that it may promote the growth of vancomycin-resistant enterococci.

Additional therapies may include probiotics such as *Saccharomyces boulardii* and *Lactobacillus rhamnosus.* These may be useful in restoring normal bowel flora.

It is typically the most severely ill patients with *C. difficile* colitis, including those whose infection does not improve with conventional therapy, who come for surgery such as subtotal colectomy and ileostomy. If a patient infected with *C. difficile* is in hemodynamically unstable condition, major surgery should be deferred and an ileostomy, cecostomy, or colostomy performed as a temporizing intervention; cardiac surgery is associated with high mortality. Resuscitation and preoperative treatment of metabolic derangements may be beneficial. Patients with *C. difficile* infection should be scheduled for surgery at the end of the surgical day so that the operating room can undergo additional cleaning to minimize the risk of transmission to subsequent patients.

13.5.6 Prognosis

C. difficile infection accounts for considerable increases in length of hospital stay and more than $1.1 billion in healthcare costs each year in the United States. The condition is a common cause of significant morbidity and even death in elderly, debilitated, and immunocompromised patients.

13.6 Infectious Diseases in Cardiac Transplant Recipients

13.6.1 Background

Each year, over 16,000 patients in the United States receive solid-organ transplants, and approximately 2500 patients received cardiac transplants. Because of advances in surgical technique, immunosuppressive therapy, and medical management, this patient population has a 1-year survival rate of 80–90%. To prevent allograft rejection, solid-organ transplant recipients commonly receive a combination of immunosuppressive agents. The mechanisms of action of immunosuppressants include blunting of general antibody responses, depression of cell-mediated immunity, downmodulation of lymphocyte and macrophage function, inhibition of cell proliferation, blocking of T-cell activation, and depletion of T-cells. Regardless of the effect, immunosuppression is variable and depends on dosage, duration of therapy, and time since transplantation. Immunosuppression is most intense in the first few months immediately after transplantation and becomes progressively less intense as immunosuppressive therapy is gradually withdrawn over time.

Immunosuppression in transplant recipients can also be affected by metabolic abnormalities, damage to mucocutaneous barriers, foreign bodies that interrupt these barriers (such as surgical incisions, chest tubes, biliary drains, endotracheal tubes, urinary catheters), and possible presence of immunomodulating viruses such as cytomegalovirus and HIV. Therefore, the resultant state of immunosuppression in the posttransplantation patient is a dynamic condition that impacts the development of infectious diseases and/or cancer.

13.6.2 Infectious Disease Occurrence

The best approach to infection control in the cardiac transplant recipient is prevention. If prevention is not possible, immediate diagnosis and treatment are essential. The challenges in managing infectious diseases in organ transplant recipients are many and include the following: (1) the spectrum of infective organisms is diverse and unusual, (2) the inflammatory response is blunted because of immunosuppressive therapy so that clinical and radiologic findings may be limited, and (3) antimicrobial coverage is complex and typically empirically based. There are three major time periods during which specific infectious disease processes occur in the posttransplantation patient: the first month, the second through sixth months, and beyond the sixth month after transplantation. In addition, these periods may be influenced by surgical factors, net level of immunosuppression present, and environmental exposures. Defining the time period after transplantation will assist the clinician in determining likely infectious processes.

During the first month after transplantation, active infections can be harbored within the allograft and are typically bacterial or fungal. In addition, anatomic defects related to surgery must be addressed if they foster infection, such as devitalized tissue and undrained fluid collections that are at high risk for microbial seeding. The only common viral infection during the first month after transplantation is reactivated herpes simplex virus infection in individuals positive for this virus before transplantation.

The period from the second through the sixth month after transplantation may be marked by unusual infections. These may be either community-acquired or opportunistic infections. Opportunistic pathogens possess very little virulence in healthy hosts, but can cause serious infections in patients with immunocompromise or immune defects. Trimethoprim-sulfamethoxazole is commonly given as prophylaxis for *Pneumocystis* pneumonia during the first 6 months after transplantation in all solid-organ graft recipients and for longer periods in heart- and lung-transplant recipients. In addition, high-dose immunosuppression may lead to reactivation disease syndromes caused by organisms present in the recipient before transplantation. TB has become especially common and occurs in 1% of the posttransplant population.

From 6 months after transplantation onward, most transplant recipients do fairly well from an infectious disease standpoint and usually only sustain infections paralleling those seen in the community at large. However, another group of patients may have chronic or progressive viral infections with hepatitis B virus, hepatitis C virus, cytomegalovirus, or Epstein-Barr virus. The most commonly occurring viral infection is varicella-zoster virus infection manifesting as herpes zoster.

Patients with chronic or recurrent rejection are generally taking high dosages of immunosuppressants and are predisposed to acquiring the opportunistic infections typically seen in posttransplantation patients during the second to sixth months. In addition, posttransplantation patients with HIV and/or AIDS must be more closely followed for evidence of infections, both common and opportunistic. HIV highly active antiretroviral therapeutic regimens must be maintained and can complicate immunosuppressive drug dosing.

13.7 *Mycobacterium chimaera* Infection

13.7.1 Background

Mycobacterium chimera, a non-tuberculosis strain usually found in soil and water, has been reported as an invasive, possibly iatrogenic cause of infection in patients who underwent cardiac surgery from 2005 to 2016. In 2015, the first reported clusters of cases were identified in Sweden and Pennsylvania, USA, in patients who had undergone open-heart surgery. The source of infection is presumed to be secondary to exposure during cardiopulmonary bypass with use of in-line heater-cooler unit (Stöckert 3T, LivaNova PLC—formerly Sorin Group Deutschland GmbH).

The results of field investigations in each respective county prompted notification of potentially exposed patients who underwent cardiac surgery during the specified time frame. Although heater-cooler devices are used to regulate patients' blood temperature during cardiopulmonary bypass through water circuits that are closed, these reports suggest that aerosolized *M. chimaera* from the devices resulted in the invasive infections. The United States Food and Drug Administration (FDA) and Centers for Disease Control (CDC) have issued alerts regarding the need to follow updated manufacturer's instructions for use of the devices, evaluate the devices for contamination, remain vigilant for new infections, and continue to monitor reports from the United States and overseas.

The CDC-performed whole-genome sequencing was completed on isolates from 11 patients and from 5 Stöckert 3T heater-cooler devices from hospitals in Pennsylvania and Iowa, two of the states where clusters of infections were identified. Samples from heater-cooler devices included swabs from the interior of the device, water drained from the devices, and air samples collected while a device was operating. Single-nucleotide polymorphisms (SNPs) were identified after comparing patient and device samples against sequence data from an *M. chimaera* reference isolate. These results strongly suggest a point-source contamination of Stöckert 3T heater-cooler devices with *M. chimaera*. A recent report from Germany noted that preliminary typing results of *M. chimaera* from heater-cooler devices from three different European countries were almost identical to samples obtained from the manufacturing site, further supporting the likelihood of point-source contamination.

Whole-genome sequencing confirms that this is a common-source outbreak, with nearly identical isolates found in Stöckert 3T heater-cooler units and patients from multiple countries. It is therefore likely that most Stöckert 3T heater-cooler units manufactured over the past decade are contaminated with the same *M. chimaera* strain, and that these contaminated Stöckert 3T heater-cooler units have been and continue to be used globally.

13.7.2 Prevention and Surveillance

Since the identification of the *M. chimaera* infections, most centers performing cardiac surgery have removed the Stöckert 2T heater-cooler device as it has been implicated as the cause for the infection outbreak. Although thousands of patients in the United States have been notified regarding potential exposure to contaminated heater-cooler devices, the number who were exposed might be much larger. Over 250,000 procedures using cardiopulmonary bypass are performed in the United States each year; Stöckert 3T heater-cooler devices represent approximately 60% of the US market. The CDC and FDA are continuing efforts to increase provider and patient awareness of the risk.

The CDC is working closely with each hospital reporting outbreaks and has formed *M. chimaera* multidisciplinary working groups. Each respective institution has issued guidance on identifying patients at risk to ensure timely diagnosis and treatment of these indolent and often unrecognized infections. FDA is continuing to gather information, issue communications, and assess the situation from both public health and regulatory perspectives. Institutional surveillance has consisted of notification to each patient who has undergone heart surgery with cardiopulmonary bypass between 2012 and 2016 with additional notations of surveillance in electronic medical records when possible.

13.7.3 Signs, Symptoms, and Diagnosis

The relatively low virulence and slow growth of *M. chimaera* present major challenges for case identification. Patients with disseminated *M. chimaera* infection contracted via contaminated 3T heater-cooler can present months to years after cardiac surgery with endocarditis and even disseminated infection. Therefore, the timeline for *M. chimaera* disease surveillance must extend at least 2–6 years after cardiac surgery.

Part of the difficulty in identifying a potential *M. chimaera* infection is that patients present with nonspecific symptoms and a variety of infection sites, and a culture for mycobacteria is usually not part of a routine diagnostic workup in patients presenting with signs of infection. Cases to date have presented with nonspecific symptoms, most commonly fatigue (90%), followed by fever (75%), sweats (60%), dyspnea (60%), weight loss (60%), and cough (50%).

Confirmation of *M. chimaera* diagnosis is via positive culture taken from site of infection—a potentially difficult task if the site is occult (i.e., cardiac graft site, bone). Histopathology demonstrates non-caseating granulomas in involved tissue, which are rarely smear positive for acid-fast bacteria (AFB). Identification of *M. chimaera* requires sequencing; therefore, non-sequencing methods may fail to identify the correct Mycobacterium species. Diagnosis has most often been made by AFB blood culture, though other sites (i.e., bone marrow) are sometimes culture positive in the setting of negative blood cultures, and polymerase chain reaction has also been valuable in some patients. The time for *M. chimaera* culture growth period is typically 6–8 weeks; therefore, diagnosis may be one of exclusion. Laboratory characteristics of disseminated *M. chimaera* include an elevated C-reactive protein; pan-negative conventional blood cultures, with anemia, lymphopenia, and thrombocytopenia; and elevated lactate dehydrogenase, creatinine, and transaminases.

13.7.4 Treatment

Optimal treatment of this infection has not been established, but typically involves combination antimicrobial therapy and, if possible, removal of involved prosthetic material. In many cases, unfortunately, the patient is too sick or the procedure too high risk for graft/valve/device explantation to be attempted, and there are no data available on the risk for reinfection of a newly placed device into the involved site. *M. chimaera* is typically treated with a prolonged course of clarithromycin, ethambutol, and rifampin.

13.7.5 Perioperative Recommendations

A multidisciplinary team of anesthesiologists, infectious disease physicians, infectious disease control nurses, microbiologists/pathologists, and cardiac surgeons should be established at each institution with any probable or confirmed outbreak of

M. chimaera. The team should work closely with the CDC to develop institutional specific guidelines for perioperative management.

Specific initiatives to treat the infected patient shield the disease from other patients and medical personnel, and meticulous cleaning regimens are ongoing and still in evolution. However, prudent infectious control processes should be put in place and may include the following:

- Patients infected with *M. chimaera* do not need contact isolation in the perioperative period.
- Continuation of *M. chimaera* antimycobacterials, as well as maintenance of usual antibiotics, is appropriate for antimicrobial prophylaxis and SSI prevention.
- Use of mycobactericidal disinfectant (not glutaraldehyde) is appropriate for cleaning operating room.
- Subsequent operations in the same operating room should have a minimum 30-min "washout" period where the room can sit idle after terminal cleaning prior to any subsequent case setup or provider activity.
- Anesthesia machine ventilator filters and carbon dioxide canister should be changed after each case.
- High-flow oxygen "washout" of anesthesia machine circuit should be performed.
- Specialized masks (i.e., N95) are not required during care of *M. chimaera*-infected patients.
- Standard/universal infection control processes should always be followed per institutional guidelines.

Bibliography

Bartlett JG. Narrative review: the new epidemic of Clostridium difficile—associated enteric disease Clostridium difficile–associated colitis. Ann Intern Med. 2006;145:758–64.

Bratzler DW, Hunt DR. The surgical infection prevention and surgical care improvement projects: national initiatives to improve outcomes for patients having surgery. Clin Infect Dis. 2006;43:322–30.

Burgess W, Margolis A, Gibbs S, Duarte RS, Jackson M. Disinfectant susceptibility profiling of glutaraldehyde-resistant nontuberculous mycobacteria. Infect Control Hosp Epidemiol. 2017;38(7):784–91.

Dellinger EP. Prophylactic antibiotics: administration and timing before operation are more important than administration after operation. Clin Infect Dis. 2007;44:929–30.

Dellinger RP, Carlet JM, Masur H, Gerlach H, Calandra T, Cohen J, Jea-Benacloche J, Keh D, Marshall JC, Parker MM, Ramsay G, Zimmerman JL, Vincent JL, Levy MM. Surviving sepsis campaign: guidelines for management of severe sepsis and shock. Intensive Care Med. 2008;34:17–60.

Furnary AP, Zerr KJ, Grunkemeier GL, Starr A. Continuous intravenous insulin infusion reduces the incidence of deep sternal wound infection in diabetic patients after cardiac surgical procedures. Ann Thorac Surg. 1999;67:352–60.

Haller S, Höller C, Jacobshagen A, Hamouda O, Sin MA, Monnet DL, Plachouras D, Eckmanns T. Contamination during production of heater-cooler units by Mycobacterium chimaera potential cause for invasive cardiovascular infections: results of an outbreak investigation in Germany, April 2015 to February 2016. Euro Surveill. 2016;21. https://doi.org/10.2807/1560-7917.ES.2016.21.17.30215.

Kohler P, Kuster SP, Bloemberg G, Schulthess B, Frank M, Tanner FC, Rössle M, Böni C, Falk V, Wilhelm MJ. Healthcare-associated prosthetic heart valve, aortic vascular graft, and disseminated *Mycobacterium chimaera* infections subsequent to open heart surgery. Eur Heart J. 2015;36:2745–53.

Kubota H, Miyata H, Motomura N, Ono M, Takamoto S, Harii K, Oura N, Hirabayashi S, Kyo S. Deep sternal wound infection after cardiac surgery. J Cardiothorac Surg. 2013;8:132.

Robinson PJ, Billah B, Leder K, Reid CM, Committee AD. Factors associated with deep sternal wound infection and haemorrhage following cardiac surgery in Victoria☆. Interact Cardiovasc Thorac Surg. 2007;6:167–71.

Sax H, Bloemberg G, Hasse B, Sommerstein R, Kohler P, Achermann Y, Rössle M, Falk V, Kuster SP, Böttger EC, Weber R. Prolonged outbreak of mycobacterium chimaera infection after open-chest heart surgery. Clin Infect Dis. 2015;61:67–75.

Toumpoulis IK, Anagnostopoulos CE, DeRose JJ, Swistel DG. The impact of deep sternal wound infection on long-term survival after coronary artery bypass grafting. Chest. 2005;127:464–71.

Postoperative Rhythm Disorders After Adult Cardiac Surgery

14

Majid Haghjoo

Abstract

New-onset arrhythmias are a common complication of cardiac surgery. Atrial fibrillation is the most common arrhythmia encountered postoperatively, although ventricular arrhythmias and conduction disturbances can also occur. Postoperative arrhythmias are an important cause of increased morbidity, prolonged hospitalization, and higher medical costs. Prophylactic pharmacological and non-pharmacological treatments are highly useful in avoiding these problems.

Keywords

Postoperative · Cardiac surgery · Rhythm disorder · Supraventricular · Ventricular · Bradycardia

Abbreviations

ACCF	American College of Cardiology Foundation
AF	Atrial fibrillation
AFL	Atrial flutter
AHA	American Heart Association
AT	Atrial tachycardia
AV	Atrioventricular
AVB	Atrioventricular block
BiA	Biatrial pacing

M. Haghjoo, M.D.
Department of Cardiac Electrophysiology, Rajaie Cardiovascular Medical and Research Center, Iran University of Medical Sciences, Tehran, Iran

A. Dabbagh et al. (eds.), *Postoperative Critical Care for Adult Cardiac Surgical Patients*, https://doi.org/10.1007/978-3-319-75747-6_14

CABG	Coronary artery bypass grafting
ESC	European Society of Cardiology
PVC	Premature ventricular complex
SND	Sinus node dysfunction
VA	Ventricular arrhythmia
VT	Ventricular tachycardia

New-onset arrhythmias are a common complication of cardiac surgery. Atrial fibrillation (AF) is the most common arrhythmia encountered postoperatively, although ventricular arrhythmias and conduction disturbances can also occur. Postoperative arrhythmias are an important cause of increased morbidity, prolonged hospitalization, and higher medical costs. Prophylactic pharmacological and non-pharmacological treatments are highly useful in avoiding these problems. This chapter discusses the incidence, prognosis, pathogenesis, preventive strategies, and management of these arrhythmias in adult patients undergoing cardiac surgery.

14.1 Supraventricular Tachyarrhythmias

14.1.1 Incidence and Prognosis

Supraventricular tachycardias are recognized as the most common arrhythmia to occur after coronary artery bypass grafting (CABG) with the reported incidence of 20–40% after CABG surgery (Creswell et al. 1993) and even higher following valvular surgery (Asher et al. 1998). AF (Fig. 14.1) and atrial flutter (AFL) (Fig. 14.2) are the most prevalent supraventricular arrhythmias; however, atrial tachycardias (AT) occurred as well. Most cases of AF occur between the second and fourth postoperative days (Almassi et al. 1997). Although this arrhythmia is usually benign and self-limiting, it may result in hemodynamic instability, thromboembolic events, a longer hospital stay, and increased healthcare costs (Hakala et al. 2002; Lahtinen et al. 2004).

14.1.2 Pathogenesis

The mechanism of postoperative AF is not well described and is probably multifactorial. It is suggested that endogenous adenosine, inflammation, and oxidative injury may play a mechanistic role in this arrhythmia (Yavuz et al. 2004; Chung et al. 2001; Korantzopoulos et al. 2006). The perioperative period is also characterized by acute ischemic reperfusion injury and delayed inflammatory response that together result in a net depletion at plasma antioxidants (De Vecchi et al. 1998). Furthermore,

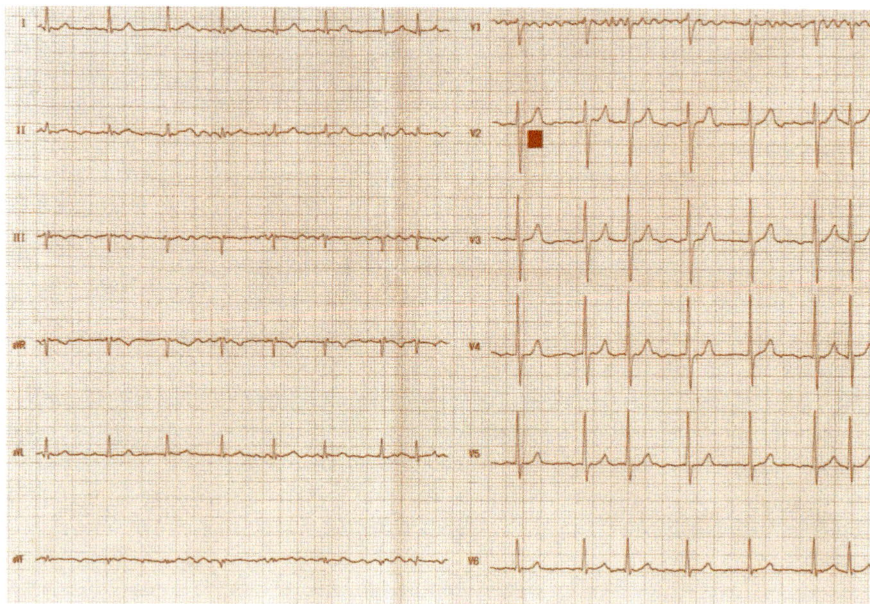

Fig. 14.1 This figure shows atrial fibrillation with undulating atrial activity and irregular ventricular response

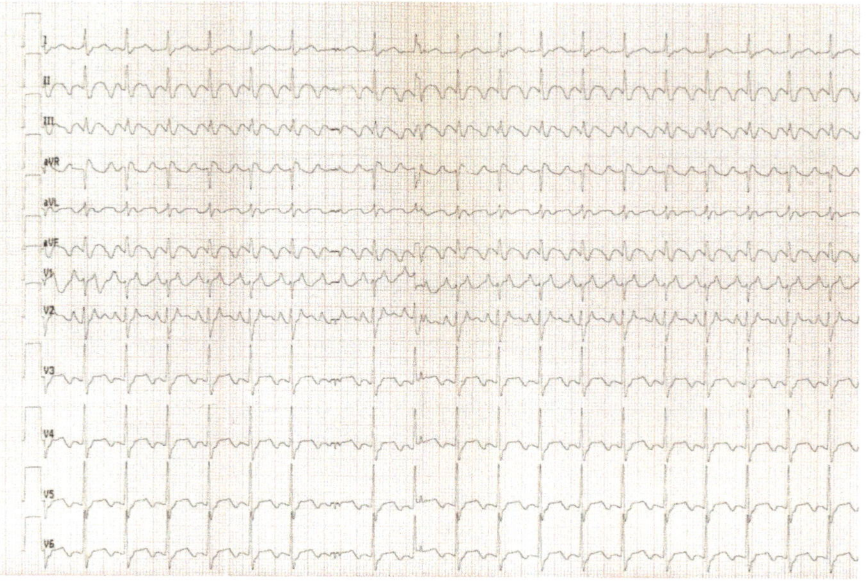

Fig. 14.2 A 12-lead electrocardiogram of atrial flutter was recorded after mitral valve replacement in a patient with severe mitral stenosis

patients undergoing cardiac surgery often have underlying atrial enlargement or increased atrial pressures that may predispose to AF. Age-related structural or electrophysiological changes also appear to lower the threshold for postoperative AF in elderly patients (Leitch et al. 1990). Other reported predisposing conditions for development of the postoperative AF included left main or proximal right coronary artery stenoses, chronic obstructive pulmonary disease, beta-blocker withdrawal, history of AF or heart failure, and preoperative electrocardiographic findings of PR interval of 185 ms or longer, P-wave duration of 110 ms or longer in lead V1, and left atrial abnormality (Passman et al. 2001; Amar et al. 2004).

Considering the peak incidence of AF in the first 2–3 days after surgery, inflammatory mechanisms have been suggested. The idea has also been supported by the efficacy of anti-inflammatory agents in decreasing the incidence of postoperative AF (Ho and Tan. 2009). However, there are other electrophysiological explanations for the higher incidence of AF in this period. Nonuniform atrial conduction is greatest on postoperative days 2 and 3, and longest atrial conduction is on day 3 (Ishii et al. 2005). Perioperative hypokalemia has been shown to be associated with postoperative AF partly via changes in atrial conduction and refractoriness (Wahr et al. 1999).

There are recent evidences indicating that minimally invasive cardiac surgery or surgery without cardiopulmonary bypass has been associated with lower incidence of postoperative AF. In a prospective randomized study, 200 patients were randomly assigned into on-pump CABG and off-pump CABG. The results of this study clearly indicated that postoperative AF occurs with lower frequency in patients who underwent off-pump beating heart surgery compared to those with on-pump CABG (Ascione et al. 2000).

14.1.3 Prophylaxis

Several pharmacological and non-pharmacological strategies have been employed to prevent postoperative AF after cardiac surgery. Efficacy of beta-blockers, amiodarone, sotalol, magnesium, and atrial pacing has been assessed in several randomized and nonrandomized clinical trials.

Because patients recovering from cardiac surgery often have enhanced sympathetic tone, the risk of postoperative AF is increased. Beta-blockers antagonize the effects of catecholamines on the myocardium and are, thus, expected to prevent AF after cardiac surgery. Multiple clinical trials and three landmark meta-analyses have shown a significant reduction in postoperative AF by beta-blocker prophylaxis in cardiac surgery patients (Crystal et al. 2002). Following these remarkable results, updated American Heart Association/American College of Cardiology Foundation (AHA/ACCF) 2006/2011 and recent European Society of Cardiology (ESC) 2010 guidelines recommended beta-blocker prophylaxis to prevent AF in cardiac surgery patients in the absence of contraindications (Fuster et al. 2011; Camm et al. 2010). Oral carvedilol, with its unique antioxidant and antiapoptotic properties, appears to be the most effective beta-blocker in the prevention of postoperative AF (Haghjoo et al. 2007). It has been demonstrated that both prophylactic oral and intravenous amiodarone are effective and safe agents in reducing the incidence of AF and its related cerebrovascular accident and postoperative ventricular tachyarrhythmia (Bagshaw et al. 2006). Currently, preoperative administration of amiodarone is deemed class IIa indication for prophylactic therapy in patients at high risk for postoperative AF in the latest AHA/ACCF and ESC guidelines for AF management (Fuster et al. 2011; Camm et al. 2010). Sotalol is a class III antiarrhythmic agent with potent beta-blocking activity. As a result, it would be a suitable drug for AF prevention after cardiac surgeries. Sotalol has been proven to be an effective agent across all the clinical trials using this drug (Pfisterer et al. 1997; Weber et al. 1998). Only issue is related to its safety profile.

Hypomagnesemia has been suggested as a cause of both supraventricular and ventricular tachycardias, and it is an independent risk factor for the development of AF in cardiac surgery patients. Therefore, it has been hypothesized that magnesium supplementation may reduce the incidence of AF after heart surgery. Several clinical trials have examined the use of intravenous magnesium sulfate for the prevention of AF after CABG (Fanning et al. 1991; Kaplan et al. 2003). A meta-analysis of eight identified randomized controlled trials revealed that the use of intravenous magnesium supplementation was associated with a significant reduction in the AF incidence after CABG (Alghamdi et al. 2005).

Overdrive atrial pacing may exert its preventive effect on postoperative AF by suppressing bradycardia-induced irregular heart rate, overdrive suppression of atrial premature beats, suppressing compensatory pauses after atrial premature beats, and resynchronizing atrial activation (Fan et al. 2003). Efficacy of right atrial, left atrial, and biatrial (BiA) pacing has been studied in several randomized studies (Archbold and Schilling 2004). It appears that BiA pacing is more effective than single-site pacing; be that as it may, available data do not permit a firm recommendation on the application of this intervention in a postoperative setting. Recently, the ESC 2010 guidelines on AF management considered BiA pacing as a class IIB recommendation for AF prevention after cardiac surgery (Camm et al. 2010). Latest AHA/ACCF and ESC recommendations for AF prevention in cardiac surgery are summarized in Table 14.1.

14.1.4 Management

Considering the self-limited course of the postoperative AF or AFL, treatment begins with pharmacological control of the heart rate (Table 14.2). Beta-blockers should be first-line agents for the rate control because of rapid onset of action and 50% likelihood of conversion to sinus rhythm. Both metoprolol and esmolol are available in intravenous (IV) formulation. Calcium-channel antagonists are less effective than beta-blockers and considered as second-line agents. Calcium-channel antagonists result in rate control of AF more rapidly than does digoxin. These latter agents may be useful when beta-blockers are contraindicated (i.e., bronchospasm).

Conversion of postoperative AF is not needed in the majority of patients after cardiac surgery because of high recurrence rate and self-limited nature. However,

Table 14.1 Recommendations for prevention of atrial fibrillation after cardiac surgery

Recommendation	Class	Level
Unless contraindicated, treatment with an oral beta-blocker to prevent postoperative AF is recommended for patients undergoing cardiac surgery	I	A
Preoperative administration of amiodarone reduces the incidence of AF in patients undergoing cardiac surgery and represents appropriate prophylactic therapy for patients at high risk for postoperative AF	IIa	A
Prophylactic administration of sotalol may be considered for patients at risk of developing AF following cardiac surgery	IIb	A
Biatrial pacing may be considered for prevention of AF after cardiac surgery	IIb	A
Corticosteroids may be considered in order to reduce the incidence of AF after cardiac surgery, but are associated with risk	IIb	B

Source: Camm et al. (2010) and Fuster et al. (2011)

Table 14.2 Antiarrhythmic medications used for rate and rhythm control in postoperative atrial fibrillation

Antiarrhythmic	Loading dose	Maintenance dose
Beta-blockers		
Esmolol	500 μg/kg IV over 1 min	50–200 μg/kg/min IV[a]
Metoprolol	5 mg IV every 5 min Max 15 mg	25–100 mg PO bid or tid
Propranolol	1 mg IV every 2–5 min Max 0.1–0.2 mg/kg	10–80 mg PO tid or qid
Calcium-channel antagonists		
Verapamil	5–10 mg IV over 1–2 min	5 μg/kg/min IV or 40–160 mg PO tid
Diltiazem	0.25 mg/kg IV over 2 min	5–15 mg/h IV or 30–90 mg PO qid
Digitalis		
Digoxin	0.25–0.5 mg IV, then 0.25 mg every 4–6 h Max 1 mg/day	0.125–0.25 mg/day

IV intravenous, *PO* orally, *bid* twice a day, *tid* three times a day, *qid* four times a day, *max* maximum

[a]After initial maintenance infusion, depending upon the desired ventricular response, the maintenance infusion may be continued at 50 μg/kg/min or increased stepwise to 100 μg/kg/min, 150 μg/kg/min, and finally to a maximum of 200 μg/kg/min with each step being maintained for 4 min

this approach may be useful in high-risk patients who are refractory to or intolerant of atrioventricular (AV) nodal blocking agents. Conversion of AF, AFL, and AT can be accomplished using electrical cardioversion, pharmacological cardioversion, and overdrive pacing (if AFL or AT present). Pharmacological cardioversion should be considered in the setting of unstable respiratory status or other contraindication for anesthesia. Drugs proven to be useful for cardioversion include procainamide, amiodarone, propafenone, ibutilide (VanderLugt et al. 1999), and dofetilide. Latter two agents carry a risk of torsades de pointes about 2–4%. This risk is higher in the setting of bradycardia, female gender, hypokalemia, and hypomagnesemia. Rapid atrial pacing using epicardial wires implanted during surgery was proved to be safe and effective in the conversion of postoperative AFL and AT. Rapid atrial pacing is highly desirable in the patients unsuitable for electrical cardioversion such as patients with chronic obstructive pulmonary disease. Electrical cardioversion is reserved for patients exhibiting acute hemodynamic instability. For elective cardioversion, anterior-posterior paddles are preferred with the posterior paddle placed at the lower tip of the scapula. It has been shown that there is a higher risk of stroke in cardiac surgery patients with AF. Accordingly, anticoagulation with heparin or oral anticoagulation is appropriate when AF persists longer than 48 h, as recommended for nonsurgical patients (Fuster et al. 2011). Recently, novel oral anticoagulants such as dabigatran, rivaroxaban, and apixaban are shown to be safe and effective in the prevention of thromboembolic events after cardiac surgery (Anderson et al. 2015). Duration of anticoagulation must be based on individual clinical situation.

14.2 Ventricular Tachyarrhythmias

14.2.1 Incidence and Prognosis

New-onset ventricular arrhythmias (VA) are uncommon after cardiac surgery (El-Chami et al. 2012). The highest incidence was observed between 3 and 5 post-operative days (Brembilla-Perrot et al. 2003). The prognosis of postoperative VAs is highly dependent on the type of arrhythmia and the severity of structural heart disease. Patients with simple premature ventricular complex (PVC) usually exhibit a benign prognosis (Huikuri et al. 1990). Complex ventricular arrhythmias, including frequent PVC and nonsustained ventricular tachycardia (VT), have no effect on short-term prognosis but predict a poor long-term prognosis if ventricular function is impaired (Smith et al. 1992; Pinto et al. 1996). The occurrence of sustained VT (Fig. 14.3) always predicts a poor short- and long-term prognosis (Tam et al. 1991). Traditionally, early (<48 h) postoperative VA was considered to have little if any long-term prognostic value and should be ignored after treating the acute episode. Recently, this traditional notion has been challenged by recent data indicating that VAs occurring within 48 h of cardiac surgery resulted in similar long-term outcomes as those occurring >48 h after surgery (El-Chami et al. 2012).

14.2.2 Pathogenesis

Etiologies for postoperative VAs include hemodynamic instability, electrolyte abnormalities, hypoxia, hypovolemia, ischemia and infarction, acute graft closure, reperfusion after cessation of cardiopulmonary bypass, and proarrhythmia caused by inotropic and antiarrhythmic drugs (Chung 2000).

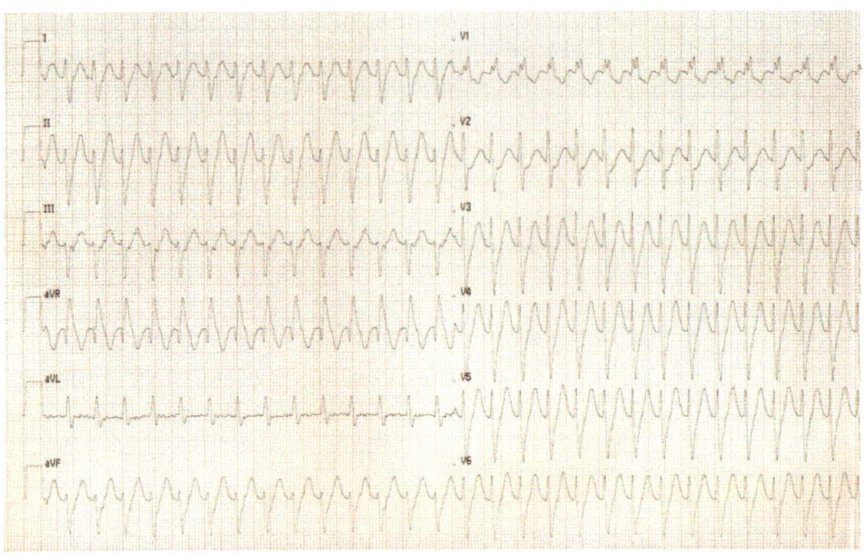

Fig. 14.3 A 12-lead electrocardiogram was recorded from a patient after coronary bypass surgery. This ECG shows wide QRS tachycardia with positive QRS complex in aVR, RBBB pattern with superior axis compatible with ventricular tachycardia

14.2.3 Prophylaxis

In contrast to atrial arrhythmia, there is no clear recommendation for prevention of VA after cardiac surgery. However, some measures such as correcting electrolyte/metabolic disturbance (especially potassium), volume replacement, better myocardial protection, and special attention to use of inotropic and antiarrhythmic drugs may be useful in reducing the incidence of postoperative VAs. In addition, it has been recently shown that off-pump surgery is protective against the VAs after cardiac surgery (El-Chami et al. 2012).

14.2.4 Management

Patients with asymptomatic and hemodynamically stable PVC and even short runs of nonsustained VT usually do not require any specific treatment. All reversible underlying causes should be corrected. In case of the symptomatic or hemodynamically significant PVC or nonsustained VT, lidocaine and overdrive pacing are recommended. For hemodynamically stable sustained VT, IV antiarrhythmic medication is the first-line treatment approach (Fogel and Prystowsky 2000). Dosages of common antiarrhythmic medications are listed in Table 14.3. Lidocaine is usually the first-choice drug and can be tried in dosage recommended in the nonsurgical setting. Procainamide is often the second choice. This drug should be used with caution or not at all in patients with renal dysfunction. In patients with left

Table 14.3 Antiarrhythmic medications for control of postoperative ventricular arrhythmia

Antiarrhythmic	Loading dose	Maintenance dose
Lidocaine	1–1.5 mg/kg up to 3 mg/kg in two divide dose 15 min apart	2–4 mg/min
Procainamide	20–50 mg/min up to 15 mg/kg	1–4 mg/min
Amiodarone	150 mg over 10 min, additional bolus of 150 mg for recurrent arrhythmia	1 mg/min for 6 h and 0.5 mg/min for 18 h

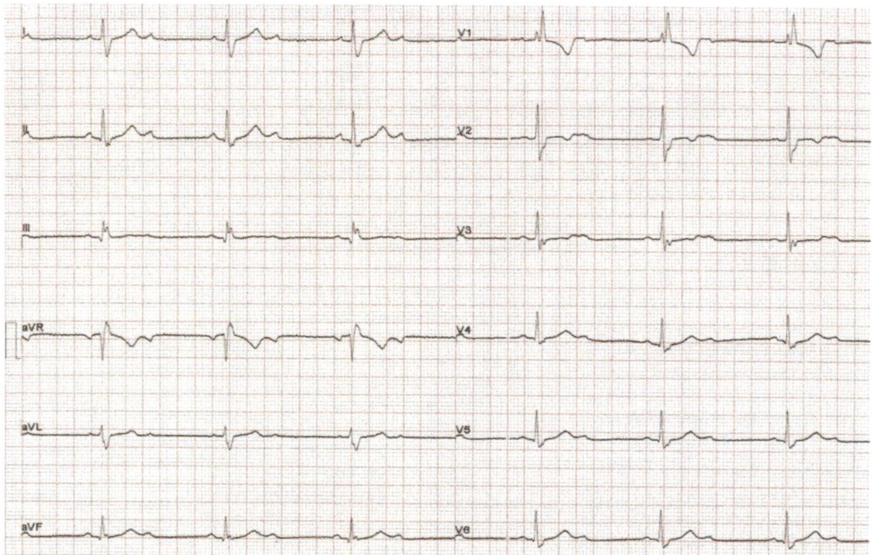

Fig. 14.4 This electrocardiogram was taken from a patient who recently underwent aortic valve replacement. Underlying rhythm is sinus with wide complex and 2:1 atrioventricular conduction

ventricular dysfunction, amiodarone is a better choice than other antiarrhythmics. In this group of the patients, overdrive ventricular pacing using epicardial wires placed at the time of surgery may be attempted. In patients with hemodynamically unstable or drug-refractory VT, electrical cardioversion or defibrillation with energy level of 200–360 J is recommended.

14.3 Bradyarrhythmias

14.3.1 Incidence and Prognosis

Bradyarrhythmias are a common complication following cardiac surgery. Permanent pacemaker is required for sinus node dysfunction (SND) or atrioventricular block (AVB) in 0.6–4.6% of patients after CABG (Goldman et al. 1984). Varying degrees of AVB (Figs. 14.4 and 14.5) are more common after valve replacement (up to 24%) than other types of cardiovascular surgery (Jaeger et al. 1994; Brodell et al. 1991).

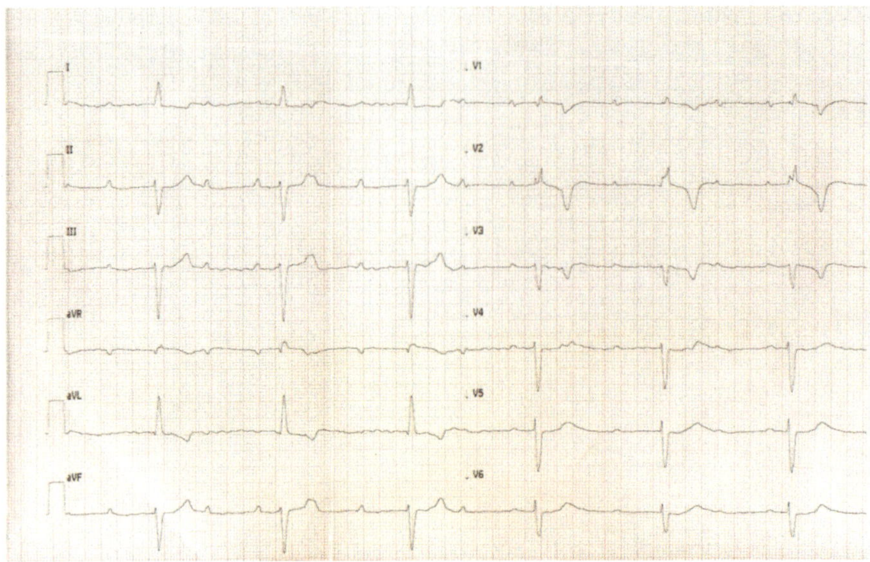

Fig. 14.5 This electrocardiogram showed complete atrioventricular block after multivalvular replacement

Bradyarrhythmia due to SND and to lesser extent AVB is relatively common after orthotopic heart transplantation and leads to permanent pacemaker implantation in up to 21% of patients with SND and 4.5% of patients with AVB (Grant et al. 1995). Improvement in postoperative bradyarrhythmia may occur in significant number of patients. Rate of recovery is less common after complete AVB than SND (Merin et al. 2009).

14.3.2 Pathogenesis

Postoperative bradyarrhythmias can be caused by incomplete washout of cardioplegia solution, antiarrhythmic drugs, or their toxicity. In addition, it may caused by trauma or surgical manipulation in the area of the AV node or bundle of His.

14.3.3 Prophylaxis

In order to reduce the incidence of postoperative conduction disorder, special attention to the anatomy of the conduction system, careful administration of sinus or AV nodal blocking agents, and complete washout of cardioplegia solution are warranted.

14.3.4 Management

According to American College of Cardiology/American Heart Association guidelines "permanent pacemaker implantation is indicated for third-degree and advanced second-degree AVB at any anatomic level associated with postoperative AVB that is not expected to resolve after cardiac surgery" (Tracy et al. 2013). Generally, it is recommended to implant a permanent pacemaker if symptomatic complete AVB or SND persists longer than 5–7 days after cardiac surgery (Merin et al. 2009). Any decision regarding timing of implantation of a permanent pacemaker will be impacted by the stability of the temporary pacing system. Therefore, in patients with no intrinsic underlying rhythm or those with failure of temporary pacing leads, permanent pacing may be performed even sooner. In patients with resolved or resolving bradyarrhythmias, electrophysiological study or exercise stress testing is useful to determine the need for permanent pacemaker implantation.

References

Alghamdi AA, Al-Radi OO, Latter DA. Intravenous magnesium for prevention of atrial fibrillation after coronary artery bypass surgery: a systematic review and meta-analysis. J Card Surg. 2005;20:293–9.

Almassi GH, Schowalter T, Nicolosi AC, et al. Atrial fibrillation after cardiac surgery. A major morbid event? Ann Surg. 1997;226:501–13.

Amar D, Shi W, Hogue CW Jr, Zhang H, et al. Clinical prediction rule for atrial fibrillation after coronary artery bypass grafting. J Am Coll Cardiol. 2004;44:1248–53.

Anderson E, Johnke K, Leedahl D, et al. Novel oral anticoagulants vs warfarin for the management of postoperative atrial fibrillation: clinical outcomes and cost analysis. Am J Surg. 2015;210:1093–103.

Archbold RA, Schilling RJ. Atrial pacing for the prevention of atrial fibrillation after coronary artery bypass graft surgery: a review of the literature. Heart. 2004;90:129–33.

Ascione R, Caputo M, Calori G, et al. Predictors of atrial fibrillation after conventional and beating heart coronary surgery: a prospective, randomized study. Circulation. 2000;102:1530–5.

Asher CR, Miller DP, Grimm RA, et al. Analysis of risk factors for development of atrial fibrillation early after cardiac valvular surgery. Am J Cardiol. 1998;82:892–5.

Bagshaw SM, Galbraith PD, Mitchell LB, et al. Prophylactic amiodarone for prevention of atrial fibrillation after cardiac surgery: a meta-analysis. Ann Thorac Surg. 2006;82:1927–37.

Brembilla-Perrot B, Villemot JP, Carteaux JP, et al. Postoperative ventricular arrhythmias after cardiac surgery: immediate- and long-term significance. Pacing Clin Electrophysiol. 2003;26:619–25.

Brodell GK, Cosgrove D, Schiavone W, et al. Cardiac rhythm and conduction disturbances in patients undergoing mitral valve surgery. Cleve Clin J Med. 1991;58:397–9.

Camm AJ, Kirchhof P, Lip GY, et al. Guidelines for the management of atrial fibrillation: the Task Force for the Management of Atrial Fibrillation of the European Society of Cardiology (ESC). Eur Heart J. 2010;31:2369–429.

Chung MK. Cardiac surgery: postoperative arrhythmias. Crit Care Med. 2000;28(Suppl):N136–44.

Chung MK, Martin DO, Sprecher D, et al. C-reactive protein in patients with atrial arrhythmias: inflammatory mechanisms and persistence of atrial fibrillation. Circulation. 2001;104:2886–91.

Creswell LL, Schuessler RB, Rosenbloom M, et al. Hazards of postoperative atrial arrhythmias. Ann Thorac Surg. 1993;56:539–49.

Crystal E, Connolly SJ, Sleik K, et al. Intervention on prevention of postoperative atrial fibrillation in patients undergoing heart surgery: a metaanalysis. Circulation. 2002;106:75–80.

De Vecchi E, Pala MG, Di Credico G, et al. Relation between left ventricular function and oxidative stress in patients undergoing bypass surgery. Heart. 1998;79:242–7.

El-Chami MF, Sawaya FJ, Kilgo P, et al. Ventricular arrhythmia after cardiac surgery: incidence, predictors, and outcomes. J Am Coll Cardiol. 2012;60:2664–71.

Fan K, Lee K, Lau CP. Mechanisms of biatrial pacing for prevention of postoperative atrial fibrillation—insights from a clinical trial. Card Electrophysiol Rev. 2003;7:147–53.

Fanning WJ, Thomas CS Jr, Roach A, et al. Prophylaxis of atrial fibrillation with magnesium sulfate after coronary artery bypass grafting. Ann Thorac Surg. 1991;52:529–33.
Fogel RI, Prystowsky EN. Management of malignant ventricular arrhythmias and cardiac arrest. Crit Care Med. 2000;28(Suppl):N165–9.
Fuster V, Ryden LE, Cannom DS, et al. 2011 CCF/AHA/HRS focused updates incorporated into the ACC/AHA/ESC 2006 guidelines for the management of patients with atrial fibrillation: a report of the American College of Cardiology Foundation/American Heart Association Task Force on Practice Guidelines. Circulation. 2011;123:e269–367.
Goldman BS, Hill TJ, Weisel RD, et al. Permanent cardiac pacing after open-heart surgery: acquired heart disease. Pacing Clin Electrophysiol. 1984;7(3):367–71.
Grant SC, Khan MA, Faragher EB, et al. Atrial arrhythmias and pacing after orthotopic heart transplantation: Bicaval versus standard atrial anastomosis. Br Heart J. 1995;74:149–53.
Haghjoo M, Saravi M, Hashemi MJ, et al. Optimal beta-blocker for prevention of atrial fibrillation after on-pump coronary artery bypass graft surgery: carvedilol versus metoprolol. Heart Rhythm. 2007;4:1170–4.
Hakala T, Pitkanen O, Hippelainen M. Feasibility of predicting the risk of atrial fibrillation after coronary artery bypass surgery with logistic regression model. Scand J Surg. 2002;91:339–44.
Ho KM, Tan JA. Benefits and risks of corticosteroid prophylaxis in adult cardiac surgery: a dose–response meta-analysis. Circulation. 2009;119:1853–66.
Huikuri HV, Yli-Mayry S, Korhonen UR, et al. Prevalence and prognostic significance of complex ventricular arrhythmias after coronary arterial bypass graft surgery. Int J Cardiol. 1990;27:333–9.
Ishii Y, Schuessler RB, Gaynor SL, et al. Inflammation of atrium after cardiac surgery is associated with inhomogeneity of atrial conduction and atrial fibrillation. Circulation. 2005;111:2881–8.
Jaeger FJ, Trohman RG, Brener S, et al. Permanent pacing following repeat cardiac valve surgery. Am J Cardiol. 1994;74:505–7.
Kaplan M, Kut MS, Icer UA, et al. Intravenous magnesium sulfate prophylaxis for atrial fibrillation after coronary artery bypass surgery. J Thorac Cardiovasc Surg. 2003;125:344–52.
Korantzopoulos P, Kolettis TM, Galaris D, et al. The role of oxidative stress in the pathogenesis and perpetuation of atrial fibrillation. Int J Cardiol. 2006;115:135–43.
Lahtinen J, Biancari F, Salmela E, et al. Postoperative atrial fibrillation is a major cause of stroke after on-pump coronary artery bypass surgery. Ann Thorac Surg. 2004;77:1241–4.
Leitch JW, Thomson D, Baird DK, et al. The importance of age as a predictor of atrial fibrillation and flutter after coronary artery bypass grafting. J Thorac Cardiovasc Surg. 1990;100:338–42.
Merin O, Ilan M, Oren A, et al. Pacing Clin Electrophysiol. 2009;32:7–12.
Passman R, Beshai J, Pavri B, et al. Predicting post-coronary bypass surgery atrial arrhythmias from the preoperative electrocardiogram. Am Heart J. 2001;142:806–10.
Pfisterer ME, Klöter-Weber UC, Huber M, et al. Prevention of supraventricular tachyarrhythmias after open heart operation by low-dose sotalol: a prospective, double-blind, randomized, placebo-controlled study. Ann Thorac Surg. 1997;64:1113–9.
Pinto RP, Romerill DB, Nasser WK, et al. Prognosis of patients with frequent premature ventricular complexes and nonsustained ventricular tachycardia after coronary artery bypass graft surgery. Clin Cardiol. 1996;19:321–4.
Smith RC, Leung JM, Keith FM, et al. Ventricular dysrhythmias in patients undergoing coronary artery bypass graft surgery: incidence, characteristics, and prognostic importance. Am Heart J. 1992;123:73–81.
Tam SK, Miller JM, Edmunds LH Jr. Unexpected, sustained ventricular tachyarrhythmia after cardiac operations. J Thorac Cardiovasc Surg. 1991;102:883–9.
Tracy CM, Epstein AE, Darbar D, et al. 2012 ACCF/AHA/HRS focused update incorporated into the ACCF/AHA/HRS 2008 guidelines for device-based therapy of cardiac rhythm abnormalities: A Report of the American College of Cardiology Foundation/American Heart Association Task Force on Practice Guidelines and the Heart Rhythm Society. J Am Coll Cardiol. 2013;61:e6-e75.

VanderLugt JT, Mattioni T, Denker S, et al. Efficacy and safety of ibutilide fumarate for the conversion of atrial arrhythmias after cardiac surgery. Circulation. 1999;100:369–75.

Wahr JA, Parks R, Boisvert D, et al. Preoperative serum potassium levels and perioperative outcomes in cardiac surgery patients. Multicenter Study of Perioperative Ischemia Research Group. JAMA. 1999;281:2203–10.

Weber UK, Osswald S, Buser P, et al. Significance of supraventricular tachyarrhythmias after coronary artery bypass graft surgery and their prevention by low-dose sotalol: a prospective double-blind randomized placebo controlled study. J Cardiovasc Pharmacol Ther. 1998;3:209–16.

Yavuz T, Bertolet B, Bebooul Y, et al. Role of endogenous adenosine in atrial fibrillation after coronary artery bypass graft. Clin Cardiol. 2004;27:343–6.

15 Fluid Management and Electrolyte Balance

Felice Eugenio Agrò, Marialuisa Vennari,
and Maria Benedetto

Abstract

Cardiac surgery is responsible for profound modification in body water distribution, electrolyte plasma concentration, and acid-base balance. Maintaining homeostasis must take into account the kind of surgery, the alterations due to anesthesia, the effects of cardiopulmonary bypass, patient's comorbidities, and his own response to surgical stress. The ideal approach to perioperative fluid management is still debated in all clinical contest and in cardiac surgery patients in particular, since a load of fluid is generally needed because of cardiopulmonary bypass priming. The debate involves the kind of fluid to use (crystalloids vs. colloids, colloid vs. colloid, balanced vs. unbalance solutions) and the amount of fluid to administer (liberal, restrictive, goal-directed therapy). In this debate economics interests have influenced literature productions and results, leading more difficult the interpretation of many results and complicating clinical application of scientific founds in routinely practice. Electrolytes are always modified after cardiac surgery. With respect to the past, the benefit of their administration (in particular calcium) has been discussed in literature. In this chapter the basis of fluid and electrolyte management in cardiac surgery patient is explained, through understanding physiology and pathophysiology and considering with critical approach literature evidences.

Keywords

Physiology of body fluids · Ionic balance · Sodium · Potassium · Calcium · Magnesium · Chloride · Bicarbonate · Osmolar balance · Fluid movement through capillary membranes · Basis of pathophysiology of fluid and electrolyte in the postoperative ICU setting of cardiac surgery · Water distribution

F. E. Agrò, M.D. (✉) · M. Vennari, M.D. · M. Benedetto, M.D.
Intensive Care and Pain Management Department, University School of Medicine Campus Bio-Medico of Rome, Rome, Italy
e-mail: f.agro@unicampus.it; m.vennari@unicampus.it; m.benedetto@unicampus.it

A. Dabbagh et al. (eds.), *Postoperative Critical Care for Adult Cardiac Surgical Patients*, https://doi.org/10.1007/978-3-319-75747-6_15

modification Electrolyte modifications · Clinical management of fluid · Which kind of fluid? · Physical and chemical properties · Crystalloids · Classification · Pharmacokinetics: distribution and duration of action · Normal saline solution · Ringer's lactate and Ringer's acetate · Latest-generation crystalloids · Potential risks and side effects · Water distribution modification · Electrolyte modifications · Clotting disorders · Hypertonic crystalloids · Colloids · Physiological properties of the main colloids · Pharmacokinetics: distribution and duration of action · Natural colloids: albumin (HA) · Composition and concentration · Pharmacokinetics: distribution, elimination, and duration of action · Potential risks and side effects · Synthetic colloids · Dextrans · Pharmacokinetics: distribution, elimination, and duration of action · Potential risks and side effects · Gelatins · Pharmacokinetics: distribution, elimination, and duration of effect · Potential risks and side effects · Hydroxyethyl starches · Pharmacokinetics: distribution, elimination, and duration of action · Potential risks and side effects · Coagulation and platelet function · Kidney dysfunction · Anaphylaxis · Storing and itching · Hypertonic colloid solutions · Comparison between crystalloids and colloids · Comparison between HES and other colloids · Comparison between balanced and unbalanced solutions · Liberal vs. restricted approach · Goal-directed fluid therapy · Clinical impact in cardiac surgery patients · Electrolyte management · Sodium · Potassium · Calcium · Magnesium

15.1 Introduction

In 1865 Claude Bernard firstly referred the human body as a "milieu interieur," provided of its own homeostasis (Bernard 1865). Homeostasis is the prerequisite of the performance of any physiologic function, and it is founded on three main systems, electrolyte system, acid-base system, and osmolar system, that are strictly interconnected. Any change in one of them is responsible of modification of both the remainders. They are responsible for body water distribution and movements of fluids and molecules. Maintaining or restoring the homeostasis acting on the three systems is the final goal of any clinical treatment, in particular in the perioperative setting of cardiac surgery. In this case, the maintenance of fluid, ionic, osmolar, and acid-base balance is the sum of complex clinic evaluations and actions, taking into account the kind of surgery, the alterations due to anesthesia, the effects of cardiopulmonary bypass, patient's comorbidities, and his own response to surgical stress (Fanzca 2012). In clinical practice clinicians are often faced with much uncertainty that should be in part overcome through an adequate knowledge of human physiology.

15.1.1 Physiology of Body Fluids

The human body is divided into two main compartments: the intracellular space (ICS) and the extracellular space (ECS). The ECS is divided into three additional compartments: the intravascular space (IVS, plasma), the interstitial space (ISS), and the transcellular space (TCS). These compartments contain the body water and are surrounded by a semipermeable membrane through which fluids pass from one space to another (Agro and Vennari 2013a) (Fig. 15.1).

The water within the body accounts for approximately 60% of body weight; it is mainly distributed in the ECS and ICS. The ICS contains nearly 55% of total body water and the ECS approximately 45% (about 15 L in a normal adult). Among the three compartments, the IVS accounts for about 15% of ECS water, the ISS for nearly 45%, and the TCS for about 40% (Agro and Vennari 2013a) (Fig. 15.2).

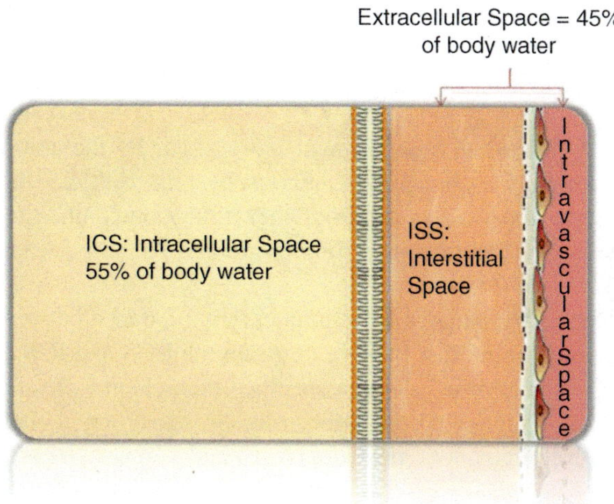

Fig. 15.1 Body compartment representation. From Agro F.E., Vennari M. "Physiology of body fluid compartments and body fluid movements." In "Body Fluid Management—From Physiology to Therapy" Agrò F.E. Springer Milan 2013, pages 1–26

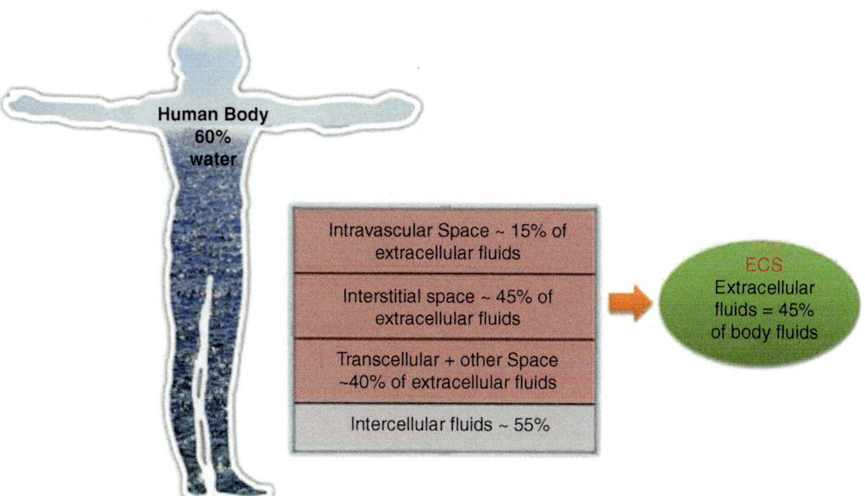

Fig. 15.2 Body water distribution. From Agro F.E., Vennari M. "Physiology of body fluid compartments and body fluid movements." In "Body Fluid Management—From Physiology to Therapy" Agrò F.E. Springer Milan 2013, pages 1–26

Table 15.1 Main properties of body fluids

Properties	Plasma	Interstitial fluid	Intracellular fluid
Colloids osmotic pressure (mmHg)	25	4	–
Osmolality (mOsmol/kg)	280	280	280
pH	7.4	7.4	7.2
Na^+ (mEqlL)	142	143	10
K^+ (mEqlL)	4	4	155
Cl^- (mEqlL)	103	115	8
Ca^{2+} (mEqlL)	2.5	1.3	<0.001

From Agro F.E., Vennari M. "Physiology of body fluid compartments and body fluid movements." In "Body Fluid Management—From Physiology to Therapy" Agrò F.E. Springer Milan 2013, pages 1–26

The TCS is a functional compartment represented by the amount of fluid and electrolytes continually exchanged (in and out) by cells with the ISS and by the ISS with the IVS (Agro and Vennari 2013a). Other fluids composing the TCS are secretions, ocular fluid, and cerebrospinal fluid (Agro and Vennari 2013a; Chappell et al. 2008).

Fluid and electrolyte balance is both an external balance between the body and its environment and an internal balance between the ECS and ICS and between the IVS and ISS. This balance is based on specific chemical and physical properties of body fluids, such as ionic composition, pH, protein content, osmotic pressure, osmolarity, and colloid osmotic pressure (Agro and Vennari 2013a) (Table 15.1).

15.1.2 Ionic Balance

Ionic balance is based on the principle of the "electric neutrality": the sum of cations must be the same of the sum of anions. In other words, the net sum of the electric charge in the body fluids is zero. Ionic composition of ICS and ECS is different, and further differences exist in the ECS between the IVS and the ISS (Table 15.1).

In clinical practice the only value directly measurable is the plasma concentration of each ion. Generally, this value is considered as a reference to evaluate the presence of electrolyte alterations. The relationship between the ionic plasmatic composition and the neutrality principle is expressed by Gamble gram (Fig. 15.3). Examining the Gamble gram is immediately evident that the sum of cations (Na^+ + K^+ + Ca^{++} + Mg^{++} + others) is 154 mEq/L and is the same of anions (Cl^- + bicarbonate + proteins + phosphates + sulfates + organic acids). Na^+ and K^+ represent the 94% of all IVS cations, while Cl^- and bicarbonate represent the 84% of all anions. Na^+, K^+, Ca^{++}, and Mg^{++} are electrolytes generally measured through laboratory exams, while bicarbonate is only calculated using Henderson-Hasselbalch equation when arterial blood sampling is performed (Gamble 1947) (see Chap. 16).

15.1.2.1 Sodium

Sodium is the most highly represented cation in the ECS, and it has a key hemodynamic role: it is the main determinant of ECS volume, contributes to renin-angiotensin-aldosterone system activation, and regulates ADH secretion. Sodium

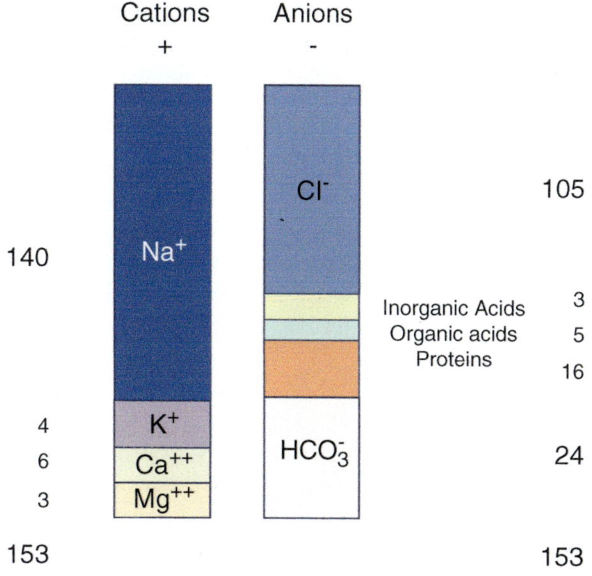

Fig. 15.3 Gamble gram. Electric neutrality principle: the sum of plasmatic cations is equivalent to the sum of plasmatic anions

concentration determines body fluid osmolarity. Changes in sodium plasma level are responsible for modification in fluid movement across the body space, determining ICS and ECS volume variation. The normal sodium concentration in plasma and the ISS is about 142 mEq/L, and it is higher than the ICS concentration (10 mEq/L) (Agro and Vennari 2013a; Miller 2009).

15.1.2.2 Potassium

Potassium is the main cation of the ICS. It plays a central role in determining the resting cell membrane potential, especially for excitable cells such as myocytes. Therefore it influences the transmission of impulses along the cardiac pacemakers (potentially predisposing to arrhythmias) and the contraction of myocardial cells. It is also involved in a variety of metabolic processes, including energy production and the synthesis of nucleic acids and proteins. The normal potassium concentration in plasma is about 4.5 mEq/L (Agro and Vennari 2013a; Miller 2009).

15.1.2.3 Calcium

Several extra- and intracellular activities are regulated by calcium action. Calcium is involved in endocrine, exocrine, and neurocrine secretion; coagulation activation; muscle contraction (it has a great inotropic effect); potential membrane depolarization; cell growth; enzymatic regulation; and in the metabolism of other electrolytes (especially potassium and magnesium). The normal calcium plasma concentration is 2–2.6 mEq/L. Calcium may circulate in the plasma bound to albumin and free from proteins. Free calcium may be ionized (physiologically active) or non-ionized (chelated with inorganic anions such as sulfate, citrate, and phosphate). The amounts of the three forms are altered by many factors, such as pH, plasma protein levels (hypoalbuminemia reduces total calcium, but not free fraction), and percentage of anions associated with ionized calcium (blood products contain citrate) (Agro and Vennari 2013a; Miller 2009).

15.1.2.4 Magnesium

Magnesium is the physiological antagonist of calcium. It plays a crucial role in neuromuscular stimulation and modulation of excitable cells activity (membrane-stabilizing activity); it also acts as a cofactor of several enzymes involved in the metabolism of three major categories of nutrients: carbohydrates, lipids, and proteins. The normal plasma concentration is about 0.85–1.25 mEq/L (Agro and Vennari 2013a; Miller 2009).

15.1.2.5 Chloride

Chloride is the most important anion of the ECS. Together with sodium, it determines the ECS volume. It is also responsible for the resting potential of the membrane and action potential, acid-base balance, and plasma osmotic pressure. The normal plasma chloride concentration is 97–107 mEq/L (Agro and Vennari 2013a; Miller 2009).

15.1.2.6 Bicarbonate

Bicarbonate is the main buffer system of the blood. It plays a crucial role in maintaining acid-base balance. Two-thirds of the CO_2 in the human body is metabolized as bicarbonate, through the action of carbonic anhydrase. The equilibrium between CO_2 and bicarbonate leads to the elimination of volatile acid. The bicarbonate buffer system is described by the following equilibrium reaction (Agro and Vennari 2013a):

$$CO_2 + H_2O \leftrightarrow H_2CO_3 \leftrightarrow HCO_3^- + H^+$$

When there is an increased concentration of H^+, the system reacts by shifting the reaction equilibrium to the left (toward the production of CO_2); while when the concentration of H^+ is reduced, the system moves to the right, resulting in the production of H^+. The bicarbonate buffer system works “in concert” with several organs (see Chap. 16). Bicarbonate has a normal plasma concentration of about 24 mmol/L (Agro and Vennari 2013a).

15.1.3 Osmolar Balance

Chemical properties of ICS and ECS are very different (Table 15.1). According to their Na^+ and glucose concentration, ICS is sweet, while ECS is salty. The principle of iso-osmolarity is crucial for body balance: ICS osmolarity and ECS osmolarity must be the same. Osmotic pressure (μ) is the force exerted by the sum of osmotically active particles (Na^+ and other electrolytes) that do not freely pass through semipermeable membranes (Agro and Vennari 2013a). According to osmotic pressure difference among the compartments, water freely passes from ICS to ECS and vice versa, in order to achieve the equilibrium (Agro and Vennari 2013a) (Fig. 15.4). In particular, water shifts from the body compartment with lower osmotic pressure to that with higher osmotic pressure. The osmotic pressure gradient between the two compartments is described as the tonicity (Agro and Vennari 2013a; Voet et al. 2001).

The osmotic pressure of the plasma is 288 ± 5 mOsm/L, and it can be measured or calculated by measuring the plasma concentrations of Na, glucose, and urea.

$$\text{Plasma osmotic pressure} = 2\times\left[\text{Na}^+\right](\text{mmol}/\text{L}) \\ +\text{urea}/2.8(\text{mg}/\text{dL})+\text{glucose}/18(\text{mg}/\text{dL})$$

The difference between measured osmolarity and calculated osmolarity is called the osmolar gap. A high osmolar gap suggests either the presence of an exogenous compound (e.g., ethanol) whose identity should be sought or the elevation of endogenous constituents that may not have been measured (e.g., proteins, keto acids, lipids) (Hendry 1961).

The main determinant of plasma osmolarity is Na^+. Sodium salts are responsible for the 95% of the whole plasma osmotic pressure. Since osmotic pressure determines water tendency to move in or out the cell, the Na^+ concentration is the main determinant of the relative volumes and hydration of the ICS and ECS (Voet et al. 2001). When the ECS osmotic pressure increases (i.e., hypernatremia), water immediately pass from ICS to ECS to restore osmotic equilibrium, leading to a

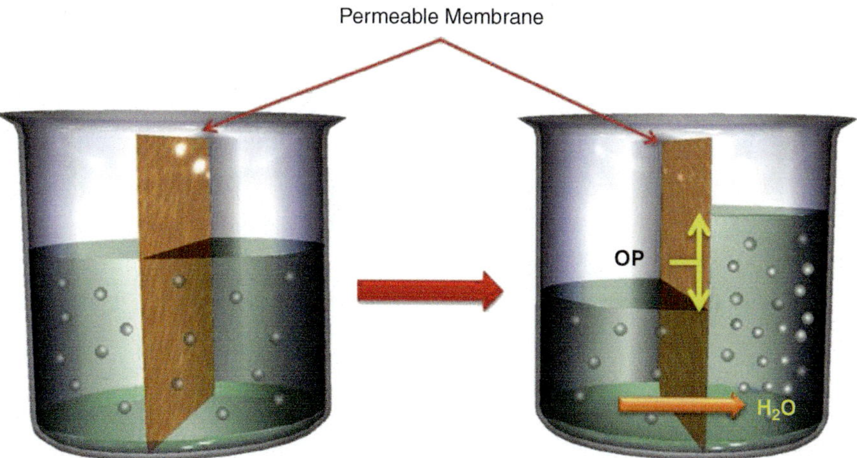

Fig. 15.4 Osmotic pressure. According to osmotic pressure, water diffusion will take place from low to high electrolytic concentration. From Agro F.E., Vennari M. "Physiology of body fluid compartments and body fluid movements." In "Body Fluid Management—From Physiology to Therapy" Agrò F.E. Springer Milan 2013, pages 1–26

reduction in ICS volume and an increase in ECS volume, while the opposite movement develops when ECS osmotic pressure is reduced (i.e., hyponatremia), with an increase in ICS volume and a reduction in ECS volume (Agro and Vennari 2013a). Sodium and water movements are further related by the mechanism of regulation of osmolarity and volemia. They are hormonal systems such as ADH, renin-angiotensin-aldosterone (RAA) system, ANP, BNP, and the thirst. Although with different threshold of sensibility (i.e., ADH is more sensible to osmolarity while RAA system to volemia), they are all enrolled both in case of osmolarity and volemia alterations (Agro and Vennari 2013a). Being the sole organ able to divide water movement from Na^+ movement, the kidney is the main target of the regulatory systems. When an increase in plasma osmotic pressure develops, ADH and the thirst promote water reabsorption and intake, while when plasma osmotic pressure reduces, the reduction in water intake and its increased kidney excretion restore normo-osmolarity (Agro and Vennari 2013a) (Fig. 15.5).

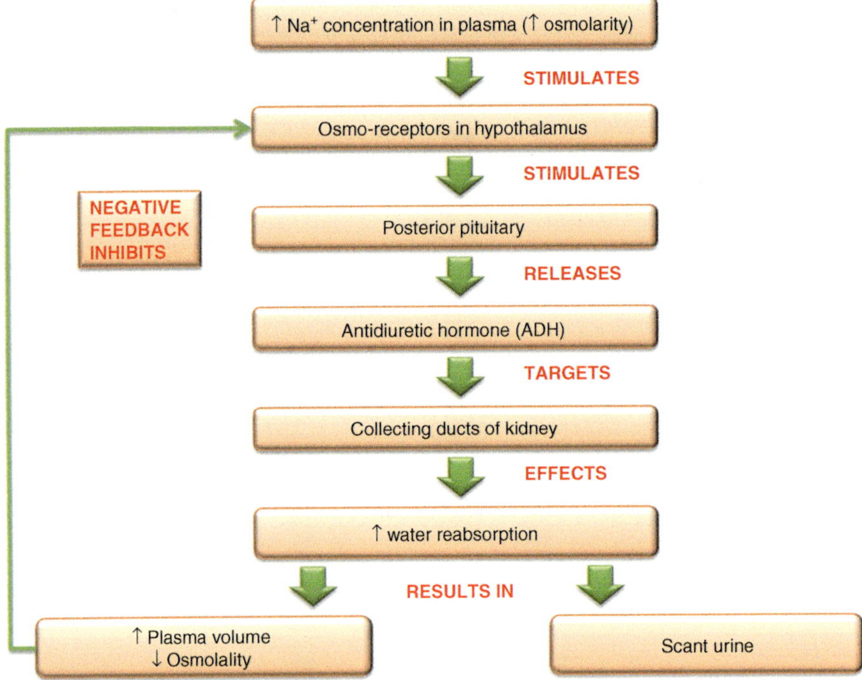

Fig. 15.5 Mechanism of ADH secretion: when fluid volume decreases, plasma sodium concentration and plasma osmolarity increase, leading to hypothalamic osmoreceptor stimulation. The hypothalamus will then stimulate the posterior pituitary gland that releases antidiuretic hormone. ADH will make renal distal tubules able to reabsorb water into the IVS in order to maintain homeostasis of fluid balance. ADH secretion is more sensible to plasma osmolarity than circulating blood. From Agro F.E., Vennari M. "Clinical treatment: the right fluid in the right quantity." In "Body Fluid Management—From Physiology to Therapy" Agrò F.E. Springer Milan 2013, pages 71–92

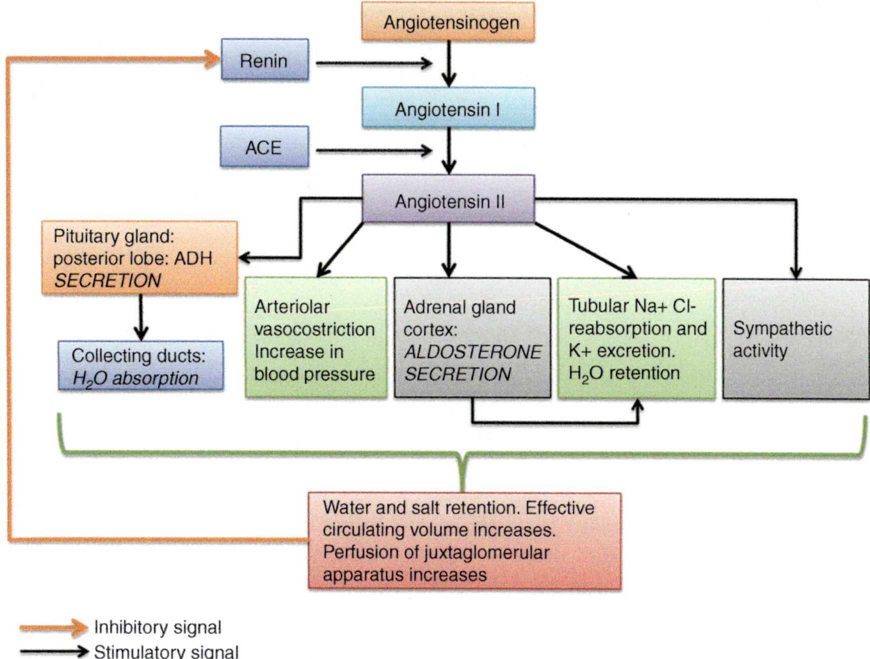

Fig. 15.6 Renin-angiotensin-aldosterone system: hypovolemia reduces perfusion of juxtaglomerular apparatus, with renin release. Circulating renin converts angiotensinogen into angiotensin I; subsequently ACE (angiotensin-converting enzyme) acts on angiotensin I converting it into angiotensin II. This hormone increases NSS activity, increases reabsorption of Na and water by the kidneys directly and through aldosterone action, and determines vasoconstriction and ADH secretion. From Agro F.E., Vennari M. "Clinical treatment: the right fluid in the right quantity." In "Body Fluid Management—From Physiology to Therapy" Agrò F.E. Springer Milan 2013, pages 71–92

The RAA system is mainly enrolled in sodium and water renal reabsorption, when a hypovolemia develops. In case of hypervolemia, the ANP and the RAA system inhibition lead to excretion of sodium and water overload (Agro and Vennari 2013a) (Fig. 15.6).

15.1.4 Fluid Movement Through Capillary Membranes

Fluid movements across capillary membrane are regulated by physical forces and specific properties of the semipermeable membranes (Agro and Vennari 2013a).

Accordingly, electrolyte and protein concentrations, as well as osmotic properties, play a crucial role, as expressed in the Starling equation:

$$Jv = K_{\mathrm{f}}\left(\left[P_{\mathrm{c}} - P_{\mathrm{i}}\right] - \sigma\left[\delta_{\mathrm{c}} - \delta_{\mathrm{i}}\right]\right).$$

According to this equation, water flow depends on six variables:

1. Capillary hydrostatic pressure (P_c)
2. Interstitial hydrostatic pressure (P_i)
3. Capillary oncotic pressure (δ_c)
4. Interstitial oncotic pressure (δ_i)
5. Filtration coefficient (K_f)
6. Diffusion coefficient (σ)

The equation states that the net filtration (Jv) is proportional to the net driving force ($[P_c - P_i] - \sigma [\delta_c - \delta_i]$). If this value is positive, water leaves the IVS (filtration). If it is negative, water enters or remains the IVS (absorption) (Fig. 15.7). A modification of only one of the forces involved in Starling equation may alter fluid movement across body compartment (Agro and Vennari 2013a).

A revised Starling model has been proposed taking into account the physical characteristics of the endothelial glycocalyx layer, the endothelial basement membrane, and the extracellular matrix (Reed and Rubin 2010).

According to this model, when the vascular barrier is intact, transcapillary movement of fluid is unidirectional, as there is no absorption of fluid from the ISS back to the IVS and drainage of the ISS is primarily due to lymphatic clearance. At supranormal capillary pressures, infusion of colloid solution preserves oncotic pressure and increases capillary pressure, thus increasing movement of fluid into the ISS, while infusion of crystalloid solutions also increases capillary pressure but by dilution decreases oncotic pressure, thus resulting in more transcapillary movement

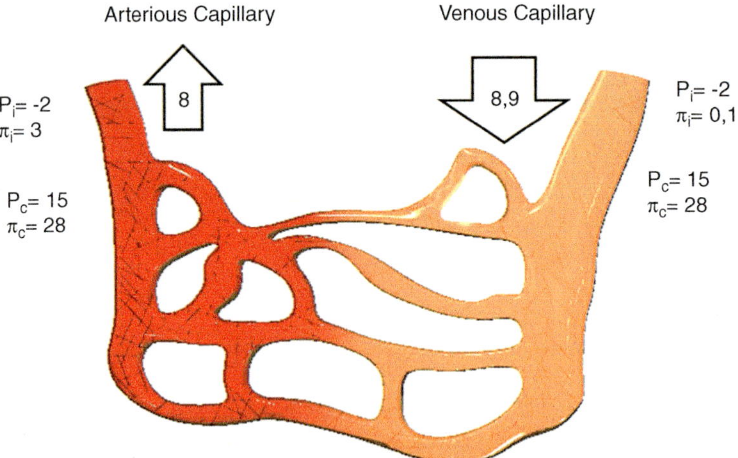

Fig. 15.7 Starling forces. On the arterial side of capillary vessels, forces putting out water overcome those putting in. On the venous side is the contrary. Modified from Agro F.E., Vennari M. "Physiology of body fluid compartments and body fluid movements." In "Body Fluid Management—From Physiology to Therapy" Agrò F.E. Springer Milan, 2013 pages 1–26

than colloids. At subnormal capillary pressures, transcapillary movement nears zero; thus, infusion of both crystalloids and colloids results in increase in capillary pressure, but no change in transcapillary movement (Lira and Pinsky 2014).

The tissues (i.e., liver and gut mucosa) that can accumulate large amounts of interstitial fluid during physiologic stress in their healthy state contain non-fenestrated capillaries. In response to physical and chemical stress, non-fenestrated capillaries change into fenestrated, resulting in both endothelial dysfunction and increased permeability. This change is largely responsible for increase in permeability leading to changes in volume kinetics, edema, and intravascular depletion due to fluid shift. This model underscores the integrity of the glycocalyx as one of the key factors involved in fluid dynamics and suggests that its restoration needs to be one of the therapeutic goals in conditions of physiologic stress. Regrettably, at this time, no specific therapies have been shown to augment glycocalyx restoration (Lira and Pinsky 2014).

15.2 Basis of Pathophysiology of Fluid and Electrolyte in the Postoperative ICU Setting of Cardiac Surgery

15.2.1 Water Distribution Modification

An adequate fluid replacement strategy, maintaining vascular barrier competence, preventing interstitial edema, and keeping microcirculation intact, is crucial to achieve an optimal outcome in CPB surgery. Blood contact with roller pumps and foreign surfaces during CPB induces shear stress and a pressure drop across the pump boot that leads to transient systemic activation of the inflammatory and hemostatic systems (Moret et al. 2014).

In patients undergoing cardiac surgery, a correct fluid management maintains an adequate circulatory volume and a proper electrolyte and acid-base balance, avoiding arrhythmic (i.e., atrial fibrillation), hemodynamic (i.e., hypotension, pulmonary edema), and other complications (Agrò et al. 2013). Hypovolemia is a frequent occurrence among cardiac surgical patients. Fluid imbalance may be due to an absolute volume deficit or to a relative volume deficit and may be associated to concurrent electrolyte and acid-base imbalance problems (Agrò et al. 2013).

Absolute volume deficits can be due to hemorrhage (i.e., coagulation and platelet impairment, surgical complications) or to severe dehydration issues (i.e., diuresis induced by mannitol often used during cardiopulmonary bypass), while relative volume deficits can be due to vasodilatation caused by sedation, systemic inflammatory response syndrome (SIRS) due to surgical stress and cardiopulmonary bypass (CPB), and rewarming. These cases may present the capillary leak syndrome that is a maladaptive response to stress leading undesirable loss of fluid and electrolytes from IVS to ISS, generating edema. The more severe form of this syndrome is the global increased permeability syndrome (GIPS) manifesting in patients with persistent systemic inflammation. It is characterized by a transcapillary albumin leakage, resulting in increasingly positive net fluid balances. GIPS may represent a third hit after the initial insult and the ischemia-reperfusion injury (Duchesne et al. 2015). In this case hypovolemia develops in the absence of obvious fluid loss, leading to a reduction in cardiac index (CI), tissue perfusion, and O_2 delivery (DO_2) with a high risk of organ failure, potentially fatal. Despite a reduction of IVS volume, fluid overload should be avoided in this setting. Markers like the extravascular lung water, capillary leak index, and pulmonary permeability index may help the clinician in guiding appropriate fluid management.

Another cause of concern is the risk of fluid overload, which may precipitate or worse the cardiac function (especially in patient with impaired ventricular contractility or compliance), leading to acute pulmonary edema and/or cardiogenic shock. These events may complicate patient management, requiring the use of inotropes and other cardiovascular active drugs. Moreover, a fluid overload may lead to interstitial edema, compression of microvasculature, and an increased oxygen diffusion distance, compromising DO_2 and O_2 diffusion to tissue (Fanzca 2012).

Fluid overload may develop secondary intra-abdominal hypertension (IAH) and abdominal compartment syndrome (ACS), leading to a reduction of the cardiac function by affecting preload, contractility, and afterload (Duchesne et al. 2015). Finally, aggressive perioperative fluid administration may cause hemodilution, with an increased need for blood products.

In order to avoid both hypovolemia and fluid overload, stabilization of the cardiovascular system through a rational fluid therapy should take into account the type of surgery and the mechanism of fluid movement among body compartments (Duchesne et al. 2015; Vretzakis et al. 2011).

According to Starling equation, ISS volume is generally maintained by lymphatic drainage. Any flux of fluid into the ISS arise its hydrostatic pressure and decrease its oncotic pressure, limiting the development of interstitial edema. In literature many works demonstrated that Starling equation does not fully explain the movement between IVS and ISS across the endothelial membrane (Fanzca 2012; Adams 2007; Hu and Weinbaum 1999; Hu et al. 2000; Levick 2004). The deviation from theory is due to a meshwork of membrane-bound, negatively charged glycoproteins and proteoglycans, called endothelial glycocalyx.

The endothelial glycocalyx is a dynamic structure continuously degraded and resynthesized. It is composed by proteins produced by endothelial cells or entrapped from the plasma. Glycocalyx is a barrier for larger molecules and probably is the main responsible for the oncotic gradient across IVS and ISS (Fanzca 2012). Moreover it prevents the endothelial adhesion of inflammatory cells, reducing the consequence of the increase of endothelial permeability. In fact, a damage of the glycocalyx leads to the passage of larger molecules from the IVS into the ISS, reducing the IVS-ISS oncotic gradient and increasing the ISS fluid volume with tissue edema. Possible tissue edema may result in an impairment of tissue oxygenation, leading to wound healing disturbances and initiation of inflammatory responses up to tissue apoptosis (Knotzer et al. 2014). Various conditions associated with cardiac surgery may potentially destroy glycocalyx: hemodilution, ischemia and reperfusion damage, and inflammation (Fanzca 2012).

Hemodilution may cause the dissolution of bound plasma protein into the flowing blood and the loss of glycocalyx (Pries et al. 1998; Rehm et al. 2001). The effect may be due to ANP increased levels in cardiac surgery and to fluid overload (Fanzca 2012; Bruegger et al. 2005).

In patients undergoing cardiac surgery with cardiopulmonary bypass, plasma level of glycocalyx component (heparin sulfate and syndecan-1) was significantly increased with respect to the preoperative levels, demonstrating a dangerous effect of ischemia on glycocalyx (Fanzca 2012; Rehm et al. 2007).

In a coronary artery animal model, the loss of glycocalyx due to ischemia leads to an increased permeability to water, albumin, and hydroxyethyl starches (Rehm et al. 2004).

Van den Berg et al. (Van den Berg et al. 2003) demonstrated in a rat model the correlation between the presence of myocardial edema and the absence of endothelial glycocalyx. Interstitial edema may be detrimental for cardiac cells resulting in impairment of function (Fanzca 2012; Dongaonkar et al. 2010).

15.2.2 Electrolyte Modifications

Strictly related to fluid management is the management of electrolyte and acid-base balance. Electrolyte alterations are frequent in the postoperative period after cardiac surgery. Polderman et al. (Polderman and Girbes 2004) compared sodium, potassium, calcium, magnesium, and phosphate levels at the admission to ICU of patient undergoing CABG vs. patients undergoing other major surgeries. Although all patients received electrolyte intraoperative supplementation, they found a higher percentage (88% vs. 20%) of patients with deficit of one or more electrolytes in the first group rather than in the second. These alterations may be due to increased kidney elimination, especially in case of furosemide and mannitol use, and intracellular shift caused by alteration of ISS, IVS, and ICS equilibrium caused by CPB, extracorporeal circulation, and stress response (SIRS) (Fanzca 2012).

15.3 Clinical Management of Fluid

The ideal approach to perioperative fluid management is still debated in cardiac surgery patients. In the clinical practice, it may be very difficult: practitioners have to taint into account surgical- related factors, such as the kind of procedure and duration, CPB duration, SIRS, and glycocalyx damage, and patient-related factors, such as cardiac disease, the presence of reduced ventricular function and its postoperative modification, the need for pharmacologic or mechanical assistance, comorbidities (renal and pulmonary dysfunctions are frequent among cardiac surgery patients), and possible complications.

The clinical and literary debate involves different specialists (anesthesiologists, intensivists, and surgeons) and concerns the establishment of the ideal fluid management in terms of kind and amount of fluid to administer.

15.3.1 Which Kind of Fluid?

The choice of the fluid to administer should be guided by the properties of the targeted body space (IVS, ISS, whole body water) (Agro and Benedetto 2013).

Different solutions are available: crystalloids, colloids, and other fluids, such as dextrose solutions, mannitol solutions, and other concentrated solutions. Each one has its specific indications and side effects (Nuevo et al. 2013).

Historically, the debate about fluid management was developed around the dispute crystalloids vs. colloids. In its course, the medical literature has largely demonstrated the difference in the pharmacokinetics and pharmacodynamics of these two classes of plasma substitutes. Consequently, crystalloids should no longer be considered as an alternative to colloids and vice versa. Instead, crystalloids and colloids must be considered as the two faces of the same coin and their use as part of an integrative fluid management (Agro and Vennari 2013b).

Recently, the historical debate crystalloid/colloid has enlarged to include colloid/colloid discussion. Nonetheless, the physical and chemical properties of the various colloids determine the different therapeutic and adverse effects. Thus, any debate about intravenous volume replacement with colloids should consider the potential side effects, involving endothelial integrity, coagulation, platelet function, and organ function (e.g., the kidneys), and not only the effect of the chosen fluid on hemodynamics (Agrò et al. 2013).

The electrolyte composition of the fluid (crystalloid or colloid) is another source of controversy. The debate on balanced, plasma-adapted solutions started in the 1970s, when their features were first described. A new definition was proposed in 2000 in "Avoiding iatrogenic hyperchloremic acidosis: Call for a new crystalloid fluid," published in *Anesthesiology*, which referred to the classic need of "a solution containing sodium bicarbonate" because it was clear that "…the predominate physiologic deficit is metabolic acidosis…" (Dorje et al. 2000). Subsequent developments were summarized in 2003 by Reid et al., (Reid et al. 2003) who highlighted that scientists and clinicians must inevitably reach a compromise in their long-standing attempts to find the ideal physiological solution.

15.3.2 Physical and Chemical Properties

Depending on their physical and chemical properties, IV solutions may be classified as balanced or unbalanced, plasma-adapted or not plasma-adapted, and isotonic, hypertonic, or hypotonic (Agro and Benedetto 2013).

A balanced plasma-adapted solution has a composition closer to plasma. It contains sodium, chloride, potassium, magnesium, and calcium in similar concentrations than plasma and metabolizable anions, and it is isotonic than plasma (same osmolarity). Except for the risk of fluid overload, the infusion of this solution reduces the incidence of side effects related to fluid management, such as metabolic acidosis, electrolytic imbalances, and cellular tone alterations (Agro and Benedetto 2013).

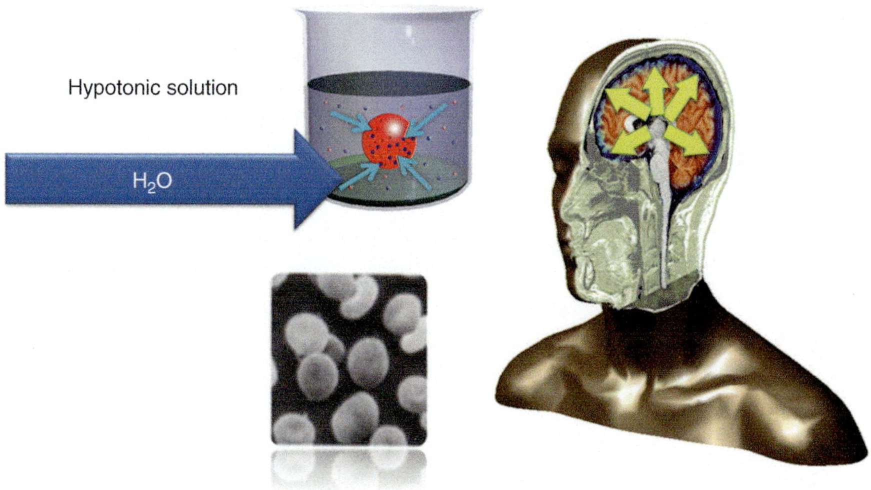

Fig. 15.8 Cellular and cerebral edema caused by hypotonic solutions. Agro F.E., Benedetto M. "Properties and composition of plasma substitutes." In "Body Fluid Management—From Physiology to Therapy" Agrò F.E. Springer Milan 2013, pages 27–36

The infusion of hypotonic or hypertonic solutions will change plasma osmolarity, resulting in a modification of body water distribution. In particular, a hypotonic solution reduces plasma osmotic pressure, moving water from the ECS to the ICS (Agro and Benedetto 2013; Williams et al. 1999). Cellular edema and lysis (i.e., hemolysis) may occur (Fig. 15.8). Larger volumes of hypotonic solutions have been known to produce a transient increase in intracranial pressure (ICP), due to cerebral edema (Agro and Benedetto 2013; Tommasino et al. 1988). The magnitude of this increase can be predicted by the reduction of plasma osmolality (Agro and Benedetto 2013; Schell et al. 1996). Patients with an osmolality below 240 mOsmol/kg will fall into a coma, with a mortality rate of 50% (Rehm et al. 2007; Arieff et al. 1976). Consequently, the infusion of large amount of hypotonic solutions should be avoided, expected specific cases (Agro and Benedetto 2013).

On the other side, hypertonic solutions increase plasma osmotic pressure, moving water from the ICS to the ECS, causing cellular dehydration and, potentially, apoptosis (Agro and Benedetto 2013) (Fig. 15.9). Many clinical settings may increase plasma osmotic pressure, with a very high mortality (Agro and Benedetto 2013). Hypovolemic shock triggers hyperglycemia with hyperosmolarity, through the release of epinephrine or through an increase in lactate blood levels (Agro and Benedetto 2013; Boyd and Mansberger 1968; Järhult 1973; Kenney et al. 1983). It has been shown that in ICU patients, non-survivors had a higher plasma osmolarity than survivors (Agro and Benedetto 2013; Holtfreter et al. 2006). Moreover, hypertonicity has been shown to make solutions more acidifying. The administration of hypertonic solution reduces strong ion difference (SID) through dilution caused by water movement from ICS to ECS (Makoff et al. 1970) (see Chap. 16).

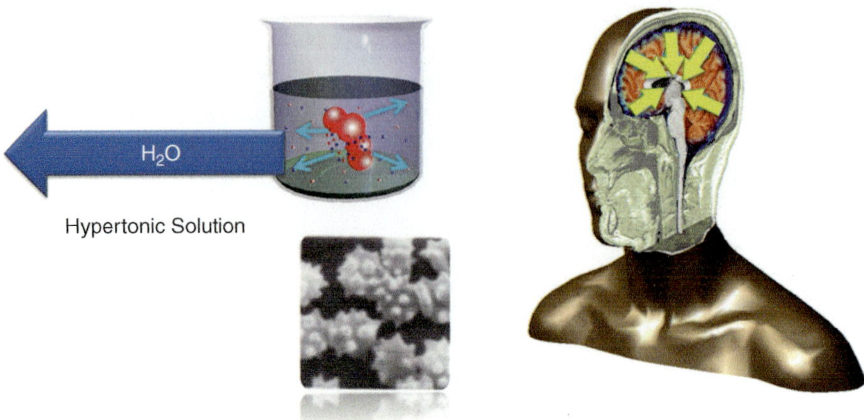

Fig. 15.9 Hypertonic solutions cause cellular dehydration, leading to apoptosis. From Agro F.E., Benedetto M. "Properties and composition of plasma substitutes." In "Body Fluid Management—From Physiology to Therapy" Agrò F.E. Springer Milan 2013, pages 27–36

15.4 Crystalloids

Crystalloids are low-molecular weight salts, dissolved in water. After the infusion, water and salt pass across the body compartment according to physiology (Nuevo et al. 2013).

15.4.1 Classification

Based on their tonicity, crystalloids are classified as hypotonic, isotonic, or hypertonic. There are different generations of crystalloids on the market (Nuevo et al. 2013) (Fig. 15.10). Many studies have focused on producing more balanced and plasma-adapted crystalloids in order to reduce side effect of their use. So far, the rational use of crystalloids remains a clinical problem (Nuevo et al. 2013).

The main properties of the most widely used crystalloids are described in Table 15.2 (Nuevo et al. 2013).

15.4.2 Pharmacokinetics: Distribution and Duration of Action

An isotonic crystalloid is distributed in the IVS (20%) but mostly in the ISS (80%). Accordingly, the efficiency of these solutions to expand the plasma volume is only 20%; the remainder is sequestered in the ISS (Agro and Benedetto 2013; Reid et al. 2003; Lamke and Liljedahl 1976; Grathwohl et al. 1996; Greenfield et al. 1989; Hauser et al. 1980; Hahn et al. 1997; Takil et al. 2002) (Fig. 15.11). Olsson et al. (2004) found that approximately 30% of infused crystalloids remain within the IVS

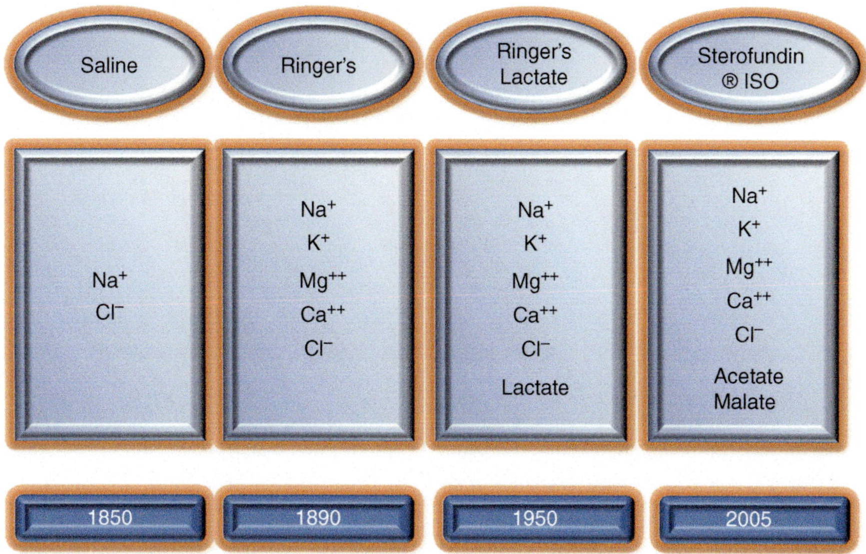

Fig. 15.10 Crystalloid generations. Modified from F.R. Nuevo, Vennari M., Agro F.E. "How to maintain and restore fluid balance: crystalloids." In "Body Fluid Management—From Physiology to Therapy" Agrò F.E. Springer Milan 2013, pages 37–46

Table 15.2 Main properties of crystalloids

Electrolyte or parameter	Plasma	0.9% NaCl	Ringer's lactate	Ringer's acetate	Sterofundin
Colloid-osmotic pressure (mmHg)	25	–	–	–	–
Osmolality (mOsm/kg)	287	308	277	256	291
Sodium (mEq/L)	142	154	131	130	145
Potassium (mEq/L)	4.5	–	5.4	5	4
Magnesium (mEq/L)	1.25	–	–	1	1
Chloride (mEq/L)	103	154	112	112	127
Calcium (mEq/L)	2.5	–	1.8	1	2.5
Bicarbonate (mEq/L)	24	–	–	–	–
Lactate (mEq/L)	1	–	28	–	–
Acetate/malate(mEq/L)	–	–	–	27/–	24–5
SID (mEq/L)	38–42	0	26	26	29

Modified from F.R. Nuevo, Vennari M., Agro F.E. "How to maintain and restore fluid balance: crystalloids." In "Body Fluid Management—From Physiology to Therapy" Agrò F.E. Springer Milan 2013, pages 37–46

for only 30 min. Crystalloids have a short-term volume effect due to their rapid movement from the IVS into the ISS (Nuevo et al. 2013). Thus, the use of crystalloids to replace severe volume deficits, following massive blood or rapid fluid loss, is not effective to restore fluid balance and blood pressure (Drummond and Petrovitch 2005). Attaining the targeted goal of adequate blood pressure requires

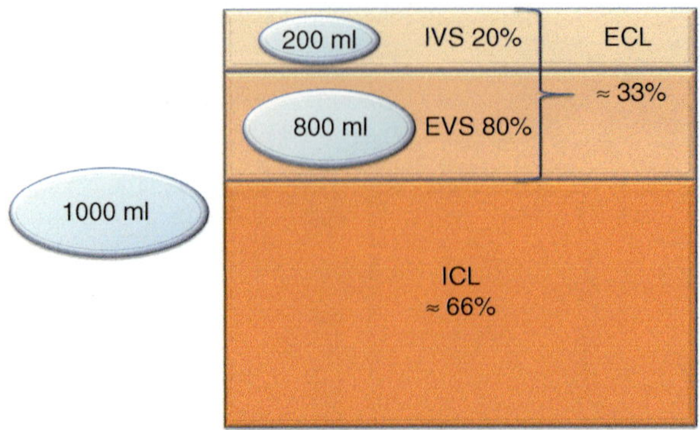

Fig. 15.11 Representation of isotonic crystalloid distribution. *IVS* intravascular space, *ISS* interstitial space, *ECS* extracellular space. Modified from F.R. Nuevo, Vennari M., Agro F.E. "How to maintain and restore fluid balance: crystalloids." In "Body Fluid Management—From Physiology to Therapy" Agrò F.E. Springer Milan 2013, pages 37–46

massive, repetitive infusions, causing the dilution of osmotically active component of plasma and a reduction in plasma oncotic pressure causing further interstitial edema and electrolyte imbalances (Fanzca 2012).

15.4.3 Normal Saline Solution

The standard 0.9% NaCl solution is also known as a normal or physiological saline solution. It contains only sodium and chloride, at the same high concentration ($Na^+ = Cl^- = 154$ mmol/L) (Nuevo et al. 2013). Consequently, its administration may cause metabolic acidosis and sodium overload. Sodium overload promotes interstitial edema, particularly in the face of the endocrine response to cardiac surgery: the cortisol- and aldosterone-induced sodium retention (Fanzca 2012). This mechanism may be further worsening in patient with kidney dysfunction or postoperative cardiac impairment (Nuevo et al. 2013). Finally, normal saline solution is slightly hypertonic (osmolality 308 mOsm/kg), potentially implying the complications of hypertonic solutions, including a higher acidifying power, especially when large amount are infused (Nuevo et al. 2013). As a result, normal saline solution is not actually normal, because it is neither isotonic, nor balanced, nor plasma-adapted (Nuevo et al. 2013).

15.4.4 Ringer's Lactate and Ringer's Acetate

Ringer's solutions are second-generation crystalloids. Compared to saline solutions, they have less sodium (130 mmol/L) and less chloride (112 mmol/L). They also contain potassium, calcium, magnesium (Ringer's acetate), and metabolizable ions: lactate (Ringer's lactate) and acetate (Ringer's acetate) (Nuevo et al. 2013).

Ringer's lactate may interfere with lactate monitoring and may precipitate or aggravate a lactic acidosis, especially in critical cardiac patients (see Chap. 16). Therefore, Ringer's acetate is generally preferred (Nuevo et al. 2013). Both Ringer's solutions are more plasma-adapted than normal saline but are nonetheless unbalanced (Nuevo et al. 2013).

15.4.5 Latest-Generation Crystalloids

The ionic composition of the latest-generation crystalloids is very close to that of plasma. They have a lower chloride content than normal saline, together with two metabolizable ions (acetate and malate) rather than the only (acetate or lactate) of Ringer's solutions (Nuevo et al. 2013). As a result, these are isotonic, balanced, and plasma-adapted solutions that reduce the risk of cellular osmotic damage (particularly cerebral), chloride and sodium excess, and dilution acidosis, with a decreased influence on lactate monitoring, lactic acidosis, and base excess (BE) (Nuevo et al. 2013, see Chap. 16).

15.4.6 Potential Risks and Side Effects

15.4.6.1 Water Distribution Modification

Over the past decades, clinicians have routinely restored fluid in the IVS with crystalloids. However, due to the rapid interstitial fluid shifts and the great distribution volume of crystalloids, large volumes must be administered. This in turn causes fluid overload, particularly interstitial edema and potential pulmonary edema (they may be deleterious for cardiac surgery patients), as well as metabolic acidosis (Nuevo et al. 2013). Finally a crystalloid volume replacement strategy may alter the plasma albumin concentration. Large-volume infusions of crystalloids can lead to albumin hemodilution effects and cause a reduction in colloid oncotic pressure (COP), yet reduced by the dilution effects of extracorporeal circulation (Fanzca 2012; Nuevo et al. 2013). The reduction of COP alters Starling forces: fluids move from IVS to ISS and remain in ISS. The result is interstitial edema up to "compartmental syndrome" and thus albumin leakage (a vicious circle is established!) with a little improvement of hemodynamics (IVS fluid has not been restored because of the shift of the infused fluid in the ISS) (Nuevo et al. 2013; Cervera and Moss 1974). In critically ill patients, a reduction in COP is associated with a mortality rate of approximately 50% (Nuevo et al. 2013; Morissette et al. 1975; Rackow et al. 1977).

15.4.6.2 Electrolyte Modifications

A large amount of crystalloid infusion may cause hyperchloremia (especially using older crystalloid generation) that alters kidney perfusion leading to sodium and chloride retention. Chloride retention brings to hyperchloremic acidosis further invalidating glomerular filtration rate, while sodium overload causes water retention (Nuevo et al. 2013). The result is a fluid overload that may precipitate the hemodynamic status of the patient, especially in the first hours after the surgery, with a weight gain that may increase mortality (Nuevo et al. 2013; Zander 2009).

15.4.6.3 Clotting Disorders

It is common knowledge that crystalloid administration is an economical means of volume replacement, with an apparently lower risk of clotting disorders (Nuevo et al. 2013). However, in two studies, Ruttmann et al. (2001, 2002) and Ng et al. (2002) have shown that in vivo dilution with crystalloids resulted in a significant potentiation of coagulation, due to a decreased concentration of antithrombin III. The resultant hypercoagulability is unrelated to the type of crystalloid. It is also associated with an increased risk of perioperative deep vein thrombosis (Nuevo et al. 2013).

15.4.7 Hypertonic Crystalloids

Hypertonic crystalloid solutions (HCS) contain higher sodium concentrations, ranging from 3 to 7.5% (Nuevo et al. 2013). According to their high osmolarity, they have a greater expanding volume effect with respect to isotonic crystalloid. HCS may improve the cardiovascular system (especially after CPB-related changes in body fluid compartments due to a capillary permeability) with only a smaller infused volume than isotonic crystalloids (4 mL/kg). However, HCS have a transient volume effect (Nuevo et al. 2013).

Jarvela et al. (2001) studied patient fluid management after CABG surgery. They found that 30 min after the infusion, 7.5% hypertonic saline determined a higher volume expansion with respect to HES 6%/120/0.7, but lower after 70 and 110 min. HES volume expansion persists for all the observation time, while 7.5% hypertonic saline volume expansion was shorter. EVS expansion was greater and faster with HCS than with 0.9% saline solution.

The hemodynamic effects of HCS can be due to the following mechanisms (Nuevo et al. 2013):

- Direct myocardial, positive inotropic effect
- Direct vasodilator effect (both the systemic and the pulmonary circulation)
- Reduced venous capacitance
- Fluid shift into the IVS from ISS

HCS have been associated with a reduction in post-injury edema at the microcirculatory level and an improvement in microvascular perfusion (Duchesne et al. 2015). Initially, there was enthusiasm in the use of HCS in case of refractory hypovolemic shock, although if HCS are not properly used, there may be life-threatening side effects (Nuevo et al. 2013).

After their infusion there is a rapid shift of water from EVS into the IVS, without a reduction in COP. An adequate volume status of both the ICS and ECS spaces is necessary to obtain this effect, such that the prolonged usage of HCS crystalloid is not recommended (Maningas and Bellamy 1986). Both Wade et al. (1997) and

Bunn et al. (2002) reported, in their meta-analyses, no significant improvement in outcome in critical patients by using HCS. They hypothesized that the combined use of HCS and colloids would be superior to isotonic fluid resuscitation. HCS infusion may be indicated in case of hyposmolarity with hyponatremia (see subsequent paragraphs).

15.5 Colloids

Colloids are high molecular weight molecules that do not dissolve completely in water, nor do they pass freely through the capillary membrane. According to their molecular size, structure, and vessel permeability, colloids determine the oncotic pressure (Bunn et al. 2002).

15.5.1 Classification

Many colloids are currently available. They include natural colloids (human albumin, HA) and synthetic colloids (dextrans, gelatins, hydroxyethyl starches), differing in their physicochemical properties, pharmacokinetics, clinical effects, and safety. Colloids also can be classified according to their electrolyte composition and tonicity. Consequently, there are balanced and unbalanced colloids, plasma-adapted and non-plasma-adapted colloids, and isotonic and hypertonic colloids (Agro et al. 2013).

15.5.2 Physiological Properties of the Main Colloids

The table below describes the main properties of some colloids used in clinical practice (Agro et al. 2013) (Table 15.3).

Table 15.3 Properties of some colloid

Electrolyte or parameter	Plasma	Venofundin 6%	Gelofusine 4%	Tetraspan 6%
Colloid-osmotic pressure (mmHg)	25	37.8	33.3	37.8
Osmolality (mOsm/kg)	287	308	274	296
Colloid molecule	Albumin	HES 130/0.42	MFGel	HES 130/0.42
Sodium (mEq/L)	142	154	154	140
Potassium (mEq/L)	4.5	–	–	4
Magnesium (mEq/L)	1.25	–	–	1
Calcium (mEq/L)	2.5	–	–	2.5
Chloride (mEq/L)	103	154	120	118
Bicarbonate (mEq/L)	25	–	–	–
Acetate/malate (mEq/L)	–	–	–	24/5

From Agro F.E., Fries D., Benedetto M. "How to maintain and restore the balance: colloids." In "Body Fluid Management—From Physiology to Therapy" Agrò F.E. Springer Milan 2013, pages 47–70

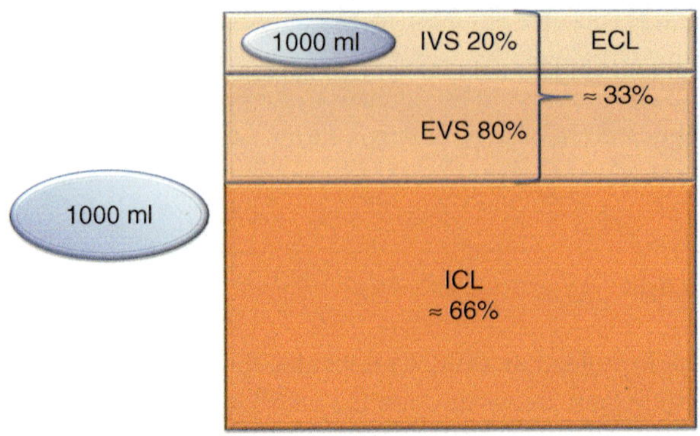

Fig. 15.12 Isotonic colloid distribution. *IVS* intravascular space, *ECS* extracellular space, *EVS* extravascular space, *ICS* intracellular space. From Agro F.E., Fries D., Benedetto M. "How to maintain and restore the balance: colloids." In "Body Fluid Management—From Physiology to Therapy" Agrò F.E. Springer Milan 2013, pages 47–70

15.5.3 Pharmacokinetics: Distribution and Duration of Action

The IVS volume expansion after the infusion of a colloid depends on the oncotic pressure and the molecular weight (MW), and the higher the oncotic pressure and the higher the MW, the greater the initial volume increase in the intravascular space (IVS) after the infusion. The duration of IVS volume expansion is influenced by MW and organ elimination (mainly the kidneys). Thus, different colloids have different duration of volume effects (Agro et al. 2013; Mitra and Khandelwal 2009).

Isotonic and iso-oncotic colloids have a lower volume-replacing power, in contrast to hypertonic and hyperoncotic colloids. Based on previous evidence, (Agro et al. 2013; Nadler et al. 1962; McIlroy and Kharasch 2003) found that, an isotonic colloid is distributed only within the IVS. The efficiency of this kind of solution to expand plasma volume is thus 100% with respect to the infused volume (Agro et al. 2013) (Fig. 15.12). However, iso-oncotic, isosmotic colloids rapidly leave the vascular tree, through extravasation or metabolism, especially during certain conditions, such as systemic inflammation, sepsis, capillary leak syndrome, and third-space syndrome, reducing the effective expansion of IVS volume (Chappell et al. 2008; Agro et al. 2013; Roberts and Bratton 1998).

15.6 Natural Colloids: Albumin (HA)

For many years, HA was considered the gold standard in hypovolemia treatment. HA is composed of 585 amino acids with a molecular mass of 69,000 daltons. It is the main plasma protein (50–60%), accounting for 80% of normal oncotic pressure. Furthermore, HA contributes to the formation of a normal anion gap and acid-base balance while being a charged protein (Agro et al. 2013).

15.6.1 Composition and Concentration

Current HA solutions consist of 96% albumin, with the remaining 4% being globulins. Different concentrations of HA are commercially available: 20% and 25% HA (hyperoncotic), 5% HA (iso-oncotic), and 4% HA (hypo-oncotic) (Agro et al. 2013).

15.6.2 Pharmacokinetics: Distribution, Elimination, and Duration of Action

A 5% HA solution can be reasonably considered for volume replacement, leading to an 80% initial volume expansion, whereas 25% HA leads to a 200–400% volume increase within 30 min. The volume effect lasts for 16–24 h (Agro et al. 2013; Mitra and Khandelwal 2009). The decrease in the plasma HA concentration is firstly due to passage from the IVS to the EVS through the transporter albondin (transcapillary exchange) and secondly to the fractional degradation rate (Agro et al. 2013; Dubois and Vincent 2007).

15.6.3 Clinical Use

There is an extensive literature about the use of HA in the treatment of acute hypovolemia, especially in cardiac surgery. In this class of patients, it is historically considered the best volume replacement solution. Additional applications are sepsis, systemic inflammatory response syndrome, and capillary leakage syndromes (Agro et al. 2013).

Based on the results of the SAFE study (Study Investigators et al. 2011), HA has been mainly used to treat low plasma protein levels. The rationale is to prevent fluid extravasation by increasing the IVS COP in patients at high risk of hypoalbuminemia (Agro et al. 2013). Low serum albumin was shown to be a marker of poor outcome, with a mortality of approximately 100% (Agro et al. 2013; Fleck et al. 1985; Marik 1993; Margarson and Soni 1998; Rubin et al. 1997).

HA is not exclusively retained in the IVS, rather, 10% of the administered dose leaves the IVS within 2 h. It is therefore likely to leak into the ISS, potentially aggravating interstitial edema and hypoalbuminemia, without clinical benefits, especially in patient with increased vessel permeability (cardiac surgery, cardiopulmonary bypass stress response, glycocalyx damages) (Lira and Pinsky 2014; Agro et al. 2013).

A meta-analysis by Russell et al. (2004) showed HA use yields good results with respect to platelet count, as well as a positive influence on oncotic pressure and postoperative weight gain in cardiac surgery patients, with respect to crystalloids. On the other side, more recent preliminary data indicate albumin is associated with increased risk of acute kidney injury after cardiac surgery (Caironi et al. 2015). HA rational use is guided by absolute and relative indications. The administration of HA is indicated in acute conditions requiring plasma expansion and in chronic conditions characterized by low albumin plasma levels (Vincent et al. 2003). There is widespread consensus in the literature and in clinic, regarding absolute indications. Relative indications refer to settings in which HA is indicated when other specific criteria are satisfied (Agro et al. 2013).

The cardiac surgery is a relative indication to HA use. In particular HA is indicated as the third choice after crystalloid and synthetic colloid administration.

Another relative indication that may be present in cardiac surgery patients is hemorrhagic shock, although in this case, it is indicated when there is no response to crystalloid and synthetic colloid administration (Agro et al. 2013).

Finally HA may be preferred over synthetic colloids for CPB priming, since it preserves oncotic pressure, prevents platelet adhesion, and likely induces less consumption of coagulation factors (Lira and Pinsky 2014).

HA dose needed may be calculated as follows (Agro et al. 2013):

$$\text{Dose}(g) = \left[\text{targeted albuminemia}(2.5\,\text{g/dL}) - \text{real albuminemia}(\text{g/dL})\right] \times \text{plasmatic volume}\ (0.8 \times \text{body weight in kg})$$

Albumin is routinely administered, albeit improperly, in post-cardiac surgery ICU patients in case of (Agro et al. 2013):

- Hypoalbuminemia in the absence of peripheral edema or acute hypotension
- Malnutrition and malabsorption
- Wound healing
- Nonhemorrhagic shock
- Diuretic-responsive ascites
- Hemodialysis
- Ischemic stroke

HA use in the cardiac surgery patient is expensive, and the clinical advantages achievable do not seem to justify its cost (Agro et al. 2013). Large, randomized clinical trials comparing the benefit of HA versus other fluids are needed to define HA distinct role in select high-risk surgical populations.

15.6.4 Potential Risks and Side Effects

Several lines of evidence explain why HA supplementation may worsen the ICU patient condition (Agro et al. 2013). In fact, after rapid volume replacement, cardiac failure may occur, causing or worsening pulmonary edema, especially in capillary leak syndrome (Agro et al. 2013; Kaminski and Williams 1990). Furthermore, HA may impact coagulation and hemostasis by enhancing antithrombin III activity and inhibiting platelet function (Agro et al. 2013; Rajnish et al. 2004). Tobias et al. (1998) found that albumin may also lead to hypocoagulability. Dietrich et al. (1990) showed an in vitro increase in bleeding time, which may increase blood loss in postsurgical patients. Finally, albumin administration may impair the efficiency of endothelial cell adhesion. The importance of this effect is uncertain, since increased plasma levels of endothelial adhesion molecules may be markers of mortality (Agro et al. 2013; Kaminski and Williams 1990).

In acute renal failure, HA may accumulate after its massive administration (Agro et al. 2013; Kaminski and Williams 1990).

HA is generally well tolerated, but immediate allergic reactions are possible, consisting of fever, nausea, vomiting, pruritus, hypotension, and even cardiorespiratory collapse (Agro et al. 2013).

15.7 Synthetic Colloids

Synthetic or artificial colloids (dextrans, gelatins, hydroxyethyl starches) are produced from biological, nonhuman molecules. Their assessment criteria include (Agro et al. 2013) (Table 15.4):

- Concentration
- Initial volume effect
- Duration of the volume effect
- Side effects

15.8 Dextrans

Dextrans are glucose polymers of different sizes, derived from *Leuconostoc mesenteroides*, a bacterium originally isolated from contaminated sugar beets (Agro et al. 2013).

Dextrans are mainly used in the United States, as they are no longer available in European countries. The most widely used dextran solutions are dextran 40 (a 10% solution with 40,000 mean MW) and dextran 70 (a 6% solution with 70,000 mean MW) (Agro et al. 2013) (Table 15.5).

Table 15.4 Comparison between therapeutic and side effects of artificial colloids

	Volemic effect		Side effect		
Colloid	Efficacy	Duration	AKI	Coag.	Anaph.
Dextrans	+++	+++	+++$_{(40)}$	+++$_{(70)}$	++
Gelatins	+	+	+	+	+++
HES with high MMW	+++	+++	++	+++	+
HES with low MMW	+++	++	+	++	+

+ mild; ++ moderate; +++ high; MMW, mean molecular weight

From Agro F.E., Fries D., Benedetto M. "How to maintain and restore the balance: colloids." In "Body Fluid Management—From Physiology to Therapy" Agrò F.E. Springer Milan 2013, pages 47–70

Table 15.5 Main properties of dextrans

Characteristics of dextran solutions	6% dextran 70	10% dextran 40
Mean molecular weight (dalton)	70,000	40,000
Volume efficacy (%)	100	175–(200)
Volume effect (hours)	5	3–4
Maximum daily dose (g/kg)	1.5	1.5

From Agro F.E., Fries D., Benedetto M. "How to maintain and restore the balance: colloids." In "Body Fluid Management—From Physiology to Therapy" Agrò F.E. Springer Milan 2013, pages 47–70

15.8.1 Pharmacokinetics: Distribution, Elimination, and Duration of Action

Dextrans are endowed with a high COP, due to their high water-binding capacity. After the infusion, dextrans lead to a 100–150% increase in the volume of the IVS (Agro et al. 2013; Mitra and Khandelwal 2009). They are mainly eliminated by the kidney, while only a small fraction transiently passes into the ISS or is eliminated by the gastrointestinal tract. In particular, smaller molecules (14,000–18,000 kDa) are excreted by the kidneys within 15 min, whereas larger molecules are excreted after several days. At 12 h from administration, 60% of dextran 40 and 30% of dextran 70 have already been eliminated (Agro et al. 2013; Mitra and Khandelwal 2009; Arthurson et al. 1964; Atik 1967).

15.8.2 Clinical Use

Dextran solutions may be suitable in post-cardiac surgery ICU patients because they have positive effects on circulation. In fact, they have been shown to adequately restore and maintain hemodynamic in case of shock and to ameliorate tissue perfusion and microcirculation. At the same degree of hemodilution, rheological effects are mainly correlated with the use of dextran 40 rather than with any other plasma substitute. Moreover, dextran protects against ischemia-reperfusion injury by reducing the harmful interactions between activated leukocytes and the microvascular endothelium (Agro et al. 2013).

15.8.3 Potential Risks and Side Effects

Despite evidence on improvement of macro- and microcirculation after infusion, dextrans are no longer used because of their side effects (Agro et al. 2013).

Dextran administration may lead to anaphylactoid reactions more frequently and more severely than other colloids. This is due to the massive production of vasoactive mediators triggered by anti-dextran antibodies. These reactions may be prevented by pretreatment of the solution with 20 mL of hapten (dextran 1000) few minutes before infusion (Agro et al. 2013; Allhoff and Lenhart 1993).

Another possible side effect is renal dysfunction and AKI, through the production of hyperviscous urines leading to swelling and vacuolization of tubular cells and tubular plugging. This is especially true in patients with advanced age, hemodynamic alterations, pre-existing renal disease, and dehydration (Agro et al. 2013; Mitra and Khandelwal 2009; Baron 2000; Moran and Kapsner 1987).

Finally, dextrans may alter platelet function, decrease factor VIII levels, and increase fibrinolysis, with significant bleeding disorders, especially after the administration of high doses (Agro et al. 2013; Mitra and Khandelwal 2009; Barron and Wilkes 2004). These side effects resulted in maximum daily dose recommendation of approximately 1.5 L.

Currently dextrans have a very limited use in the clinical practice, especially in ICU patients who present many risk factors for the development of dextran side effects (Agro et al. 2013).

15.9 Gelatins

Gelatins are polydispersed peptides derived from bovine collagen. Three types of gelatins are currently available: cross-linked or oxypolygelatins (e.g., Gelofundiol), urea-cross-linked gelatins (e.g., Haemaccel), and succinylated or modified fluid gelatins (e.g., Gelofusine) (Table 15.6). Their average MW is 30–35,000 daltons, and they are based on unbalanced, hypotonic solutions. In particular, polygelines are dispersed in a 3.5% polyelectrolyte solution generally containing Na^+ 145 mEq/L, K^+ 5.1 mEq/L, Ca^{2+} 6.25 mEq/L, and Cl^- 145 mEq/L. Thus, they may increase serum calcium, in particular after large-volume infusions. Succinylated gelatins are dispersed in a 4% polyelectrolyte solution generally containing Na^+ 154 mEq/L, K^+ 0.4 mEq/L, Ca^{2+} 0.4 mEq/L, and Cl^-120 mEq/L (effective SID = 34). Their low chloride content reduces the risk of hyperchloremic acidosis and may be helpful in patients with acid-base alterations (see Chap. 16). They are compatible with blood transfusions because of their low calcium content (Agro et al. 2013; Mitra and Khandelwal 2009).

Table 15.6 Main properties of gelatins

Characteristics of gelatin solutions	Succinylated gelatins	Cross-linked gelatins	Urea-cross-linked gelatins
Concentration (%)	4.0	5.5	3.5
Mean molecular weight (dalton)	30,000	30,000	35,000
Volume efficacy (%)	80	80	80
Volume effect in hours	1–3	1–3	1–3
Osmolarity (mOsm/L)	274	296	301

From Agro F.E., Fries D., Benedetto M. "How to maintain and restore the balance: colloids." In "Body Fluid Management—From Physiology to Therapy" Agrò F.E. Springer Milan 2013, pages 47–70

15.9.1 Pharmacokinetics: Distribution, Elimination, and Duration of Effect

Gelatins have similar IVS volume-expanding power and a half-life of about 2.5 h. After 24 h post administration, 13% remains in the IVS, 16% has passed into the ISS, 71% is rapidly cleared by the kidneys, and a small amount has been cleaved by proteases in the reticuloendothelial system (RES). Notably, the volume expansion is lower than the infused volume (about 70–80%). Gelatins have the shortest duration of effect than any other colloids. Therefore, repeated infusions are required and allowed by their rapid elimination, as there are no dose limitations, in contrast to other colloids (Agro et al. 2013; Mitra and Khandelwal 2009; Barron and Wilkes 2004).

15.9.2 Potential Risks and Side Effects

In ICU patients and in patients with severe hemorrhagic shock, who need large intravascular volume replacement, gelatin solutions are still widely adopted because of the lack of accumulation in the reticuloendothelial system (RES), the unlimited dose, and the absence of significant side effects on kidney function. Conversely, they are the second most frequent cause of anaphylactic shock in cardiac surgery patients, following antibiotics (Agro et al. 2013; Barron and Wilkes 2004).

Historically gelatins have been considered safer than other colloid with respect to bleeding. However, recently, there has been evidence of platelet dysfunction and clotting disorders (Agro et al. 2013). In a study comparing the effects of progressive hemodilution with gelatins, saline, hydroxyethyl starches, and albumin on blood coagulation, significant changes in the thromboelastogram were found after the infusion of gelatin solutions (Adamson 2008). Nonetheless, in clinical practice, they seem to impair fibrin polymerization less than the "modern" medium-molecular weight starches (Agro et al. 2013).

15.10 Hydroxyethyl Starches

Hydroxyethyl starches (HES) are modified natural polysaccharides derived from amylopectin, a highly branched starch similar to glycogen, derived from maize or potatoes. Polymerized D-glucose units are connected by 1–4 linkages with one 1–6 branching linkage every 20 glucose units. Natural starches cannot be used in clinical routine since they are rapidly hydrolyzed by circulating α-amylases (Fig. 15.13). HES are obtained by replacing the hydroxyl groups of natural starches with hydroxyethyl groups at the C2, C3, and C6 carbon positions of anhydroglucose residues. A greater solubility and less amylase degradation are obtained, especially for hydroxyethyl groups at the C2 position (Agro et al. 2013; Mitra and Khandelwal 2009).

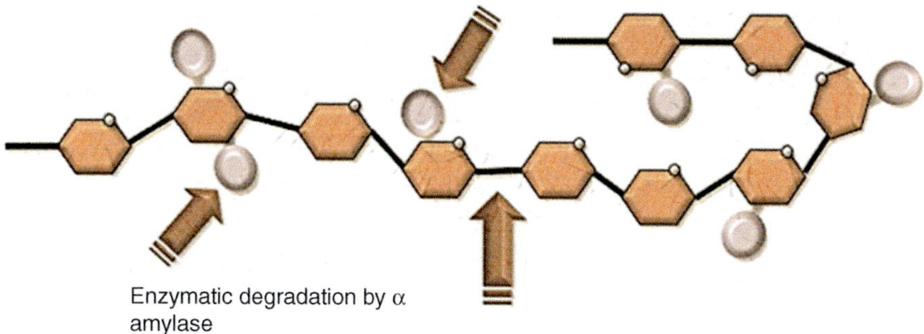

Fig. 15.13 Effect of α-amylases on natural starches. From Agro F.E., Fries D., Benedetto M. "How to maintain and restore the balance: colloids." In "Body Fluid Management—From Physiology to Therapy" Agrò F.E. Springer Milan 2013, pages 47–70

15.10.1 Classification

The first HES was produced in the 1970s in the United States. Since then, further generations have been produced. HES are designated by a series of numeric parameters (e.g., HES 10% 200/0.5/5) reflecting their pharmacokinetics. The first number relates to the solution concentration, the second represents the mean MW (MMW), the third is the molar substitution rate (MSR), and the fourth is the C2/C6 ratio. Thus, HES may be classified according to (**Agro et al.** 2013):

- Concentration (3%, 6%, 10%)
- MMW (low molecular weight, 70 kDa; medium molecular weight, 130–270 kDa; high molecular weight, > 450 kDa)
- MSR (low MS, 0.4–0.5; high MS, 0.62–0.7)
- C2/C6 ratio

The volume expansion power of HES is firstly influenced by concentration. HES at 6% concentration are iso-oncotic and have a 100% volume-expanding power (1 L of fluid infused = 1 L of plasma volume expansion). HES at 10% concentration are hyperoncotic and have a volume-expanding power > 100% (1 L of fluid infused = > 1 L of plasma volume expansion) (Agro et al. 2013; Mitra and Khandelwal 2009; Dubois and Vincent 2007).

HES are polydispersed solutions made up of different-sized molecules. Particles with a low MW (45–70 kDa) have a rapid enzymatic degradation and a fast renal excretion, because their size is under the renal threshold. Particles with high MW (>70 kDa) have a longer half-life, according to both their size and their rate of enzymatic degradation. The combined effect of the particles with different metabolism influences duration of volemic effect after HES infusion (Agro et al. 2013; Barron and Wilkes 2004).

The MSR is the rate of the total number of hydroxyethyl groups to the total number of glucose units. The MSR impacts human α-amylase degradation and thus the breakdown of the starch: the higher the MSR, the slower the degradation, the longer the volume effect, and the higher the incidence of side effects (Agro et al. 2013; Mitra and Khandelwal 2009; Barron and Wilkes 2004).

The quotient of the total number of hydroxyethyl groups on carbon atom 2 and the total number of hydroxyethyl groups on carbon atom 6 yields the C2:C6 ratio (Fig. 15.14). For example, a C2:C6 ratio of 9 is to 1 means that substitution with hydroxyethyl groups at position C2 is nine times higher than at position C6 (Agro et al. 2013; Barron and Wilkes 2004). The C2 hydroxyethyl group hinders the action of α-amylase, delaying HES degradation and increasing the volume-expanding power. A higher C2:C6 ratio means lower α-amylase degradation, with a longer and greater volume effect (Agro et al. 2013; Mitra and Khandelwal 2009; Barron and Wilkes 2004).

HES can also be classified according to the electrolyte features of the carrier solution, yielding balanced or unbalanced, plasma-adapted or non-plasma-adapted HES solutions (Agro et al. 2013).

Three successive generations of HES have been commercialized (Agro et al. 2013) (Table 15.7):

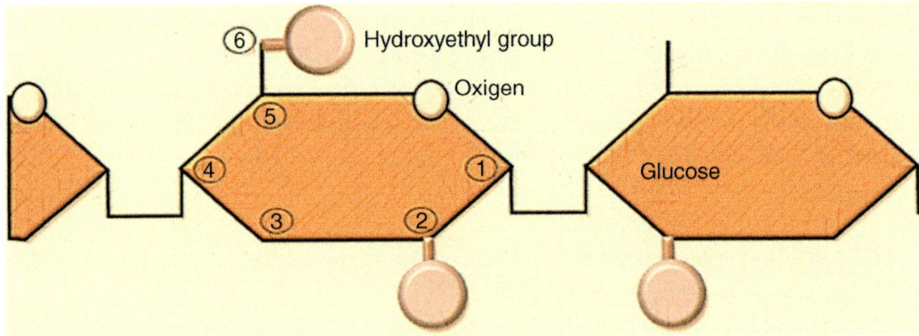

Fig. 15.14 Representation of the C2:C6 ratio. From Agro F.E., Fries D., Benedetto M. "How to maintain and restore the balance: colloids." In "Body Fluid Management—From Physiology to Therapy" Agrò F.E. Springer Milan 2013, pages 47–70

Table 15.7 Comparison between HES generation properties

Concentration	Origin	Solvent	Mean molecular weight (MMW)	Molar substitution rate (MSR)	C2/C6 ratio
3% (hyponcotic)	Potato-derived HES	Unbalanced	Low = 70 KD	Low:<0.5	9:1
6% (normoncotic)	Waxy maize-derived HES	Balanced	Medium 130–370 KD	Medium = 0.5	6:1
10% (hyperoncotic)	–	–	High >450 KD	High: >0.5	4:1

From Agro F.E., Fries D., Benedetto M. "How to maintain and restore the balance: colloids." In "Body Fluid Management—From Physiology to Therapy" Agrò F.E. Springer Milan 2013, pages 47–70

- First generation: MW > 450 kDa, MS > 0.7, and high C2:C6 ratio
- Second generation: lower MW (200 kDa), MS (0.5), and lower C2:C6 ratio
- Third generation: MW = 130 kDa, MS < 0.5, and lower C2:C6 ratio

Thus, HES widely differ with respect to the extent and duration of their volume-expansion power and their side effects (Agro et al. 2013).

15.10.2 Pharmacokinetics: Distribution, Elimination, and Duration of Action

The water-binding capacity of HES varies between 20 and 30 mL/g (Agro et al. 2013; Mitra and Khandelwal 2009). As previously described, small molecules are rapidly excreted by the kidney (up to 50% of the administered dose within 24 h), whereas larger molecules are retained for longer amounts of time. The oncotic effect of HES is due solely to the number of particles, and not their size. While renal elimination of the small molecules reduces the oncotic power, this is compensated by the enzymatic degradation of the large molecules. Consequently, the expanding power of HES is greater than that of other synthetic colloids, particularly gelatins (Agro et al. 2013). The duration of the volume effect equals the time interval of HES retention in the vascular bed, usually 8–12 h. A minor amount of the small molecules passes into the ISS, for later redistribution and elimination. Another fraction is trapped by RES, which slowly break down the starch (tissue storage) (Agro et al. 2013; Mitra and Khandelwal 2009). Thus, HES can be detected for several days after their infusion (Solanke et al. 1971; Lehmann et al. 2007; Wilkes et al. 2001).

As mentioned, there are potato- and maize-derived HES. They have the same oncotic power and plasma-expanding effects, even if the former have a more rapid elimination due to their lower amylopectin content (about 80%) (Agro et al. 2013; Wilkes et al. 2001).

In the subsequent HES generations, MMW, MSR, and the C2:C6 ratio have been modified to allow α-amylase degradation, to reduce the retention of residual fractions, and to prolong the volume effect, with less accumulation and side effects (Agro et al. 2013; Mitra and Khandelwal 2009) (Table 15.8).

HES molecules are generally dispersed in unbalanced, non-plasma-adapted solutions (first, second, and third generations). The first balanced HES solution (Hextend) had high MMW (550 kDa) and MS (0.7). However, it resulted in tissue storage, impaired coagulation, and platelet dysfunction. Consequently, the fourth-generation HES have a lower MMW and MSR and are dissolved in balanced solutions (Agro et al. 2013) (Fig. 15.15). At the state of the art, newest-generation HES, such as 6% HES 130/0.42, have the best clinical profile. It is available in two different carrier solutions: 0.9% saline solution (Venofundin) and a solution very similar to plasma (Tetraspan) (Agro et al. 2013).

Table 15.8 Properties of different HES

Properties	HES 70/0.5	HES 130/0.4	HES 200/0.5	HES 200/0.5	HES 200/0.62	HES 400/0.7
Concentration (%)	6	6	6	10	6	6
Mean molecular weight (KD)	70	130	200	200	200	450
Volume effect in hours	1–2	2–3	3–4	3–4	5–6	5–6
Volume efficacy (%)	100	100	100	130	100	100
Molar substitution rate	0.5	0.4	0.5	0.5	0.62	0.7
C2–C6 ratio	4:1	9:1	6:1	6:1	9:1	4.6:1

From Agro F.E., Fries D., Benedetto M. "How to maintain and restore the balance: colloids." In "Body Fluid Management—From Physiology to Therapy" Agrò F.E. Springer Milan 2013, pages 47–70

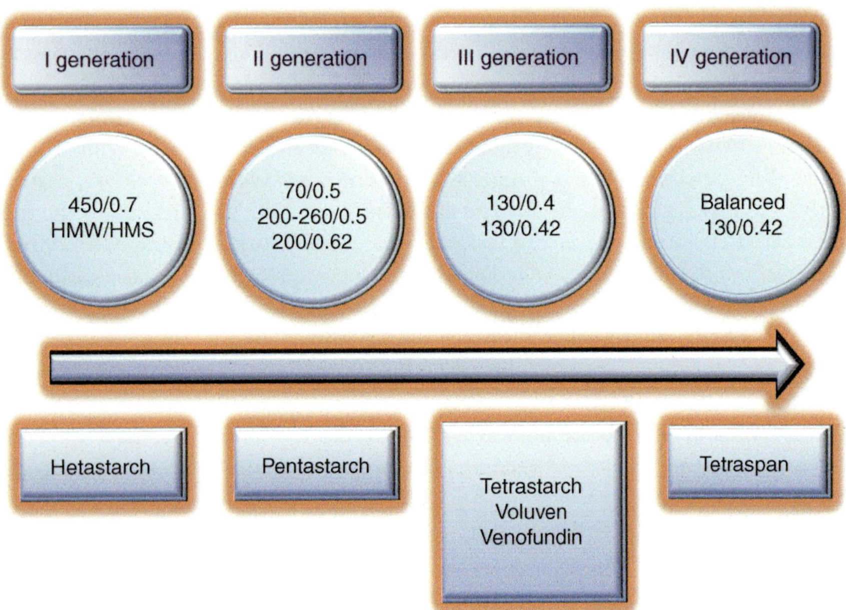

Fig. 15.15 The four HES generations. From Agro F.E., Fries D., Benedetto M. "How to maintain and restore the balance: colloids." In "Body Fluid Management—From Physiology to Therapy" Agrò F.E. Springer Milan 2013, pages 47–70

15.10.3 Clinical Use

In cardiac surgery patients, HES have been widely used for correcting hypovolemia and in CPB priming. The rationale of HES use in the postoperative setting of cardiac surgery is due to their improvement of the macro- and microcirculation in hypovolemic patients. Their effects are determined by the high hemodilutional power in combination with a specific action on red cells, platelets, plasma viscosity, and endothelium. A lower blood viscosity means a reduced vascular resistances, increased venous return, and improved CI. This ameliorates tissue perfusion and oxygenation, with fewer infectious complications, especially in ICU patients (Agrò et al. 2013).

The first- and second-generation HES demonstrated good hemodynamic effects but were the cause of important side effects involving renal function, coagulation, platelet function, and tissue storage and frequently causing pruritus (Agrò et al. 2013).

HES with a lower MMW and a lower MSR (third and fourth generations) are safer in terms of kidney injury, even at higher doses, than older HES generation. In fact, HES 6% 130/0.4 may confer protection in ischemic/toxic renal injury, at least compared to HES 6% 200/0.5. This is an important highlight considering that acute renal failure is a frequent complication in cardiac surgery patients, especially after CPB (Agrò et al. 2013).

Third-generation HES result in improved tissue oxygenation in patients undergoing major abdominal surgery. In particular, patients treated with HES in 0.9% NaCl experienced greater dilution and hyperchloremic acidosis than patients treated with HES in balanced solutions (Agro et al. 2013; Dieterich et al. 2006).

The preservation of endothelial function and the maintenance of endothelial integrity using HES 6%/130/0.4 were also reported. HES solutions with a narrow range of MMW were shown to be effective in reducing capillary edema in an animal model. Furthermore, an improvement in tissue oxygenation secondary to HES infusion has been demonstrated. One explanation for these results is a direct effect of HES on inflammation (e.g., via a reduction in NF-κB release) (Agrò et al. 2013; Traumer et al. 1992; Tian et al. 2004; DeJonge and Levi 2001).

These observations point to potential beneficial effects of HES in reducing systemic stress and the inflammatory response due to surgery and CPB, which may cause glycocalyx damage and capillary leak syndrome, with interstitial and pulmonary edema, increased VO_2, and reduced DO_2 and O_2 tissue diffusion. Thus, modern HES preparations can be expected to reduce cardiovascular changes that may alter or precipitate disturbances in the hemodynamic and metabolic equilibrium of cardiac surgery patients. Larger studies are needed to confirm HES anti-inflammatory effects on cardiac surgery outcomes (Fanzca 2012; Agrò et al. 2013; Agro et al. 2013).

15.10.4 Potential Risks and Side Effects

HES side effects are cause of matter in literature, particularly in cardiac surgery patients that are at increased risk to develop bleeding, renal failure, and alteration of colloids volume effect. The development of one of these features may affect their survival (Fanzca 2012; Agro et al. 2013).

15.10.4.1 Coagulation and Platelet Function

One concern regarding HES use in cardiac surgery is their association with coagulation and platelet disturbances and, consequently, a greater bleeding risk with an increased transfusional need. There is a broad debate about whether HES coagulation and platelet effects have an actual clinical impact (Agrò et al. 2013).

Observed decreases in von Willebrand factor, fibrinogen levels, and thrombin generation presumably alter the coagulation time, clot formation time, and maximum clot firmness, as shown on intrinsic thromboelastography (Agro et al. 2013). Previous reports in the literature showed a severe increase in the bleeding risk with high MMW and MSR HES (i.e., heptastich, MW 450 kDa, MSR, 0.7). This is due to a von Willebrand-like syndrome, with decreased factor VIII activity and reduced levels of von Willebrand factor antigen and factor VIII-related ristocetin cofactor. HES also impair fibrin polymerization, although HES with a medium MMW and a low MS probably do not strongly affect the coagulation system (Agro et al. 2013; DeJonge and Levi 2001; Sanfelippo et al. 1987; Treib et al. 1999; Madjdpour et al. 2005).

The effect of HES on platelet function during cardiac surgery is an additional concern of HES use.

HES with a high MMW, high MSR, and high C2/C6 ratio (e.g., HES 450/0.7 or HES 200/0.62) alter platelet function to a greater extent than HES with a lower MMW and a lower MSR, as mentioned above for coagulation (Agro et al. 2013; Kozek-Langenecker 2005; Strauss et al. 2002; Haynes et al. 2004). Franz et al. (2001) studied the effects of IV infusion of saline solution and four HES preparations with different MWW and MSR on platelet function. HES 450/0.7, HES 200/0.6, and HES 70/0.5 prolonged platelet function analyzer (PFA)-100 closure times. All of the tested HES preparations reduced platelet GPIIb/IIIa expression. By contrast, the newest-generation HES seem to have reduced negative effects on platelets. Stogermuller et al. (2000) reported that expression of platelet GP IIb/IIIa was reduced after the infusion of non-balanced HES 200. However, according to in vitro studies, GP IIb/IIIa expression increases with high MMW and high MSR HES in a balanced solution. This unexpected result was obtained with a solvent containing calcium chloride dihydrate (2.5 mmol/L) (Agro et al. 2013; Stögermüller et al. 2000). HES in balanced plasma-adapted solutions were shown to have fewer effects on platelets. Many reports confirmed the importance of the solvent in determining potential adverse effects of HES solutions (Agro et al. 2013; Stögermüller et al. 2000). Gallandat et al. (2000) found that in cardiac surgery patients, new-generation HES increase von Willebrand factor levels to a greater extent than HES 200/0.5, resulting in a reduction of bleeding risk and transfusional need. Similar results were found in patients undergoing orthopedic surgery and major surgery (Agro et al. 2013).

However, negative effects of modern HES preparations on coagulation and platelets have also been reported. For example, Scharbert et al. (2004) found an impairment of platelet function by HES 130 similar to that of HES 200 in patients with chronic back pain undergoing epidural anesthesia. Nevertheless, HES 130 produced a not clinically significant platelet alteration. Similar results were reported for minor elective surgery (Agro et al. 2013). Finally, in a recent meta-analysis, the use of third- vs. second-generation HES was not related to clinical (and statistically significant) differences in patients with blood loss after surgery (Agro et al. 2013; Raja et al. 2011).

15.10.4.2 Kidney Dysfunction

Another clinical concern about HES use is the risk of kidney damage. All colloids can induce kidney injury. The most likely mechanism of renal dysfunction is a tubular obstruction caused by hyperoncotic urine formation with the storage of colloidal molecules filtered by the glomeruli. This mechanism is further impaired by a condition of dehydration. Another suggested mechanism is an increase in plasma oncotic pressure, with secondary renal macromolecules accumulation. Adequate hydration using crystalloids may prevent this injury (Agro et al. 2013).

The proposed risk factors for HES-related kidney dysfunction are:

- Age (older patients have a higher risk)
- Hypovolemia
- Previous kidney alterations (chronic or acute injury due to other causes)
- Others comorbidities (such as diabetes and other conditions causing direct or indirect renal alterations)

Clinical evidences of the renal effects of HES are not uniform, and there is still intense debate in the literature as to whether there is truly a critical creatinine level for HES administration. The debate leads to a large controversy, when many of the original data published by Joachim Boldt showing outcome benefits of HES were discovered to be falsified, resulting in subsequent retraction of these studies and to a revision of meta-analysis after this retrying. Several randomized controlled trials and meta-analysis have raised alarming concerns about the HES adverse effects on mortality but also on increased incidence of renal injury or failure with higher need for renal replacement therapy (RRT) in critically ill patients. It is unknow if these findings could be exteded to the perioperative setting, where a variety of distinct patient populations is encountered; these concerns (in particular reported in VISEP, CHEST, and 6S studies) have resulted in the negative advice given by the EMA in 2013 with regard to the use of HES solutions in patient care, limiting their use in hemorrhagic shock when crystalloid alone is not adequate. The US Food and Drug Administration also communicated a serious warning with respect to HES use (Ghijselings and Rex 2014; Serpa Neto et al. 2014; Mutter et al. 2013).

Despite the fact that these different studies were all published in prestigious journals, they all contain some methodological biases that have been focused in literature, since the publication of warning and limitation to HES (De Hert and De Baerdemaeker 2014; Wiedermann 2014). An inappropriate daily positive fluid balance was likely an important source of heterogeneity in the trials reporting HES130/0.4 associated with excess mortality in septic patients (Ma et al. 2015). Other biases are the reduced number of patients in which a difference in the HES group was found (i.e., 30 vs. 7000 patients in CHEST study), the much larger HES doses (in some cases in excess of recommendations or common practice) used (VISEP, 6S study), and the inclusion of studies with a wide range of HES used (first- and second-generation HES, together with third generation) (Vincent et al. 2013). Furthermore in the three studies (VISEP, 6S, CHEST), the starting was delayed after diagnosis of severe sepsis, when the majority of patients have already completed the initial stabilization (hemodynamic goals achieved, according to Surviving Sepsis Campaign), implying that the patients randomized to the HES group were tested for a non-indicated drug compared to the rational and well-established strategy for fluid maintenance with crystalloids in stable patients (De Hert and De Baerdemaeker 2014; Wiedermann 2014; Ma et al. 2015; Vincent et al. 2013).

Patient with renal failure at randomization were included in the studies, while they should be excluded (De Hert and De Baerdemaeker 2014; Wiedermann 2014; Ma et al. 2015; Vincent et al. 2013).

It is very likely that the higher incidence of RRT simply reflects the situation that more patients received this therapy, but not that this therapy was indeed required. Instead, an independent analysis of the data even indicates that due to an improved kidney function and no differences in RRT, CHEST shows an advantage over HES (De Hert and De Baerdemaeker 2014; Vincent et al. 2013). Finally, in the three studies, patients who had renal failure at randomization were anyway included in the study. In 508 patients of the saline group who had received HES prior to randomization, 30% of the patients were septic, and in this subgroup, no difference in mortality, renal failure, or need for renal replacement therapy was observed (De Hert and De Baerdemaeker 2014; Wiedermann 2014; Ma et al. 2015; Vincent et al. 2013). The major studies supporting limited HES use present issues about treatment strategies, ignoring contraindications and maximum recommended daily doses, overinterpretation of results, and selective biased analysis of data (De Hert and De Baerdemaeker 2014; Wiedermann 2014; Ma et al. 2015; Vincent et al. 2013).

The use of last-generation HES in elective surgery patients is associated with reduced fluid accumulation and no clinically relevant difference in bleeding or AKI rate as compared with crystalloid use alone. As they provide no benefit, older starch preparations should not be used (Heßler et al. 2015).

The Colloids Compared to Crystalloids in Fluid Resuscitation of Critically Ill Patients study, which included 3000 patients, showed a less positive fluid balance and lower 90-day mortality rates in colloid-treated than in crystalloid-treated patients, and the colloids administered were primarily synthetic (Vincent et al. 2013).

Recent trials that supported HES clinical use restriction have clearly characterized the toxic effects of HES solutions but do not inform on potential benefit. None of the intravenous fluids currently available may be entirely safe, especially when given in large amounts. All fluids should be considered as drugs, and no drug is risk-free. Indeed, one can consider that even oral fluids have their risks: beer, wine, and nonalcoholic beverages, such as coffee and sugar-containing beverages, should all be taken only in moderation, and even water can be harmful if taken in excess (Mutter et al. 2013; De Hert and De Baerdemaeker 2014; Wiedermann 2014; Ma et al. 2015; Vincent et al. 2013).

The type of HES administered (higher MMW and MS) and the total amount infused per kg of body weight have been shown to have an important role in the possibility of side effect manifestation. An increased incidence of kidney dysfunction has been reported in patients treated with high MMW and high MS HES (Agro et al. 2013; Vincent et al. 2013). When used in the proper indication, it has been shown that 6% HES 130/0.4 could have a superior risk/benefit ratio and improved outcome compared to crystalloids (Vincent et al. 2013).

The history of HES has impressively shown that infusion therapy must be adjusted on a scientifically founded basis, whether in intensive care medicine, perioperative medicine, or emergency medicine. Large prospective studies with clinically relevant endpoints are urgently needed (Heßler et al. 2015).

15.10.4.3 Anaphylaxis

All colloidal plasma substitutes can cause anaphylactic/anaphylactoid reactions due to specific or non-specific histamine release. In a trial comprising approximately 20,000 patients, Laxenaire et al., (Rehm 2013) found a decreased incidence of anaphylaxis with HES compared to other colloids. Histamine release seems to be induced by the starch itself; thus, it is unlikely that recent modifications of the MMW, MS, or C2/C6 ratio are the cause of the increased anaphylactic power (Agro et al. 2013).

15.10.4.4 Storing and Itching

HES are stored in either the reticuloendothelial or mononuclear phagocyte system, depending on their chemical features, without causing phagocyte dysfunction. High MMW HES have an elevated rate of storage, especially after prolonged or repetitive administrations. By contrast, in animal studies, the newest-generation HES were found to cause less storage, even after multiple uses (Agro et al. 2013). One day after the infusion of HES 130/0.4, the percentage remaining in the plasma is approximately 2%, rather than the 8% after the infusion of HES 200/0.5 (Agro et al. 2013). Moreover, in a prospective crossover study on healthy volunteers, HES 130/0.42 showed minimal accumulation after repeated administration, whereas HES 200/0.5 was stored in significant amounts (Laxenaire et al. 1994).

Itching reportedly occurs after prolonged administration of large amounts of HES, especially the older generation ones. In some cases, pruritus has been reported after a single large HES dose (≥ 2 L). Itching induced by HES has a late onset (weeks or even months after their administration) and is long-lasting. It is due to storage of the material in small peripheral nerves (Agro et al. 2013). In a prospective multicenter study, 500 patients were observed 3–9 weeks postoperatively; no differences were found in terms of itching between patients treated with HES and control patients (Agro et al. 2013; Waitzinger et al. 2003).

15.11 Hypertonic Colloid Solutions

In a recent study, the hemodynamic effects of hypertonic colloids (7.2% HES, HC) were compared with Ringer's solution, after CABG (Metze et al. 1997). At 15 min from the infusion, they were shown to significantly increase CI with a lower infused volume. Systemic and pulmonary resistances were lower in the HC group at short (15 min), intermediate (60 min), and longer time (180 min) after the infusion. HC and crystalloid groups did not differ in mean blood loss.

The use of 7.5% HES was shown to have a positive effect on hemodynamics with reduced fluid requirements and few effects on postoperative bleeding after CABG (Sirvinskas et al. 2007).

15.12 Comparison Between Crystalloids and Colloids

The previous paragraphs evidenced the crucial need to restore IVS volume in the cardiac surgery patients.

Theoretically, we expect greater advantages in blood volume expansion with isotonic colloids than with isotonic crystalloids (Agro and Vennari 2013b) (Fig. 15.16).

Crystalloids are mainly distributed in the ISS, with less effectiveness in maintaining plasma volume, because they do not contain oncotic particles (Agro and Vennari 2013b). (Their duration of action is short, with large volume needed for a specific target volume expansion (Agro and Vennari 2013b; Habicher et al. 2011). Their infusion dilutes plasma proteins, thus reducing the COP. Consequently, there is a diffusion of fluids from the IVS to the ISS. This fluid shift increases when vascular permeability is altered, increasing interstitial edema. A relationship between the administration of high fluid volumes and increased mortality has been reported in cardiac surgery patients (Agrò et al. 2013; Rackow et al. 1983).

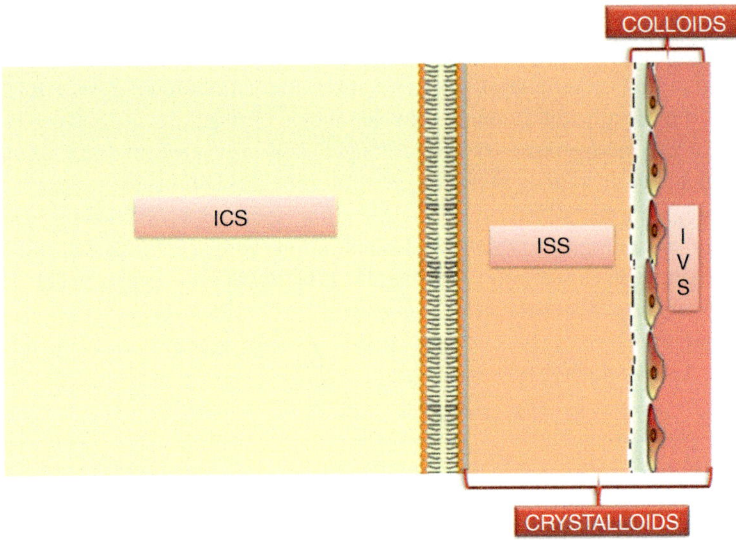

Fig. 15.16 Comparison between colloids and crystalloids distribution. Modified from Agro F.E., Vennari M. Clinical treatment: the right fluid in the right quantity. From: "Body Fluid Management—From Physiology to Therapy" Agrò F.E. Springer Milan 2013, pages 71–92

According to the literature, the use of crystalloids for volume stabilization in patients with circulatory shock is related to a higher risk of altered lung function because of pulmonary edema (fluid overload, referred to as "Da Nang lung" based on the large number of cases in the Vietnam war) (Agrò et al. 2013; Pradeep et al. 2010). In particular, the use of crystalloids seems to be less appropriate in patients with reduced myocardial function. Animal studies on acute normovolemic hemodilution with Ringer's lactate vs. HES demonstrated that HES group presented a significative increase in CI. Moreover, the microscopic study of left ventricular wall revealed the destruction of myofilaments, and mucosal gastric pH was significantly reduced (index of hypoperfusion) in the Ringer's lactate group (Stein et al. 1975). Cardiopulmonary bypass with crystalloids has also been associated with postoperative myocardial edema and cerebral dysfunction with respect to colloids (Otsuki et al. 2007; Lasks et al. 1977). On the other hand, Ringer's solutions were found to not increase water pulmonary volume with respect to dextran 70, after CABG procedures, with no difference on PO_2/FiO_2 (Iriz et al. 2005). Similar result was found in a more recent study comparing 0.9% saline, 4% gelatin, 6% HES 200/0.5, and 5% albumin in a sample of major vascular surgery: no difference was found in PaO_2/FIO_2 ratio and in pulmonary leak index among the groups (Karanko et al. 1987).

Colloids are distributed in the IVS, with a larger increase in plasma volume because they contain oncotic particles. They have a longer duration of action, with smaller volumes needed for a specific target volume expansion than crystalloids (Agrò et al. 2013; Verheij et al. 2006a, b; Ernest et al. 2001). If endothelial permeability is intact, colloids are retained in the IVS, with a subsequent increase of the plasma oncotic pressure and the diffusion of fluids from the ISS to the IVS (Agro and Vennari 2013b) (Fig. 15.16). Colloids have a "contest volume effect": in hypovolemic patients, they have a volume effect >90% of the volume infused; in normovolemic patients, two-thirds of the infused volume shifts to the ISS within minutes (Chappell et al. 2008). Consequently, they should be used only in hypovolemia, even when there is capillary membrane damage. In fact, in this case, hypovolemia is connected to the shift into the ISS of protein-rich fluids, with a plasma COP reduction. Colloids that are able to increase COP are needed (Chappell et al. 2008; Dorje et al. 2000).

In 2006, Verheij et al. (2006b) showed that volume expansion and CI were significantly higher after colloid infusion than after the administration of crystalloids, following cardiac surgery. They found colloids were approximately five times as efficient in expanding the IVS volume with respect to saline 0.9%. Ley et al. (Ley et al. 1990) compared fluid replacement with crystalloids or colloids in patients undergoing coronary artery bypass or valve substitution. Patients treated with HES showed a reduced length of ICU stay than patients treated with normal saline solution. In addition, they required fewer fluid infusions after surgery and showed better hemodynamic performance than the crystalloid group (Agrò et al. 2013). Despite this evidence, colloids have been associated with coagulopathy and platelet dysfunction, predisposing cardiac surgery patients to postoperative bleeding (in particular when high MW molecules and CPB are involved) and to anaphylaxis

Table 15.9 Comparison between crystalloid and colloid effects

Crystalloids	Colloids
Facilitate fluid overload	Less time in intensive care
Lower and short time volemic effect	Less fluids after surgery
Pulmonary edema	Better hemodynamic performance
Less indicated in patients with reduced myocardial function	Anaphylactic reactions
Hemodilution	Coagulopathy
Suggested for continuous loss	Suggested for temporary loss

(especially gelatins), which may cause tubular damage with renal dysfunction (Agrò et al. 2013; Mahmood et al. 2009).

In case of acute hemorrhage, how fluid resuscitation has to be performed is still controversial. Although the forced administration of crystalloids and colloids has been and still is practiced, nowadays there are good arguments that a cautious infusion of crystalloids may be initially sufficient, since no large prospective randomized clinical trials have showed an improvement in survival after an aggressive fluid resuscitation. Fluid resuscitation is thought to boost bleeding by increasing blood pressure and dilutional coagulopathy. Nevertheless, national and international guidelines recommend that fluid resuscitation should be applied at the latest when hemorrhage causes hemodynamic instability. In acute and possibly rapidly progressing hypovolemic shock, colloids can be used (Roessler et al. 2014).

The third- and fourth-generation HES are safe and effective if used correctly and within prescribed limits. If fluid resuscitation is applied with ongoing reevaluation of the parameters which determine oxygen supply, it should be possible to keep fluid resuscitation restricted without causing undesirable side effects and also to administer a sufficient quantity so that survival of patients is ensured (Roessler et al. 2014). At the state of the art, balanced crystalloids are suggested for continuous losses (*perspiratio insensibilis* and urinary output 0.5–1 mL/kg/h), while colloids are suggested for temporary losses (IVS loss, such as due to hemorrhage) (Agrò et al. 2013; Agro and Vennari 2013b; Rehm et al. 2017).

A comparison between crystalloid and colloid effect is presented in the table below (Table 15.9).

15.13 Comparison Between HES and Other Colloids

In literature there is a large production concerning the use of colloids in cardiac patient, their hemodynamic, and side effects (Agrò et al. 2013).

Verheij (Verheij et al. 2006b) found no significant difference in hemodynamic state and COP registration after the infusion of 6% HES 450/0.7, 5% HA, or 6% dextran. For the same solutions, Jones (Jones et al. 2004) demonstrated no significant differences in hemodynamic power. On the other hand, Niemi (Niemi et al. 2008) found that CI and DO_2 increase immediately after the infusion (at ICU arrival) of 6% HES 130/0.4, whereas over a more long term (2 and 18 h after ICU arrival), the increase of CI was comparable in HES and 4% HA groups. This finding might be related to a greater plasma-expanding effect of HES compared to HA, due to a higher in vivo molecular weight. This hypothesis is supported by a higher hemodilution instantly after HES infusion. Moreover, the positive immediate effect of HES on CI may be due to HES capacity of blunt to the CPB-induced inflammatory process and endothelial activation. In fact, the effect of HES on DO_2 seems to be higher with respect to hemodilution due to HES expanding effect (Niemi et al. 2008; Feng et al. 2006). According to this study, HA seems to have a delayed hemodynamic effect with respect to HES solutions after cardiac surgery leading to a reduced DO_2 and a higher incidence of metabolic acidosis (BE more negative) (Agrò et al. 2013; Niemi et al. 2008).

In 2006, Palumbo (Palumbo et al. 2006) found that after the infusion of crystalloids, CVP does not significantly change and that CI significantly increases after the infusion of 6% HES 130/0.4, but not after the infusion of 20% HA. In addition, Van der Linden (Van der Linden et al. 2004) showed that the quantity of colloids necessary to maintain target values of CI, SvO_2, and diuresis did not significantly change between 6% HES 200/0.5 and 3.5% urea-linked gelatin during and after cardiac surgery. COP and rescue colloid administration were similar too.

Another issue is the hemodynamic effects of the different HES, depending on their metabolism. The enzymatic degradation of HES has two opposing effects on volemic expansion: a reduction in volume expansion, because it improves renal excretion, and an increase in hemodynamic power, by increasing the number of active osmotic particles (Agro and Vennari 2013b). Most studies report similar hemodynamic effects between HES with higher MMW and MSR and HES with lower MMW and MSR (Dorje et al. 2000; Gandhi et al. 2007; Ickx et al. 2003). However, according to a report on a small sample population (20 patients), plasma volume expansion induced by an HES with low MMW and MSR (HES 130/0.4) is longer-lasting than that achieved with the infusion of an HES with high MMW and MSR (HES 670/0.75) (Agro and Vennari 2013b; James et al. 2004).

The effect of a solution on coagulation per volume infused is an important factor to consider in choosing the solution to administer.

There is some evidence that HES affects coagulation to a greater extent than gelatins in cardiac surgery (Agrò et al. 2013; Niemi et al. 2006). Specifically, there is greater blood loss and an increased need for blood products in patients treated with HES 200/0.5 (Agrò et al. 2013; Van der Linden et al. 2004). In contrast, the high-dose administration of newer HES (6% HES 130/0.4) was comparable to gelatin with regard to blood loss (Van der Linden et al. 2005; Ooi et al. 2009). Although the difference among HES has been confirmed by a study in non-cardiac surgery patient in which high MW HES showed more negative effect on coagulation than low MW HES (Brunkhorst et al. 2008); in a study on CABG patients, the maximum dose (50 mL/kg) of 6% HES 130/0.4 showed the same effect on coagulation and blood requirement with respect to 33 mL/kg of 6% HES 200/0.5 (Sirvinskas et al. 2007).

The rationale for HA use in cardiac surgery patients is the minimal effect on coagulation (Agrò et al. 2013). A recent study demonstrated a reduction in postoperative transfusion requirement in patient who has undergone off-pump CABG and was treated with 1 L of HA with respect to those treated with 1 L of first-generation HES (Hecth-Dolkin et al. 2009). HA was shown to have lower effect on coagulation at thromboelastometry rather than 4% succinylated gelatin or 6% HES 200/0.5 after cardiac surgery. Absolute drainage loss and transfusion requirements were not significantly different between the groups (Niemi et al. 2006). The same study group confirmed the increased coagulation impairment after the infusion of 15 mL/kg of either 6% HES 200/0.5 or 6% HES 130/0.4 with respect to 4% albumin at 15 mL/kg, although drain blood loss and transfusion requirements did not differ between the groups over the study period (Sirvinskas et al. 2007; Ickx et al. 2003).

A restricted meta-analysis to compare HES 130/0.4 and HA infusion did not reveal significant difference in the volume of perioperative lost blood, confirming that third-generation HES preparations may seem to be safer due to their lower MW, rapid turnover, and conceivable reduced impact on coagulation competence (Rasmussen et al. 2016). HA shows reduced effects at thromboelastometry, which does not correlate with an effective clinical benefit (bleeding and transfusion requirement) (Sirvinskas et al. 2007). Moreover there are several studies demonstrating the lack of effect of HA on patient outcome in the critically ill (Agrò et al. 2013). These evidences and the costs of HA have determined a reduction of its use in the management of cardiac surgery patients.

Literature suggests that newer-generation HES and gelatins have few and comparable effects on coagulation, risk of postoperative bleeding, and transfusion requirement, but gelatins have a higher incidence of anaphylaxis, while HES are safer when infused at sub-maximum doses.

Since HES was introduced to the market, there is ongoing debate on their renal effects. At the state of the art, literature is lacking about colloid effects on renal function (Sirvinskas et al. 2007). In an isolated renal perfusion model in which tubular damage occurs, HES were shown to impair kidney function (Hüter et al. 2009). However, different results emerged from studies on the latest-generation HES: compared to gelatins, third- and fourth-generation HES exhibit positive effects on both the inflammatory response and endothelial integrity, with reduced renal effects and a decrease in the total volume of colloid required (Agrò et al. 2013).

Gelatins cause greater kidney damage than HES, when compared to third- and fourth-generation HES (Agrò et al. 2013). Allison and colleagues (Allison et al. 1999) studied the influence of gelatin and HES 6% 200/0.5 on the renal excretion of albumin. Excretion was significantly higher in the gelatin group, consistent with a better integrity of vascular membranes in the HES-treated patients. In a study on aortic aneurysm surgery patients, 6% HES of 200/0.62 or HES 130/0.4 and 4% gelatin were compared with respect to renal effects (Mahmood et al. 2007). HES were shown to improve renal function and reduced renal injury compared with gelatins. In another study on septic patient, HES 200/0.6 with a maximum dose of 33 mL/kg HES (cumulative dose of 80 mL/kg) and 3% gelatin with no dose limitation were compared. HES correlated to a significantly higher rate of AKI; however, no increase in renal replacement therapy was shown. Further similar studies found a negative effect of HES administration on renal function. The need for replacement therapy correlated to cumulative dose, which was often exceeded (Metze et al. 1997; Ickx et al. 2003).

On the other side, other studies relieved no renal effect using HES in patient who has undergone kidney transplantations or with pre-existing renal damage (Deman et al. 1999; Jumgheinrich et al. 2002).

On the base of evidence, it is not possible to recommend the use of modern HES in cardiac surgery patient with respect to renal effect (Drt et al. 2010). However, newest-generation HES seems to be safer with respect to renal dysfunction, and there is no study demonstrating a severe renal effect after use, especially when limiting dose is respected (Agrò et al. 2013; Otsuki et al. 2007).

In Ooi et al.'s recent prospective, randomized, single-blinded, controlled study, HES 6% 130/0.4 at a maximum dose of 30 mL/kg/d is safe with regard to blood loss, transfusion requirements, and renal function in patient who has undergone CABG procedures. They suggested the use of HES 6% 130/0.4 instead of gelatins (Ooi et al. 2009).

15.14 Comparison Between Balanced and Unbalanced Solutions

When evaluating the effects of different volume replacement strategies, the electrolytic composition has to be taken into account. There has been a recent surge in the literature comparing different solutions, in particular chloride-liberal versus chloride-restricted solutions. Notably, evidence accumulates that the most commonly used fluid (NS) has no advantage over balanced solutions, increases the risk of acute kidney injury, and should therefore be abandoned (Lira and Pinsky 2014; Kampmeier et al. 2014). Hyperchloremic acidosis caused by non-balanced nor non-plasma-adapted solutions can alter kidney sensitivity to vasoconstrictors, leading to increased vascular tone and a reduction in glomerular filtration. Moreover acidosis may worsen the hemodynamic status of cardiac patients and facilitate infection development (Agrò et al. 2013; Base et al. 2011) (see Chap. 16).

The routine use of solutions with a supraphysiologic chloride content and a low strong ion difference (SID, see Chap. 16) may be associated with adverse outcomes, especially among critically ill patients. Balanced and plasma-adapted solutions avoid hyperchloremic acidosis, with a lower risk of kidney injury, even in cardiac surgery patients, as well as a reduced bleeding risk and inflammatory response; they present a SID closer to plasma (see Chap. 16) and may improve the likelihood of survival (Agrò et al. 2013).

Several studies now have shown perioperative mortality and morbidity (especially AKI incidence) benefits of balanced solutions over NS, and growing evidence exists suggesting greater benefit in critically ill patients (Agrò et al. 2013).

Clotting disturbances can be avoided or reduced by dissolving HES in balanced, plasma-adapted solutions. Furthermore, there is growing evidence that the use of balanced solutions reduces the need for blood products because of the improved coagulation status (Agrò et al. 2013; Roche et al. 2002; Martin et al. 2002).

15.15 How Much Fluid?

The second main concern of the debate on fluid management is "how much to fill" the patient? In fact, although there are many evidences about the benefits of fluid administration in restoring and maintaining an adequate IVS volume, the risk to develop congestive heart failure with interstitial edema, respiration complication, and wound healing delay remains in case of excessive fluid administration (Agrò et al. 2013; Agro and Vennari 2013b). Moreover, in the daily practice, practitioners have to face with the lack of consensus guidelines and the limited equipment for hemodynamic monitoring. As a consequence, it is not surprising that the need for rescue therapy in shock patient, with congestive heart failure, and prolonged mechanical ventilation is yet too frequent both in operating room than in ICU (Sirvinskas et al. 2007).

In a 50-year ongoing debate, literature proposed many strategies for perioperative fluid management in cardiac surgery patient (Agrò et al. 2013; Agro and Vennari 2013b).

15.15.1 Liberal vs. Restricted Approach

Historically, there have been two main approaches to fluid management: liberal and restrictive. Studies used different references to establish the nature (liberal or restrictive) of fluid administration. As a consequence, literature may appear contradictory.

Considering a normal water assumption of 25–35 mL/kg, a patient with no particular fluid loss should be treated with 1.75–2.75 L/die (Powell-Tuck et al. 2008). According to this basal requirement, a fluid strategy may be considered (Varadhan and Lobo 2010):

- Liberal, when more of 2.75 L/die of fluid is administered
- Restrictive when less of 1.75 L/die is administered

In the liberal approach, fluid replacement has been funded on the estimation of preoperative loss due to fasting; intraoperative loss due to perspiratio insensibilis, urine output, and bleeding; and anticipated postoperative loss due to fluid shifting in the third space (Fanzca 2012; Shires et al. 1961). According to this approach, surgical patient is hypovolemic before the starting of the procedure because of fasting and intestinal cleaning preparation (when necessary); the perspiration has a great increase when the continuity of the skin is interrupted by the surgical procedure; the third-space shifting is the natural response to surgical stress, and it is responsible for an effective ECS (Jenkins et al. 1975; Campbell et al. 1990; Holte and Kehlet 2002). Finally, the kidney is able to eliminate any fluid overload (Watenpaugh et al. 1992). As a consequence, a preoperative fluid load is needed (Chappell et al. 2008; Holte and Kehlet 2002; Maharaj et al. 2005) as the administration of about 20 mL/kg/h of IV fluids (Bamboat and Bordeianou 2009).

Although the use of a liberal approach was supported by some studies demonstrating an improvement of tissue perfusion and oxygenation and the reduction of inflammatory response and of organ failure risk (Maharaj et al. 2005; Arkilic et al. 2003; Mythen and Webb 1995; Holte et al. 2004; Lobo et al. 2010; Hiltebrand et al. 2007), it has been related with a fluid overload potentially impacting on patient outcomes (Nisanevich et al. 2005; Lobo et al. 2002). Hypervolemia elicits the release of atrial natriuretic peptides that damage the endothelial glycocalyx layer (Hahn 2015). A mathematical model demonstrated that using a liberal approach causes a massive retention of fluid in the stressed tissues, especially when infusion overcomes 10 mL/kg/h, with reduced or no impact on IVS volume (Tatara and Tashiro 2007). Moreover in a normal organism, the surgical stress increases the capacity of fluid overload elimination, but not in a proportional way to the administration. As a consequence, if administration is excessive, fluids will accumulate (Holte et al. 2007a).

Lowell et. al found that at ICU admission, 40% of surgery patients presented an increase of total body water of 10% or more (Lowell et al. 1990). This fluid overload may need days to be eliminated, determining a body weight gain. The gain is mainly due to interstitial edema responsible for heart failure; pulmonary edema and ARDS; increased abdominal pressure, with possible development of compartmental syndrome; tissue hypoperfusion and hypoxia, slowing down of wound healing and increased risk of dehiscence; ileus; and MOF (Reid et al. 2003; Watenpaugh et al. 1992; Lobo et al. 2001; Balogh et al. 2003; Shandall et al. 1985; Sheridan et al. 1987; Lobo 2004). Finally fluid and sodium overload causes cellular membrane hyperpolarization, neurotransmitter metabolism alteration, and mitochondrial dysfunction (Petty and Ashbaugh 1971).

At the state of the art, it is not clear if a liberal fluid administration is the cause of the consequence of fluid shift in the third space. In an animal model, the surgical damage (mechanical and inflammatory) has been shown as the first cause of fluid shift that is increased by abundant fluid administration (Chan et al. 1983). However, literature on major abdominal surgery demonstrated liberal approach may augment the risk of complication development, increase hospital stay, and worsen outcomes (Nisanevich et al. 2005; Brandstrup 2006; Brandstrup et al. 2003).

Moreover, evidence demonstrated that Shire theory premises were not very correct. In fact, it has been shown that preoperative fasting does not produce a significative reduction in IVS volume (Jacob et al. 2008); basal perspiratio is 0.5 mL/kg/h, and during surgery it is no more than 1 mL/kg/h (Lamke et al. 1977); the stress response to surgery is responsible of an inappropriate increase of ADH and aldosterone levels, determining an overload of water and sodium; finally a "primitive" third space does not exist (Chappell et al. 2008). These evidences suggest the use of a restrictive approach to fluid management, first proposed by Moore (Moore et al. 1955). Many studies demonstrated that a restrictive management (defined as a contained infusion respected liberal approach) reduces the risk of complications and hospital stay, favoring wound healing and postoperative recovery of organ function (especially abdominal) and lowering the incidence of cardiopulmonary events, with no cases of prerenal AKI (Chappell et al. 2008; Nisanevich et al. 2005; Lobo et al.

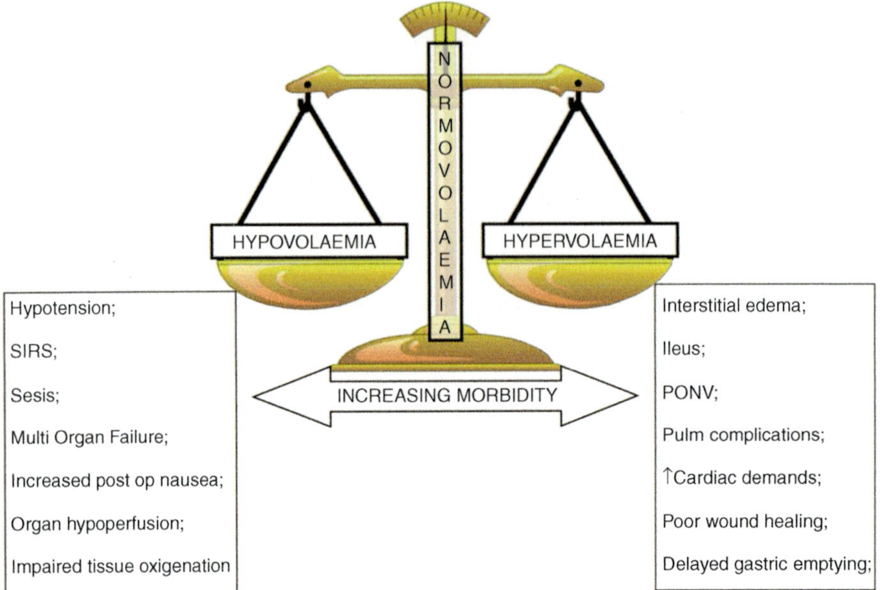

Fig. 15.17 Liberal and restrictive approaches: consequences on morbidity

2002; Moyer 1950). On the other hand, when a real restrictive administration is realized (infusion <1.75 L/die), perioperative morbidity increased (Vermeulen et al. 2009; Holte et al. 2007b). In fact, a restrictive management may cause hypovolemia with hypoperfusion and DO_2 reduction, increasing the risk of organ damage. Moreover, there is an increase viscosity of body fluids potentially leading to microcirculation alteration and microthrombosis, pulmonary mucus concentration with bronchial obstruction, and atelectasis development (MacKay et al. 2006) (Fig. 15.17).

The discussion about the ideal fluid management in the cardiac surgery patient remains still opened, because works are widely different and no studies have been conducted on cardiac surgical population. However, the evidence that both perioperative fluid restriction and liberal fluid administration can have deleterious effects and lead to increased morbidity and mortality is undiscussed (Schindler and Marx 2016). For this reason, in the last two decades, a guided fluid management has been emphasized as an alternative to both fluid management approaches (Sirvinskas et al. 2007). It consists on the administration of fluids according to the evaluation of physiologic parameters and hemodynamic variables. This approach is called goal-directed therapy (Williams et al. 1999).

15.15.2 Goal-Directed Fluid Therapy

In cardiac surgery patient, a rational fluid administration is one of the main tools useful to optimize tissue perfusion, avoiding hypo- and hypervolemia with respect to these patients who have a reduced tolerance (Sirvinskas et al. 2007).

Goal-directed therapy (GDT) is a complex strategy for fluid infusions aimed at optimizing tissue perfusion and oxygenation. Through hemodynamic monitoring, GDT allows physicians to administer fluids and/or use other therapies, such as inotropic or vasoactive drugs, only to those patients who need them, in order to assure sufficient DO_2 to fulfill the metabolic requirement of the particular patient. With GDT, hemodynamic management is therefore personalized (Agro and Vennari 2013b).

15.15.2.1 Physiological Basis

Management of both critically ill and major surgery patients is mainly aimed at assuring adequate tissue perfusion and oxygenation. A continuous supply of oxygen is needed because it is indispensable for aerobic metabolism (Agro and Vennari 2013b).

Physiologically adequate DO_2 is assured by cardiovascular and respiratory systems, and it corresponds to the quantity (in mL) of oxygen per minute carried to the tissues (Agro and Vennari 2013b; Lees et al. 2009).

DO_2 is defined by the following equation (Agro and Vennari 2013b):

$$DO_2\left(\text{mL}/\text{min}\right) = \text{cardiac output}\left(\text{CO}\right) \times \text{arterial oxygen content}\left(\text{CaO}_2\right) \quad (15.1)$$

DO_2 physiologically corresponds to 900–1100 mL/min or to 500–600 mL/min/m^2 if reported as body surface area (DO_2I) (Agro and Vennari 2013b).

Considering the factors in determining CO and CaO_2, Eq. (15.1) can be rewritten as (Agro and Vennari 2013b):

$$DO_2\left(\text{mL}/\text{min}\right) = \left(\text{HR} \times \text{SV}\right) \times \left[\left(1.34 \times \text{Hb} \times \text{SaO}_2\right) + \left(0.003 \times \text{paO}_2\right)\right] \quad (15.2)$$

where:

- HR is the heart rate.
- SV is the stroke volume.
- 1.34 is the number of mL of oxygen carried by hemoglobin at 100% saturation.
- Hb is the amount of hemoglobin in g/dL.
- SaO_2 is the arterial O_2 saturation in arterial blood.
- 0.003 is the solubility coefficient of oxygen.
- PaO_2 is the partial O_2 pressure of arterial blood.

Thus, oxygen delivery can be improved by modifying:

- SV, by using inotropic or vasoactive drugs (post-load) and fluid administration (preload)
- Hb, by the transfusion of red cells
- SaO_2 and paO_2, by O_2 therapy and in some cases by mechanical ventilation (Agro and Vennari 2013b)

Oxygen demand-consumption (VO_2) is the quantity (in mL) of oxygen consumed by the tissue per minute. It depends on the metabolic state, and it is increased by surgical stress and critical conditions. VO_2 may be described by the following relationship (**Agro and Vennari** 2013b):

$$VO_2\left(\text{mL}/\text{min}\right) = \text{cardiac output}\left(\text{CO}\right) \times [\text{arterial } O_2 \text{ content}\left(\text{Ca}O_2\right) \\ -\text{venous } O_2 \text{ content}\left(\text{Cv}O_2\right) \tag{15.3}$$

Equation (15.3) can be rewritten as (Agro and Vennari 2013b):

$$VO_2\left(\text{mL}/\text{min}\right) = \left(\text{FC} \times \text{SV}\right) \times \begin{bmatrix} \left(1.34 \times \text{Hb} \times \text{Sa}O_2\right) + \left(0.003 \times \text{pa}O_2\right) - \\ \left(1.34 \times \text{Hb} \times \text{Sv}O_2\right) + \left(0.003 \times \text{pv}O_2\right) \end{bmatrix} \tag{15.4}$$

where:

- CO and CaO_2 are described by the same factor as in Eq. (15.2).
- SvO_2 is the saturation of mixed venous blood.
- PvO_2 is the partial O_2 pressure in mixed venous blood (Agro and Vennari 2013b).

VO2 is about 200–300 mL/min (110–160 mL/min/m^2 if reported as body surface area) at basal metabolism (Agro et al. 2013). Under stress conditions it may increase four- to sixfold.

O_2 extraction (O_2ER) is the fraction of DO_2 released to the tissues per minute (Agro and Vennari 2013b). It is a tissue oxygenation index, expressed as:

$$O_2ER = VO_2 / DO_2 \tag{15.5}$$

Under basal conditions, the ratio is 0.25, but it can increase in order to assure VO_2. In fact, normally, VO_2 is maintained despite wide-ranging DO_2 values, through an increase of O_2ER. Below a critical value of DO_2 (critical DO_2), O_2ER can no longer increase, and VO_2 becomes flow dependent (Agro and Vennari 2013b). Tissue hypoxia appears, and anaerobic metabolism starts. The tissue hypoxia causes unbalance between ATP production and ATP demand. A reduction in cAMP and cGMP levels activates the endothelium, reducing its barrier function and causing the release of pro-inflammatory cytokines, leading to capillary leak syndrome. Disruption of the endothelial barrier exposes the blood to procoagulant factors and leukocyte adhesion molecules. Leukocytes and complement are activated, leading to a systemic inflammation with organ hypoperfusion and failure (multi-organ failure). The detection and prevention of tissue hypoxia is therefore crucial, especially in cardiac surgery patient (Agro and Vennari 2013b; Lamke et al. 1977).

A rational approach to fluid therapy (GDT) is the most readily available and simplest tool to assure adequate DO_2. Some patients have reduced compensatory mechanisms when VO_2 increases, because of comorbidities (cardiovascular or pulmonary diseases), and thus have a higher probability of reaching the critical DO_2 under stress conditions, such as surgery. Cardiac surgery patient are high-risk patients who are likely to benefit from a GDT approach (Agro and Vennari 2013b).

15.15.2.2 Hemodynamic Variables in GDT

The rational approach to fluid administration in GDT is based on the prediction of fluid responsiveness. Fluid-responder patients are those who, according to Starling's law, will benefit from fluid loading in terms of hemodynamic stability and DO_2 (Agro and Vennari 2013b). It was been shown that if fluid responsiveness is not assessed, only 40–72% of critically ill patients respond to fluid therapy with a significant increase in stroke volume (Michard and Teboul 2002). It is immediately evident that fluid responsiveness is not evaluable on the bases of the sole clinic (Grebe et al. 2006). In fact, clinic parameters change after the real modification of volemia, determining a tardive hypovolemia treatment, potentially fatal for cardiac surgery patients (Grebe et al. 2006; Grocott et al. 2005).

Defined hemodynamic variables are necessary to evaluate volume status and to test fluid responsiveness. These can be divided into static and dynamic. Static variables indicate hemodynamic status at a specific time, for the preload value at that time. An example of static variable is the value of CI obtained in a single thermodilution. Dynamic variables indicate hemodynamic changes in response to a periodic variation in preload. Static indexes are comparable to a picture, while dynamic ones to a movie. Dynamic variables are better indicators of fluid responsiveness than static ones (Williams et al. 1999; Grocott et al. 2005).

Historically, filling pressures (CVP, MAP, and PCWP) were used to guide intravascular volume therapy. In cardio-surgical ICU, CVP is the most used (87% of intensivists), followed by MAP (84%) and PCWP (30%) (Kastrup et al. 2007). Many studies have shown that CVP does not adequately reflect preload and fails to predict fluid responsiveness (Williams et al. 1999; Kastrup et al. 2007; Cavallaro et al. 2008; Marik et al. 2008). In one study PCWP was found to adequately predict fluid responsiveness in 19 patients undergone CABG (Bennett-Guerrero et al. 2002). Other studies found a significant CVP and PCWP increase after a fluid challenge, but they do not correlate to an increase in SV (Wiesenack et al. 2001; Brock et al. 2002). Moreover, pressure parameters are altered by intra-abdominal pressure variation, modification of cardiac compliance, pulmonary resistance, and cardiac pathologies (Bennett-Guerrero et al. 2002). As a result they are not very reliable and useful in cardiac surgery patient who present at less one of these conditions (Sirvinskas et al. 2007; Wittkowski et al. 2009; Michard et al. 2003; Hofer et al. 2005a; Reuter et al. 2002a; Reuter et al. 2002b; Sakka et al. 2009; Breukers et al. 2009a; Breukers et al. 2009b; Goedje et al. 2000).

Pulse wave analysis allows the assessment of other functional hemodynamic parameters, such as stroke volume variation (SVV), pulse pressure variation (PPV), and continuous CI (Agro and Vennari 2013b). Intermittent transpulmonary thermodilution can be used to calibrate pulse wave analysis, enhancing the reliability of CI measurements, according to the monitoring system applied (Agro and Vennari 2013b).

Pulse pressure is defined as the difference between systolic and diastolic pressure for each heartbeat. PPV corresponds to the variation in pulse pressure at different heartbeats induced by variations of the intrathoracic pressure due to mechanical ventilation (Agro and Vennari 2013b) (Fig. 15.18). A PPV cutoff value of 12% has been shown to be useful to identify responder patients (PPV > 12%) and non-responder patients (PPV < 12%) (Auler et al. 2008). In a study on CABG patients comparing PEEP and fluid infusion effects on hemodynamics, PPV was found to be the best predictor of fluid responsiveness with respect to PCWP and other variables (Bendjelid et al. 2004). PPV use in guiding volume therapy has been demonstrated, suggesting a possible improvement in outcome after high-risk surgery (Lopes et al. 2007).

SVV is based on cyclic changes in the SV due to intrathoracic pressure during mechanical ventilation (Dorje et al. 2000) (Fig. 15.19).

$$SVV = (SV\,max - SV\,min) / SV\,mean$$

It is conceptually similar to PPV, but more precise and reliable (Agro and Vennari 2013b). SVV has been found to consistently predict fluid responsiveness, with threshold values of 11–13% (Agro and Vennari 2013b; Marik et al. 2009; Benes et al. 2010). SVV may indicate the actual position on the Frank-Starling curve. When the heart operates on the ascending limb of the Frank-Starling curve, the intrathoracic pressure induces large changes in preload and SV (SVV > 13%),

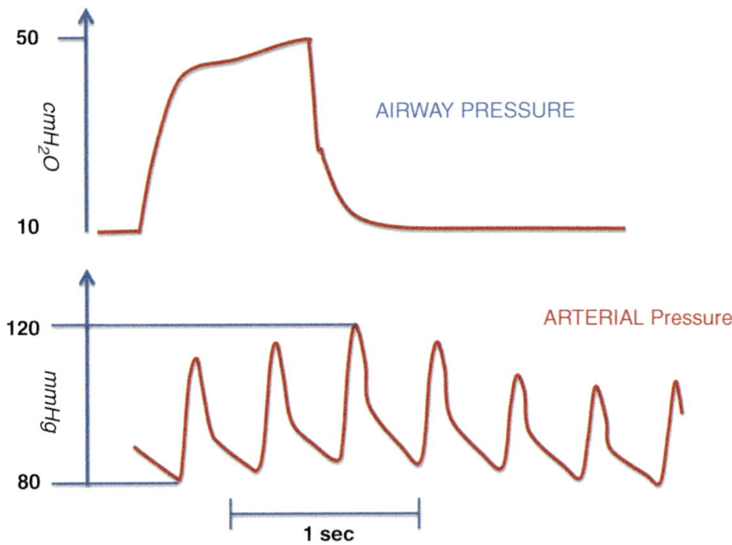

Fig. 15.18 PPV and intrathoracic pressure. In the inspiratory phase of mechanical ventilation, the intrathoracic pressure increases, reducing preload and consequently increasing PPV. In expiration, intrathoracic pressure decreases, increasing preload and consequently reducing reduction in PPV. Agro F.E., Vennari M. Clinical treatment: the right fluid in the right quantity. From: "Body Fluid Management—From Physiology to Therapy" Agrò F.E. Springer Milan 2013, pages 71–92

indicating a preserved preload reserve and an improvement after fluid administration (fluid responders). By contrast, at the plateau of the Frank-Starling curve, small changes in SV are observed (SVV < 13%), representing a lower preload reserve and a minimal or no improvement after fluid administration (fluid non-responders) (Fig. 15.20). In this case inotropes may be required (Agro and Vennari 2013b). In a study on 20 patients who have undergone cardiac surgery, SVV modification correlated to CI changes (Reuter et al. 2002b).

However, there are some limitations that may exclude a valid use of SVV (Reid et al. 2003):

- Right ventricular failure
- Arrhythmias
- Spontaneous breathing

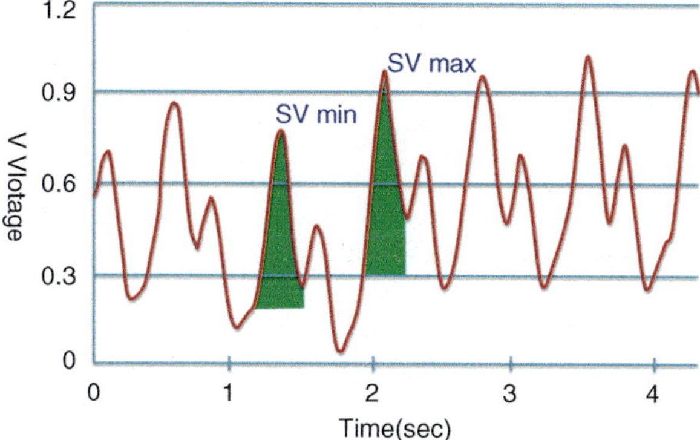

Fig. 15.19 Pulse wave analysis and SVV: the area under the curve corresponds to the SV. Knowing the HR, CI may be calculated continuously. Agro F.E., Vennari M. Clinical treatment: the right fluid in the right quantity. From: "Body Fluid Management—From Physiology to Therapy" Agrò F.E. Springer Milan 2013, pages 71–92

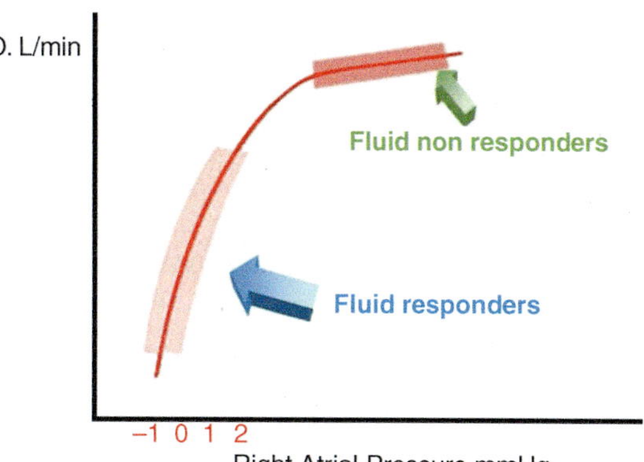

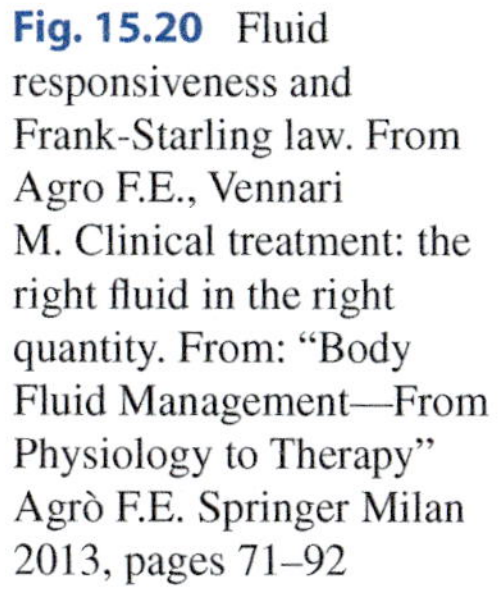

Fig. 15.20 Fluid responsiveness and Frank-Starling law. From Agro F.E., Vennari M. Clinical treatment: the right fluid in the right quantity. From: "Body Fluid Management—From Physiology to Therapy" Agrò F.E. Springer Milan 2013, pages 71–92

- Ratio heart rate/respiratory rate < 3.6
- Low tidal volume (<8 mL/kg)

In fact, Reuter et al. (Reuter et al. 2003) demonstrated that tidal volume may affect reliability of SVV value in cardiac surgery patient. In a similar population, SVV was found to be reduced by high blood pressure value and increased by high airway pressure, without effective change in volemic status (Sirvinskas et al. 2007).

Both high PPV and SVV are indicators of hypovolemia, indicate fluid responsiveness, and correlate to the CI increase after fluid challenge administration (Wiesenack et al. 2003; Hofer et al. 2005b). This evidence was confirmed in a study on off-pump CABG patients, in which both SVV and PPV strongly correlated to CI improvement after a fluid challenge, with respect to filling pressure (Belloni et al. 2008). As a consequence, dynamic parameters such as PPV and SVV are able to adequately distinguish fluid-responder and fluid non-responder patients and are suitable to guide fluid management in the perioperative period of cardiac surgery, with respect to filling pressure (Benes et al. 2010; Carl et al. 2000).

GEDV (global end-diastolic volume) is a volumetric parameter easily obtainable through transpulmonary thermodilution. It may index to body surface (GDVI) (Wittkowski et al. 2009). It has been shown as a better marker of cardiac preload than CVP (Agro and Vennari 2013b). This evidence was confirmed by a study where GEDVI was compared to PAC pressure through echocardiography: it correlated with ventricular preload (Hofer et al. 2005a). However, it is a static parameter that does not allow the evaluation of cardiac responsiveness to fluid loading (Agro and Vennari 2013b).

ITBV (intrathoracic blood volume) is another volumetric index of preload (ITBVI). In cardiac surgery patient with hypovolemia, ITBV has been shown to significantly correlate to SV increase after a fluid challenge, with respect to CVP and PCWP (Brock et al. 2002). These results are confirmed by many studies on cardiac surgery patients (Sirvinskas et al. 2007; Wiesenack et al. 2001; Brock et al. 2002; Reuter et al. 2002a, b). Moreover in another study on cardiac surgery patient, a filling pressure-guided management was compared to a management based on ITBVI, CI, MAP, HR, and $ScvO_2$ use. The first group showed a longer ICU and hospital stay, with respect to the second group (Smetkin et al. 2009).

In case of left ventricular failure or acute lung injury, the EVLW (extravascular lung water, index of lung edema) can be used. EVLW is an independent predictor of survival (Agro and Vennari 2013b). In GDT, the use of EVLW accelerates the resolution of lung edema, whether due to increased vascular permeability or to an increase in hydrostatic pressure (Agro and Vennari 2013b).

In cardiac surgery patients, the use of a goal-directed protocol (GEDV >800 mL/m^2, EVLW = 10–12 mL/kg) resulted in an enhanced postoperative outcome (Agro and Vennari 2013b; Goepfer et al. 2007).

Left ventricular end-diastolic area (LVEDA) is the most popular echocardiographic parameter (measured with transesophageal probe) used to assess preload, very easy to measure, and reliable with respect to other sophisticated parameters.

Literature evidenced that LVEDA is a valid parameter to guide fluid management in cardiac surgery patient and to evaluate fluid responsiveness (LVDA increase in fluid responder after the challenge) (Goepfer et al. 2007; Cheung et al. 1994). LVEDA correlates with SVV and ITBV (Tousignant et al. 2000; Buhre et al. 2001). In patients who have undergone cardiac surgery, LVEDA showed a better predictive capacity to fluid responsiveness than filling pressure (Wiesenack et al. 2005). As a consequence, its use is suitable in this kind of patients (Sirvinskas et al. 2007).

Literature has showed that volumetric parameters are superior to conventional filling pressures to assess cardiac preload and might prove helpful in guiding fluid therapy in cardiac surgical patients (Sirvinskas et al. 2007).

15.15.2.3 Monitoring Systems in GDT

The use of GDT requires hemodynamic assessment and monitoring. The ideal system should be simple, noninvasive or hardly invasive, safe, or precise, allowing immediate therapeutic intervention. Unfortunately, this system has not yet been invented. Many systems have been proposed for hemodynamic assessment, especially recently (Agro and Vennari 2013b). All these systems have to be compared to the Swan-Ganz or pulmonary artery catheter (PAC), which remains the gold standard, despite its limits. In fact, many clinical trials showed that PAC is not suitable for GDT in the routine perioperative setting (Agro and Vennari 2013b). Its use is further discouraged by the invasiveness of the procedure, which exposes patients to complications. In addition, PAC cannot be used without adequate training and experience. Finally, its performance mainly refers to filling pressure values (PVC, PCWP), which have been found to be not so effective in clinical practice. Consequently, its fame in the literature and in clinics has decreased over the years (Agro and Vennari 2013b). Moreover, less invasive systems with similar precision have been introduced. Modern technologies provide filling volume values that are more reliable as preload and fluid responsiveness indices (Agro and Vennari 2013b; Lees et al. 2009). Current and less invasive flow monitoring techniques include Doppler technologies or arterial pressure waveform analysis.

The esophageal Doppler (ED) allows measurement such as LVEDA and the blood velocity at the level of the descending aorta. The flow time in the descending aorta, corrected for HR (FTc normally 330–360 ms), corresponds to the SV. According to the chosen probe, the correspondence is obtained through a monogram calculated from comparative studies performed with a PAC or through the measurement of the vessel cross section. At lower velocities, hypovolemia should be suspected. FTc correlates with LVEDA (Agro and Vennari 2013b; DiCorte et al. 2000). ED requires shorter operator training than other systems and does not require calibration, but it is difficult to use in awake patients and in a prolonged monitoring; finally its results may be operator-dependent. GDT using ED was shown to improve patient outcomes (Agro and Vennari 2013b; Chytra et al. 2007) and has shown that the optimization of fluid management using ED in trauma patients reduces blood lactate levels, the incidence of infections, and the duration of ICU and hospital stay. A meta-analysis showed that patients undergoing major abdominal surgery, who received ED-oriented GDT, had a reduction in complications, requirement of inotropes, ICU admissions, and hospital stay, with a rapid organ function recovery (Agro and Vennari 2013b; Abbas and Hill 2008).

New monitoring devices, assessing dynamic and volumetric parameters, are PiCCO system and PiCCO2 Pulsion Medical Systems, Munich, Germany; Flotrac, Edwards Life Systems; and LiDCOrapid, LIDCO, London, UK.

These devices use transpulmonary thermodilution and/or pulse wave analysis. When the methodologies are used in combination, the validity of pulse pressure analysis depends on periodic recalibration through thermodilution (Agro and Vennari 2013b; Marik et al. 2011; Reuter et al. 2010). These systems require invasive arterial lines and a central venous catheter, but they are less invasive than PAC.

The PiCCO system needs a modified arterial catheter with a temperature and pressure sensor. It must be positioned in a central artery through femoral, brachial, axillary, or radial access (Sirvinskas et al. 2007). The PiCCO system lets a continuous monitoring of SV, SVV, and CI, while it yields static parameters such as the GEDV/GEDVI, ITBV/ITBVI, and EVLW through thermodilution methodology (Michard et al. 2003). The PiCCO system uses a single-indicator thermodilution. It has been shown as reliable in many studies on cardiac and non-cardiac patients, although determining a slight overestimation (Sirvinskas et al. 2007). SVV evaluated by the PiCCO plus system (an evolution of PiCCO) adequately indicates fluid-responder patients in various clinical settings (Agro and Vennari 2013b).

Another system based on pulse wave analysis is the FloTrac/Vigileo system. It uses Langewouters' algorithm to perform the wave analysis and does not require thermodilution for calibration. Consequently, it can be used only with a normal invasive arterial line connected to the FloTrac sensor (Agro and Vennari 2013b). A study on 40 patients undergoing cardiac surgery compared the SVV measured with FloTrac/Vigileo and the PiCCO plus and found no significant difference in the prediction of fluid responsiveness (Dorje et al. 2000; Hofer et al. 2008). In high-risk patients undergoing major abdominal surgery, Benes et al. found that intraoperative fluid optimization through the FloTrac/Vigileo system decreased the incidence of postoperative complications, reducing hospitalization time (Agro and Vennari 2013b; Benes et al. 2010). The FloTrac/Vigileo system may be used with the Presep catheter (Edwards Life Science, Irvine, CA). It is a central catheter that allows S_CVO_2 continuous monitoring. The limits of Vigileo involve the validity of the wave pressure analysis and SVV values only in mechanically ventilated patients (Agro and Vennari 2013b).

A new, noninvasive monitor for the measurement of continuous CI is the Nexfin HD (Bmeye) monitor. It measures CI continuously completely noninvasively by an inflatable finger cuff. The Nexfin HD using volume clamp technology continuously measures finger blood pressure and converts the value into a blood pressure wave of the brachial artery. The truly noninvasive nature of the Nexfin HD allows the measurement of CI and can be used in awake, not mechanically ventilated patients (Agro and Vennari 2013b).

15.15.2.4 Clinical Impact in Cardiac Surgery Patients

GDT has been demonstrated to reduce length of ICU stay, ameliorating outcomes (Sirvinskas et al. 2007). Since 1988 many studies on different monitoring systems have demonstrated GDT benefits in non-cardiac major surgery patients, maintaining a $DO_2 \geq 600$ mL/min/m^2 (Dorje et al. 2000; Otsuki et al. 2007; Hofer et al. 2008; Shoemaker et al. 1988; Pearse et al. 2005a; Pearse et al. 2005b; Giglio et al. 2009).

Considering a cardiac surgery population, only one study using PAC demonstrated that an S_VO_2-oriented management may improve morbidity and hospital stay length (Polonen et al. 2000).

In a more recent study on 30 cardiac surgery patients, using FloTrac and Presep system to optimize CI, SVV, and DO_2, there was no significant improvement on outcome with respect to standard management, probably due to the small sample (Kapoor et al. 2008).

The ICU use of esophageal Doppler flowmetry (aimed at maintaining a stroke index above 35 mL/m^2) has been found to reduce the length of hospital stay in cardiac surgery patient (McKendry et al. 2004). Moreover comparing 40 cardiac surgery patients treated with a GEDVI, ITBVI, CI, and MAP-guided algorithm, with a historic sample treated with standard approach, the GDT group presented a shorter duration of mechanical ventilation and a reduced need for intensive therapies and catecholamines (Goepfert et al. 2007). In a similar study conducted in off-pump coronary artery bypass patients, it was shown that GDT determined an increased use of dobutamine and colloids, correlating with a reduction of the length ICU and hospital stay (Smetkin et al. 2009).

Recently studies evaluating fluid resuscitation in the septic patient (ProCESS and ARISE trials) found no difference in outcome of sepsis patients treated in an emergency department with early GDT versus two types of usual care, with a large amount of fluid administered in GDT, suggesting that EGDT does not yield survival benefit. On the other side in the perioperative literature, GDT resulted in more conservative volume resuscitation, reflecting a more vasoconstrictive patient status rather than sepsis. Furthermore, studies comparing GDT with liberal strategies showed improved outcomes with GDT. It is probably not just the amount of volume, but mostly the ability to stabilize the patient with the needed volume that defines outcome. Fluid administration should be used only in volume-responsive patients and only when end-organ perfusion goals are not met, on the basis of dynamic parameters of hemodynamic monitoring, individualized to each patient (Lira and Pinsky 2014).

Volume responsiveness is not the only parameter of GDT, but also responsiveness to vasoconstrictor and inotropic agent should be considered: the goals of therapy are to make the patient stable. Obviously, understanding pathophysiologic factors (comorbidities, type of surgical procedure or stress, patient status at the beginning of the treatment) needs to be incorporated into the treatment plan for each patient (Lira and Pinsky 2014).

The present evidences suggest GDT as a useful clinical tool to improve cardiac surgery fluid management during ICU stay, favorably impacting on outcomes (Sirvinskas et al. 2007).

15.16 Electrolyte Management

15.16.1 Sodium

In the cardiac surgery patient, sodium overload is the most common alteration due to fluid administration and to the surgical stress response (increased level of aldosterone and cortisol). In this case it is accompanied by hypervolemia and fluid overload, with interstitial edema (Fanzca 2012). Hypernatremia may be also due to a loss of hypotonic fluids. Renal losses may be caused by furosemide use, osmotic diuresis (severe hyperglycemia, uremia, mannitol overdose), pre-existing renal diseases, and the development of ATN (polyuric phase). In these cases sodium losses are associated to water losses, with a reduction of IVS fluid and the presence of sign and symptoms of hypovolemia (Agro and Vennari 2013a). Less frequently hypernatremia may be due to a loss of free body water (hypernatremia due to sodium concentration). In this case EVS volume is preserved. The most frequent cause of normovolemic hypernatremia is the lack of an adequate restore of perspiratio insensibilis, especially when it is increased (i.e., patients with fever) (Agro and Vennari 2013a). A possible flowchart for hypernatremia diagnosis is presented below (Fig. 15.21).

Thirst is one of the first symptoms of hypernatremia, observable in awake patients. Other symptoms are lethargy, reduction of consciousness, up to coma and

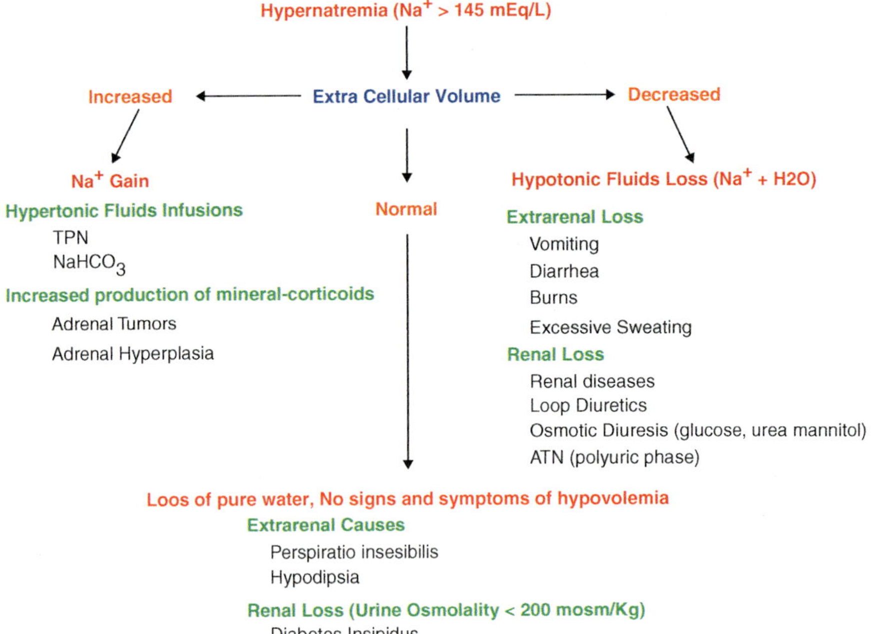

Fig. 15.21 Flowchart for hypernatremia diagnosis

convulsions, peripheral edema, myoclonus, ascites and/or pleural effusion, tremor and/or rigidity, and increased reflexes (Agro and Vennari 2013a). If hypernatremia develops slowly, it is well tolerated because the brain is able to regulate its own volume in response to ECS fluid and osmolarity changes. Acute and severe hypernatremia may lead to a shift of water from the ICS, causing brain shrinkage and tearing of the meningeal vessels, with the risk of intracranial hemorrhage, especially when patient has started therapy with LMWH (Agro and Vennari 2013a; Miller 2009).

Hypernatremia management is based on normal osmolarity and volume restoration. It includes the administration of hypotonic crystalloids or dextrose solutions. The rate of correction depends on the symptoms and the development of hypernatremia (acute, subacute, or chronic). Chronic hypernatremia needs more care in the treatment. In fact the brain has yet developed compensation mechanism, and a too rapid correction may lead to cerebral edema (Agro and Vennari 2013a).

As a general rule, it is reasonable to have an initial sodium target of 145 mEq/L, with a rate of correction of plasmatic [Na+], not greater than 1–0.5 mEq/h (Agro and Vennari 2013a).

A useful formula to establish the rate of infusion for an adequate corrected is reported:

$$\frac{0.5\,\mathrm{mEq/h}}{\left(\mathrm{Infused}\left[\mathrm{Na}\right]-\mathrm{Measured}\left[\mathrm{Na}\right]\right)\mathrm{in\ mEq/L/Total\ body\ water}\times 1000}=\mathrm{mL/h}$$

where:

- 0.5 mEq/L is the recommendable rate of [Na+] correction.
- Infused [Na] is the concentration of sodium in the solution chosen for the correction.
- Measured [Na] is the sodium plasma concentration of the patient.
- Body water is calculated as

$$\mathrm{Total\ body\ water}=\left(\mathrm{correction\ factor\ x\ body\ weight\ in\ kg}\right)+1$$

Correction factor:

- 0.6 men and children
- 0.5 women
- 0.5 old men
- 0.45 old women

In the postoperative period, many cardiac surgery patients may present a reduction of sodium plasma levels, due to a shift of water from ICS to IVS rather than a reduction in total body sodium content. The shift is caused by hyperglycemia (diluting hyponatremia) triggered by the surgical stress response, the reduction in insulin production and insulin resistance, and an overload in the bypass pump prime

(Fanzca 2012; Kutschen et al. 1985). A similar mechanism may be triggered by mannitol overdose. In these cases, hyponatremia is accompanied by hypertonicity (plasma osmolarity >300 mosm/L) (Agro and Vennari 2013a).

Other causes responsible for hyponatremia in the ICU cardiac surgery patient are associated with a reduction of plasma osmolarity (true hyponatremia). In this case IVS volume may be normal, increased, or reduced (Agro and Vennari 2013a).

Advanced heart failure, severe hypovolemia, and hepatic complications with ascites alter ADH release and the kidneys' capacity to dilute urines, leading to hyponatremia with IVS volume reduction and interstitial edema development. The use of diuretics (especially if inappropriate) and the development of SIADH due to cerebral complications or prolonged mechanical ventilation may cause normo-hypervolemic hyponatremia without edema.

Hyponatremia with hypovolemia may be due to cerebral salt wasting (cerebral complications), hypokalemia, renal losses, and extrarenal losses. The most frequent cause of renal losses in the cardiac surgery patient is diuretic use and the development of ATN. Possible extrarenal losses are PONV, gastric suction, and diarrhea (i.e., related to enteral nutrition in long-stay patient). In the critical patient, frequent causes of hypovolemic hyponatremia are third-space syndromes.

Hyponatremia symptoms depend on the severity of the sodium deficit. Clinical features are weakness, nausea, vomiting, modification of consciousness (agitation, confusion, coma, and seizures), visual alteration, cramps, and myoclonus. When the sodium level falls below 123 mEq/L, cerebral edema occurs. At a sodium concentration of 100 mEq/L, cardiac symptoms develop. In diluting hyponatremia, an increase in IVS volume can lead to pulmonary edema, hypertension, and heart failure (Agro and Vennari 2013a).

Sodium level alterations are related to an increased risk of postoperative delirium, especially in patients with pre-existing hyponatremia (Fitzsimons and Agnihotri 2007).

A possible flowchart for hyponatremia diagnosis is showed in the flowchart below (Fig. 15.22).

The first-line treatment of hyponatremia is the elimination of the underlying cause. The second-line treatment is correction of the sodium deficit, generally through intravenous sodium administration (0.9% saline solution or other hypertonic saline solutions). The dose of sodium required to correct hyponatremia may be calculated using the following formula (Agro and Vennari 2013a):

$$\text{Sodium deficit}\left(\text{mEq}\right)=\left(130\,\text{mEq}-\text{measured serum Na mEq}\right)\times\text{Total body water}$$

The rate of infusion of the chosen fluid may be calculated according to the same formula explained for hypernatremia. A recommendable initial [Na] target is 125–130 mEq/L. A slow rate (maximum rate = 0.5 mEq/L/h) of correction is always indicated, because rapid correction can cause central pontine myelinolysis, especially in case of chronic hyponatremia. For this reason it is suggested to use a velocity rate correspondent to the half of the obtained value. In case of hypervolemia, it

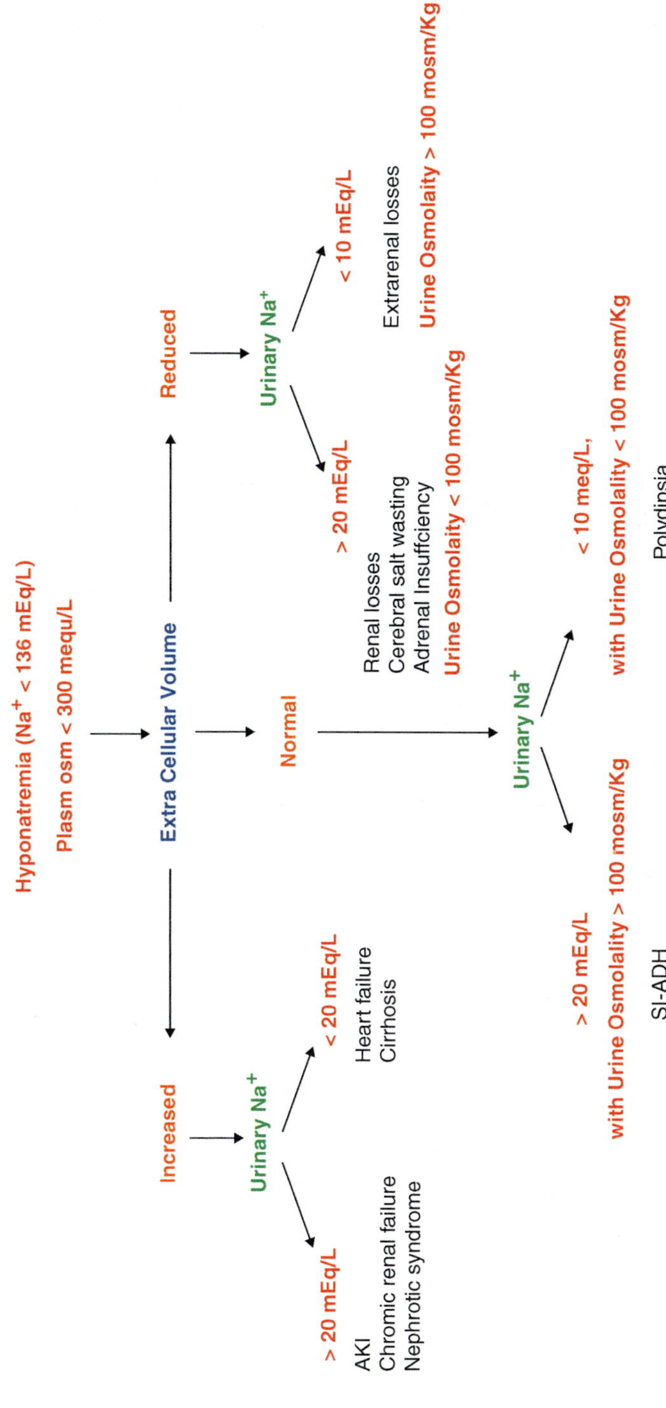

Fig. 15.22 Flowchart for hyponatremia diagnosis

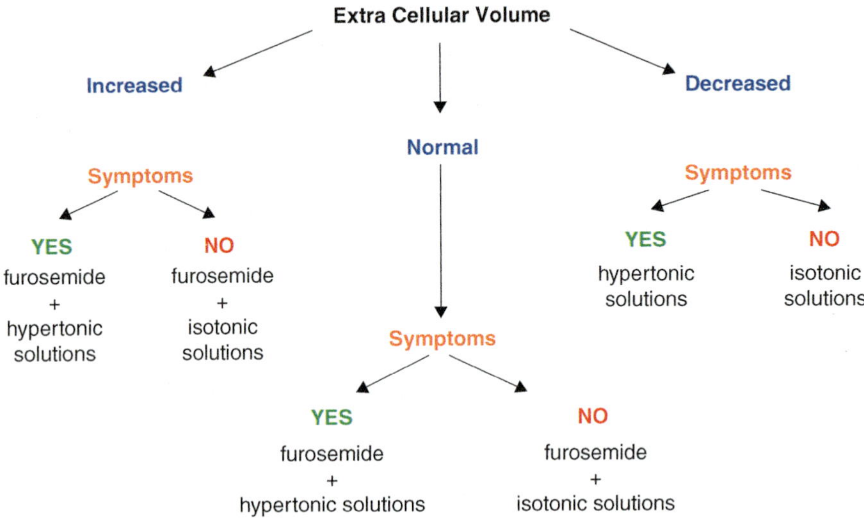

Fig. 15.23 Flowchart for hyponatremia management

may be preferred to utilize water restriction and a diuretic, such as furosemide (Agro and Vennari 2013a).

A possible flowchart for hyponatremia management is showed below (Fig. 15.23).

15.16.2 Potassium

Maintaining adequate potassium levels is crucial for bypass pump separation and to prevent postoperative dysrhythmias. In the perioperative setting, many factors may affect potassium plasma levels in different directions. Generally factors determining a reduction of potassium levels are predominant; as a consequence potassium loss must be adequately prevented and managed (Fanzca 2012).

Hyperkalemia may be the consequence of an increase in total potassium body stores or of a shift of potassium from the ICS to the ECS (Agro and Vennari 2013a).

In the cardiac surgery patient, an increase in [K^+] is commonly due to ICS shift caused by acidemia, hypoinsulinemia, hemolysis, and potassium IV load due to cardioplegia (Fanzca 2012).

In case of postoperative ATN, hyperkalemia often reflects a reduced renal excretion of potassium due to reduced tubular secretion, rather than a reduced glomerular filtration. Adrenal dysfunction (due to disease or drugs), with reduced aldosterone production, can lead to potassium retention (Agro and Vennari 2013a). Muscular weakness, up to paralysis, is one of the main manifestations of hyperkalemia. Cardiac signs are increased automaticity and repolarization of the myocardium, leading to ECG alterations and arrhythmias. Mild hyperkalemia may appear with T waves and a prolonged P-R interval; severe hyperkalemia may cause a wide QRS complex, asystole, or ventricular fibrillation Agro and Vennari 2013a.

The management of hyperkalemia includes heart protection and facilitating in ICS redistribution of potassium. Rapid-effect therapies are the administration of calcium gluconate, insulin with glucose (considering patients with glycemia), and correction of acidemia through bicarbonate administration or hyperventilation. In acute and severe case (often associated with AKI and the development of postoperative complication such as sepsis), CRRT may be indicated considering other electrolytes and acid-base status. Additional therapies are resin exchange, diuretics, aldosterone agonists, and β-adrenergic agonists. They act in a long term, and their use is suitable in long-stay ICU patients who have developed a chronic condition determining hyperkalemia (Agro and Vennari 2013a).

Cardiac surgery patient often presents hypokalemia, which may be caused by an absolute deficiency of total body potassium stores or by an abnormal shift of potassium from the ECS to the ICS (despite a normal total potassium) (Agro and Vennari 2013a).

In the perioperative setting, a reduction in potassium level is due to augmented catecholamine production with increase skeletal uptake; diuresis caused by hypothermia, furosemide, and mannitol use during CPB; and increased cortisol and aldosterone levels due to surgical stress. Other causes may be gastrointestinal loss or renal losses due to diuretic or the development of acute renal damage. Hypokalemia is always associated with metabolic alkalosis (see acid-base paragraph) (Fanzca 2012; Agro and Vennari 2013a).

Hypokalemia signs and symptoms depend on the potassium level. Arrhythmias (frequently, atrial fibrillation and premature ventricular beat) and other electrocardiographic abnormalities (sagging of the ST segment, T wave depression, and U-wave elevation) appear at potassium concentrations <3 mEq/L (Agro and Vennari 2013a).

The rate of potassium administration (generally potassium chloride) must be adjusted considering the distribution within the ECS. The administration rate is limited to 0.5–1.0 mEq/kg/h (Agro and Vennari 2013a).

15.16.3 Calcium

Hypocalcemia is frequent during the intraoperative period. Hypocalcemia refers to free ionized calcium levels in the plasma. It develops when calcium concentrations are low but plasma protein levels are normal. As a consequence, it is necessary to know if the calcium values measured is the total plasma value (in this case it should be adjusted for albumin value) or the ionized fraction (Agro and Vennari 2013a).

In the cardiac surgery patients, hypocalcemia is generally limited, and it is caused by citrate use, hemodilution, increase of albumin-binding fraction, and hypomagnesemia. In these cases hypocalcemia is treated in order to normalize calcium level and to uptake its effects on the myocardium (protection and inotropism) and vessels (vasopressor) (Fanzca 2012). In the ICU setting, the most frequent cause of hypocalcemia is hypoalbuminemia. Other causes are the development of postoperative renal dysfunctions, hyperventilation, blood transfusion (citrate chelation), and septic complications (the pathogenesis of the mechanisms correlating sepsis and hypocalcemia is not fully understood) (Fanzca 2012).

The main clinical manifestations of hypocalcemia are due to the increased cardiac and neuromuscular excitability and to the reduced contractile force of cardiac and vascular smooth muscle. Tetanic syndrome, a result of increased neuromuscular excitability, is characterized by numbness (especially around the mouth, lips, and tongue) and muscle spasms, particularly in the hands, feet, and face (characteristic are Chvostek and Trousseau signs). Regarding the cardiovascular alterations, hypocalcemia causes prolongation of the PQ interval, which predisposes patients to the onset of severe ventricular arrhythmias. Hypocalcemia may also lead to hypotension.

Nervous symptoms are due to the impaired mental status (Agro and Vennari 2013a).

The treatment of hypocalcemia should be causal but should also be aimed at quickly increasing the serum calcium concentration. It may be corrected by administering 10% calcium chloride (1.36 mEq/mL) or calcium gluconate (0.45 mEq/mL) (Agro and Vennari 2013a). The role of calcium administration has been discussed in literature. In particular, there is concern about the exacerbation of ischemia-reperfusion damage. In fact, in ischemic cells, there are high calcium levels due to the impairment of ATP-calcium pump and to a reverse activity of Na^+-Ca^{2+} pump. Finally calcium transport is impaired by the oxidative stress. Intracellular hypercalcemia leads to mitochondrial dysfunction and cellular death. Calcium administration may further increase calcium flux into cardiac cells, accelerating this process (Fanzca 2012). In patient who have undergone CABG, De Hert et al. (Fanzca 2012; Dehert et al. 1997) found a transient improvement (<10 min) in systolic function, associated with a diastolic dysfunction (reduced myocardial compliance), when calcium was administered early after bypass separation. However, in a subsequent study the reduction of diastolic function after CABG was not related to calcium administration (Fanzca 2012; Ekery et al. 2003). Moreover calcium has been shown to reduce adrenaline effect in the postoperative period and in animal studies to increase the negative inotropic effect of protamine (Fanzca 2012; Zaloga et al. 1990; David et al. 2001). Evidence suggest that the use of calcium at the time or before the reperfusion has benefit which cannot be obtained using other agent, although implying potentially adverse effect (Fanzca 2012).

Hypercalcemia is less frequent in the immediate postoperative period of cardiac surgery. It is generally related to an overtreatment of hypocalcemia, while in the long-stay ICU patient, it may be due to the development of renal dysfunction or increased bone reabsorption (immobilization) (Agro and Vennari 2013a).

Main symptoms of hypercalcemia may be remembered using the rhyme “groans (constipation), moans (psychic moans, e.g., fatigue, lethargy, depression), bones (bone pain, especially in hyperparathyroidism), stones (kidney stones), and psychiatric overtones (including depression and confusion)." Other symptoms are anorexia, fatigue, vomiting, and nausea. ECG alterations, such as a short QT interval or widened T wave, are suggestive of hypocalcemia. Symptoms are common at high calcium concentration (>3 mEq/L). Severe hypocalcemia (>4 mEql/L) is a medical emergency. It may lead to coma and cardiac arrest (Agro and Vennari 2013a).

Hypercalcemia management involves increased diuresis and plasma dilution. Accordingly, diuretics and saline solutions are used, because sodium reduces calcium reabsorption by the kidneys. In patient with a chronic cause or status leading to hypocalcaemia, other possible treatments are calcitonin, bisphosphonate, and glucocorticoids. In all patients rapid mobilization and physiotherapy after the surgery is fundamental to maintain bone balance (Agro and Vennari 2013a).

15.16.4 Magnesium

Hypomagnesemia is frequent in the postoperative period after cardiac surgery. It may be triggered by hyperaldosteronism (heart failure, stress response), by calcium alteration (hypercalcemia), and by the use of drugs such as diuretics or adrenergic drugs (Agro and Vennari 2013a). The effects of magnesium deficits are neuromuscular excitability disorders (related to the concurrent development of hypercalcemia), such as involuntary contraction of the facial muscles, cramps, tetany, and arrhythmias, or other symptoms mainly related to metabolism, such as morning fatigue. Hypomagnesemia may lead to hypertension, coronary vasoconstriction, and arrhythmias (Fanzca 2012; David et al. 2001; Kimura et al. 1989). It may also be characterized by an alteration of consciousness, as demonstrated by confusion, hallucinations, and epilepsy.

Magnesium supplementation has been demonstrated to reduce the reperfusion injury, by blocking calcium ingress in myocardial cells and acting as a free radical scavenger (Fanzca 2012; Booth et al. 2003). In fact, in animal studies, magnesium use has been related to a reduction of infarct size. The timing of administration appears to be very important: no effects have been found when administration is realized early after the reperfusion (Fanzca 2012; Garcia et al. 1998; Ravn et al. 1999). Literature also demonstrated that after CABG, magnesium supplementation reduces the risk of postoperative arrhythmiasS, improves the short-term neurological function, and may have a significant opioid-sparing effect (Fanzca 2012; Herzog et al. 1995; England et al. 1992).

Magnesium inhibits platelet function with a prolongation of bleeding time at 24 h after cardiac surgery. However a correlation of this effect with an increase of postoperative blood losses is not clear (Fanzca 2012; Mille et al. 2005). On the other side, a recent study demonstrated reduced postoperative bleeding and transfusional need after CABG, in patient receiving magnesium (Fanzca 2012; Gries et al. 1999; Dabbagh et al. 2010).

Hypermagnesemia is less frequent in cardiac surgery patient. The most common and probable cause is kidney failure. Hemolysis, hypocalcemia, adrenal insufficiency, diabetic ketoacidosis, lithium intoxication, and hyperparathyroidism are other predisposing conditions. Hypermagnesemia is characterized by weakness, hypocalcemia, nausea and vomiting, hypotension, breathing symptoms, and arrhythmias up to asystole (Agro and Vennari 2013a).

In severe cases, the first-line hypomagnesemia management is the administration of calcium gluconate, since calcium is the natural antagonist of magnesium. Subsequently, according to renal function, diuretics or dialysis is needed (Agro and Vennari 2013a).

Conclusion

A perfect fluid management for perioperative treatment of cardiac surgery patient is still lacking.

One of the first goals is to contain the IVS losses to a minimum using the cell savage technique and reducing the need for colloids (with their side effect!) (Fanzca 2012).

Preload assessment and DO_2 optimization by assessing fluid responsiveness represent the main goal in cardiac surgery patients. The best approach is using GDT to measure preload and to restore it in patients with reduced circulating volume (fluid responders) while using a continuous infusion of fluid to compensate urinary loss and perspiration, being mindful of glycocalyx alterations caused by cardiac surgery and that may generate tissue edema (Fanzca 2012). Colloids are needed when a fast hemodynamic improvement is necessary (Agro and Vennari 2013b). The volume effect of colloids depends on the IVS volume and hydration state of the patient. Giving fluids, not before but when hypovolemia occurs, seems to be more rational because the volume effects of colloids are more effective (Chappell et al. 2008; Dubois and Vincent 2007). Treating relative hypovolemia with colloids in patients undergoing surgery or in the critically ill who need sedation ignores the indirect vasodilator effect of anesthetic drugs. Thus, when vascular tone is restored, a relative hypervolemia can occur, potentially causing postoperative pulmonary edema (Dubois and Vincent 2007).

Crystalloids are needed to compensate urinary and perspiration losses, avoiding overload (Agro and Vennari 2013b).

Possible future strategies could be aimed to protect and rapidly restore the endothelial glycocalyx (Fanzca 2012).

It is of prime importance that intravenous fluids should be treated as drugs: their administration should be realized taking into account strict indications and the necessary precautions with respect to side effects and potential adverse reactions.

Fluid therapy should be individualized on the basis of the available evidence and the clinical context, considering that currently available data is evaluated in an objective manner with respect to the underlying physiology and pathophysiology of fluid treatment in various disease states (see HES debate). Only in this way can evidence-based clinical recommendations be provided (Raghunathan et al. 2013).

References

Abbas SM, Hill AG. Systematic review of the literature for the use of oesophageal Doppler monitor for fluid replacement in major abdominal surgery. Anaesthesia. 2008;63:44–51.

Adams HA. Volumen und Flüssigkeitsersatz—Physiologie, Pharmakologie und klinischer Einsatz. Anästh Intensivmed. 2007;48:448–60.

Adamson JW. New blood, old blood, or no blood? N Engl J Med. 2008;358:1295–6.

Agro FE, Benedetto M. Properties and composition of plasma substitutes. In: Agrò FE, editor. Body fluid management—from physiology to therapy. 1st ed. Milan: Springer; 2013.

Agro FE, Vennari M. Physiology of body fluid compartments and body fluid movements. In: Agrò FE, editor. Body fluid management—from physiology to therapy. 1st ed. Milan: Springer; 2013a.

Agro FE, Vennari M. Clinical treatment: the right fluid in the right quantity. In: Agrò FE, editor. Body fluid management—from physiology to therapy. 1st ed. Milan: Springer; 2013b.

Agrò FE, Fries D, Vennari M. Cardiac Surgery. In: Agrò FE, editor. Body fluid management—from physiology to therapy. 1st ed. Milan: Springer; 2013.

Agro FE, Fries D, Benedetto M. How to maintain and restore the balance: colloids. In: Agrò FE, editor. Body fluid management—from physiology to therapy. 1st ed. Milan: Springer; 2013.

Allhoff T, Lenhart FP. Severe dextran-induced anaphylactic/anaphylactoid reaction in spite of hapten prophylaxis. Infusionsther Transfusionsmed. 1993;20:301–6.

Allison KP, Gosling P, Jones S, et al. Randomized trial of hydroxyethyl starch versus gelatin for trauma resuscitation. J Trauma. 1999;47:1114–21.

Arieff AI, Llach F, Massry SG. Neurological manifestations and morbidity of hyponatremia: correlation with brain water and electrolytes. Medicine. 1976;55:121–9.

Arkilic CF, Taguchi A, Sharma N, et al. Supplemental perioperative fluid administration increases tissue oxygen pressure. Surgery. 2003;133:49–55.

Arthurson G, Granath K, Thoren L, et al. The renal excretion of LMW dextran. Acta Clin Scand. 1964;127:543–51.

Atik M. Dextran-40 and dextran-70, a review. Arch Surg. 1967;94:664–7.

Auler JOJ, Galas F, Hajjar L, et al. Online monitoring of pulse pressure variation to guide fluid therapy after cardiac surgery. Anesth Analg. 2008;106:1201–6.

Balogh Z, McKinley BA, Cocanour CS, et al. Supranormal trauma resuscitation causes more cases of abdominal compartment syndrome. Arch Surg. 2003;138:633–42.

Bamboat ZM, Bordeianou L. Perioperative fluid management. Clin Colon Rectal Surg. 2009;22(1):28–33.

Baron JF. Adverse effects of colloids on renal function. In: Vincent JL, editor. Yearbook of intensive care and emergency medicine. 1st ed. Berlin: Springer; 2000.

Barron ME, Wilkes NRJ. A systematic review of the comparative safety of colloids. Arch Surg. 2004;139:552–63.

Base EM, Standl T, Lassnigg A, et al. Efficacy and safety of hydroxyethyl starch 6% 130/0.4 in a balanced electrolyte solution (Volulyte) during cardiac surgery. J Cardiothorac Vasc Anesth. 2011;25(3):407–14.

Belloni L, Pisano A, Natale A, et al. Assessment of fluid responsiveness parameters for off-pump coronary artery bypass surgery: a comparison among LiDCO, transesophageal echocardiography, and pulmonary artery catheter. J Cardiothorac Vasc Anesth. 2008;22:243–8.

Bendjelid K, Suter PM, Romand JA. The respiratory change in preejection period: a new method to predict fluid responsiveness. J Appl Physiol. 2004;96:337–42.

Benes J, Cytra I, Altmann P, et al. Intraoperative fluid optimization using stroke volume variation in high risk surgical patients: result of prospective randomized study. Crit Care. 2010;14:R118.

Bennett-Guerrero E, Kahn RA, Moskowitz DM, et al. Comparison of arterial systolic pressure variation with other clinical parameters to predict the response to fluid challenges during cardiac surgery. Mt Sinai J Med. 2002;69:96–100.

Bernard C. Introdution à l'étude de la médecine expérimentale. Paris: J. B. Baillière et fils; 1865.

Booth J, Philips-Bute B, McCants C, et al. Low serum magnesium level predicts major adverse cardiac events after coronary artery bypass graft surgery. Am Heart J. 2003;145:1108–13.
Boyd DR, Mansberger AR Jr. Serum water and osmolal changes in hemorrhagic shock: an experimental and clinical study. Am Surg. 1968;34:744–9.
Brandstrup B. Fluid therapy for the surgical patient. Best Pract Res Clin Anaesthesiol. 2006;20:265–83.
Brandstrup B, Tønnesen H, Beier-Holgersen R, et al. Effects of intravenous fluid restriction on postoperative complications: comparison of two perioperative fluid regimens: a randomized assessor-blinded multicenter trial. Ann Surg. 2003;238:641–8.
Breukers RM, de Wilde RBP, van den Berg PCM, et al. Assessing fluid responses after coronary surgery: role of mathematical coupling of global end-diastolic volume to cardiac output measured by transpulmonary thermodilution. Eur J Anaesthesiol. 2009a;26:954–60.
Breukers RM, Trof RJ, de Wilde RBP, et al. Relative value of pressures and volumes in assessing fluid responsiveness after valvular and coronary artery surgery. Eur J Cardiothorac Surg. 2009b;35:62–8.
Brock H, Gabriel C, Bibl D, et al. Monitoring intravascular volumes for postoperative volume therapy. Eur J Anaesthesiol. 2002;19:288–94.
Bruegger D, Jacob M, Rehm M, et al. Atrial natriuretic peptide induces shedding of endothelial glycocalyx in coronary vascular bed of guinea pig hearts. Am J Physiol Heart Circ Physiol. 2005;289:H1993–9.
Brunkhorst FM, Engel C, Bloos F, et al. Intensive insulin therapy and pentastarch resuscitation in severe sepsis. N Engl J Med. 2008;358:125–39.
Buhre W, Buhre K, Kazmaier S, et al. Assessment of cardiac preload by indicator dilution and transesophageal echocardiography. Eur J Anaesthesiol. 2001;18:662–7.
Bunn F, Roberts I, Tasker R, Akpa E. Hypertonic versus isotonic crystalloid for fluid resuscitation in critically ill patients (Cochrane Review). Cochrane Database Syst Rev. 2002;3:CD002045.
Caironi P, Langer T, Gattinoni L. Albumin in critically ill patients: the ideal colloid? Curr Opin Crit Care. 2015;21(4):302–8.
Campbell IT, Baxter JN, Tweedie IE, et al. IV fluids during surgery. Br J Anaesth. 1990;65:726–9.
Carl M, Alms A, Braun J, et al. Die intensivmedizinische Versorgung herzchirurgischer Patienten: Hämodynamisches Monitoring und Herz-Kreislauf-Therapie S3-Leitlinie der Deutschen Gesellschaft für Thorax-, Herz- und Gefäbchirurgie (DGTHG) und der Deutschen Gesellschaft für Anästhesiologie und Intensivmedizin (DGAI). Thorac Cardiovasc Surg. 2000;55:130–48.
Cavallaro F, Sandroni C, Antonelli M. Functional hemodynamic monitoring and dynamic indices of fluid responsiveness. Minerva Anestesiol. 2008;74:123–35.
Cervera AL, Moss G. Crystalloid distribution following haemorrhage and haemodilution: mathematical model and prediction of optimum volumes for equilibration at normovolemia. J Trauma. 1974;14:506–20.
Chan ST, Kapadia CR, Johnson AW, et al. Extracellular fluid volume expansion and third space sequestration at the site of small bowel anastomoses. Br J Surg. 1983;70:36–9.
Chappell D, Jacob M, Hofmann-Kiefer K, et al. A rational approach to perioperative fluid management. Anesthesiology. 2008;109:723–40.
Cheung AT, Savino JS, Weiss SJ, et al. Echocardiographic and hemodynamic indexes of left ventricular preload in patients with normal and abnormal ventricular function. Anesthesiology. 1994;81:376–87.
Chytra I, Pradl R, Bosman R, et al. Esophageal Doppler-guided fluid management decreases blood lactate levels in multiple-trauma patients: a randomized controlled trial. Crit Care. 2007;11(1):R24.
Dabbagh A, Rajaei S, Shamsolhrar M. The effect of intravenous magnesium sulfate on acute postoperative bleeding in elective coronary artery bypass surgery. J Perianesth Nurs. 2010;25:290–5.
David J, Vivien B, Lecarpentier Y, et al. Extracellular calcium modulates the effects of protamine on rat myocardium. Anesth Analg. 2001;92:817–23.
De Hert S, De Baerdemaeker L. Why hydroxyethyl starch solutions should NOT be banned from the operating room. Anaesthesiol Intensive Ther. 2014;46(5):336–41.

Dehert S, Ten Broeke P, De Mulder P, et al. Effect of calcium on left ventricular function early after cardiopulmonary bypass. J Cardiothorac Vasc Anesth. 1997;11:846–9.
DeJonge E, Levi M. Effects of different plasma substitutes on blood coagulation: a comparative review. Crit Care Med. 2001;29:1261–7.
Deman A, Peeters P, Sennesael J. Hydroxyethyl starch does not impair immediate renal function in kidney transplant recipient. A retrospective, multicenter analysis. Nephrol Dial Transplant. 1999;14:1517–20.
DiCorte CJ, Latham P, Greilich PE, et al. Esophageal Doppler monitor determinations of cardiac output and preload during cardiac operations. Ann Thorac Surg. 2000;69:1782–6.
Dieterich HJ, Weissmuller T, Rosenberger P, et al. Effect of hydroxyethyl starch on vascular leak syndrome and neutrophil accumulation during hypoxia. Crit Care Med. 2006;34:1775–82.
Dietrich G, Orth D, Haupt W, et al. Primary hemostasis in hemodilution-infusion solutions. Infusionstherapie. 1990;17:214–6.
Dongaonkar R, Stweart R, Geisller H, Laine G. Myocardial microvascular permeability, interstitial oedema, and compromised cardiac function. Cardiovasc Res. 2010;87:331–9.
Dorje P, Adhikary G, Tempe DK. Avoiding iatrogenic hyperchloremic acidosis: call for a new crystalloid fluid. Anesthesiology. 2000;92:625–6.
Drt A, Mutter T, Ruth C, et al. Hydroxyethyl starch (HES) versus other fluid therapies: effects on kidney function. Cochrane Database Syst Rev. 2010;1:CD007594.
Drummond JC, Petrovitch CT. Intraoperative blood salvage: fluid replacement calculation. Anesth Analg. 2005;100:645–9.
Dubois MJ, Vincent JL. Colloid fluids. In: Hahn RG, Prough DS, Svensen CH, editors. Perioperative fluid therapy. 1st ed. New York: Wiley; 2007.
Duchesne JC, Kaplan LJ, Balogh ZJ, Malbrain ML. Role of permissive hypotension, hypertonic resuscitation and the global increased permeability syndrome in patients with severe hemorrhage: adjuncts to damage control resuscitation to prevent intra-abdominal hypertension. Anaesthesiol Intensive Ther. 2015;47(2):143–55.
Ekery D, Davidoff R, Orlandi Q, et al. Imaging and diagnostic testing: dysfunction after coronary artery bypass grafting: a frequent finding of clinical significance not influenced by intravenous calcium. Am Heart J. 2003;145:896–902.
England M, Gordon G, Salem M, et al. Magnesium administration and dysrhythmias after cardiac surgery. A placebo controlled double-blind randomized trial. JAMA. 1992;268:2395–402.
Ernest D, Belzberg AS, Dodek PM. Distribution of normal saline and 5% albumin infusions in cardiac surgical patients. Crit Care Med. 2001;29:2299–302.
Fanzca RY. Perioperative fluid and electrolyte management in cardiac surgery: a review. J Extra Corpor Technol. 2012;44:20–6.
Feng X, Yan W, Liu X, et al. Effects of hydroxyethyl starch 130/0.4 on pulmonary capillary leakage and cytokines production and nF-kappaB activation in ClP-induced sepsis in rats. J Surg Res. 2006;135:129–36.
Fitzsimons M, Agnihotri A. Hyponatremia and cardiopulmonary bypass. J Cardiothorac Vasc Anesth. 2007;86:1883–7.
Fleck A, Raines G, Hawker F, et al. Increased vascular permeability. Major cause of hypoalbuminaemia in disease and injury. Lancet. 1985;1:781–3.
Franz A, Bräunlich P, Gamsjäger T, et al. The effects of hydroxyethyl starches of varying molecular weights on platelet function. Anesth Analg. 2001;92:1402–7.
Gallandat Huet RCG, Siemons AW, Baus D, et al. A novel hydroxyethyl starch (VoluvenR) for effective perioperative plasma volume substitution in cardiac surgery. Can J Anaesth. 2000;47:1207–15.
Gamble J. Chemical anatomy, physiology and pathology of extracellular fluid. Cambridge: Harvard University Press; 1947.
Gandhi SD, Weiskopf RB, Jungheinrich C, et al. Volume replacement therapy during major orthopedic surgery using Voluven® (hydroxyethyl starch 130/0.4) or hetastarch. Anesthesiology. 2007;106:1120–7.

Garcia L, Dejong S, Martin S, et al. Magnesium reduces free radicals in an in vivo coronary occlusion reperfusion model. J Am Coll Cardiol. 1998;32:536–9.

Ghijselings I, Rex S. Hydroxyethyl starches in the perioperative period. A review on the efficacy and safety of starch solutions. Acta Anaesthesiol Belg. 2014;65(1):9–22.

Giglio MT, Marucci M, Testini M, et al. Goal-directed haemodynamic therapy and gastrointestinal complications in major surgery: a meta-analysis of randomized controlled trials. Br J Anaesth. 2009;103:637–46.

Goedje O, Seebauer T, Peyerl M, et al. Hemodynamic monitoring by double-indicator dilution technique in patients after orthotopic heart transplantation. Chest. 2000;118:775–81.

Goepfer MS, Reuter DA, Akyiol D, et al. Goal-directed fluid management reduces vasopressor and catecholamine use in cardiac surgery patients. Intensive Care Med. 2007;33:96–103.

Grathwohl KW, Bruns BJ, LeBrun CJ, et al. Does haemodilution exist? Effects of saline infusion on hematologic parameters in euvolemic subjects. South Med J. 1996;89:51–5.

Grebe D, Sander M, von Heymann C, et al. Fluid therapy—pathophysiological principles as well as intra- and perioperative monitoring. Anasthesiol Intensivmed Notfallmed Schmerzther. 2006;41:392–8.

Greenfield RH, Bessen HA, Henneman PL. Effect of crystalloid infusion on hematocrit and intravascular volume in healthy, no bleeding subjects. Ann Emerg Med. 1989;18:51–5.

Gries A, Bode C, Gross S, et al. The effect of intravenously administered magnesium on platelet function in patient after cardiac surgery. Anesth Analg. 1999;88:1231–9.

Grocott MP, Mythen MG, Gan TJ. Perioperative fluid management and clinical outcomes in adults. Anesth Analg. 2005;100:1093–106.

Habicher M, Perrino AJ, Spies CD, et al. Contemporary fluid management in cardiac anesthesia. J Cardiothorac Vasc Anesth. 2011;25(6):1141–53.

Hahn RG. Must hypervolaemia be avoided? A critique of the evidence. Anaesthesiol Intensive Ther. 2015;47(5):449–56.

Hahn RG, Drobin D, Stähle L. Volume kinetics of Ringer's solution in female volunteers. Br J Anaesth. 1997;78:144–8.

Hauser CJ, Shoemaker WC, Turpin I, et al. Oxygen transport responses to colloids and crystalloids in critically ill surgical patients. Surg Gynecol Obstet. 1980;150:811–6.

Haynes GH, Havidich JE, Payne KJ. Why the Food and Drug Administration changed the warning label for hetastarch. Anesthesiology. 2004;101:560–1.

Hecth-Dolkin M, Barkan H, Tahara A, et al. Hetastarch increases the risk of bleeding complications in patients after off-pump coronary by-pass surgery. J Thorac Cardiovasc Surg. 2009;138:703–11.

Hendry EB. Osmolarity of human serum and of chemical solutions of biological importance. Clin Chem. 1961;7:156–64.

Herzog W, Schlossberg M, MacMurdy K, et al. Timing of magnesium therapy affects experimental infarct size. Circulation. 1995;92:2622–6.

Heßler M, Arnemann PH, Ertmer C. To use or not to use hydroxyethyl starch in intraoperative care: are we ready to answer the 'Gretchen question'? Curr Opin Anaesthesiol. 2015;28(3):370–7.

Hiltebrand LB, Pestel G, Hager H, et al. Perioperative fluid management: comparison of high, medium and low fluid volume on tissue oxygen pressure in the small bowel and colon. Eur J Anaesthesiol. 2007;24:927–33.

Hofer CK, Furrer L, Matter-Ensner S, et al. Volumetric preload measurement by thermodilution: a comparison with transoesophageal echocardiography. Br J Anaesth. 2005a;94:748–55.

Hofer CK, Müller SM, Furrer L, et al. Stroke volume and pulse pressure variation for prediction of fluid responsiveness in patients undergoing off-pump coronary artery bypass grafting. Chest. 2005b;128:848–54.

Hofer CK, Senn A, Weibel L, et al. Assessment of stroke volume variation for prediction of fluid responsiveness using the modified FloTrac™ and PiCCOplus™ system. Crit Care. 2008;12:R82.

Holte K, Kehlet H. Compensatory fluid administration for preoperative dehydration: does it improve outcome? Acta Anaesthesiol Scand. 2002;46:1089–93.

Holte K, Klarskov B, Christensen DS, et al. Liberal versus restrictive fluid administration to improve recovery after laparoscopic cholecystectomy: a randomized doubleblind study. Ann Surg. 2004;240:892–9.

Holte K, Hahn RG, Ravn L, et al. Influence of a "liberal" versus "restrictive" intraoperative fluid administration on elimination of a postoperative fluid load. Anesthesiology. 2007a;106:75–9.

Holte K, Foss NB, Andersen J, et al. Liberal or restrictive fluid administration in fasttrack colonic surgery: a randomized, double-blind study. Br J Anaesth. 2007b;99:500–8.

Holtfreter B, Bandt C, Kuhn SO, et al. Serum osmolality and outcome in intensive care unit patients. Acta Anaesthesiol Scand. 2006;50:970–7.

Hu X, Weinbaum S. A new view of Starling's hypothesis at the micro-structural level. Microvasc Res. 1999;58(3):281–304.

Hu X, Adamson RH, Liu B, Curry FE, Weinbaum S. Starling forces that oppose filtration after tissue oncotic pressure is increased. Am J Physiol Heart Circ Physiol. 2000;279(4): H1724–36.

Hüter L, Simon TP, Weinmann L, et al. Hydroxyethylstarch impairs renal function and induces interstitial proliferation, macrophage infiltration and tubular damage in an isolated renal perfusion model. Crit Care. 2009;13:R23.

Ickx BE, Bepperling F, Melot C, et al. Plasma substitution effects of a new hydroxyethyl starch HES 130/0.4 compared with HES 200/0.5 during and after extended acute normovolaemic haemodilution. Br J Anaesth. 2003;91:196–202.

Iriz E, Kolbakir F, Akar H, et al. Comparison of hydroxyethyl starch and ringer as prime solution regarding S-100beta protein levels and informative cognitive tests in cerebral injury. Ann Thorac Surg. 2005;79:666–71.

Jacob M, Chappel D, Conzen P, et al. Blood volume is normal after overnight fasting. Acta Anaesthesiol Scand. 2008;52:522–9.

James MF, Latoo MY, Mythen MG, et al. Plasma volume changes associated with two hydroxyethyl starch colloids following acute hypovolaemia in volunteers. Anaesthesia. 2004;59:738–42.

Järhult J. Osmotic fluid transfer from tissue to blood during hemorrhagic hypotension. Acta Physiol Scand. 1973;89:213–26.

Jarvela K, Koskinen M, Kaukinen S, et al. Effects of hypertonic saline (7.5%) on extracellular fluid volumes compared with normal saline (0.9%) and 6% hydroxyethyl starch after aortocoronary bypass graft surgery. J Cardiothorac Vasc Anesth. 2001;15:210–5.

Jenkins MT, Giesecke AH, Johnson ER. The postoperative patient and his fluid and electrolyte requirements. Br J Anaesth. 1975;47:143–50.

Jones SB, Whitten CW, Monk TG. Influence of crystalloid and colloid replacement solutions on hemodynamic variables during acute normovolemic hemodilution. J Clin Anesth. 2004;16:11–7.

Jumgheinrich C, Scharpf R, Wargenau M, et al. The pharmacokinetics and tolerability of an intravenous infusion the new hydroxyethyl starch 130/04 (6% 500 ml) in mild to severe renal impairment. Anaesth Analg. 2002;95:544–51.

Kaminski MV, Williams SD. Review of the rapid normalization of serum albumin with modified total parenteral nutrition solutions. Crit Care Med. 1990;18:327–35.

Kampmeier T, Rehberg S, Ertmer C. Evolution of fluid therapy. Best Pract Res Clin Anaesthesiol. 2014;28(3):207–16.

Kapoor PM, Kakani M, Chowdhury U, et al. Early goal-directed therapy in moderate to high-risk cardiac surgery patients. Ann Card Anaesth. 2008;11:27–34.

Karanko MS, Klossner JA, Laaksonen VO. Restoration of volume by crystalloid versus colloid after coronary artery bypass: hemodynamics, lung water, oxygenation, and outcome. Crit Care Med. 1987;15:559–66.

Kastrup M, Markewitz A, Spies C, et al. Current practice of hemodynamic monitoring and vasopressor and inotropic therapy in post-operative cardiac surgery patients in Germany: results from a postal survey. Acta Anaesthesiol Scand. 2007;51:347–58.

Kenney PR, Allen-Rowlands CF, Gann DS. Glucose and osmolality as predictors of injury severity. J Trauma. 1983;23:712–9.

Kimura T, Yasue H, Sukaino N, et al. Effects of magnesium on isolated human coronary arteries. After CABG it has been shown as a predictor of major cardiac events. Circulation. 1989;79:118–24.

Knotzer H, Filipovic M, Siegemund M, Kleinsasser A. The physiologic perspective in fluid management in vascular anesthesiology. J Cardiothorac Vasc Anesth. 2014;28(6):1604–8.

Kozek-Langenecker SA. Effects of hydroxyethyl starch solutions on hemostasis. Anesthesiology. 2005;103:654–60.

Kutschen F, Galletti P, Hahn C, et al. Alterations of insulin and glucose metabolism during cardiopulmonary bypass under normothermia. J Thorac Cardiovasc Surg. 1985;89:97–106.

Lamke LO, Liljedahl SO. Plasma volume changes after infusion of various plasma expanders. Resuscitation. 1976;5:93–102.

Lamke L, Nilsson G, Reithner H. Water loss by evaporation from the abdominal cavity during surgery. Acta Chir Scand. 1977;143:279–84.

Lasks H, Standeven J, Balir O, et al. The effects of cardiopulmonary by-pass with crystalloid and colloid hemodilution on myocardial extravascular water. J Thorac Cardiovasc Surg. 1977;73:129–38.

Laxenaire M, Charpentier C, Feldman L. Reactions anaphylactoides aux subitutes colloidaux du plasma: incidence, facteurs de risque, mecanismes. Ann Fr Anest Reanim. 1994;13:301–10.

Lees N, Hamilton M, Rhodes A. Clinical review: goal-directed therapy in high risk surgical patients. Crit Care. 2009;13:231. https://doi.org/10.1186/cc8039.

Lehmann G, Marx G, Forster H. Bioequivalence comparison between hydroxyethyl starch 130/0.42/6:1 and hydroxyethyl starch 130/0.4/9:1. Drugs R D. 2007;8:229–40.

Levick JR. Revision of the Starling principle. New views of tissue fluid balance. J Physiol. 2004;557:704.

Ley SJ, Miller K, Skov P, et al. Crystalloid versus colloid fluid therapy after cardiac surgery. Heart Lung. 1990;19:31–40.

Lira A, Pinsky MR. Choices in fluid type and volume during resuscitation: impact on patient outcomes. Semin Cardiothorac Vasc Anesth. 2014;18(3):252–9.

Lobo DN. Sir David Cuthbertson medal lecture. Fluid, electrolytes and nutrition: physiological and clinical aspects. Proc Nutr Soc. 2004;63:453–66.

Lobo DN, Stanga Z, Simpson JAD, et al. Dilution and redistribution effects of rapid 2- litre infusions of 0.9% (w/v) saline and 5% (w/v) dextrose on haematological parameters and serum biochemistry in normal subjects: a double-blind crossover study. Clin Sci (Lond). 2001;101: 173–9.

Lobo DN, Bostock KA, Neal KR, et al. Effect of salt and water balance on recovery of gastrointestinal function after elective colonic resection: a randomised controlled trial. Lancet. 2002;359:1812–8.

Lobo DN, Stanga Z, Aloysius MM, et al. Effect of volume loading with 1 liter intravenous infusions of 0.9% saline, 4% succinylated gelatin (Gelofusine) and 6% hydroxyethyl starch (Voluven) on blood volume and endocrine responses: a randomized, threeway crossover study in healthy volunteers. Crit Care Med. 2010;38:464–70.

Lopes MR, Oliveira MA, pereira VO. Goal-directed fluid management based on pulse pressure variation monitoring during high-risk surgery: a pilot randomized controlled trial. Crit Care. 2007;11:R100.

Lowell JA, Schifferdecker C, Driscoll DF, et al. Postoperative fluid overload: not a benign problem. Crit Care Med. 1990;18:728–33.

Ma PL, Peng XX, Du B, et al. Sources of heterogeneity in trials reporting hydroxyethyl starch 130/0.4 or 0.42 associated excess mortality in septic patients: a systematic review and meta-regression. Chin Med J. 2015;128(17):2374–82.

MacKay G, Fearon K, McConnachie A, et al. Randomized clinical trial of the effect of postoperative intravenous fluid restriction on recovery after elective colorectal surgery. Br J Surg. 2006;93:1469–74.

Madjdpour C, Dettori N, Frascarolo P, et al. Molecular weight of hydroxyethyl starch: is there an effect on blood coagulation and pharmacokinetics? Br J Anaesth. 2005;94:569–76.

Maharaj CH, Kallam SR, Malik A, et al. Preoperative intravenous fluid therapy decreases postoperative nausea and pain in high risk patients. Anesth Analg. 2005;100:675–82.
Mahmood A, Gosling P, Vohra RK. Randomized clinical trial comparing the effects on renal function of hydroxyethyl starch or gelatin during aortic aneurysm surgery. Br J Surg. 2007;94:427–33.
Mahmood A, Gosling P, Barclay R, et al. Splanchnic microcirculation protection by hydroxyethyl starches during abdominal aortic aneurysm surgery. Eur J Vasc Endovasc Surg. 2009;37:319–25.
Makoff DL, da Silva JA, Rosenbaum BJ, et al. Hypertonic expansion: acid-base and electrolyte changes. Am J Phys. 1970;218:1201–7.
Maningas PA, Bellamy RF. Hypertonic sodium chloride solutions for the prehospital management of traumatic hemorrhagic shock: a possible improvement in the standard of care? Ann Emerg Med. 1986;15:1411–4.
Margarson MP, Soni N. Serum albumin: touchstone or totem? Anaesthesia. 1998;53:789–803.
Marik PE. The treatment of hypoalbuminemia in the critically ill patient. Heart Lung. 1993;22:166–70.
Marik PE, Baram M, Vahid B. Does central venous pressure predict fluid responsiveness? A systematic review of the literature and the tale of seven mares. Chest. 2008;134:172–8.
Marik PE, Cavallazzi R, Vasu T, et al. Dynamic changes in arterial waveform derived variables and fluid responsiveness in mechanically ventilated patients: a systematic review. Crit Care Med. 2009;37:2642–7.
Marik PE, Cecconi M, Hofer CF. Cardiac output monitoring: an integrative perspective. Crit Care. 2011;15:214.
Martin G, Bennett-Guerrero E, Wakeling H, et al. A prospective, randomized comparison of thrombelastographic coagulation profile in patients receiving lactated Ringer's solution, 6% hetastarch in a balanced-saline vehicle, or 6% hydroxyethyl starch in saline during major surgery. J Cardiothorac Vasc Anesth. 2002;16:441–6.
McIlroy DR, Kharasch ED. Acute intravascular volume expansion with rapidly administered crystalloid or colloid in the setting of moderate hypovolemia. Anesth Analg. 2003;96(6):1572–7.
McKendry M, McGloin H, Saberi D, et al. Randomised controlled trial assessing the impact of a nurse delivered, flow monitored protocol for optimisation of circulatory status after cardiac surgery. BMJ. 2004;329:258.
Metze D, Reimann S, Szepfalusi Z, et al. Persistent pruritus after hydroxyethyl starch infusion therapy: a result of long-term storage in cutaneous nerves. Br J Dermatol. 1997;136:553–9.
Michard F, Teboul J-L. Predicting fluid responsiveness in ICU patients: a critical analysis of the evidence. Chest. 2002;121:2000–8.
Michard F, Alaya S, Zarka V, et al. Global end-diastolic volume as an indicator of cardiac preload in patients with septic shock. Chest. 2003;124:1900–8.
Mille S, Crystal E, Garfinkle K, et al. Effects of magnesium in atrial fibrillation after cardiac surgery: a meta analysis. Heart. 2005;91:618–23.
Miller RD. Miller's anesthesia. 7th ed. London, UK: Churchill Livingstone; 2009.
Mitra S, Khandelwal P. Are all colloids same? How to select the right colloid? Indian J Anaesth. 2009;53(5):592.
Moore FD, Steenburg RW, Ball MR, et al. Studies in surgical endocrinology. The urinary excretion of 17-hydroxycorticoids, and associated metabolic changes, in cases of soft tissue trauma of varying severity and in bone trauma. Ann Surg. 1955;141:145–74.
Moran M, Kapsner C. Acute renal failure associated with elevated plasma oncotic pressure. N Engl J Med. 1987;317:150–3.
Moret E, Jacob MW, Ranucci M, Schramko A. Albumin-beyond fluid replacement in cardiopulmonary bypass surgery: why, how, and when? Semin Cardiothorac Vasc Anesth. 2014;18(3):252–9.
Morissette M, Weil MH, Shubin H. Reduction in colloid osmotic pressure associated with fatal progression of cardiopulmonary failure. Crit Care Med. 1975;3:115–7.
Moyer CA. Acute temporary changes in renal function associated with major surgical procedures. Surgery. 1950;27:198–207.
Mutter TC, Ruth CA, Dart AB. Hydroxyethyl starch (HES) versus other fluid therapies: effects on kidney function. Cochrane Database Syst Rev. 2013;7:CD007594.

Mythen MG, Webb AR. Preoperative plasma volume expansion reduces the incidence of gut mucosal hypoperfusion during cardiac surgery. Arch Surg. 1995;130(4):423–9.
Nadler SB, Hidalgo JU, Bloch T. Prediction of blood volume in normal human adults. Surgery. 1962;51:224–32.
Ng KFJ, Lam CCK, Chan IC. In vivo effect of haemodilution with saline on coagulation: a randomized controlled tril. Br J Anaesth. 2002;88:475–80.
Niemi TT, Suojaranta-Ylinen RT, Kukkonen SI, et al. Gelatin and hydroxyethyl starch, but not albumin, impair hemostasis after cardiac surgery. Anesth Analg. 2006;102:998–1006.
Niemi T, Schramko A, Kuitunen A, et al. Haemodynamics and acid-base equilibrium after cardiac surgery: comparison of rapidly degradable hydroxyethyl starch solutions and albumin. Scand J Surg. 2008;97:259–65.
Nisanevich V, Felsenstein I, Almogy G, et al. Effect of intraoperative fluid management on outcome after intraabdominal surgery. Anesthesiology. 2005;103:25–32.
Nuevo FR, Vennari M, Agro FE. How to maintain and restore fluid balance: crystalloids. In: Agrò FE, editor. Body fluid management—from physiology to therapy. 1st ed. Milan: Springer; 2013.
Olsson J, Svense'n CH, Hahn RG. The volume kinetics of acetated Ringer's solution during laparoscopic cholecystectomy. Anesth Analg. 2004;99:1854–60.
Ooi JS, Ramzisham AR, Zamrin MD. Is 6% hydroxyethyl starch 130/0.4 safe in coronary artery bypass graft surgery? Asian Cardiovasc Thorac Ann. 2009;17:368–72.
Otsuki D, Fantoni D, Margarido C, et al. Hydroxyethyl starch is superior to ringer as a replacement fluid in pig model of acute normovolemic haemodilution. Br J Anaesth. 2007;98:29–37.
Palumbo D, Servillo G, D'Amato L, et al. The effects of hydroxyethyl starch solution in critically ill patients. Minerva Anestesiol. 2006;72:655–64.
Pearse R, Dawson D, Fawcett J, et al. Changes in central venous saturation after major surgery, and association with outcome. Crit Care. 2005a;9:R694–9.
Pearse R, Dawson D, Fawcett J, et al. Early goal-directed therapy after major surgery reduces complications and duration of hospital stay. A randomised, controlled trial [ISRCTN38797445]. Crit Care. 2005b;9:R687–93.
Petty TL, Ashbaugh DG. The adult respiratory distress syndrome. Clinical features, factors influencing prognosis and principles of management. Chest. 1971;60(3):233–9.
Polderman K, Girbes R. Severe electrolyte disorders following cardiac surgery. A prospective controlled observational study. Crit Care. 2004;8:459–66.
Polonen P, Ruokonen E, Hippelainen M, et al. A prospective, randomized study of goal-oriented hemodynamic therapy in cardiac surgical patients. Anesth Analg. 2000;90:1052–9.
Powell-Tuck J, Gosling P, Lobo DN et al. (2008) British consensus guidelines on intravenous fluid therapy for adult surgical patients. GIFTASUP. http://www.bapen.org.uk/pdfs/bapen_pubs/giftasup.pdf. Accessed 1 April 2010.
Pradeep A, Rajagopalam S, Kolli HK, et al. High volumes of intravenous fluid during cardiac surgery are associated with increased mortality. HSR Proceedings in Intensive Care and Cardiovascular. Anesthesia. 2010;2:287–96.
Pries AR, Secomb TW, Sperandi M, Gaehtgens P. Blood flow resistance during hemodilution. Effect of plasma composition. Cardiovasc Res. 1998;37:225–35.
Rackow E, Fein AI, Leppo J. Colloid osmotic pressure as a prognostic indicator of pulmonary oedema and mortality in the critically ill. Chest. 1977;72:709–13.
Rackow EC, Falk JL, Fein IA, et al. Fluid resuscitation in circulatory shock: a comparison of the cardio-respiratory effects of albumin, hetastarch, and saline solutions in patients with hypovolemic and septic shock. Crit Care Med. 1983;11:839–50.
Raghunathan K, Shaw AD, Bagshaw SM. Fluids are drugs: type, dose and toxicity. Curr Opin Crit Care. 2013;19(4):290–8.
Raja SG, Akhtar S, Shahbaz Y, et al. In cardiac surgery patients does Voluven® impair coagulation less than other colloids? Interact Cardiovasc Thorac Surg. 2011;12:1022–7.
Rajnish KJ, et al. Albumin: an overview of its place in current clinical practice. J Indian An. 2004;53:592–607.

Rasmussen KC, Secher NH, Pedersen T. Effect of perioperative crystalloid or colloid fluid therapy on hemorrhage, coagulation competence, and outcome: a systematic review and stratified meta-analysis. Medicine (Baltimore). 2016;95(31):e4498.

Ravn H, Moeldrup U, Brookes C, et al. Intravenous magnesium reduces infarct size after ischemia/reperfusion injury combined with a thrombogenic lesion in the left anterior descending artery. Arterioscler Thromb Vasc Biol. 1999;19:569–74.

Reed RK, Rubin K. Transcapillary exchange: role and importance of the interstitial fluid pressure and the extracellular matrix. Cardiovasc Res. 2010;87:211–7.

Rehm M. Limited applications for hydroxyethyl starch: background and alternative concepts. Anaesthesist. 2013;62(8):644–55.

Rehm M, Haller M, Orth V, et al. Changes in blood volume and hematocrit during acute preoperative volume loading with 5T albumin or 6% hetastarch solutions in patients before radical hysterectomy. Anesthesiology. 2001;95:849–56.

Rehm M, Zahler S, Lotsc M, et al. Endothelial glycocalyx as an additional barrier determining extravasation of 6% hydroxyethyl starch or 5% albumin solutions in the coronary vascular bed. Anesthesiology. 2004;100:1211–23.

Rehm R, Bruegger D, Christ F, et al. Shedding of the endothelial glycocalyx in patients undergoing major vascular surgery with global and regional ischemia. Circulation. 2007;116:1896–906.

Rehm M, Hulde N, Kammerer T, Meidert AS, et al. State of the art in fluid and volume therapy: a user-friendly staged concept. Anaesthesist. 2017;66(3):153–67.

Reid F, Lobo DN, Williams RN, et al. (Ab)normal saline and physiological Hartmann's solution: a randomized double-blind crossover study. Clin Sci. 2003;104:17–24.

Reuter DA, Felbinger TW, Moerstedt K, et al. Intrathoracic blood volume index measured by thermodilution for preload monitoring after cardiac surgery. J Cardiothorac Vasc Anesth. 2002a;16:191–5.

Reuter DA, Felbinger TW, Kilger E, et al. Optimizing fluid therapy in mechanically ventilated patients after cardiac surgery by on-line monitoring of left ventricular stroke volume variations. Comparison with aortic systolic pressure variations. Br J Anaesth. 2002b;88:124–6.

Reuter DA, Bayerlein J, Goepfert MS, et al. Influence of tidal volume on left ventricular stroke volume variation measured by pulse contour analysis in mechanically ventilated patients. Intensive Care Med. 2003;29:476–80.

Reuter DA, Huang C, Edrich T, et al. Cardiac output monitoring using indicator dilution techniques: basic, limits and perspectives. Anesth Analg. 2010;110:799–811.

Roberts JS, Bratton SL. Colloid volume expanders. Problems, pitfalls and possibilities. Drugs. 1998;55(5):621–30.

Roche AM, James MF, Grocott MP, et al. Coagulation effects of in vitro serial haemodilution with a balanced electrolyte hetastarch solution compared with a saline-based hetastarch solution and lactated Ringer's solution. Anaesthesia. 2002;57:950–5.

Roessler M, Bode K, Bauer M. Fluid resuscitation in hemorrhage. Anaesthesist. 2014;63(10):730–44.

Rubin H, Carlson S, DeMeo M, et al. Randomized, double-blind study of intravenous human albumin in hypoalbuminemic patients receiving total parenteral nutrition. Crit Care Med. 1997;25:249–52.

Russell JA, Navickis RJ, Wilkes MM. Albumin versus crystalloid for pump priming in cardiac surgery: meta-analysis of controlled trials. J Cardiothorac Vasc Anesth. 2004;18:429–37.

Ruttmann TG, James MFM, Lombard EM, et al. Haemodilution-induced enhancement of coagulation is attenuated in vitro by restoring antithrombin III to predilution concentration. Anaesth Intesive Care. 2001;29:489–93.

Ruttmann TG, James MFM, Finlayson J, et al. Effects on coagulation of intravenous crystalloid or colloid in patients undergoing peripheral vascular surgery. Br J Anaesth. 2002;89:226–30.

Sakka SG, Becher L, Kozieras J, et al. Effects of changes in blood pressure and airway pressures on parameters of fluid responsiveness. Eur J Anaesthesiol. 2009;26:322–7.

Sanfelippo MJ, Suberviola PD, Geimer NF. Development of a von Willebrand-like syndrome after prolonged use of hydroxyethyl starch. Am J Clin Pathol. 1987;88:653–5.

Scharbert G, Deusch E, Kress HG, et al. Inhibition of platelet function by hydroxyethyl starch solutions in chronic pain patients undergoing peridural anesthesia. Anesth Analg. 2004;99:823–7.

Schell RM, Applegate RL, Cole DJ. Salt, starch, and water on the brain. J Neurosurg Anesthesiol. 1996;18:179–82.

Schindler AW, Marx G. Evidence-based fluid management in the ICU. Curr Opin Anaesthesiol. 2016;29(2):158–65.

Serpa Neto A, Veelo DP, Peireira VG, et al. Fluid resuscitation with hydroxyethyl starches in patients with sepsis is associated with an increased incidence of acute kidney injury and use of renal replacement therapy: a systematic review and meta-analysis of the literature. J Crit Care. 2014;29(1):185.e1–7.

Shandall A, Lowndes R, Young HL. Colonic anastomotic healing and oxygen tension. Br J Surg. 1985;72:606–9.

Sheridan WG, Lowndes RH, Young HL. Tissue oxygen tension as a predictor of colonic anastomotic healing. Dis Colon Rectum. 1987;30:867–71.

Shires T, Williams J, Borwn F. Acute change in extracellular fluids associated with major surgical procedures. Ann Surg. 1961;154:803–10.

Shoemaker WC, Appel PL, Kram HB, et al. Prospective trial of supranormal values of survivors as therapeutic goals in high-risk surgical patients. Chest. 1988;94:1176–86.

Sirvinskas E, Sneider E, Svagzdiene M, et al. Hypertonic hydroxyethyl starch solution for hypovolaemia correction following heart surgery. Perfusion. 2007;22:121–7.

Smetkin AA, Kirov MY, Kuzkov VV, et al. Single transpulmonary thermodilution and continuous monitoring of central venous oxygen saturation during off-pump coronary surgery. Acta Anaesthesiol Scand. 2009;53:505–14.

Solanke TF, Khwaja MS, Kadomemu EL. Plasma volume studies with four different plasma volume expanders. J Surg Res. 1971;11:140–3.

Stein L, Berand J, Morisette M. Pulmonary edema during volume infusion. Circulation. 1975;52:483–9.

Stögermüller B, Stark J, Willschke H, et al. The effect of hydroxyethylstarch 200 kD on platelet function. Anesth Analg. 2000;91:823–7.

Strauss RG, Pennell BJ, Stump DC. A randomized, blinded trial comparing the hemostatic effects of pentastarch versus hetastarch. Transfusion. 2002;42:27–36.

Study Investigators SAFE, Finfer S, McEvoy S, et al. Impact of albumin compared to saline on organ function and mortality of patients with severe sepsis. Intensive Care Med. 2011;37(1):86–96.

Takil A, Eti Z, Irmak P, et al. Early postoperative respiratory acidosis after large intravascular volume infusion of lactated Ringer's solution during major spine surgery. Anesth Analg. 2002;95:294–8.

Tatara T, Tashiro C. Quantitative analysis of fluid balance during abdominal surgery. Anesth Analg. 2007;104:347–54.

Tian J, Lin X, Guan R, et al. The effects of hydroxyethyl starch on lung capillary permeability in endotoxic rats and possible mechanisms. Anesth Analg. 2004;98:768–74.

Tobias MD, Wambold D, Pilla MA, et al. Differential effects of serial hemodilution with hydroxyethyl starch, albumin, and 0.9% saline on whole blood coagulation. J Clin Anesth. 1998;8:366–71.

Tommasino C, Moore S, Todd MM. Cerebral effects of isovolemic hemodilution with crystalloid or colloid solutions. Crit Care Med. 1988;16:862–8.

Tousignant CP, Walsh F, Mazer CD. The use of transesophageal echocardiography for preload assessment in critically ill patients. Anesth Analg. 2000;90:351–5.

Traumer LD, Brazeal BA, Schmitz M, et al. Pentafraction reduces the lung lymph response after endotoxin administration in the ovine model. Circ Shock. 1992;36:93–6.

Treib J, Baron JF, Grauer MT, et al. An international view of hydroxyethyl starches. Intensive Care Med. 1999;25:258–68.

Van den Berg B, Vink H, Spaan J. The endothelial glycocalyx protects against myocardial edema. Circ Res. 2003;92:592–4.

Van der Linden PJ, De Hert SG, Daper A, et al. 3.5% urea-linked gelatin is as effective as 6% HES 200/0.5 for volume management min cardiac surgery patients. Can J Anaesth. 2004;51:236–41.

Van der Linden PJ, De Hert SG, Deraedt D, et al. Hydroxyethyl starch 130/0.4 versus modified fluid gelatin for volume expansion in cardiac surgery patients: the effects on perioperative bleeding and transfusion needs. Anesth Analg. 2005;101:629–34.

Varadhan KK, Lobo DN. A meta-analysis of randomised controlled trials of intravenous fluid therapy in major elective open abdominal surgery: getting the balance right. Proc Nutr Soc. 2010;69:488–98.

Verheij J, van Lingen A, Raijmakers PGHM, et al. Effect of fluid loading with saline or colloids on pulmonary permeability, oedema and lung injury score after cardiac and major vascular surgery. Br J Anaesth. 2006a;96:21–30.

Verheij J, van Lingen A, Beishuizen A, et al. Cardiac response is greater for colloid than saline fluid loading after cardiac or vascular surgery. Intensive Care Med. 2006b;32:1030–8.

Vermeulen H, Hofland J, Legemate DA, et al. Intravenous fluid restriction after major abdominal surgery: a randomized blinded clinical trial. Trials. 2009;10:50.

Vincent JL, Kellum JA, Shaw A, Mythen MG. Should hydroxyethyl starch solutions be totally banned? Crit Care. 2013;17(5):193.

Vincent JL, Dubois MJ, Navickis RJ, et al. Hypoalbuminemia in acute illness: is there a rationale for intervention? A meta-analysis of cohort studies and controlled trials. Ann Surg. 2003;237:319–34.

Voet D, Voet JG, Pratt CW. Fundamentals of biochemistry. New York: Wiley; 2001.

Vretzakis G, Kleitsaki A, Aretha D, Karanikolas M. Management of intraoperative fluid balance and blood conservation techniques in adult cardiac surgery. Heart Surg Forum. 2011;14:E28–39.

Wade CE, Kramer GC, Grady JJ, Fabian TC, Younes RN. Efficacy of hypertonic 7.5% saline and 6% dextran-70 in treating trauma: a meta-analysis of controlled clinical studies. Surgery. 1997;122:609–16.

Waitzinger J, Bepperling F, Pabst G, et al. Hydroxyethyl starch (HES) [130/0.4], a new HES specification: pharmacokinetics and safety after multiple infusions of 10% solution in healthy volunteers. Drugs R D. 2003;4:149–5.

Watenpaugh DE, Yancy CW, Buckey JC, et al. Role of atrial natriuretic peptide in systemic responses to acute isotonic volume expansion. J Appl Physiol. 1992;73:1218–26.

Wiedermann CJ. Reporting bias in trials of volume resuscitation with hydroxyethyl starch. Wien Klin Wochenschr. 2014;126(7–8):189–94.

Wiesenack C, Prasser C, Keyl C, et al. Assessment of intrathoracic blood volume as an indicator of cardiac preload: single transpulmonary thermodilution technique versus assessment of pressure preload parameters derived from a pulmonary artery catheter. J Cardiothorac Vasc Anesth. 2001;15:584–8.

Wiesenack C, Prasser C, Rodig G, et al. Stroke volume variation as an indicator of fluid responsiveness using pulse contour analysis in mechanically ventilated patients. Anesth Analg. 2003;96:1254–7.

Wiesenack C, Fiegl C, Keyser A, et al. Continuously assessed right ventricular end diastolic volume as a marker of cardiac preload and fluid responsiveness in mechanically ventilated cardiac surgical patients. Crit Care. 2005;9:R226–33.

Wilkes NJ, Woolf R, Mutch M, et al. The effect of balanced versus saline-based hetastarch and crystalloid solutions on acid-base and electrolyte status and gastric mucosal perfusion in elderly surgical patients. Anesth Analg. 2001;93:811–6.

Williams EL, Hildebrand KL, McCormick SA, et al. The effect of intravenous lactated Ringer's solution versus 0.9% sodium chloride solution on serum osmolality in human volunteers. Anesth Analg. 1999;88:999–1003.

Wittkowski U, Spies C, Sander M, et al. Haemodynamic monitoring in the perioperative phase. Available systems, practical application and clinical data. Anaesthesist. 2009;58(764–778):780–66.

Zaloga G, Strikland R, Butterworth J, et al. Calcium attenuates epinephrine's betaadrenergic effects in postoperative surgery patients. Circulation. 1990;81:196–200.

Zander R. Fluid Management. Melsungen: Bibliomed, Medizinische Verlagsgesellschaft mbH; 2009.

Acid-Base Balance and Blood Gas Analysis

16

Felice Eugenio Agrò, Marialuisa Vennari, and Maria Benedetto

Abstract

Cardiac surgery patients may develop alterations of acid-base balance due to cardiac pathology, comorbidities, type and duration of surgery, and CPB. Acid-base status evaluation through ABG is the base for an adequate perioperative treatment. ABG interpretation needs more useful tool than those proposed by Henderson-Hasselbalch approach, such as anion gap, standard base excess, and strong ions difference, in order to identify the underlying acid-base disorders. In this chapter, the physiology and pathophysiology of acid-base balance in cardiac patients and their consequence on perioperative management are described; an overview on ABG interpretation and its relation with diagnostic hypothesis and therapeutic management are presented.

Keywords

The descriptive approach · The semiquantitative approach · The quantitative approach · Relation among fluid · Electrolyte and acid-base balance · Basis of pathophysiology acid-base balance in the postoperative ICU setting of cardiac surgery · Fluid and electrolyte management consequences on acid-base balance · Hyperchloremic acidosis · Dilution acidosis · Metabolizable anions and base excess · Crystalloids and acid-base status · Colloids and acid-base status · Maintaining acid-base balance · Arterial blood gas analysis interpretation · Boston rules · Base excess · Standard base excess · Anion gap · Stewart approach · Metabolic acidosis · Metabolic alkalosis · Respiratory acidosis · Respiratory alkalosis

F. E. Agrò, M.D. (✉) · M. Vennari, M.D. · M. Benedetto, M.D.
Postgraduate School of Anesthesia and Intensive Care, Anesthesia, Intensive Care and Pain Management Department, University School of Medicine Campus Bio-Medico of Rome, Rome, Italy
e-mail: f.agro@unicampus.it; m.vennari@unicampus.it; m.benedetto@unicampus.it

A. Dabbagh et al. (eds.), *Postoperative Critical Care for Adult Cardiac Surgical Patients*, https://doi.org/10.1007/978-3-319-75747-6_16

16.1 Introduction

"The most significant and the most conspicuous property of blood is the extraordinary ability to neutralize large amounts of acids or bases without losing its neutral reaction" (Henderson 1908).

Acid-base balance represents a complex system through which the body maintains a neutral pH (7.38–7.42), in order to prevent protein degradation and alterations of all biochemical reactions, leading to death. Our body has to fight against acidity: there are many acids produced by proteic, glicidic, and lipidic metabolisms; the energetic systems generate 15.000–20.000 mEq of CO_2 per day; a normal diet determines the formation of 50–100 mEq of H^+. Althouh the cospicious production of acids, normally free H^+ plasma concentration is very low (0.00004 mEq/L), and pH homeostasis is guaranteed. The body has three system opposing acids and base concentration blood variation: blood buffer systems, lungs, and kidneys, with different times of action (Agro and Vennari 2013; Kellum and Weber 2009) (Table 16.1).

Blood buffer systems have an immediate action time. They are present in a total amount lower than produced acids (2.400 mEq/L). This difference entails the need for a continuous renovation of buffer systems.

The most important blood buffer is the HCO_3^-/H_2CO_3 system. Its main role is imputable to three factors: it represents the 65% of whole buffer power of our body; it has an ubiquitarious distribution (ISS, ICS, plasma, red cells, bones); it has a pathway of elimination and pathway of renovation (Rose 1995).

Other buffer systems are hemoglobin, plasma proteins, and phosphate systems.

Hemoglobin lies the H^+ (carbaminohemoglobin) formed by the diffusion of CO_2 from plasma into erythrocytes (formation and dissociation of H_2CO_3 for combination with H_2O), while bicarbonate returns in the plasma (Rose 1995).

Other plasma proteins, present as anion, may buffer H^+ excess, exchanging Ca^{2+} with H^+: the aminic group NH_2^- lies H^+, becoming NH_3 and releasing Ca^{2+} (acidosis increases free Ca^{2+}) (Rose 1995). Finally, phosphate ions act as buffer system in similar way as bicarbonate, but they are present in very low concentration in the ECS with respect to bicarbonate, while are very important in maintaining ICS pH (Rose 1995):

$$H_2PO_4^- \leftrightarrow H^+ + HPO_4^{2-} \leftrightarrow N_2HPO_4$$

The kidney and lung eliminate acids or base in excess, permitting a regeneration of blood buffer systems. When the primitive cause of an acid-base alteration is respiratory, a metabolic compensation develops (see Chap. 14): the kidney

Table 16.1 Body compensatory system and time of action

Homeostatic system	Action time
Blood buffer systems	Immediate (fraction of second)
Lung (ventilation regulation)	1–15 min
Kidney (alkaline or acid urine elimination)	Hours–days

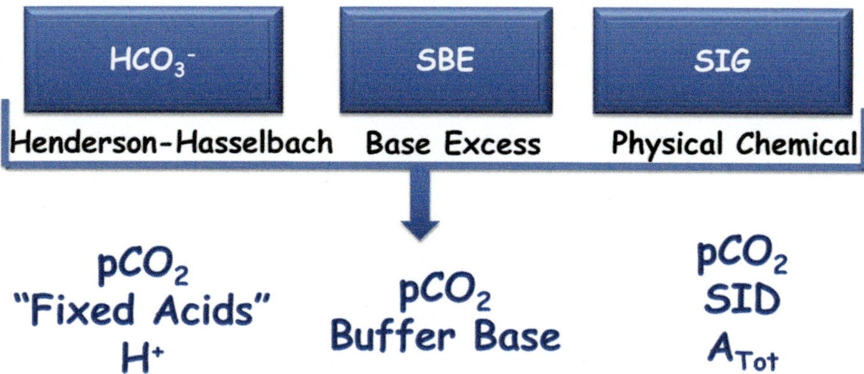

Fig. 16.1 The three possible approaches to acid-base balance system description. Some factors (i.e., p CO_2) are considered by all the approach. Modified from Agro F.E., Vennari M. "Physiology of body fluid compartments and body fluid movements." In "Body Fluid Management—From Physiology to Therapy" Agrò F.E. Springer Milan 2013, pages 1–26

eliminates exceeding H^+ and not volatile acids, regenerating bicarbonate through their production (from amino-acid metabolism) and their increased reabsorption from proximal tubules (acid urine excretion) or increasing bicarbonate elimination and H^+ reabsorption (alkaline urine excretion). When the primitive alteration is metabolic, a respiratory compensation develops (see bicarbonate section): hyperventilation leads to CO_2 elimination when metabolic acidosis occurs, while hypoventilation generates CO_2 retention when metabolic alkalosis develops. The lung acts in some minutes, while the kidney in some hours (8–12 h) (Agro and Vennari 2013; Rose 1995).

There are three approaches to interpreting acid-base balance physiology. They use distinct variables derived from a set of master equations that can be transferred from one approach to the other two (Agro and Vennari 2013; Kellum 2000) (Fig. 16.1).

16.2 The Descriptive Approach

The traditional descriptive approach is based on arterial pH, pCO_2, and bicarbonate measurements. This approach originated at the end of the nineteenth century, when Henderson revisited the law of mass action from an acid-base equilibrium perspective (Agro and Vennari 2013; Kellum 2005a). The result was:

$$\left[H^+\right] = Ka \cdot [HA] / \left[A^-\right]$$

where $[H^+]$ is the hydrogen ion concentration in solution, HA is a weak acid, A^- is a strong base, and Ka is the dissociation constant of the acid. Henderson's equation revealed that when $[HA] = [A^-]$, $[H^+]$ does not change as a result of small variations in the amount of acid or base in the solution (Agro and Vennari 2013).

For the H_2CO_3/HCO_3^- system, the relation is:

$$\left[H^+\right] = Ka \cdot \left[H_2CO_3\right] / \left[HCO_3^-\right]$$

Considering that H_2CO_3 is CO_2 dissolved in water the relation may be rewritten:

$$\left[H^+\right] = Ka \cdot \left[pCO_2\right] / \left[HCO_3^-\right]$$

In 1917, K.A. Hasselbalch applied Henderson's equation to the main physiological buffer system (CO_2/HCO_3^-) using logarithms, giving rise to the Henderson-Hasselbalch equation (Agro and Vennari 2013; Kellum 2005b):

$$pH = pKa + \log\left(\left[HCO_3^-\right] / \left[pCO_2\right]\right)$$

The pCO_2 value describes the respiratory contribution (CO_2 elimination/retention) to acid-base imbalances, while the metabolic contribution (acid overproduction, accumulation, reduced metabolism) is described by the bicarbonate concentration in the blood. When pCO_2 is increased, H^+ production increases and a respiratory acidosis develops, while when pCO_2 is reduced, H^+ production reduces, leading to a respiratory alkalosis. On the other hand when bicarbonate reduces, free H^+ increases and a metabolic acidosis develops, while when bicarbonate increases, free H^+ reduces, causing metabolic alkalosis.

Since the 1940s, researchers have recognized the limitations of this approach to acid-base physiology: blood bicarbonate concentration is useful in determining the type of acid-base abnormality, but it is not able to quantify the amount of acid or base excess-deficit in the plasma, unless pCO_2 is held constant. This observation promoted more researches, in order to quantify the metabolic component (Agro and Vennari 2013; Kellum 2005a).

16.3 The Semiquantitative Approach

In 1957, K.E. Jörgensen and P. Astrup developed a tool to calculate bicarbonate concentration, in which fully oxygenated whole blood was equilibrated with a pCO_2 of 40 mmHg at 37 °C. This measurement was called standard bicarbonate. However, subsequent studies determined the role of the other plasma buffer systems (albumin, hemoglobin, and phosphates), which were not considered either using the bicarbonate concentration or the standard bicarbonate method (Agro and Vennari 2013; Astrup et al. 1960).

In 1948, Singer and Hastings defined the sum of the nonvolatile weak acid the "buffers" and bicarbonates as the "buffer base" (Agro and Vennari 2013; Siggaard-Andersen 1962). This led to several revisions of the method to calculate changes in the buffer base, including the base excess (BE) methodology (Agro and Vennari 2013; Kellum 2005a; Kellum 2005b; Astrup et al. 1960; Siggaard-Andersen 1962; Grogono et al. 1976; Severinghaus 1976).

BE is the quantity of metabolic acidosis or alkalosis, defined as how much base or acid should be added to an in vitro whole blood sample to reach a pH of 7.40, while the pCO_2 is maintained at 40 mmHg. The most widely used formula for calculating BE is the equation of Van Slyke (Agro and Vennari 2013; Kellum 2005a; Siggaard-Andersen 1977; Wooten 1999; Brackett et al. 1965):

$$\text{BE} = \left(\text{HCO}_3^- \text{-}24.4 + [2.3 \times \text{Hb} + 7.7] \times [\text{pH-}7.4]\right) \times (1\text{-}0.023 \times \text{Hb})$$

where HCO_3 and hemoglobin (Hb) are expressed in mmol/L.

Subsequently the standard base excess (SBE) was developed (Siggaard-Andersen and Fogh-Andersen 1995). SBE is the BE corrected for the buffer effect of hemoglobin (assuming a mean extracellular hemoglobin concentration of 50 g/L), and it better quantifies the acid-base status in vivo with respect to BE (Agro and Vennari 2013; Brackett et al. 1965; Prys-Roberts et al. 1966):

$$\text{SBE} = 0.93 \times \left\{\left[\text{HCO}_3^-\right] + 14.84 \times (\text{pH-}7.4)\text{-}24.4\right\}$$

16.4 The Quantitative Approach

Another approach to acid-base pathophysiology is the calculation of the anion gap (AG), which is the difference in the main measured plasma anion and cation concentrations (Astrup et al. 1960; Fanzca 2012):

$$\left[\left(\text{Na}^+ + \text{K}^+\right)\text{-}\left(\text{Cl}^- + \text{HCO}_3^-\right)\right] = 8\text{-}16 \text{ mEq / L.}$$

The AG corresponds to the difference between non-measured anions and cations:

$$\left[\left(\text{Ca}^{2+} + \text{Mg}^{2+}\right) - \left(\text{PO}_4^{3-} + \text{SO}_4^{2-} + \text{organic anions} + \text{proteins}\right)\right].$$

Generally, AG values indicate a variation in the concentration of organic acids (lactic acidosis, ketoacidosis). In fact, when their levels increase, the produced H^+ consumes bicarbonate, reducing AG values, while the organic anions maintain electric neutrality of the plasma (Agro and Vennari 2013). A possible limit of the AG is the wide variability in both plasma albumin concentrations and renal function with respect to phosphate storage, especially in critically ill patients (Agro and Vennari 2013; Kellum 2005a).

In the 1980s, P. Stewart introduced a new approach finalized to identify dependent and independent variable enrolled in H^+ concentration determination (pH) (Agro and Vennari 2013). This approach was based on (Agro and Vennari 2013; Kellum 2005a):

- The law of mass conservation
- The electric neutrality
- Water dissociation constant

Stewart's approach considers three independent variables (Agro and Vennari 2013; Kellum 2005a):

- The strong ion difference (SID)
- Total weak acid concentration (Atot)
- pCO_2

The relationship between SID, pCO_2, and Atot is the only determinant of pH and of $[HCO_3^-]$ that are dependent variables (Morgan 2005).

SID is the difference in the total amount of strong (totally dissociated) anions and cations (Fig. 16.2):

$$\mathrm{SID} = \left(\left[\mathrm{Na}^+\right]+\left[\mathrm{K}^+\right]+\left[\mathrm{Ca}^{2+}\right]+\left[\mathrm{Mg}^{2+}\right]\right)\text{-}\left(\left[\mathrm{Cl}^-\right]+\left[\mathrm{A}^-\right]+\left[\mathrm{SO}_4^{2-}\right]\right)$$

Considering water electric neutrality and water constant dissociation, it is possible to demonstrate two fundamental principles (Mercieri and Mercieri 2006):

- SID is the independent variable influencing H^+ and OH^- concentrations
- SID may vary only adding or reducing strong ions

As a consequence, H^+ or OH^- variations are index of a primary SID modification, and the *primum movens* of acid-base alteration is the variation of strong ion concentration. If strong anions increase with respect to strong cations, SID will be negative and H^+ are increased with respect to OH^-: H^+ concentration is the same of

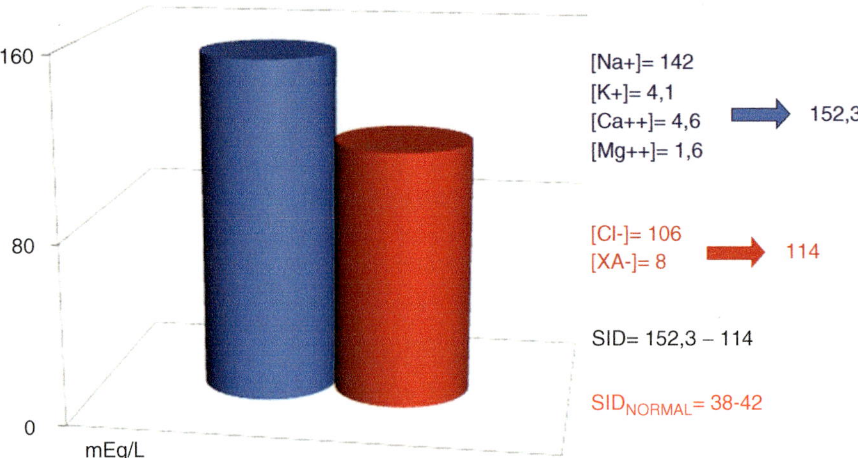

Fig. 16.2 SID representation. SID, Strong ion difference; XA-, dissociated organic acids. Modified from Agro F.E., Vennari M. "Physiology of body fluid compartments and body fluid movements." In "Body Fluid Management—From Physiology to Therapy" Agrò F.E. Springer Milan 2013, pages 1–26

the opposite of SID value (electroneutrality principle), while OH^- are inversely related to the opposite of SID value (Mercieri and Mercieri 2006):

$$[H^+] = -[SID]$$
$$[OH^-] = -K'w / [SID]$$

On the other hand, if strong cations prevail on strong anion, SID is positive. In this case, OH^- are higher than H^+ and OH^- are the same of SID value (electroneutrality principle), while H^+ are inversely related to SID (Mercieri and Mercieri 2006).

$$[OH^-] = [SID]$$
$$[H^+] = K'w / [SID]$$

SID is physiologically positive (38–42 mEq/L). To preserve electric neutrality, it must be balanced by a corresponding excess of negative charges, represented by dissociated weak acid such as HCO_3^-, proteins (especially albumin), phosphate, and minimal concentrations of CO_3^{2-} and OH^-. Generally, proteins, phosphates, and other nonvolatile acids are indicated as A^- (Kellum 2005a; Mercieri and Mercieri 2006; Kellum et al. 1995).

As a consequence (Mercieri and Mercieri 2006):

$$SID = bicarbonate + A^-$$

The SID value obtained with this formula is called effective SID (eSID) vs. the apparent SID (aSID), obtained by the calculus of the sum of strong anions and strong cations. When there is a difference between aSID and eSID, a strong, non-measured anion is present (i.e., lactate, ketoacidosis), and it is causing a consumption of buffer systems (bicarbonate and A^-), with a reduction of eSID (Mercieri and Mercieri 2006).

The difference between aSID and eSID is defined as SID gap (SIG) and is an index for strong anions not measurable (XA^-) (Fencl et al. 2000):

$$SIG = XA^- = aSID\text{-}eSID = 6\text{-}10 \text{ mEq} / L$$

In body fluid compartments, there are varying concentrations of nonvolatile weak acids. In plasma they are represented by inorganic phosphate and albumin. The same applies to ISS, although total concentrations here are very small. In red cells the predominant source is hemoglobin (Morgan 2005).

The undissociated form of weak acids (HA) is neutral; the dissociated form (A^-) is negative. Their concentrations reflect the law of mass conservation:

$$([Atot] = [A^-] + [HA])$$

and the dissociation equilibrium:

$$([H^+] \times [A^-] = Ka \times [HA)].$$

Table 16.2 The six equations of Stewart's approach

Physical and chemical law	Equation
Water constant dissociation	$[H^+] \times [OH^-] = K'w$
Weak acid constant dissociation	$[H^+] \times [A^-] = Ka \times HA$
Mass conservation law	$[HA] + [A^-] = Atot$
Acid carbonic constant dissociation	$\left[H^+\right] \times \left[HCO_3^-\right] = Kc \times pCO_2$
Bicarbonate constant dissociation	$\left[H^+\right] \times \left[CO_3^{2-}\right] = Kc \times \left[HCO_3^-\right]$
Electric neutrality	$SID + \left[H^+\right] - \left[H^+\right] - \left[HCO_3^-\right] - \left[CO_3^{2-}\right] - \left[A^-\right] - \left[OH^-\right] = 0$

As a consequence A^-, HA, and H^+ may vary with pH, but Atot remains the same and is the independent variable influencing other parameters (Mercieri and Mercieri 2006).

When CO_2 is present in water solution, four kinds of molecules originate: dissolved CO_2, H_2CO^3, HCO_3^-, and CO_3^{2-}. Each of these species is involved in chemical reaction in our body resulting in acid-base balance (Mercieri and Mercieri 2006).

Adding CO_2 to a solution (body fluids) containing strong ions and weak acids, Stewart needed six equations to describe acid-base balance modification (Table 16.2).

Knowing the independent variables (pCO_2, SID, Atot), the system may be solved for the remaining unknown variables ($[A^-]$, $[HCO_3^-]$, $[OH^-]$, $[CO_3^{2-}]$, [HA],and [H+]) (Morgan 2005).

Resolving the system for pH ($-\log [H^+]$), a resultant is a simplified equation that may be written as (Mercieri and Mercieri 2006):

$$pH = pK1 + \log\left\{SID + -\left[ATOT / \left(1 + 10p^{Ka-pH}\right)\right]\right\} / pCO_2$$

When $SID = HCO_3^-$ and $Atot = 0$, the equation becomes the same of Henderson-Hasselbalch (Mercieri and Mercieri 2006):

$$pH = pK1 + \log\left[HCO_3^-\right] / pCO_2.$$

16.5 Relation Among Fluid, Electrolyte, and Acid-Base Balance

In Chap. 14 and in the previous paragraphs has been evidenced that body homeostasis is mainly based on three principles (Fig. 16.3):

- The electroneutrality principle (ionic)
- The iso-osomolarity principle (osmolar)
- The neutrality principle (acid-base)

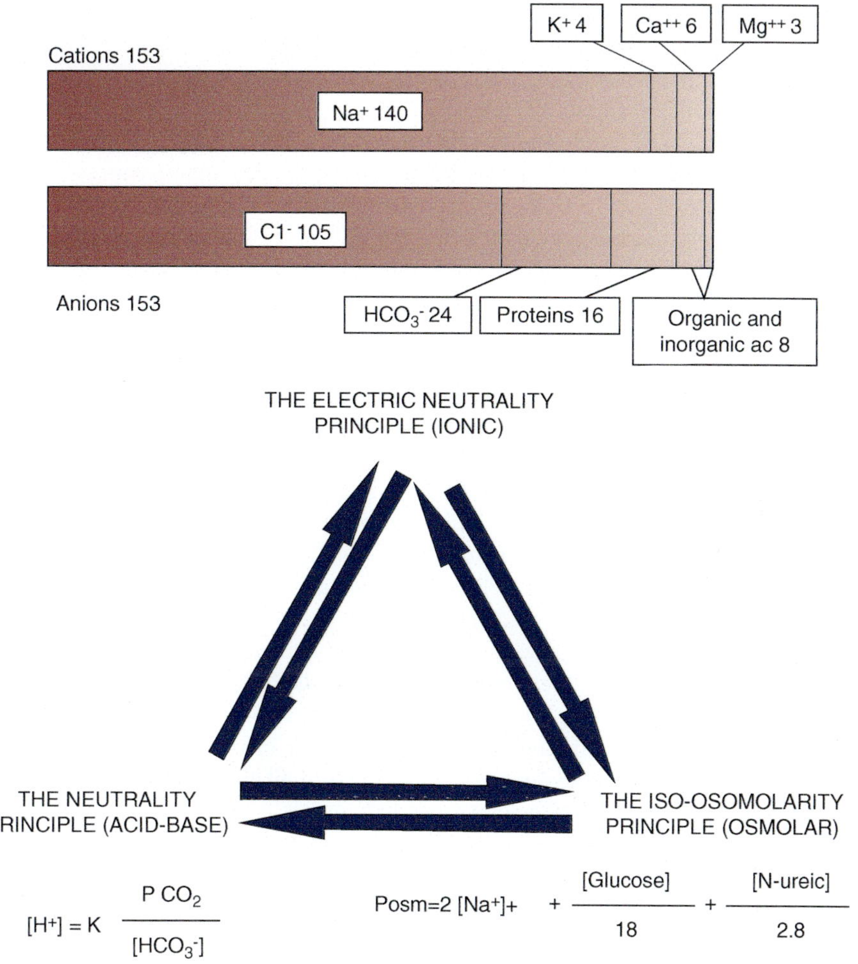

Fig. 16.3 Relation among the ionic, acid-base, and osmolar balances

These three principles are strictly interconnected as is immediately evidenced from Stewart's approach to acid-base balance.

Hydro-electrolytic and acid-base balances are related by bicarbonate: it is present in the Gamble gram and in the Henderson-Hasselbalch equation. Variation of bicarbonate plasma levels may affect the electroneutrality and the neutrality principles. Hydrogen ions are also present in the Gamble ionogram and in the Henderson-Hasselbalch equation.

Osmolar and hydro-electrolytic balances are mainly connected by sodium, present in Gamble gram and osmolarity equation, where sodium concentration is multiplied by two. As a consequence, little sodium variation may have great influences on osmolarity. Generally sodium is contained in the plasma as salts such as $NaHCO_3$ or NaCl. The relation between sodium and anions evidences other interconnections between osmotic, electrolytic, and acid-base balance.

If bicarbonates are reduced, other anions have to increases in order to maintain electric neutrality. Chloride and bicarbonates are strictly related, and their sum must be constant in any moment: if one of them increases, the other reduces and vice versa, in a rate of 1:1. In order to maintain electric neutrality, when both chloride and bicarbonates are reduced, there should be increases of other anions (see Gamble gram and AG) (Sgambato and Prozzo 2003; Vulterini et al. 1992).

Finally, all acid-base interventions, including fluid administration, act through SID (electrolyte, osmolarity) or Atot or in combination (Morgan 2005; Sgambato and Prozzo 2003).

The clinical consequences of the relations between the three systems are presented in some example.

1. In case of diarrhea, bicarbonate will be reduced. With respect to electroneutrality principle, a hypo-bicarbonatemia causes hyperchloremia. It is also responsible for a variation in Henderson-Hasselbalch equation with an increase in hydrogen ion concentration and the development of metabolic acidosis.
2. In case of vomitus, there is a loss of HCl. In order to respect electric neutrality, chloride reduction is replaced by bicarbonate increase. Hydrogen ion loss and rising bicarbonate will determine a metabolic alkalosis (accompanied by hypochloremia). In case of prolonged vomitus, to restore fluid and chloride deficit, fluids are administered. The restoration of chloride levels determines a reduction of bicarbonate and, consequently, a correction of alkalosis.
3. Bicarbonate is present in the plasma as sodium salt. As a consequence, any variation in bicarbonate levels will modify sodium and osmolar balance and vice versa. For example, when bicarbonate ($NaHCO_3$) is administered to correct a severe metabolic acidosis, osmolarity increases potentially developing hypervolemia. Moreover, sodium overload determines a reduction of other cations (K^+ or Ca^{2+}).

16.6 Basis of Pathophysiology of Acid-Base Balance in the Postoperative ICU Setting of Cardiac Surgery

Maintaining acid-base balance during and after cardiac surgery is essential for the success of the surgery, especially for procedure requiring prolonged bypass time. Cardiac surgery patients are at high risk for developing arrhythmias: the presence of a neutral pH is necessary to prevent them and to obtain a response to pharmacological and electric treatments.

Acid-base status is considered as an index of adequate perfusion of tissue (i.e., lactate increase, adequate renal compensation) and may modify blood flux distribution. Moreover pH and pCO_2 variation may influence Hb curve dissociation reducing Hb saturation (acidosis, pCO_2 increases) or reducing Hb capacity to transfer O_2 to tissue (alkalosis, pCO_2 decreases) (Agrò et al. 2013).

Literature demonstrated in experimental and clinical studies the influence of pH on vascular tone resulting in possible blood flux redistribution and blood pressure alteration (Celotto et al. 2008). Both modification of ECS pH (pHe) and ICS pH (pHi) may cause these alterations, through many proposed mechanisms: neurotransmitter release, prostanoids, purines, smooth cells hyperpolarization, NO, and changes in intracellular calcium concentration (Franco-Cereceda et al. 1993; Aalkjaer and Poston 1996; Ishizaka and Kuo 1996). Moreover, acid-base balance alterations have been related to endothelium activity modification, with different effects according to the type of considered vessel (Celotto et al. 2008).

On the other hand, cardiac surgery is responsible for profound alteration in acid-base system. The mechanism at the base of these modifications is different, causing an impact on acid-base balance in opposite directions (Dobell et al. 1960; Beecher and Murphy 1950; Gibbon et al. 1950; Puyau et al. 1962). Some of these mechanisms depend on the type of oxygenator and the type of blood flow during the CPB duration, the kind and the duration of postoperative mechanical ventilation, hypotension and or cardiac acute failure in the perioperative setting (need for inotropes and/or vasoactive drugs, bleeding, ECMO), the kind of fluid used for priming and for liquid management (balanced vs. unbalanced), temperature modifications (hypothermia reduces buffer system dissociation, determining a "natural alkaline shift," while CO_2 becomes more soluble and pCO_2 is decreased), hemolysis, and the need for postoperative ECMO (Fanzca 2012; Ito et al. 1957; Coffin and Ankeney 1960; Litwin et al. 1959; Kirklin et al. 1956).

The more frequent alteration of acid-base equilibrium in cardiac patients is metabolic acidosis (Fanzca 2012). It is thought to be due to pre-existing respiratory alkalosis, increased lactate levels, hypoxia, and hypoperfusion (Dobell et al. 1960; Beecher and Murphy 1950; Gibbon et al. 1950; Puyau et al. 1962; Ito et al. 1957). Acidosis induces systemic vasodilatation (included coronary) and pulmonary vasoconstriction (Fanzca 2012). Although vasodilatation may have positive effect, such as an increase in coronary blood flow, its consequence may be detrimental in patient presenting a cardiac dysfunction after the surgery (Celotto et al. 2008; Clancy and Gonzalez 1975; Ely et al. 1982). Moreover, acidosis reduces the responsiveness to catecholamines, decreasing pharmacological effectiveness of the treatment of postoperative hemodynamic instability and further precipitating patients' conditions. Pulmonary vasoconstriction may increase pulmonary resistance and decompensate the hemodynamic and respiratory status of cardiac surgery patients (Celotto et al. 2008).

A persistent acidosis may indicate an organ damage/failure still latent such as renal or hepatic due to preoperative severe hypoperfusion, a shock eventually combined with pre-existing alterations.

16.7 Fluid and Electrolyte Management Consequences on Acid-Base Balance

The previous chapter evidenced the relation among fluid administration and modification of acid-base status, according to fluid properties. Moreover, Stewart's approach underlined the role of electrolyte in maintaining or modifying acid-base balance. As a consequence, the debate on SID of infused solution has adjunct to literature discussion.

16.7.1 Hyperchloremic Acidosis

When establishing fluid therapy, both acid-base and electrolyte iatrogenic disorders must be avoided. Generally, metabolic acidosis with hyperchloremia is the most frequent induced alteration (Agro and Vennari 2013). Many available solutions do not contain Atot (anions), leading to a dilution of ECS Atot and, consequently, to a metabolic alkalosis. However, this effect is commonly overwhelmed by the increase of the SID with the infusion, contributing to acidosis development (Morgan 2005). Clinical studies have revealed that chloride excess causes a specific splanchnic and renal vasoconstriction, interferes with cellular exchanges, and reduces the glomerular filtration rate (GFR), leading to sodium and water retention (Agro and Vennari 2013; Quilley et al. 1993; Wilcox 1983). Hyperchloremia is generally associated with metabolic acidosis and may cause a further reduction in GFR (Agro and Vennari 2013; Wilcox 1983). It has been shown that balanced and plasma-adapted solutions help to avoid hyperchloremic acidosis while assuring the same volume effect as unbalanced solutions and potentially reducing morbidity and mortality (Agro and Vennari 2013; Zander 2006).

16.7.2 Dilution Acidosis

Currently available solutions used throughout the world do not contain the physiological buffer base bicarbonate because it cannot be incorporated into polyelectrolyte solutions, since carbonate precipitation would occur (Agro and Vennari 2013). For this reason, any fluid infusion may cause "dilution" acidosis, i.e., a dilution of the HCO_3^- concentration, while the CO_2 partial pressure (buffer acid) remains constant (Agro and Vennari 2013; Shires and Holman 1948; Asano et al. 1966). Metabolic acidosis may have catastrophic consequences, especially in patients with pre-existing acidosis (i.e., patient with reduced CI and hypoperfusion) (Agro and Vennari 2013).

16.7.3 SID

In the recent literature, the classic view of dilution acidosis has been reviewed. In fact, according to Stewart approach, bicarbonate is a dependent variable, while the

SID of the infused solutions is the determinant of acid-base effects. When SID of used fluid is zero such as saline solutions with [Cl^-] = [Na^+], dextrose, mannitol, or water, the administration of large volume leads to a reduction (dilution) of SID, causing metabolic acidosis, independently from plasma [Cl^-] variations (Makoff et al. 1970; Miller and Waters 1997; Storey 1999; Figge et al. 1998).

In order to avoid iatrogenic alteration of acid-base balance, an infused solution should reduce SID (acidifying power) in a minimal rate, necessary to counteract the Atot dilution alkalosis. As a consequence, the concept of balanced solution should be extended considering SID and, particularly, the need for a SID lower than plasma, but higher than zero (Morgan 2005). The ideal SID value is 24 mEq/L. It means that 24 mEq/L of the strong anion Cl^- should be replaced by other anions, such as metabolizable anions (Morgan 2005; Morgan et al. 2004).

16.7.4 Metabolizable Anions and Base Excess

Bicarbonate absence was compensated, adjunncting in vitro OH^-, HCO_3^- and CO_3^{2-} as component of i.v. fluids. It was immediately evident that they rapidly equilibrate with CO_2 (Morgan 2005). To overcome this problem, metabolizable anions were used. Metabolizable anions are organic anions that may be converted to HCO_3^- by tissues. The main metabolizable anions are gluconate, malate, lactate, citrate, and acetate. In i.v. fluids, the most frequently used metabolizable ions are acetate, malate, and lactate (Agro and Vennari 2013).

Acetate and malate are contained in plasma in very low concentrations. They may be metabolizable in all tissues, especially in muscles, liver, and heart (Agro and Vennari 2013; Lundquist 1962). Acetate is an early-onset (within 15 min) alkalizing anion, while malate has a slower action (Agro and Vennari 2013; Mudge et al. 1949; Knowles et al. 1974; Akanji et al. 1989).

The most commonly used metabolizable anion is lactate, which is normally produced in the human body. In fact, lactate is the main product of anaerobic glycolysis. It is metabolizable only by the liver (Agro and Vennari 2013). However, the use of lactate has been a cause of debate in clinical practice and in the literature, especially with respect to patients with pre-existing lactic acidosis. This condition is a manifestation of disproportionate tissue lactate formation, with respect to hepatic lactate metabolism (Agro and Vennari 2013; Johnson et al. 1969; Levraut et al. 1998). Lactate levels are major criteria in the routine evaluation of critically ill patients (Beecher and Murphy 1950; Gibbon et al. 1950; Puyau et al. 1962; Ito et al. 1957; Coffin and Ankeney 1960; Litwin et al. 1959; Kirklin et al. 1956; Clancy and Gonzalez 1975; Ely et al. 1982); indeed, changes in lactate concentration can provide an early and objective evaluation of patient responsiveness to therapy (Agro and Vennari 2013; Abramson et al. 1993; Bakker et al. 1996; Cowan et al. 1984; Falk et al. 1985; Friedman et al. 1995; Henning et al. 1982; McNelis et al. 2001; Vincent et al. 1983; Rivers et al. 2001). Furthermore, plasma lactate levels in the first 24–48 h have a high predictive power for mortality in patients with various forms of shock, including cardiac, hemorrhagic, and septic (Agro and Vennari 2013). In these situations, the administration of lactate-containing fluids may exacerbate the already existing lactic acidosis and interfere with lactate monitoring for diagnostic purpose (Agro and Vennari 2013; Levraut et al. 1998; Weil and Afifi 1970). According to these evidences, common sense suggests that in ICU patients, any use of lactate-containing solutions should be avoided (Agro and Vennari 2013).

Another indicator of acidosis is base excess (BE). Since 1990, clinical trials have demonstrated that evaluating BE at the time of admission of critically ill patients is indeed the best prognostic indicator for mortality, complication rate, and transfusion needs (Agro and Vennari 2013). Persistent base excess disorders above or below 4 mmol/L differ with respect to mortality rates: 9% and 50%, respectively (Agro and Vennari 2013; Kincaid et al. 1998).

Balanced, plasma-adapted solutions reduce the risk of acidosis and BE alterations (Agro and Vennari 2013).

16.7.5 Crystalloids and Acid-Base Status

The composition of widely used crystalloids is discussed in Chap. 14 (see Table 14.3).

Normal saline solution is a solution with SID = 0, and literature has extensively demonstrated it causes metabolic acidosis, especially after large amount of infusion during normovolemic hemodilution or for cardiopulmonary bypass (Morgan 2005; Morgan et al. 2004; Scheingraber et al. 1999; McFarlane and Lee 1994; Prough and Bidani 1999; Rehm et al. 2000; Hayhoe et al. 1999; Liskaser et al. 2000; Himpe et al. 2003; Beers 2006). In addition to renal effects (discussed in Chap. 14), metabolic acidosis inhibits cardiac contractility, adrenoceptor function, and coagulation (Fanzca 2012).

Considering a stable and normal plasma lactate concentration of 2 mEq/L, Ringer's lactate and Ringer's acetate SID is 27 mEq/L. As a consequence, they are slight alkalinizing solutions, reducing metabolic acidosis risk, typical of first-generation crystalloids (Morgan 2005; Reid et al. 2003; Traverso et al. 1986; Waters et al. 2001).

Both Ringer solutions are more plasma-adapted than normal saline, but are nonetheless unbalanced.

The latest-generation crystalloids are isotonic, balanced, and plasma-adapted solutions that reduce the risk of chloride excess and dilution acidosis, with a decreased influence on lactate monitoring, lactic acidosis, and base excess (BE). They have a SID higher than zero but lower than plasma (SID ~ 29 mEq/L) and, like Ringer's solutions, have an alkalinizing power (Morgan 2005).

16.7.6 Colloids and Acid-Base Status

As for crystalloids, SID value of each colloid is an important feature to consider before the administration. For colloids the possible effect of their SID is reduced by two factors: the lower amount infused with respect to crystalloids and their possible contribution to Atot (the colloidal molecules may be weak acid) (Finfer et al. 2004; Liskaser and Story 1999). As a consequence, Atot dilution alkalosis is reduced, as long as colloidal molecules persist in the EVS (Morgan 2005). However, after the infusion, weak acid colloids with SID > 0 such albumin and gelatins presented a tendency to induce metabolic acidosis similar to 0.9% saline solution and other colloids with SID = 0 (Morgan 2005).

Currently available HA solutions are prepared as NaCl solutions (SID = 0), which can lead to metabolic acidosis and hyperchloremia and interfere with sodium and water excretion, thus impairing renal function, especially in hypovolemic shock patients. In acute renal failure, HA may accumulate after its massive administration (Morgan 2005).

Succinylated gelatins are dispersed in a 4% polyelectrolyte solution generally containing Na^+ 154 mEq/L, K^+ 0.4 mEq/L, Ca^{2+} 0.4 mEq/L, and Cl^-120 mEq/L (effective SID = 34). Their low chloride content reduces the risk of hyperchloremic acidosis and may be helpful in patients with acid-base alterations.

Recent balanced HES presented SID closer to the ideal value (24 mmEq/L). They have been demonstrated to reduce the risk of iatrogenic metabolic acidosis and potentially improve gastric mucosal blood flow, with a possible impact on endotoxemia survival (Wilkes et al. 2001; Kellum 2002). In a prospective, randomized, double-blind study of cardiac surgery patients, a balanced HES 130/0.4 preparation was compared to an unbalanced HES 130/0.4: while the hemodynamic status did not differ between the two groups, the base excess was significantly less negative in the balanced than in the unbalanced HES group (Base et al. 2011).

16.8 Maintaining Acid-Base Balance

16.8.1 Arterial Blood Gas Analysis Interpretation

The evaluation of seriated arterial blood gases (ABG) analysis appears as indispensable to guide the postoperative management of the cardiac surgery patients and to permit a precocious diagnosis of tissue hypoperfusion and DO_2 modification. In fact, ABG gives direct information about the main determinant of DO_2 (pO_2, SpO_2, and Hb) and indirect information about CI, tissue perfusion and oxygenation (lactic acidosis, hypoxic acidosis). Moreover it allows the identification of ionic, osmolar, and acid-base alterations. In particular acid-base alterations are often cause of matter in clinical practice; they should be unrecognized and have catastrophic impact on patients.

According to acid-base perspective, ABG interpretation may use one of the approaches previously presented (Henderson-Hasselbalch, BE, AG, or Stewart approach) or more of one of them, in order to better understand the contemporary ionic and osmolar alterations and the cause of acid-balance disturbance.

Studying ABG, it is important to taint in account that pH, pCO_2, and pO_2 are measured while HCO_3^- and BE values are calculated.

To evaluate the acid-base state of the patient, the first value to consider is pH.

A pH < 7.38 indicates acidemia; pH > 7.42 indicates alkalemia. According to the presence of buffer and compensatory systems, pH may be normal, but the other parameters may be changed indicating alkalosis or acidosis. This situation is the more frequent in the clinical practice and requires a profound knowing of physiology and of the meaning of the different parameters obtainable with ABG.

In clinical practice, it is useful to only consider pCO_2 and bicarbonate values. This use should be disapproved in order to avoid disagreeable mistake. In fact an increased pCO_2 (> 40 mmHg) may suggest a respiratory acidosis or the compensation for a metabolic alkalosis, while a reduced pCO_2 (< 40 mmHg) may indicate a respiratory alkalosis or the compensation for a metabolic acidosis. At the same time a reduced HCO_3^- (< 24 mEq/L) may suggest a metabolic acidosis or the compensation for a respiratory alkalosis, while an increased HCO_3^- (> 24 mEq/L) may indicate a metabolic alkalosis or the compensation for respiratory acidosis (Fig. 16.4).

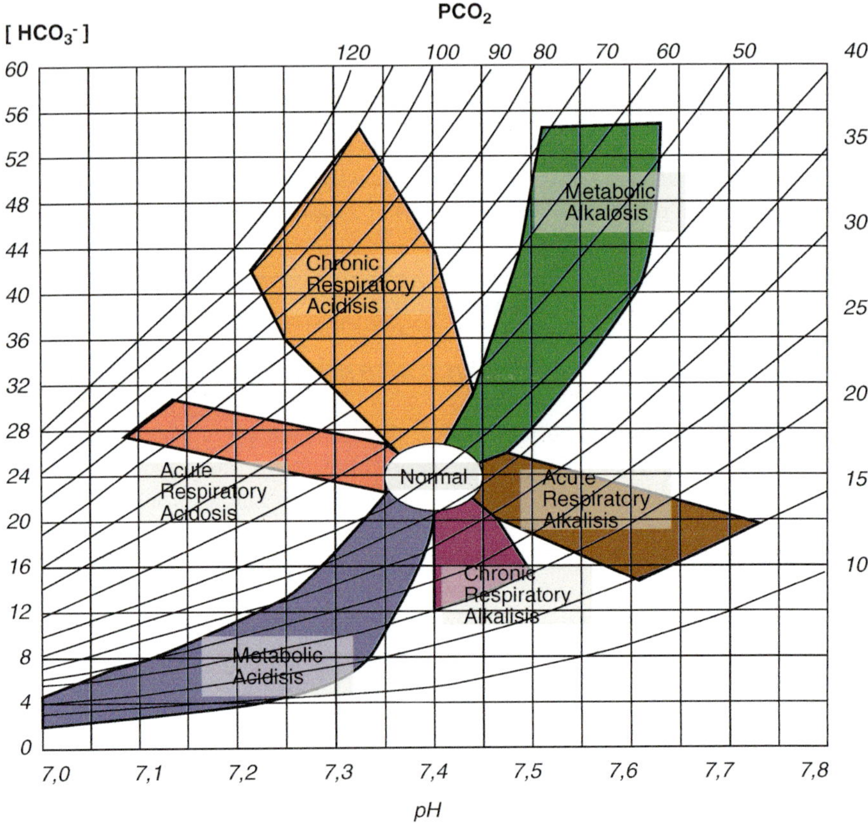

Fig. 16.4 A Graphic tool to rapidly identify acid-base patient disorders knowing pH, $[HCO_3^-]$, and pCO_2

Acid-base disorders of different origins may be contemporarily present (i.e., a metabolic acidosis due to hypoperfusion with a respiratory alkalosis due to hyperventilation). To better understand the number, the nature, and the gravity of the acid-base disturbance, other factors may be considered. The time of development of the observed alteration may be helpful. In fact, if an alteration appeared a few hours ago, it is improbable that bicarbonate variation may represent a renal compensation; it is more probable if it represents an underlying metabolic disturbance.

The evaluation of Boston rules, BE, AG, and SID may be more useful to solve the "ABG enigma."

An eight-step approach to ABG acid-base status interpretation:

1. pH (acidosis or alkalosis?)
2. pCO2 (same or opposite direction with respect to pH?)
3. $HCO3^-$ (same or opposite direction with respect to pH?)
4. Compensation (Boston rules)
5. AG
6. Delta gap (if AG increased)
7. SID-SBE
8. Electrolytes

16.8.2 Boston Rules

Boston rules are mathematical relation between bicarbonate and pCO_2 values, based on the observation of patients with note and compensate (normal pH) acid-base alterations.

In case of metabolic acidosis, pCO_2 should reduce 1.5 mmHg for each 1 mEq/L of HCO_3^- reduction. If pCO_2 is lower with respect to the expected value, there is a contemporary respiratory alkalosis; if it is higher, there is a contemporary respiratory acidosis (Beers 2006).

In case of metabolic alkalosis, pCO_2 should increase 0.7 mmHg for each 1 mEq/L of HCO_3^- increasing. If pCO_2 is lower with respect to the expected value, there is a contemporary respiratory alkalosis; if it is higher, there is a contemporary respiratory acidosis (Beers 2006).

In case of acute respiratory acidosis, HCO_3^- should increase 1 mEq/L for each 10 mmHg of pCO_2 increasing; in case of chronic acidosis, the increase should be 4 mEq/L. If the bicarbonate is lower with respect to the expected value, there has been not enough time for the development of compensation, or there is a contemporary metabolic acidosis, while if it is higher, there is an underlying metabolic alkalosis (Beers 2006).

In case of acute respiratory alkalosis, bicarbonate should reduce 1 mmEq/L for each 10 mmHg of pCO_2 decreasing, while in case of chronic respiratory alkalosis, the reduction should be 5 mmEq/L. If bicarbonate is lower with respect to the expected value, there is a contemporary metabolic acidosis, while if it is higher,

Table 16.3 Bicarbonate and pCO_2 variation according to Boston rules

pH	Disorder	HCO_3	PCO_2	Compensation evaluation	Comment
≤ 7.38 acidosis	Metabolic	≤ 24 mEq/L	↓ 1.5 mmHg for each 1 mEq/L of HCO_3 ↓	pCO_2 value higher	Respiratory acidosis
				pCO_2 value lower	Respiratory alkalosis
	Respiratory	↑ 1 mEq/L (acute), ↑ 4 mEq/L(chronic) for each 10 mmHg of pCO_2 ↑	≥ 40 mmHg	HCO_3 value higher	Metabolic alkalosis
				HCO_3 value lower	No time for compensation or metabolic acidosis
≥ 7.42 alkalosis	Metabolic	≥ 24 mEq/L	↑0.7 mmHg for each 1 mEq/L of HCO_3↑	pCO_2 value higher	Respiratory acidosis
				pCO_2 value lower	Respiratory alkalosis
	Respiratory	↓ 1 mEq/L (acute), ↓ 4 mEq/L(chronic) for each 10 mmHg of pCO_2 ↓	≤ 40 mmHg	HCO_3 value higher	No time for compensation or metabolic alkalosis
				HCO_3 value lower	Metabolic acidosis

there is a contemporary metabolic alkalosis or little time to develop compensation (Beers 2006) (Table 16.3).

16.8.3 Base Excess (BE) and Standard Base Excess (SBE)

A positive BE (> +2) suggests an alkalosis (metabolic), while a negative BE (< −2) suggests an acidosis (metabolic).

SBE is a practical tool to replace SID at bedside (Morgan et al. 2000; Schlichtig et al. 1998a; Schlichtig et al. 1998b). Normally it ranges in −3/+3 mEq/L, and it represents the change in SID value needed to restore acid-base balance. If SBE < −3, there is a metabolic acidosis (SID increased), while if SBE > +3, there is a metabolic alkalosis (Vulterini et al. 1992). In case of acidosis, SBE corresponds to the theoretical $NaHCO_3$ dose (in mmol/L) per liter of ECS water, needed to normalize acid-base balance, while in case of alkalosis, it corresponds to the theoretical dose of HCl (Fanzca 2012).

16.8.4 Anion Gap

An increased AG (> 16 mEq/L) indicates a metabolic acidosis due to the presence of non-measurable acids such as the organic lactate acid (ABG also reports lactate values) or other inorganic acids (i.e., phosphate retention in kidney dysfunctions) (Beers 2006).

A normal AG may indicate a metabolic acidosis due to HCO_3^- reduction (i.e., dilution acidosis, renal loss such as postoperative NTA) or to increased Cl^- (fluid infused, hyperchloremia). According to the electroneutrality principle, the AG remains stable because HCO_3^- variations are compensated by Cl^- and vice versa: metabolic acidosis with normal AG is always hyperchloremic.

In order to complete the evaluation of patient acid-base asset, it is important to consider the rate between the difference of patient AG with respect to the normal AG (AG gap) and the difference of normal bicarbonate with respect to the patient bicarbonate (bicarbonate gap). This ratio is defined as delta gap, and it may suggest the presence of more than one acid-base disturbance (Beers 2006):

$$\begin{aligned}\text{Delta gap} &= (\text{Measured AG} - \text{Normal AG}) / (\text{Normal } HCO_3^- - \text{Measured } HCO_3^-)\\ &= (\text{Measured AG} - 12) / (24 - \text{measured } HCO_3^-)\\ &= \text{D AG} / \text{D } HCO_3^-\end{aligned}$$

If the only alteration is the metabolic acidosis with AG, the delta gap value should be 1, reflecting the buffering of non-measurable acids. If delta gap value is <1, bicarbonate reduction is due to the presence of other acids rather than non-measurable: there is another cause of metabolic acidosis with normal AG and hyperchloremia should be present. When the delta gap value is >1, the reduction of bicarbonate is contrasted by a factor leading their increase: there is a contemporary metabolic acidosis (Beers 2006).

Using AG for ABG interpretation, it is fundamental to establish the plasma levels of proteins (especially albumin), non-measured cation (Ca^{2+} and Mg^{2+}), and measured cation (especially Na^+) levels, the presence of renal dysfunction with possible increased uremia, and the lipidic asset.

In fact, AG may be increased by hyperalbuminemia (rare in ICU patients) and uremia (increased anions) or by hypocalcemia and hypomagnesemia (reduced cations), while it may be reduced by hypoalbuminemia (frequent in ICU post bypass patient) or by hypermagnesemia and hypercalcemia (increased cations). Finally AG may result negative (artifact) in case of severe hypernatremia or hyperlipidemia.

16.8.5 Stewart Approach and SID

According to Stewart approach $([SID]+[H^+]=[HCO_3^-]+[A^-]+[CO_3^{2-}]+[OH^-])$, acid-base alterations are due to modification of independent variables. As a consequence, respiratory unbalance is caused by pCO_2 modification, while metabolic alteration is imputable to SID and/or Atot modification.

SID decreases in metabolic acidosis and increases in metabolic alkalosis (Kellum 2005a; Fanzca 2012). In fact, a reduction of SID value (strong anions > strong cations; SID < 38 mEq/L) leads to H^+ increase in order to maintain electric neutrality. SID reductions may be due to an increase of organic acids such as lactate or ketones, a loss of cations (i.e., diarrhea), an alteration of Cl^- excretion by the kidney (i.e., development of postoperative AKI), Cl^- overload (unbalanced solution use), or intoxication (i.e., salicylates). Another cause of SID reduction in postoperative ICU patients may be phosphate retentions (H^+ will increase to compensate) caused by renal dysfunction, especially in patients with chronic renal diseases (Fanzca 2012; Morgan 2005).

The reduction of SID (H^+ increase) will be compensated by homeostatic alkalinizing reactions:

- Kidney increase Cl^- excretion (strong anions reduce, SID increases, and H^+ reduce)
- Association of weak acid such as phosphate and proteins with formation of HA until 3–4 mEq/L (in severe cases)
- Hyperventilation: pCO_2 decreases of 1.2 mmHg for each 10 mEq/L of SID reduction

On the other hand, an increase of SID value (strong cations > strong anions; SID > 42 mEq/L) causes alkalosis leading to H^+ reduction in order to respect electric neutrality. SID increases may be due to loss of anions (vomitus diuretics) and cation administration (i.e., transfusions, excess of unbalanced i.v. fluids). Generally the more frequent cause is hypochloremia. In cardiac surgery ICU patients, SID increase may be due to hypoalbuminemia leading to reduction of Atot (Fanzca 2012; Morgan 2005).

The increase of SID (H^+ reduction) will be compensated by homeostatic acidifying reactions:

- Kidney retains Cl^- (strong anions increase, SID reduces, and H^+ increases)
- Na^+ shift into cell (strong cations reduce, SID reduces, and H^+ increases)
- Dissociation of weak acid with formation of A^- and H^+
- Hypoventilation: pCO_2 increases of 0.7 mmHg for each 10 mEq/L of SID increase

The value of Atot depends primarily by plasmatic proteins and in minimal part by other weak acids. An increase of its value is caused by an increase in plasma proteins or phosphate levels. The increase of Atot has the same effect of a decrease in SID: it causes metabolic acidosis. By contrast, hypoalbuminemia causes metabolic alkalosis, as a SID increases (Fanzca 2012; Morgan 2005).

In case of respiratory acidosis the increase of H^+ is compensated by an increase of SID (determining H^+ decrease) due to a reduction of Cl^-. In acute cases, the shift of Cl^- in the red cells is the most rapid mechanism of compensation, and Cl^- reduce 1 mEq/L for each increase of 10 mmHg of pCO_2 value. In chronic cases Cl^- is eliminated by kidney and its reduction is 3–4 mEq/L for each 10 mmHg of pCO_2 increase. These modifications are accompanied by HCO_3^- increase (Henderson 1908; Morgan 2005; Brackett et al. 1969).

In case of respiratory alkalosis, the H^+ reduction is compensated by SID reduction (determining H^+ increase) due to a reduced renal excretion of Cl^- and in

Table 16.4 Metabolic disorders according to Stewart approach

Metabolic acidosis	↓SID and ↓SIG RTA, TPN, normal saline, anion exchange resins, diarrhea, and loss of pancreatic secretions	↓SID and ↑SIG Ketoacidosis, lactic acidosis, salicylate, methanol
Metabolic alkalosis	↑ SID Loss of Cl^-: vomitus, gastric drainage, diuretics, posthypercapnia, villous adenoma with diarrhea, mineralocorticoid excess, Cushing, Liddle, Bartter, liquorice Sodium excess: Ringer, TPN, transfusions	↓A_{tot} Hypoalbuminemia (nephrotic syndrome, cirrhosis)

minimal part to lactate production for glycolysis activation in red cells and liver, caused by the movement of the dissociation curve of Hb (Table 16.4).

With respect to other approaches, Stewart evidences the role of renal regulation of Cl^- in maintaining the acid-base homeostasis. As a consequence, it is crucial in postoperative cardiac surgery patients to maintain an adequate renal function and to avoid any factor causing renal dysfunction or precipitating pre-existing alterations (Fanzca 2012; Morgan 2005).

Evidence confirmed the points suggested by Stewart approach demonstrating genetic modification of Cl^- membrane channel, and transporters are enrolled in the development of chronic acid-base alterations (i.e., Bartter syndrome, renal tubular acidosis, Gitelman syndrome) *(Brackett et al.* 1969*; Rodriguez-Soriano* 2000*; Choate et al.* 2003*; Bates et al.* 1997*; Shaer* 2001*).*

16.9 Metabolic Acidosis

Metabolic acidosis is the most frequent acid-base alteration in cardiac surgery patients (and generally in all postsurgical patients) in the ICU setting. It may have many causes that should be contemporary present (Fanzca 2012; Morgan 2005).

Hemodynamic instability (development of mechanical and arrhythmic postoperative complications, hemorrhage, impairment of cardiac function, vasodilatation, and capillary leakage due to postoperative SIRS) may cause tissue hypoperfusion with the manifestation of a lactic acidosis (Fanzca 2012; Morgan 2005; Beers 2006).

Lactic acidosis may be present in patients who develop hepatic damages, especially in patients with chronic hepatic disease in whom the surgery stress may induce liver insufficiency or when a pre-existing or acute cardiac failure may cause a hepatic dysfunction due to stasis (Fanzca 2012; Morgan 2005; Beers 2006).

Another cause may be due to the development of intestinal ischemia, especially in multi-district vasculopathic patients and in long-stay ICU patient (Fanzca 2012; Morgan 2005; Beers 2006).

In diabetic patients, a strict control of glycemia levels may cause ketoacidosis, which should be considered also in patient with anamnesis positive for alcoholism or prolonged fasting.

In ICU patients there often is a hyperchloremic acidosis caused by i.v. fluid infusion, especially when large amounts are needed and unbalanced or plasma-adapted solutions are used (Fanzca 2012; Morgan 2005; Beers 2006).

A severe and prolonged reduction of diuresis and the development of postoperative AKI (especially ATN) may also be cause of metabolic acidosis due to altered Cl^- and bicarbonate excretion and reduced lactate and other nonvolatile acid clearance, especially in patients with pre-existing or precipitating renal dysfunction (Beers 2006).

In complicated, long-stay ICU patients, the need for enteral nutrition, gastric aspiration, and the development of gastrointestinal dysfunction such as diarrhea may be other causes of metabolic acidosis with normal AG (Beers 2006).

As long as a mild metabolic acidosis develops, clinical manifestations are strictly related to the cause. When a severe acidosis appears (pH < 7.2) or a mild acidosis rapidly develops, symptoms such as nausea, vomiting, and malaise may be observed in the awake patients. The clinical characteristic of metabolic acidosis is hyperpnea due to the respiratory compensation; other manifestations are due to lower pH and are caused by acidosis cardiac effects (hypotension, shock, and arrhythmias) and cerebral effects (metal status impairment up to coma) (Beers 2006).

ABG values for metabolic acidosis are showed in Table 16.5.

According to the management of all acid-base alterations, the treatment of metabolic acidosis is to eliminate the underlying cause or causes. As a consequence, an adequate integration between ABG information, patient clinic, patient anamnesis, and therapy in course is fundamental.

The use of i.v. bicarbonate is generally indicated when acidemia (especially severe academia) is developing. Sodium bicarbonate use may be more useful in some cases and even deleterious in others.

When acidemia is the consequence of a loss of bicarbonate or to inorganic acids (AG normal, Cl^- increased, HCO_3^- reduced), the use of i.v. bicarbonate is considered appropriate to restore plasma levels. When acidemia is due to organic non-measurable acids (more frequently lactic acidosis), the use of bicarbonate is controversial: it may be helpful to avoid deleterious consequence of acidity (i.e., protein denaturation), but may cause other deleterious mechanisms (Fanzca 2012; Morgan 2005; Beers 2006).

Table 16.5 Metabolic acidosis: ABG values

Parameter	Variation
pH	≤ 7.38
HCO_3^-	<24 mEq/L
pCO_2	Reduced: 1.5 mmHg for each 1 mEq/L HCO_3^- reduction
BE	< −2 mEq/L
AG	>16 mEq/L: lactic acidosis Normal: hyperchloremic acidosis
Delta gap	<1: Two causes of metabolic acidosis
SID	< 38 mEq/L If SIG > 10 mEq/L: lactic acidosis If SIG < 6 mEq/L: hyperchloremic acidosis
Lactate	>4 mEq/L: lactic acidosis
Electrolyte	Hyperkalemia (H^+/K^+ exchange) or hypokalemia (K^+ depletion)

Bicarbonate reacts with H^+ producing H_2CO_3 and finally CO_2 that is eliminated through the lungs. In patient under mechanical ventilation, clinicians may modify ventilator parameters in order to optimize the clearance of pCO_2. In patients in spontaneous breathing and in those with pulmonary complication (i.e., postoperative pneumonia, pleural effusion in case of cardiac insufficiency, pulmonary edema), to increase VCO_2 may be more difficult even using invasive and noninvasive ventilation. As a consequence pCO_2 retentions with respiratory acidosis may develop aggravating the patient status. The overproduction of CO_2 may aggravate intracellular acidosis because the infused bicarbonate does not pass across the cellular membrane, while the obtained CO_2 freely pass. It reacts with endocellular water finally producing H^+ (Fanzca 2012; Morgan 2005; Beers 2006).

In case of lactic acidosis, if liver metabolism is preserved, lactate is metabolized to bicarbonate. Adding more exogenous bicarbonate may induce metabolic alkalosis responsible for the shift of Hb saturation curve, reducing the releasing of O_2 to tissue. This modification may be deleterious when lactic acidosis is the consequence of a hypoxia of a hypoperfusion, causing organ impairment (first of all cardiac). Bicarbonate may also reduce portal flux and the efficiency of hepatic lactate clearance (Fanzca 2012; Morgan 2005; Beers 2006).

Sodium bicarbonate administration may depress cardiac function worsening the hemodynamic status of postoperative ICU patient, especially when there has just been a cause of cardiac failure.

Considering that with bicarbonate sodium is administered too, the development of hypernatremia and hyperosmolarity is possible, especially when large amounts of sodium bicarbonate are used (Fanzca 2012; Morgan 2005; Beers 2006). Finally the administration of exogenous bicarbonate reduces free ionized Ca^{2+} and K^+ levels that may be deleterious in patients with hypokalemic acidosis (generally due to renal loss of salts) (Fanzca 2012; Morgan 2005; Beers 2006).

In a mechanically ventilated patient, hyperventilation may be used without bicarbonate administration in order to compensate metabolic acidosis. The consequence is the induction of a respiratory alkalosis that may reduce the hepatic clearance of lactate with a reduction of portal flux, potentially generating liver hypoxia and increase of lactate production (Fanzca 2012; Morgan 2005; Beers 2006).

In case of postoperative AKI, the use of CRRT should be precociously considered (Fanzca 2012; Morgan 2005; Beers 2006).

In any case bicarbonate is generally used when $pH < 7.2$, bicarbonate is <12 mEq/L, and hyperkalemia develops with difficulties to control its value with other treatments, when acidosis is symptomatic, or when the patient is waiting for CRRT (Fanzca 2012; Morgan 2005; Beers 2006).

Sodium bicarbonate amount (bicarbonate deficit) may be calculated according to bicarbonate value (Beers 2006):

$$\mathrm{HCO_3^-\ deficit} = 0.4\,\mathrm{body\ weight} \times \left(\mathrm{goal\ HCO_3^-} - \mathrm{measured\ HCO_3^-}\right)$$

or BE (Beers 2006):

$$\mathrm{HCO_3^-\ deficit} = \mathrm{BE}\left(\mathrm{mEq/L}\right) \times \mathrm{body\ weight}/4.$$

16.10 Metabolic Alkalosis

Metabolic alkalosis is less frequent with respect to metabolic acidosis in cardiac surgery patients. Generally it is due to a predominance of bicarbonate levels caused by retention, acid loss (renal and gastrointestinal), intracellular H^+ shift, and/or alkali administration (Beers 2006).

In ICU setting, metabolic alkalosis is generally caused by acid losses and may be due to secondary hyperaldosteronism caused by hypovolemia, heart failure, renal artery stenosis (polivasculopathic patients), cirrhosis (patients with hepatic diseases), or renal impairment; HCl and KCl losses due to PONV (especially when high doses of opioid are needed); or gastric suction. Hypokalemia and hypomagnesemia are other causes of metabolic alkalosis because K^+ and Mg^+ renal reabsorption is realized through H^+ exchange (Fanzca 2012; Morgan 2005; Beers 2006). However, the most frequent cause of metabolic alkalosis in postoperative ICU patients is the use of diuretics (especially furosemide in continuous infusion). Furosemide may lead to metabolic alkalosis through different mechanisms: hyperaldosteronism due to hypovolemia, Cl^- losses, and hypokalemia (Fanzca 2012; Morgan 2005; Beers 2006).

Other causes of metabolic alkalosis are due to bicarbonate retention overload, such as post-hypercapnic persistent elevation of bicarbonate, generally associated with K^+, Cl^-, and volume depletion; lactate or ketoacidosis conversion to bicarbonate (augmented after bicarbonate administration for acidosis); and $NaHCO_3$ loading (Fanzca 2012; Morgan 2005; Beers 2006).

A cause of metabolic alkalosis may be the administration of some kind of antibiotics such as carbapenicillin, penicillin, and ticarcillin. It should be considered in ICU patient with a prolonged therapy with them (generally complicated, long-stay patients) or with a recent story of protracted use of them (Fanzca 2012; Morgan 2005; Beers 2006).

When a metabolic alkalosis persists during the time, it indicates an increased renal reabsorption of bicarbonates. The more frequent stimuli for bicarbonate reabsorption are hypovolemia (GFR reduction) and hypokalemia. In fact, in case of hypovolemia, the kidney increases Na^+ (and water) reabsorption to restore IVS volume. Sodium is reabsorbed as NaCl or $NaHCO_3$. Maintaining IVS volume is more vital than correct alkalemia, and as a consequence $NaHCO_3$ will be reabsorbed till IVS volume is restored. This mechanism is present only if hypovolemia is caused by acid fluid losses (vomitus, gastric suction, diuretics). Hypokalemia leads to a shift of H^+ from ECS to ICS, with stimulus (intracellular acidosis) to H^+ secretion and HCO_3 reabsorption in tubular cells. Frequently two or more causes of metabolic alkalosis may coexist: for example, the use of diuretic may cause hypovolemia and hypokalemia (Fanzca 2012; Morgan 2005; Beers 2006; Narins and Gardner 1981; Adrogue and Madias 1998; Worthley 2003).

As long as a mild metabolic alkalosis is present the main clinical features are related to the underlying cause. Severe alkalosis causes the increase of Ca^{2+} binding to proteins, leading to hypocalcemia with neuromuscular excitability, lethargy to coma, delirium, seizures, and tetanus. Alkalemia reduces the thresholds for arrhythmias and angina development (Fanzca 2012; Morgan 2005; Beers 2006).

ABG values for metabolic alkalosis are showed in Table 16.6.

In some case the Cl^- urinary concentration may be used to distinguish metabolic alkalosis Cl^- responsive and not Cl^- responsive (Beers 2006):

Urinary $Cl^- < 15$ mEq/L metabolic alkalosis Cl^- responsive:

- Vomitus, gastric suction
- Diuretics
- Posthypercapic

Urinary $Cl^- > 20$ mEq/L metabolic alkalosis not Cl^- responsive:

- Hyperaldosteronism
- Hypokalemia

The treatment of metabolic alkalosis depends on the cause. Metabolic alkalosis involving Cl^- losses responds to administration of fluid containing NaCl. Generally 0.9% saline solution is used. In order to avoid other electrolytic disorders, the infusion of a balanced solution may be suggested. It is recommendable to start the infusion at a rate of 50–100 mL/h and to subsequently increase the rate, according to the estimated and measured losses (Fanzca 2012; Morgan 2005; Beers 2006).

When metabolic alkalosis is not Cl^-responsive, the correction of K^+ and Mg^{2+} levels is needed. According to Stewart approach K^+ deficit should be replaced using KCl. In fact in case of hypokalemia the deficit is manly in the ICS: the administered

Table 16.6 Metabolic alkalosis: ABG values

Parameter	Variation
PH	≥ 7.42
HCO_3^-	> 24 mEq/L
pCO_2	– Increased: 0.7 mmHg for each 1 mEq/L of HCO_3^- increasing
BE	> +2 mEq/L
AG	Normal
Delta gap	>1 contemporary metabolic acidosis and metabolic alkalosis
SID	>42 mEq/L
Lactate	Normal
Electrolyte	Hypokalemia, hypomagnesemia, hypocalcemia, hypochloremia

K^+ moves into cells, while Cl^- remains in ECS reducing SID (and SBE), with an acidifying effect (Fanzca 2012; Morgan 2005; Beers 2006).

The correction of volume, Cl^-, and/or K^+ depletion leads to K^+/H^+ exchange, restoring H^+ plasma levels and reducing Na^+ (and consequently HCO_3^-) reabsorption.

Patient with post-hypercapnic alkalosis or furosemide-induced alkalosis may be treated with acetazolamide that increases HCO_3^- kidney excretion, with caution to PO_4^- and K^+ kidney losses. Acetazolamide is also useful in case of secondary hyperaldosteronism, in which metabolic alkalosis is related to volume overload (Fanzca 2012; Morgan 2005; Beers 2006).

In case of severe alkalosis (pH > 7.5), a rapid correction is needed. In this case HCl use may be indicated. HCl 0.1–0.2 normal may be safe to use through a central line. The dose may be calculated as:

$$\begin{aligned} HCO_3^- \text{ excess} &= 0.4 \text{ body weight}\left(\text{measured } HCO_3^- - \text{goal } HCO_3^-\right) \\ &= 0.4 \text{ body weight}\left(\text{measured } HCO_3^- - 24\right). \end{aligned}$$

An infusion rate of 0.1–0.2 mmol/Kg/h is recommended with frequent ABG sample needed.

CRRT may be indicated in severe case, especially if a contemporary fluid overload is present (Fanzca 2012; Morgan 2005; Beers 2006).

16.11 Respiratory Acidosis

Respiratory acidosis is due to CO_2 accumulation caused by a reduced elimination or an increased production.

A reduction in CO_2 elimination is caused by hypoventilation. Frequent cause of hypoventilation in cardiac surgery in the ICU settings may be caused by sedation effects (during weaning from MV and in the immediate post-extubation period), neuromuscular blocker effects (fast-track protocols or long-stay patients with protracted curarization), postoperative pain, and the development complications such as cerebral complications or abdominal complications (ascites, abdominal distension), cardiac failure with pulmonary edema and/or pleural effusion, pneumothorax (postcentral line positioning or MV related), pneumonia (VAP), and atelectasis. Other cause of hypoventilation may be due to patient's comorbidity such as COPD, OSAS, and restrictive pulmonary diseases. These diseases may cause chronic acidosis that may be associated to acute causes (Fanzca 2012; Morgan 2005; Beers 2006).

Frequent causes of CO_2 overproduction may be hypovolemia, sepsis, and an inadequate artificial nutrition (long-stay patient) with an excess of calories. On the other hand, malnutrition may cause muscular weakness (Fanzca 2012; Morgan 2005; Beers 2006).

Finally it is fundamental to remember the detrimental effect of a prolonged MV on respiratory muscles and its effects during MV weaning attempts and the role of

Table 16.7 Respiratory acidosis: ABG values

Parameter	Variation
PH	≤ 7.38
HCO_3^-	> 24 mm Eq/L Acute acidosis 1 mEq/L for each 10 mmHg of CO_2 increasing Chronic acidosis 4 mEq/L for each 10 mmHg of CO_2 increasing
pCO_2	>45 mmHg
AG	Normal
SID	Normal
Lactate	Normal
Electrolyte	Hyperkalemia (H^+/K^+ exchange)

oxygen administration resulting in hyperoxemia and subsequent hypoventilation (Fanzca 2012; Morgan 2005; Beers 2006).

Clinical presentation of respiratory acidosis depends on the gravity of the disturbance and the time of development. Typical manifestations of rapid and mild-severe acidosis are cerebral, and they include headache, anxiety, confusion, lethargy, and coma. Mild or chronic acidosis is generally better tolerated and may be associated with sleep alterations, daytime sleepiness, and tremors. Other symptoms may be those of hypoxemia that frequently accompanies hypercapnia. Patients may also present dyspnea, bradipnea, and use of accessory respiratory muscles. Many clinical manifestations of respiratory acidosis are not observable in the sedated patient. Respiratory acidosis is associated with hyperkalemia potentially leading to arrhythmias (Fanzca 2012; Morgan 2005; Beers 2006).

ABG values for respiratory acidosis are showed in Table 16.7.

In order to better understand the underlying cause of a respiratory acidosis, it should be useful to calculate the alveolar-artery (A-a) O_2 gradient:

$$\text{A-a gradient} = \text{FiO}_2 - \left(\text{paO}_2 + 5/4\ \text{paCO}_2\right) = 10\ \text{mmHg}$$

A normal gradient indicates an extrapulmonary cause, while an increased gradient indicates a pulmonary alteration (Beers 2006).

Treatment is based on the management of the underlying cause and the increase of alveolar ventilation. In particular, in the case of a chronic acidosis, it is needed to remove or reduce precipitating factors such sedative or analgesic drugs, the adequate use of PS ventilation and PEEP for alveolar recruitment before the extubation, a praecox respiratory gymnastic, and the preventive use of NIV. In patients who develop hypercapnia after extubation (with negative anamnesis), it is needed to immediately search for the cause and when necessary using NIV before TI. The goal is the achievement of a normal pCO_2, excepted for patient with chronic acidosis in which the goal is the hypercapnic status before decompensation. Moreover, in these cases, clinicians should avoid a too-rapid pCO_2 reduction resulting in a post-hyperkapnic alkalosis (the kidney is slower than the lung) and in a rapid variation of cerebral pH that may cause seizures and death (Beers 2006).

16.12 Respiratory Alkalosis

Respiratory alkalosis is caused by an increase of alveolar ventilation. Many stimuli may lead to hyperventilation as a physiologic response: hypoxemia, hypotension, severe anemia, and metabolic acidosis. These causes are often present in the cardiac surgery patient in the ICU setting, especially in complicated cases (Fanzca 2012; Morgan 2005; Beers 2006).

Other causes leading to respiratory alkalosis are fever and sepsis, pain (insufficient analgesic administration), anxiety and agitation (postoperative delirium, central complication), COPD, and pulmonary embolism (Fanzca 2012; Morgan 2005; Beers 2006).

Finally the most frequent cause of respiratory alkalosis in the ICU patients is iatrogenic: mechanical ventilation. It may be the cause of pseudorespiratory alkalosis: in cases of hypoperfusion-hypoxemia, the underlying metabolic acidosis is masked by a CO_2 elimination over the normal rate and due to the mechanical control of alveolar ventilation. This alteration may be detected studying the arterial-venous difference in pCO_2, pH, and the other ABG markers of metabolic acidosis such as AG and SID (Fanzca 2012; Morgan 2005; Beers 2006).

Clinical manifestations of respiratory alkalosis are related to the rapidity of development and to the gravity of hypocapnia. Tachypnea and dyspnea are often the only presentation. Other signs and symptoms are mainly cerebral and are due to the change in central cerebral flux and pH: diziness, paresthesias, cramps, and syncope.

ABG values for respiratory alkalosis are showed in Table 16.8.

Respiratory alkalosis is not life-threatening, and as a consequence, no intervention is required to directly correct the pH. Treatment is based on the management of the underlying cause. For this reason, it is important to recognize the potentially severe causes, such as pulmonary embolism, and their immediate management. In ICU setting where patients are in VM, the first-line treatment is to reduce ventilation, excluding other possible causes of respiratory alkalosis (Fanzca 2012; Morgan 2005; Beers 2006).

Table 16.8 Respiratory alkalosis: ABG values

Parameter	Variation
PH	≥ 7.42
HCO_3^-	< 24 mEq/L Acute alkalosis 1 mmEq/L for each 10 mmHg of CO_2 decreasing Chronic alkalosis 4 mmEq/L. for each 10 mmHg of CO_2 decreasing
pCO_2	< 35 mmHg
AG	Normal
SID	Normal
Lactate	Normal
Electrolyte	Hypokalemia and hypophosphatemia (K+ and PO_4^- intracellular shift), hypocalcemia (increased protein binding), hyperchloremia (to compensate HCO_3^- reduction)

Conclusion

Critical care practitioners should consider the acid-base status of a patient before any therapeutic maneuver, especially in choosing the i.v. fluid to administer.

Literature discussed about the need for balanced pH solutions, especially in cardiac surgery patients. Although it is necessary to avoid solutions with very low or very high pH (especially for rapid infusion), the administration of solutions with different pH may have the same effect on the basis of their electrolytic composition, according to their SID (Fanzca 2012).

Older generation of i.v. fluids has a SID = 0 and reduced plasma SID, resulting in metabolic acidosis, while modern fluids present a SID higher than zero, but lower than plasma (26–29 mEq/L), resulting in a mild alkalinizing effect. In the recent literature the need for solution with a balanced SID (ideal value +24) has been evidenced, although no commercially available solutions present the ideal SID value (Morgan 2005).

In a modern view, a balanced, plasma-adapted solution should have a qualitative and quantitative composition closer than plasma and contain metabolizable anions in order to have a SID closer as possible to +24 mEq/L.

References

Aalkjaer C, Poston L. Effects of pH on vascular tension: which are the important mechanisms? J Vasc Res. 1996;33:347–59.

Abramson D, Scalea TM, Hitchcock R, et al. Lactate clearance and survival following injury. J Trauma. 1993;35:584–9.

Adrogue HJ, Madias NE. Medical progress: management of life-threatening acid-base disorders—second of two parts. Engl J Med. 1998;338:107–11.

Agro FE, Vennari M. Physiology of body fluid compartments and body fluid movements. In: Agrò FE, editor. Body fluid management—from physiology to therapy. 1st ed. Milan: Springer; 2013.

Agrò FE, Fries D, Vennari M. Cardiac surgery. In: Agrò FE, editor. Body fluid management—from physiology to therapy. 1st ed. Milan: Springer; 2013.

Akanji AO, Bruce MA, Frayn KN. Effect of acetate infusion on energy expenditure and substrate oxidation rates in non-diabetic and diabetic subjects. Eur J Clin Nutr. 1989;43:107–15.

Asano S, Kato E, Yamauchi M, et al. The mechanism of the acidosis caused by infusion of saline solution. Lancet. 1966;1:1245–6.

Astrup P, Jorgensen K, Siggaard-Andersen O. Acid-base metabolism: new approach. Lancet. 1960;1:1035–9.

Bakker J, Gris P, Coffermils M, et al. Serial blood lactate levels can predict the development of multiple organ failure following septic shock. Am J Surg. 1996;224:97–102.

Base EM, Standl T, Lassnigg A, et al. Efficacy and safety of hydroxyethyl starch 6% 130/0.4 in a balanced electrolyte solution (Volulyte) during cardiac surgery. J Cardiothorac Vasc Anesth. 2011;25(3):407–14.

Bates CM, Baum M, Quigley R. Cystic fibrosis presenting with hypokalemia and metabolic alkalosis in a previously healthy adolescent. J Am Soc Nephrol. 1997;8:352–5.

Beecher HK, Murphy AJ. Acidosis during thoracic surgery. J Thorac Surg. 1950;19:50.

Beers MH. Acid-base regulation and disorders. In: Beers MH, editor. The Merck manual XVIII. Readington, NJ: Whitehouse Station; 2006.

Brackett NC, Cohen JJ, Schwartz WB. Carbon dioxide titration curve of normal man. N Engl J Med. 1965;272:6–12.
Brackett NCJ, Cohen JJ, Schwartz WB. Carbon dioxide titration curve of normal man. N Engl J Med. 1969;272:6–12.
Celotto AC, Capellini VK, Baldo CF, et al. Effects of acid-base imbalance on vascular reactivity. Braz J Med Biol Res. 2008;41(6):439–45.
Choate KA, Kahle KT, Wilson FH, et al. WNK1, a kinase mutated in inherited hypertension with hyperkalemia, localized to diverse Cl transporting epithelia. Proc Natl Acad Sci U S A. 2003;100:663–8.
Clancy RL, Gonzalez NC. Effect of respiratory and metabolic acidosis on coronary vascular resistance. Proc Soc Exp Biol Med. 1975;148:307–11.
Coffin LH, Ankeney JL. The effect of extracorporeal circulation upon acid-base equilibrium in dogs. Arch Surg. 1960;80:447.
Cowan BN, Burns HJ, Boyle P, et al. The relative prognostic value of lactate and haemodynamic measurements in early shock. Anaesthesia. 1984;39:750–5.
Dobell ARC, Gutelius JR, Murphy DR. Acidosis following respiratory alkalosis in thoracic operations with and without heart lung bypass. J Thorac Surg. 1960;39:312.
Ely SW, Sawyer DC, Scott JB. Local vasoactivity of oxygen and carbon dioxide in the right coronary circulation of the dog and pig. J Physiol. 1982;332:427–39.
Falk JL, Rachow EC, Leavy J, et al. Delayed lactate clearance in patients surviving circulatory shock. Acute Care. 1985;11:212–5.
Fanzca RY. Perioperative fluid and electrolyte management in cardiac surgery: a review. J Extra Corpor Technol. 2012;44:20–6.
Fencl V, Jabor A, Kazda A, et al. Diagnosis of metabolic acid-base disturbances in critically ill patients. Am J Respir Crit Care Med. 2000;162:2246–51.
Figge J, Jabor A, Kazda A, et al. Anion gap and hypoalbuminemia. Crit Care Med. 1998;26:1807–10.
Finfer S, Bellomo R, Boyce N, et al. A comparison of albumin and saline for fluid resuscitation in the intensive care unit. N Engl J Med. 2004;350:2247–56.
Franco-Cereceda A, Kallner G, Lundberg JM. Capsazepine sensitive release of calcitonin gene-related peptide from Cfibre afferents in the guinea-pig heart by low pH and lactic acid. Eur J Pharmacol. 1993;238:311–6.
Friedman C, Berlot G, Kahn RJ, et al. Combined measurement of blood lactate concentrations and gastric intramucosal pH in patients with severe sepsis. Crit Care Med. 1995;23:1184–93.
Gibbon JH, Allbritten FP, Stayman JW, Judd JM. A clinical study of respiratory exchange during prolonged operations with an open thorax. Ann Surg. 1950;132:611.
Grogono AW, Byles PH, Hawke W. An in vivo representation of acid-base balance. Lancet. 1976;1:499–500.
Hayhoe M, Bellomo R, Lin G, et al. The aetiology and pathogenesis of cardiopulmonary bypass-associated metabolic acidosis using polygeline pump prime. Intensive Care Med. 1999;25:680–5.
Henderson LJ. The theory of neutrality regulation in the animal organism. Am J Phys. 1908;21:427.
Henning RJ, Weil MH, Weiner F. Blood lactate as a prognostic indicator of survival in patients with acute myocardial infarction. Circ Shock. 1982;9:307–15.
Himpe D, Neels H, De Hert S, et al. Adding lactate to the prime solution during hypothermic cardiopulmonary bypass: a quantitative acid–base analysis. Br J Anaesth. 2003;90:440–5.
Ishizaka H, Kuo L. Acidosis-induced coronary arteriolar dilation is mediated by ATPsensitive potassium channels in vascular smooth muscle. Circ Res. 1996;78:50–7.
Ito I, Faulkner WR, Kolff WJ. Metabolic acidosis and its correction in patients undergoing open heart operation; experimental basis and clinical results. Cleve Clin Q. 1957;24:193.
Johnson V, Bielanski E, Eiseman B. Lactate metabolism during marginal liver perfusion. Arch Surg. 1969;99:75–9.
Kellum JA. Determinants of blood pH in health and disease. Crit Care. 2000;4:6–14.
Kellum JA. Fluid resuscitation and hyperchloremic acidosis in experimental sepsis: improved short-term survival and acidbase balance with Hextend compared with saline. Crit Care Med. 2002;30:300–5.

Kellum JA. Clinical review: reunification of acid–base physiology. Crit Care. 2005a;9:500–7.

Kellum JA. Making strong ion difference the euro for bedside acid-base analysis. Intensive Care Emerg Med. 2005b;14:675–85.

Kellum JA, Weber PAW. Stewart's textbook of acid-base. 2nd ed. London: Lulu Enterprises; 2009.

Kellum JA, Kramer DJ, Pinsky MR. Strong ion gap: a methodology for exploring unexplained anions. J Crit Care. 1995;10:51–5.

Kincaid EH, Miller PR, Meredith JW, et al. Elevated arterial base deficit in trauma patients: a marker of impaired oxygen utilisation. J Am Coll Surg. 1998;187:384–92.

Kirklin JW, Donald DE, Harshbarger HG, et al. Studies in extra- corporeal circulation: applicability of gibbon type pump-oxygenator to human intracardiac surgery-forty cases. Ann Surg. 1956;144:2.

Knowles SE, Jarrett IG, Filsell OH, et al. Production and utilization of acetate in mammals. Biochem J. 1974;142:401–11.

Levraut J, Ciebiera JP, Chave S, et al. Mild hyperlactatemia in stable septic patients is due to impaired lactate clearance rather than overproduction. Am J Respir Crit Care Med. 1998;157: 1021–6.

Liskaser F, Story DA. The acid–base physiology of colloid solutions. Curr Opin Crit Care. 1999;5:440–2.

Liskaser FJ, Bellomo R, Hayhoe M, et al. Role of pump prime in the etiology and pathogenesis of cardiopulmonary bypass-associated acidosis. Anesthesiology. 2000;93:1170–3.

Litwin MS, Panico FG, Rubini C, et al. Lacticacidemia in extracorporeal circulation. Ann Surg. 1959;149:188.

Lundquist F. Production and utilization of free acetate in man. Nature. 1962;193:579–80.

Makoff DL, da Silva JA, Rosenbaum BJ, et al. Hypertonic expansion: acid-base and electrolyte changes. Am J Phys. 1970;218:1201–7.

McFarlane C, Lee A. A comparison of Plasmalyte 148 and 0.9% saline for intraoperative fluid replacement. Anaesthesia. 1994;49:779–81.

McNelis J, Marini CP, Jurkiewicz A, et al. Prolonged lactate clearance is associated with increased mortality in the surgical intensive care unit. Am J Surg. 2001;182:481–5.

Mercieri A, Mercieri M. L'approccio quantitativo di Stewart all'equilibrio acido-base. G Ital Nefrol. 2006;3:280–90.

Miller LR, Waters JH. Mechanism of hyperchloremic nonunion gap acidosis. Anesthesiology. 1997;87:1009–10.

Morgan TJ. Clinical review: the meaning of acid–base abnormalities in the intensive care unit—effects of fluid administration. Crit Care. 2005;9:204–11.

Morgan TJ, Clark C, Endre ZH. The accuracy of base excess: an in vitro evaluation of the van Slyke equation. Crit Care Med. 2000;28:2932–6.

Morgan TJ, Venkatesh B, Hall J. Crystalloid strong ion difference determines metabolic acid-base change during acute normovolemic hemodilution. Intensive Care Med. 2004;30:1432–7.

Mudge GH, Manning JA, Gilman A. Sodium acetate as a source of fixed base. Proc Soc Exp Biol Med. 1949;71:136–8.

Narins RG, Gardner LB. Simple acid-base disturbances. Med Clin North Am. 1981;65(321):360.

Prough DS, Bidani A. Hyperchloremic metabolic acidosis is a predictable consequence of intraoperative infusion of 0.9% saline. Anesthesiology. 1999;90:1247–9.

Prys-Roberts C, Kelman GR, Nunn JF. Determinants of the in vivo carbon dioxide titration curve in anesthetized man. Br J Anesth. 1966;38:500–50.

Puyau FA, Fowler REL, Novick R, et al. The acid-base vector of open-heart surgery. Circulation. 1962;26:902–12.

Quilley CP, Lin YS, McGiff JC. Chloride anion concentration as a determinant of renal vascular responsiveness to vasoconstrictor agents. Br J Pharmacol. 1993;108:106–108.

Rehm M, Orth V, Scheingraber S, et al. Acid–base changes caused by 5% albumin versus 6% hydroxyethyl starch solution in patients undergoing acute normovolemic hemodilution: a randomized prospective study. Anesthesiology. 2000;93:1174–83.

Reid F, Lobo DN, Williams RN, et al. (Ab)normal saline and physiological Hartmann's solution: a randomized double-blind crossover study. Clin Sci. 2003;104:17–24.

Rivers E, Nguyen B, Havstad S, et al. Early goal-directed therapy in the treatment of severe sepsis and septic shock. N Engl J Med. 2001;345:1368–77.
Rodriguez-Soriano J. New insight into the pathogenesis of renal tubular acidosis-from functional to molecular studies. Pediatr Nephrol. 2000;14:1121–36.
Rose DB. Fisiologia clinica dell'equilibrio acido-base e dei disordini elettrolitici. Milano: McGraw-Hill Libri Italia; 1995.
Scheingraber S, Rehm M, Sehmisch C, Finsterer U. Rapid saline infusion produces hyperchloremic acidosis in patients undergoing gynecologic surgery. Anesthesiology. 1999;90:1265–70.
Schlichtig R, Grogono AW, Severinghaus JW. Current status of acid-base quantitation in physiology and medicine. Anesthesiol Clin North Am. 1998a;16:211–33.
Schlichtig R, Grogono AW, Severinghaus JW. Human $PaCO_2$ and standard base excess compensation for acid-base imbalance. Crit Care Med. 1998b;26:1173–9.
Severinghaus JW. Acid-base balance nomogram–a Boston-Copenhagen détente. Anesthesiology. 1976;45:539–41.
Sgambato F, Prozzo S. Gap anionico: un ponte tra i due equilibri. Giorn Ital Med Int. 2003;2(1):20–7.
Shaer AJ. Inherited primary renal tubular hypokalemic alkalosis: a review of Gitelman and Bartter syndromes. Am J Med Sci. 2001;322:316–32.
Shires GT, Holman J. Dilution acidosis. Ann Intern Med. 1948;28:557–9.
Siggaard-Andersen O. The pH-log PCO2 blood acid-base nomogram revised. Scand J Clin Lab Invest. 1962;14:598–604.
Siggaard-Andersen O. The van Slyke equation. Scand J Clin Lab Invest. 1977;146:15–20.
Siggaard-Andersen O, Fogh-Andersen N. Base excess or buffer base (strong ion difference) as measure of a non-respiratory acid-base disturbance. Acta Anaesthesiol Scand. 1995;107:123–8.
Storey DA. Intravenous fluid administration and controversies in acid–base. Crit Care Resusc. 1999;1:151–6.
Traverso LW, Lee WP, Langford MJ. Fluid resuscitation after an otherwise fatal hemorrhage: 1. Crystalloids solutions. J Trauma. 1986;26:168–75.
Vincent JL, DuFaye P, Beré J, et al. Serial lactate determinations during circulatory shock. Crit Care Med. 1983;11:449–51.
Vulterini S, Colloca A, Chiappino MG, Bolignari P. L'equilibrio acido-base ed il suo studio mediante il dosaggio degli elettroliti del sangue venoso. Milan: Ediz Instr. Laboratory; 1992.
Waters JH, Gottleib A, Schoenwald P, et al. Normal saline versus lactated Ringer's solution for intraoperative fluid management in patients undergoing abdominal aortic aneurysm repair: an outcome study. Anesth Analg. 2001;93:817–22.
Weil MH, Afifi AA. Experimental and clinical studies on lactate and pyruvate as indicators of the severity of acute circulatory failure (shock). Circulation. 1970;41:989–1001.
Wilcox CS. Regulation of renal blood flow by plasma chloride. J Clin Invest. 1983;71:726–35.
Wilkes NJ, Woolf R, Mutch M, et al. The effects of balanced versus saline-based hetastarch and crystalloid solutions on acid-base and electrolyte status and gastric mucosal perfusion in elderly surgical patients. Anesth Analg. 2001;93:811–6.
Wooten EW. Analytic calculation of physiological acid-base parameters in plasma. J Appl Physiol. 1999;86:326–34.
Worthley LIG. Acid–base balance and disorders. In: Bersten AD, Soni N, editors. Oh's intensive care manual. 5th ed. Edinburgh: Butterworth-Heinemann; 2003.
Zander R. Infusion fluids: why should they be balanced solutions? Eur J Hospital Pharmacy Practice. 2006;12:60–2.

Postoperative Pain Management in Adult Cardiac Surgery

17

Ali Dabbagh

Abstract

Postoperative pain management is not only a medical concern but also among the human rights; this challenging issue would be much more difficult in post-operative period of cardiac surgery patients in whom the burden of the cardiac disease and the complex perioperative events impose their heavy shadow on the decision-making process for selection of analgesic remedies for acute pain suppression.

In this chapter, a brief discussion about the pathologic mechanisms of pain and their possible risk factors and potential mechanisms is presented first, and then, analgesia methods are discussed in two main categories: pharmacologic methods (including opioids, alpha 2 agonists, nonsteroidal anti-inflammatory drugs "NSAIDs," paracetamol, ketamine, $MgSO_4$, gabapentin, pregabalin, multimodal analgesia, and patient-controlled analgesia) and non-pharmacologic interventions (mainly infiltration of local anesthetics, intercostal nerve block, intrapleural infiltration of local anesthetics, and neuraxial blocks, "paravertebral, intrathecal, thoracic epidural").

Keywords

Postoperative pain · Acute pain management · Patient satisfaction and patients' expectations · Anticipated pain and experienced pain · Etiologic factors aggravating pain · "Chronic thoracic chest pain" or "chronic leg pain" · Analgesic methods Pharmacologic alternatives · Opioids · Fentanyl · Sufentanil · Alfentanil Remifentanil · Alpha 2 agonists · Nonsteroidal anti-inflammatory drugs (NSAIDs) Paracetamol · Ketamine · Gabapentin · Pregabalin · Magnesium sulfate

A. Dabbagh, M.D.
Cardiac Anesthesiology Department, Anesthesiology Research Center, Faculty of Medicine, Shahid Beheshti University of Medical Sciences, Tehran, Iran
e-mail: alidabagh@sbmu.ac.ir

A. Dabbagh et al. (eds.), *Postoperative Critical Care for Adult Cardiac Surgical Patients*, https://doi.org/10.1007/978-3-319-75747-6_17

Patient-controlled analgesia · Regional anesthetic techniques Intrapleural infiltration of local anesthetics · Neuraxial block · Paravertebral block · Spinal Epidural Intrathecal

17.1 Introduction: The Effects of Acute Postoperative Pain and the Benefits of Acute Pain Management in Postoperative Period

Today, a considerable number of patients experience acute postoperative pain, and it has been demonstrated that between 30 and 80% of patients complain of acute "moderate to severe postsurgical pain"; so, the health-care team still have to consider postoperative pain as a challenge of care. Still acute postoperative pain management is among the highest priorities, both for the patients and the health-care team. According to the NIH report, the annual pain-related health-care costs in the United States were more than one hundred billion dollars ($100,000,000,000) in 1998, estimated to be more than doubled now. According to the 13th World Congress on Pain in Montreal, Quebec, Canada, "Access to Pain Management is a Fundamental Human Right"; it has been mentioned in Article 3: "The right of all people with pain to have access to appropriate assessment and treatment of the pain by adequately trained health care professionals," while there are millions of patients who tolerate pain and experience the unpleasant sensation of acute pain, due to acute, chronic, or cancer pain. Improper or incomplete treatment of acute pain potentially leads to chronic pain in a considerable number of patients; the ultimate outcome would be "irreversible changes in the nervous system" ending in "progressive biopsychosocial epiphenomena" with further impairments, incapacities, and chronic health (Dolin et al. 2002; Popping et al. 2008a, b; International Pain Summit of the International Association for the Study of Pain 2011; Chou et al. 2016).

Besides, the quality of "acute postoperative pain management" is an important and considerable index in patient outcome; proper management of acute postoperative pain could potentially prevent a number of unwanted hemodynamic, neuroendocrine, hemostatic, and immunologic side effects, possibly decreasing the prevalence of postoperative morbidities (Peters et al. 2007; Caputo et al. 2011; Zheng et al. 2017).

In 2012, the American Society of Anesthesiologists has published the updated version of "the American Society of Anesthesiologists' Practice Guideline for Acute Pain Management in the Perioperative Setting." According to this guideline, "Anesthesiologists and other healthcare providers should use standardized, validated instruments to facilitate the regular evaluation and documentation of pain intensity, the effects of pain therapy, and side effects caused by the therapy." Also, the guideline emphasizes that "Anesthesiologists responsible for perioperative analgesia should be available at all times to consult with ward nurses, surgeons, or other involved physicians" (2012). Also, the guideline released by American Society of Pain's expert panel declares that "Safe and effective postoperative pain management should be on the basis of a plan of care tailored to the individual and the surgical procedure involved, and multimodal regimens are recommended in many situations" (Chou et al. 2016).

In this chapter, a brief explanation of the pathophysiologic pain mechanisms is described first. Then, different pharmacologic and non-pharmacologic approaches of acute pain management are discussed with an explanation about the methods of use, their potential risks, and benefits.

17.2 The Effects of Acute Postoperative Pain and the Benefits of Acute Pain Management in Postoperative Period

Acute postoperative pain imposes undesirable perioperative surgical stress response; the effects of perioperative insults to the body cause modifications in a number of body systems including the immune system and its inflammatory components and, also, the metabolic and neurohormonal systems; the collective response is called "the stress response," which would directly and indirectly affect many of the body organs. The sympathetic system is affected by the effects of acute pain, though age and sex could significantly influence the sympathetic response, although other studies suggest a much more important role for factors such as the severity of surgical lesion and "surgical trauma" than the amount of sympathetic tone severity (Liu and Wu 2007; Ledowski et al. 2011, 2012; Wolf 2012; Bigeleisen and Goehner 2015).

Suppressing acute postoperative pain would alter patient satisfaction, prevent unnecessary patient discomfort, and decrease the duration of postoperative hospital length of stay, patient costs, overall morbidity, and even mortality; most are alleviated after adequate postoperative pain management. Hence, postoperative analgesia is a major indicator of postoperative care needing "early aggressive perioperative care" (Bigeleisen and Goehner 2015; Stephens and Whitman Stephens and Whitman 2015a, b).

Acute postoperative pain in adult cardiac surgery has some special features compared with the other patients, both regarding the patient factors and the analgesic methods, while often severe and undertreated which might cause severe and prolonged chronic pain; hence, the pain management strategy should be "tailored" to each patient in order to have satisfactory results. However, the newly adopted fast-track anesthesia approach in cardiac surgeries necessitates more aggressive postoperative pain management in these patients. Multimodal analgesic methods are highly effective and possibly *the best technique* in the management of acute postoperative pain. However, this approach has very important considerations due to the specific type of cardiac procedures. For example, neuraxial analgesia has its own considerations due to the coagulation disturbances after administration of anticoagulation and antiplatelet agents, to be discussed later in this chapter (Schwann and Chaney 2003; Bigeleisen and Goehner 2015; Stephens and Whitman 2015a, b; Guimaraes-Pereira et al. 2016a; Alzahrani 2017; Correll 2017; Guimaraes-Pereira et al. 2017; Liu et al. 2017a; Sangesland et al. 2017; Monico and Quiñónez 2017; Dabbagh 2014).

17.3 Patient Satisfaction and Patients' Expectations

When dealing with pain in cardiac surgery patients, it should be considered that cardiac surgery patients usually expect a greater amount of postoperative pain than the real pain. So, when they make a comparison between *anticipated pain* and *experienced pain* (which is the actual pain), the patients usually express an acceptable and high level of satisfaction, although they really experience severe pain. So, there is a good level of *patient satisfaction* in such patients in the postoperative period. However, the health-care team should describe all aspects of postoperative pain with each patient, especially the potential for occurrence of chronic pain syndromes and its risk factors before the surgery. Of course, the different activities of the patients have different pain thresholds. One study demonstrated the following decreasing order of postoperative pain in cardiac surgical patients: "coughing, moving or turning in bed, getting up, deep breathing or using the incentive spirometer, and resting," while the pain intensity was decreased after removal of chest tubes. Also, the patients expect the health-care team to help them improve the tolerance of acute pain in order to gain their normal life (Azzopardi and Lee 2009; Ravven et al. 2013; Stenman et al. 2016).

17.4 The Pathophysiology of Acute Pain in Cardiac Surgery Patients

It should be always considered as an alerting note that in patients undergoing cardiac surgery, the acute postoperative pain could be due to residual ischemia and/or incomplete revascularization; so, acute postoperative pain in these patients should always lead the health-care team to a very important differential diagnosis: residual ischemia. *This differentiation is so much important.* After ruling out the above condition, we would focus on the most common source of acute postoperative pain in these patients which is mainly with a myofascial origin and originates from many sources, most commonly originates from the chest wall (including the muscles, bony structures, tendons, and ligaments) (Guimaraes-Pereira et al. 2016a; Guimaraes-Pereira et al. 2017).

Usually in patients undergoing surgical procedures, the perioperative surgical stress response will increase to its uppermost levels just in the immediate postoperative period when it produces its many major pathophysiologic effects (including postoperative pain). This is the same after cardiac surgery with even more severe degrees of stress response due to the nature of cardiac surgery patients; most of them often tolerate the imposed inflammatory response due to cardiopulmonary bypass.

In patients undergoing cardiac surgery, there are great homeostatic disturbances which could lead to a number of great pathophysiologic changes in many of the major organ systems, including (but not limited to) the cardiovascular system, the lungs, the gastrointestinal system, the urinary system, the endocrine system, improved oxygen consumption, the immunologic system, and, finally, the central nervous system; these unwanted effects of cardiac surgery may lead to substantial postoperative morbidity and possibly to increased mortality. On the other hand, there are many studies that have clearly demonstrated potentially improved clinical benefits after adequate postoperative analgesia, which is due to increased level of stability in hemodynamic, metabolic, immunologic, and homeostatic factors and also more levels of stress response attenuation (Guimaraes-Pereira et al. 2016a, 2017; Correll 2017).

17.5 The Etiologic Factors Aggravating Pain After Cardiac Surgery

The following are the possible etiologic risk factors for acute pain in this patient population and their pain sources:

- Incision site pain after sternotomy or thoracotomy
- Intraoperative tissue retraction and surgical dissection
- The arterial and venous vascular cannulation sites
- The site of vein harvesting
- The chest and abdominal sites for chest tubes
- A few other factors

Usually the pain location varies being a function of time; in other words, during the early postoperative days (usually the 3 postoperative days), the pain is mainly in the thoracic area, while afterward, it immigrates to the legs (i.e., the location of vein harvesting in CABG patients) and would be dominant there up to the end of the first postoperative week. During this transition, the type of pain will often change from a radicular chest pain to osteoarticular type leg pain at the end of the 1st week.

The etiology for thoracic pain is usually the injuries of the rib cage, which is a very common source of postoperative pain in cardiac surgery. It will produce *an unexplained* postoperative non-incisional pain which is the physical result of sternal retraction. In clinical evaluation, the patients often have normal routine CXR, and the potential rib fracture (usually the posterior or lateral parts of the lower ribs) could be mainly detected in bone scans. These fractures are due to sternal retraction during the surgical procedure, which causes posterior or lateral rib fracture; also, there is the possibility for brachial plexus injury *leg pain*: leg pain due to vein-graft harvesting could be also problematic in cardiac surgery patients. This phenomenon, limited to patients with conventional saphenous vein harvesting, usually occurs in the *late postoperative days*; the possible explanation for this delayed presentation of pain could be patient mobilization in the 3rd or 4th postoperative days, while there is a decrease in sternotomy-related pain which would unmask the leg pain. There is current evidence that demonstrates the minimally invasive vein-graft harvesting method (endoscopic harvesting) "reduces" the intensity and duration of postoperative leg pain.

There are a number of underlying factors including gender, age, and some ethnic groups; young age, prolonged surgical duration, and anatomical surgery location increase the chance of acute postoperative pain. Acute postoperative pain has been demonstrated to be much more severe in patients below 60 years (compared with those above 60). Also, it is experienced much more severely in women compared with men, though chronic discomfort after discharge is seen more frequently in men (Gallagher et al. 2004; Peters et al. 2007; Ferasatkish et al. 2008; van Gulik et al. 2011; Papadopoulos et al. 2013; Chou et al. 2016; Guimaraes-Pereira et al. 2016a, 2017; Correll 2017; Zheng et al. 2017).

17.6 Chronic Pain in Cardiac Surgery Patients

Chronic pain is a relatively frequent finding after cardiac surgery; its incidence has been reported to be about 20–55%; and some other recent studies have demonstrated even higher prevalence rates for chronic pain. Chronic pain and its related depressive states could affect the clinical outcome of cardiac surgical patients. Even patient sleep pattern, physical and emotional status, and daily activities might be affected by chronic postoperative pain; neuropathic pain is a very common finding in most patients with chronic postoperative pain after cardiac surgery. Chronic pain after cardiac surgery is mainly due to "chronic thoracic chest pain" or "chronic leg pain"; so, in one way, sternotomy could induce chronic pain in a number of patients with many referrals to pain clinics for managing chronic post-sternotomy pain mainly in the thoracic area; on the other hand, a number of patients undergoing CABG would refer for relief of chronic leg pain due to cardiac harvesting. These painful events should be differentiated from residual cardiac pain. Many studies have assessed post-cardiac surgery chronic pain to elucidate the related mechanisms, risk factors, and their treatment; a summary is presented here (Peters et al. 2007; Chou et al. 2016; Guimaraes-Pereira 2016; Guimaraes-Pereira et al. 2016a, b, 2017; Correll 2017).

The following are among the most possible risk factors for occurrence of postoperative chronic pain:

- Patients undergoing extensive surgical procedures (e.g., CABG plus valve surgery is associated with increased incidence of postoperative chronic pain than CABG alone)
- Prolonged time of the procedure (especially surgeries more than 3 h)
- Severe acute postoperative pain (with numeric rating scale3 ≥ 4)
- Patients with ASA classifications> III
- Any underlying history of preoperative or postoperative depression
- Any underlying history for psychological vulnerability: preoperative or postoperative
- Non-elective operations
- Redo operations needing sternotomy

- Increased needs for analgesic use during the first few postoperative days
- Female patients

Chronic chest pain: although may be rare, this type of chronic pain could be *problematic*; it is usually manifested as *prolonged and severe chest wall pain*, which presents as a persistent pain after cardiac surgery. It is often localized to the arms, shoulders, or legs. The clinician should differentiate this type of pain from residual cardiac diseases which cause cardiac pain, due to possible *residual ischemia or graft failure*. This syndrome is neuropathic in origin, would cause significant morbidity and discomfort for the patients, and occurs occasionally; but it is really difficult to treat. It is more frequent in the thoracic area after CABG, due to its etiologic factors discussed in the next paragraph. The patients who have severe acute pain in the first 10 days after surgery or who have "negative beliefs" about treatment of acute pain with opioids are at increased risk for chronic pain.

There are a great number of possible factors mentioned as etiologies for chronic pain in cardiac surgery patients, which might contribute to the appearance of chronic postoperative pain and postoperative neuropathies including:

- Physical effects of sternotomy
- Surgical dissection and harvesting of the IMA, either skeletonized or pedicled
- Direct damage to the trauma to the thoracic nerve branches including the anterior rami of intercostal nerve branch nerves
- Pressure of the retractor
- Surgical tissue destruction, fractures of the ribs
- Separation of the costochondral junction
- The surgical scar formation
- Postoperative infection of the sternum
- Sternal stainless steel wire sutures
- Inappropriate positioning of the body organs or suboptimal positioning of the arms before start of the surgical procedure
- Intraoperative or postoperative injury to the brachial plexus
- The pressure effects of rib fracture fragments
- Placement of central venous catheter

Among the above etiologies, IMA harvesting (either skeletonized or not) has been reported to cause neuropathic pain with a burning and sharp feature, which aggravates at night and would increase in severity by *stretching*, since it is due to neuritis of IMA harvest. Harvesting of IMA (thermal or mechanical injury) causes a number of dysesthesia areas presented as numbness and/or hypersensitivity located on the anterior chest region. It may even become so much worse that it would be aggravated by *usual daily activities* like putting on the clothes or showering. The patients would usually complain of the following words for describing the pain: "annoying, persistently recurring, dull, cutting and sharp, exhausting, tender, and tight." The temporal nature of pain is almost reported as brief, transient, and intermittent (Bruce et al. 2003; Dick et al. 2011; Hakim and Narouze 2015).

Chronic leg pain: chronic pain may also occur in the leg, primarily due to postoperative neuralgia of the saphenous nerve which happens after saphenous vein harvesting for CABG. It is more prevalent in the younger patients, while the correlation of severity of acute post-op pain and development of chronic pain syndromes is still vague (Bruce et al. 2003; Dick et al. 2011; Hakim and Narouze 2015).

17.7 Different Analgesic Methods

The American Society of Anesthesiologists' Practice Guideline for Acute Pain Management in the perioperative setting defines acute pain as "pain that is present in a surgical patient after a procedure. Such pain may be the result of trauma from the procedure or procedure related complications" and "pain management in the perioperative setting refers to actions before, during, and after a procedure that are intended to reduce or eliminate postoperative pain before discharge" (2012).

Preoperative pain management techniques: according to the guideline text, it is very important to start the analgesic approaches from the preoperative period. Also, preoperative expectations of the patients would influence postoperative patient satisfaction level. The preoperative patient preparation steps include (but are not limited to) the following (Aslan et al. 2009; Guo et al. 2012; Chou et al. 2016):

- Reducing underlying pain and anxiety by effective treatments.
- Restoring or adjusting those medications which are used by the patients and their abrupt discontinuation could provoke signs or symptoms of withdrawal.
- Administration of multimodal analgesic pain management program as preoperative medications before the operating room.
- Application of patient and family education programs, which could be as pain control techniques and behavioral adaptations.

Perioperative pain management techniques: among all the pain management techniques used during the perioperative period, the following are the most common; however, these are not the only options:

- Neuraxial administration of opioid analgesics (including epidural and intrathecal administration of analgesics and local anesthetics).
- Peripheral regional analgesic techniques (including intercostal blocks, intrapleural, plexus blocks, paravertebral block, local anesthetic infiltration into the incisions).
- Patient-controlled analgesia (PCA) with systemic opioids and NSAIDs.
- Traditional intravenous administration of analgesics (especially opioid analgesics, with their prototype being morphine); however, intravenous opioids have

their well-known side effects, including nausea, vomiting, pruritus, urinary retention, respiratory depression, and delayed tracheal extubation; other agents like NSAIDs and α-adrenergic agents could also be added.

17.8 Pharmacologic Alternatives Used for Treatment of Acute Cardiac Surgery Patients

17.8.1 Opioids

Morphine was detected by Friedrich Sertürner in 1803–1806, and its analgesic activity was used afterward (Klockgether-Radke 2002; Rachinger-Adam et al. 2011). However, the routine clinical administration of opioids for acute pain suppression began in the 1960s, when administration of very high doses of intravenous opioids (especially morphine) was a standard care for cardiac anesthesia. However, in the following years, it was elucidated that even administration of very large intravenous doses of opioids could not induce complete anesthesia (including full unconscious state and amnesia); so, other inhalational or intravenous anesthetics were added to the anesthetic regimens for surgical anesthesia.

17.8.1.1 Opioid Receptors

The clinical effects and side effects of the opioid agents are classified – like many other drugs – based on their receptors; the opioids interact with many different body systems through these receptors. The current opioid receptors are classified as three distinct ones, μ, κ, and δ, and the analgesic effects of opioids in the central nervous system (both at the spinal and supraspinal level) are exerted through these receptors. Primarily, the μ receptor is classified as μ1 and μ2; however, μ1 is a high-affinity receptor mainly with supraspinal analgesia, while μ2 is a low-affinity receptor predominantly with spinal anesthesia. The μ agonists cause a dose-related respiratory depression which would mainly act via μ2 receptor activities. However, kappa (κ) receptors have potential analgesic role both at the spinal and supraspinal level with possibly lower drug side effects and complications related to μ receptors, though pure κ agonists have little effect on respiration. The third type of opioid receptors known as delta (δ) receptors presents modulatory role than analgesic role, both at the spinal level δ1 and supraspinal level δ2. Peripheral terminals for opioid receptors have been also demonstrated with their special role in some clinical findings like pruritus, also cardioprotection, and wound healing. However, it seems that the greatest advantage of peripheral terminals of opioid receptors would possibly be used as a common practice in near future, in such a way that we would be able to administer opioids peripherally without the fear of their risks on the CNS; the latter clinical use of peripheral opioid receptors has now appeared practically in some tissues like joints, bone, and teeth for postoperative pain relief; possibly other surgical operations (like cardiovascular) would be able to use these new molecules of analgesics; the peripheral role of opioid receptors seems to be a result of peripheral interaction/counteraction between opioid receptors and different ingredients of the immune system including but not limited to dendritic cells and toll-like receptors (Leung Leung 2004a, b; Rachinger-Adam et al. 2011; Xu et al. 2015b; Floettmann et al. 2017; Hong et al. 2017; Oehler et al. 2017; Tejada et al. 2017; Zhang et al. 2017).

17.8.1.2 Opioid Effects on the Body Systems

Analgesics and sedatives (especially opioids) have many important interactions with body homeostasis including the body stress modulating systems like "hypothalamus-pituitary-adrenal (HPA) axis and the extrahypothalamic brain stress system"; so, opioids could have many beneficial effects in counteracting the unwanted effects of surgical stress response after cardiac surgery, which would help the body in maintenance of homeostasis; however, opioid-related adverse drug events affect the postoperative recovery (Rachinger-Adam et al. 2011; Barletta 2012; Camilleri et al. 2017).

Opioids are used extensively for suppression of acute postoperative pain in cardiac surgery and are known as the "gold standard" of pharmacologic acute pain suppression, mainly as intravenous and/or neuraxial routes. Morphine has more effective analgesic properties than the other opioids. Pharmacologically speaking, opioids have two distinct locations for their analgesic effects, supraspinal and spinal, i.e., neuraxial. Neuraxial administration of hydrophilic opioids (e.g., morphine sulfate) could create excellent postoperative analgesia, lasting at least 24 h for intrathecal and 48 h for epidural route with a number of clinical benefits; however, a very high degree of vigilance is needed to prevent possible side effects, mainly respiratory complications, hypoventilation and apnea being the most lethal ones. A maximum dose of 300 μg intrathecal morphine sulfate is considered the safety margin for prevention of postoperative respiratory depression. Morphine, used in different modes, has many potential benefits compared with other analgesic drugs (Whiteside et al. 2005; Vosoughian et al. 2007; Dabbagh et al. 2011; Mugabure Bujedo 2012; Walker and Yaksh 2012; Mahler 2013; Yamanaka and Sadikot 2013).

Respiratory system: opioids cause *respiratory depression* which could be known as the most important side effect of these very potent analgesics. The main mechanism is decreased sensitivity of the brain respiratory center to arterial pressure of CO_2, in which its mechanism is through decreased sensitivity of both medullary and peripheral chemoreceptors. Rostral ventromedial medulla is the region implicated in pain modulation and homeostatic regulation. Opioids could inhibit the chemoreceptors through the μ receptors especially μ_2 receptor, while their respiratory depressant effect in medulla is exerted through μ and δ receptors. It has been demonstrated that among the many CNS neurotransmitters involved in respiratory depression, the major neuroexcitatory and neuroinhibitory transmitters are glutamate and GABA, respectively. A third mechanism of obstructive apnea due to airway obstruction of opioids has been mentioned as the mechanism of opioid-induced apnea. The clinical steps in this process as follows are the steps of the effect of opioids on respirations:

1. Decreased respiratory rate.
2. Decreased tidal volume would happen after respiratory rate decrease.
3. Disturbed rhythmic function and generation of the respiration.

4. Change in the pattern of respiration from normal regular breath to irregular gasping pattern of spontaneous ventilation; this pattern is the characteristic pattern for the patients with diagnosis of opioid overdose.
5. Decreased sensitivity to hypoxia leading to decreased ventilator drive to hypoxia.
6. Finally, apnea.

The opioid compound with active metabolites (e.g., morphine-6-β-glucuronide) has increased respiratory depressant effects. Also, elderly patients are at higher risk of respiratory depression after opioid administration, since their central respiratory center is more sensitive to the respiratory depressant effects of opioids than the younger patients. Besides, when other anesthetics (like benzodiazepines, barbiturates, or inhalation anesthetics) are used simultaneously, the respiratory depressant effects of opioids would be more severe. And finally, genetic, environmental, and demographic factors may play a role in the severity of opioid-induced respiratory depression (Ozaki et al. 2001; Yamanaka and Sadikot 2013; Chen et al. 2017a; Pergolizzi et al. 2017; Xie et al. 2017).

Cardiovascular system: the opioids and their metabolites, including morphine, improve the analgesic effects of opioids in treatment of acute pain in patients with a history of ischemic heart disease undergoing major surgical operations. In patients undergoing cardiac surgery with extracorporeal circulation, due to increased volume of drug distribution, the required dose is increased. There are also studies that demonstrate the cardioprotective effects of opioids (Bodnar 2012; Tanaka et al. 2014; Geng et al. 2017; Gunther et al. 2017; Owusu Obeng et al. 2017; Phillips et al. 2017).

Other systems are also affected by the effects of opioids:

Immune system: opioid as demonstrated induces immunomodulation, both acquired and innate immunity, which can even affect the surgical outcome of the patients. The role of the immune system changes in creation of acute and chronic pain is negligible. Among many cellular structures and receptors, the role of toll-like receptor subtypes in many fields, including their interactions with opioids and their role in myocardial ischemia and acute coronary syndrome, has gained a great importance during the last years (Saadat et al. 2012; Chen et al. 2017a; Oehler et al. 2017; Plein and Rittner 2017; Tejada et al. 2017; Xie et al. 2017).

Gastrointestinal tract: opioids, especially morphine, decrease the mobility of the GI tract ending not only in constipation but also at times aggravate the centrally mediated nausea and vomiting, which are well-recognized unwanted side effect of opioids in all patients especially in the old age. The treatment of opioid-induced bowel dysfunction is not yet satisfactory, though a number of traditional laxatives (bulking laxatives, stimulant agents, etc.) or newer prokinetic agents like "prucalopride and lubiprostone" have been tested with different clinical results. Prucalopride is a selective, high-affinity agonist of 5-HT(4) receptor used for treatment of chronic constipation, and lubiprostone is a prostaglandin E_1 derivative which could increase the activity of chloride channels in the apical aspect of epithelial cells to produce a very high chloride content fluid secretion inside the bowel lumen, leading to softened stool and increased motility and defecation. On the other hand, opioids have a wide range of interactions with the "super active" immune system of the bowels, at times leading to aggravation of colon diseases (Cuthbert 2011; Smith et al. 2012; Dabbagh and Rajaei 2013; Valdez-Morales et al. 2013; Anselmi et al. 2015; Talebi and Dabbagh 2017).

Urinary retention: the opioid agents, especially morphine, could induce urinary retention which is accompanied with increased bladder pressure and urinary bladder sphincter pressure; also, histological damage of bladder and the sphincter of bladder are possible. There are some clinical risk factors for increased risk of urinary retention like male sex and intrathecal morphine use; possibly the use of continuous peripheral nerve block could decrease the chance of this complication (Griesdale et al. 2011; Holzer 2012; Pergolizzi et al. 2017).

Cell growth and cell death: the opioid agents have some effects in suppressing the cell growth. This might be at times against the tumor cells; however, in the recent years, there is an increasing concern regarding the apoptotic effects of anesthetics including opioids (Djafarzadeh et al. 2012; Dabbagh and Rajaei 2013; Eftekhar-Vaghefi et al. 2015; Chen et al. 2017a, b; Pergolizzi et al. 2017; Xie et al. 2017).

Other effects: there are a number of other side effects of opioids, namely, nausea and vomiting, pruritus, and urinary retention, which could be decreased by concomitant use of adjuvant analgesic agents, leading to decreased side effects of opioids while maintaining adequate postoperative analgesia. Opioids also affect appetite, thermoregulation, and mental features of the patients (Chen et al. 2017a; Pergolizzi et al. 2017; Xie et al. 2017).

17.8.1.3 Opioid Compounds

Currently, opioids are classified as two main groups: natural agents and synthetic agents; morphine is the prototype of opioid agents and known as the gold standard (i.e., the benchmark of opioid analgesics). More detailed description of these agents is presented in the "Cardiovascular Pharmacology" chapter.

Morphine is the prototype opioid agonist and the most popular analgesic used in patients after cardiac surgery. Also, many synthetic and semisynthetic opioid compounds are made by simple modifications of morphine. Morphine is a lipid-soluble agent and for therapeutic purposes has been changed to some compounds like morphine sulfate which are more water-soluble. Morphine has 30–40% plasma protein binding and has primarily hepatic metabolism being conjugated to water-soluble glucuronides like morphine-3-glucuronide and morphine-6-glucuronide. Elimination half-life of morphine is 2–3 h but would be increased in liver diseases like liver cirrhosis, though the half-life of morphine is normal in renal disease. Morphine has also extrahepatic clearance through the gut, brain, and kidneys, which comprises about 30% of the total clearance of the drug (Bosilkovska et al. 2012; Hughes et al. 2012; Ishii et al. 2012; Swartjes et al. 2012; et al. 2012).

Synthetic opioid agents: currently, we have four main synthetic opioid agonists used in clinic for acute pain management in anesthesia and/or analgesia: fentanyl, sufentanil, alfentanil, and remifentanil. These compounds are synthetic chemical derivatives of phenylpiperidine, which are chemical derivatives of meperidine.

Fentanyl, sufentanil, alfentanil, and remifentanil are very fast-equilibrating agents; alfentanil and remifentanil equilibrate "very fast" having an equilibrium half-life of just 1 min in order to equilibrate between plasma and CNS; fentanyl and sufentanil have a half-life of about 6 min for such an equilibration followed by methadone's half-life being 8 min; however, the equilibration half-life of morphine is very much longer, 2 to 3 h, and morphine-6-glucuronide (an active metabolite of morphine) near 7 h; it means that alfentanil, remifentanil, fentanyl, and sufentanil have a higher speed for reaching from plasma to their effect site (mainly CNS) compared with morphine and its metabolites (Ing Lorenzini et al. 2012; Scott 2016; Ziesenitz et al. 2018).

Another concept considered important for opioid infusions used as acute pain management is the context-sensitive half-life (CSHL) considered as the time interval from discontinuation of the infusion until gaining a plasma level of the drug half as much of the time of infusion discontinuation; of course the infusion should be discontinued after gaining a steady-state plasma level of the drug; among some other indicators of pharmacokinetic and pharmacodynamics, "time to equilibrate after start of infusion" and "CSHL" are two very important factors that could help us choose a more appropriate analgesic in acute postoperative pain management. In this regard, remifentanil and alfentanil have both short "plasma-CNS equilibration time" and short CSHL; the lowest CSHL among all the opioids belongs to remifentanil; also, due to their metabolism, none of these four compounds would impose much considerable problem due to drug overdosage in patients with *renal impairment*; studies have shown that administering infusion of short-acting opioids could decrease the time necessary for postoperative mechanical ventilation and help earlier ventilator weaning, so they could decrease the "ICU length of stay" (Servin 2003, 2008; Servin and Billard 2008; Ziesenitz et al. 2018).

Fentanyl is a very potent opioid being about 80–120 times more potent than morphine, though its receptor affinity is three times more than morphine. Since fentanyl is highly lipid-soluble (about 150 times more lipid-soluble than morphine), it can bypass the blood-brain barrier (BBB) so much faster than the water-soluble morphine, hence, creating its analgesic effects more rapidly than morphine (either administered as IV, IM, intrathecal, or other routes).

Fentanyl is metabolized by the liver and does not have an active metabolite. This is why its clearance is not impaired in renal diseases, but prolonged effects of the drug are well anticipated in liver diseases. Another interesting issue regarding fentanyl is that the drug undergoes active storage in the lungs; so, nearly two-thirds of fentanyl is inactivated in the first pass of the lung. CYP3A4 inhibitors and inducers have considerable interaction of fentanyl metabolism (Kuip et al. 2017; Ziesenitz et al. 2018).

Bolus doses of fentanyl create their analgesic effect so soon without much residual effects. On the other hand, the effects of infusion doses of fentanyl are not much similar. In other words, due to its high lipophilicity, fentanyl infusion leads to accumulated amounts of drug in adipose tissues, and when the infusion is disconnected, the infused amounts of fentanyl are released into plasma. This is why the effects of prolonged fentanyl infusion are not offset immediately after discontinuation of the infusion; this is especially very important after prolonged infusion of the drug, which could lead to very prolonged drug effects after long-time infusion. Pharmacologically speaking, context-sensitive half-time of fentanyl increases along with the saturation of inactive sites.

However, it is recommended to use fentanyl infusion as the following dosage for having adequate sedation while preventing prolonged residual effects (George et al. 2010; Scott 2016; Ziesenitz et al. 2018).

- Start fentanyl administration drug with a primary bolus dose of 1–2 μg/Kg of the drug.
- At the same time, start an IV infusion of 1–3 μg/Kg/h.
- Depending on patient needs, adjust the infusion dose, especially if the patient has a history of preoperative drug use.
- Adding patient-controlled analgesia (PCA) route with a dose of 0.1–1 μg/Kg for each bolus (depending on patient needs) and a lock time interval about 15 min to the background IV infusion for the relatively awake patient leads to excellent analgesia with good satisfaction and cooperation with limited side effects.
- This method mandates extreme cautious and close monitoring regarding respiratory depression, including respiratory rate, pulse oximeter, end-tidal CO_2, etc.
- Fentanyl is accumulated in patients with hepatic impairment due to drug accumulation, though this is not a major problem in patients with renal impairment.

Sufentanil is another opioid synthetic compound which is about five to ten times more potent than fentanyl. Being extremely lipid-soluble with a very high plasma protein-binding capacity, sufentanil is metabolized mainly in the liver. So, sufentanil pharmacokinetics (like fentanyl and alfentanil) is not very much affected in patients with renal disease; however, its effects are significantly prolonged in patients with hepatic disease due to impaired hepatic metabolism and the resulting drug accumulation. Prolonged infusions of sufentanil are offset much sooner than comparable analgesic doses of fentanyl or alfentanil. This is why IV sufentanil infusions do not demonstrate as much long sedation effects as fentanyl. Of course, the clinical effects of alfentanil are presented sooner than sufentanil and fentanyl; i.e., the time lag between plasma levels and effect site (CNS) is shorter in alfentanil (about 1 min) compared with sufentanil (about 6 min) and fentanyl (about 7 min); however, CSHL of sufentanil is shorter than alfentanil and of course fentanyl; the CSHL order after 3 h of IV infusion is sufentanil (30 min), alfentanil (50–60 min), and fentanyl (250 min) in increasing order; in other words, after discontinuation of equivalent doses of IV infusion, the drug effects would disappear first in sufentanil, then alfentanil, and, finally, fentanyl; this effect is mainly due to larger sufentanil volume of distribution. Of course, as discussed later, the effects of remifentanil would disappear very much sooner than all the other three compounds; vide infra (Bosilkovska et al. 2012; Jeleazcov et al. 2012; Zhang et al. 2015a).

Alfentanil is another opioid compound similar to fentanyl but five to ten times less potent than fentanyl. Its clinical effects are presented very shortly, 1 min after IV administration, mainly due to its very high lipid solubility which could bypass the BBB very fast; its lipid solubility is even more than fentanyl. So, alfentanil pharmacokinetics (like fentanyl and sufentanil) is not very much affected in patients with renal disease; however, its effects are significantly prolonged in patients with hepatic disease due to impaired hepatic metabolism and the resulting drug accumulation. As mentioned in the previous paragraph, its CSHL is shorter than fentanyl and longer than sufentanil (Jeleazcov et al. 2012; Ziesenitz et al. 2018).

Remifentanil is the newest version of synthetic opioids, being a potent mu agonist, having an analgesic potency "equal to fentanyl and 20–30 times more potent than alfentanil." However, remifentanil has a very short start time lag (1 min); more importantly, it has the shortest possible time (among all the opioids) for its effects to be offset after discontinuation of drug infusion. The following are among the most important pharmacological and clinical features of remifentanil (Servin 2003, 2008; Komatsu et al. 2007; Servin and Billard 2008; Olofsen et al. 2010; Ing Lorenzini et al. 2012; Hoshijima et al. 2016):

- Time interval from start of drug administration until presentation of its clinical effects is about 1 min (i.e., very fast onset).
- Its CSHL being as short as 3–5 min irrespective of the duration of IV infusion (the shortest CSHL among all the opioid compounds).
- The drug must be used as a continuous infusion as long as the patient has pain.
- The opioid effects of the drug, including respiratory depression, are offset in just 3–5 min after discontinuation of infusion irrespective of the duration of the infusion.
- Acute postoperative pain management in patients under anesthesia using remifentanil as the main opioid mandates considering an appropriate agent as soon as the remifentanil infusion is set off, or remifentanil infusion with its analgesic dose (and not the anesthetic dose) should be continued postoperatively.
- The main mechanism of remifentanil metabolism is *rapid hydrolysis* by nonspecific esterase found both in tissue and plasma, which takes a very short time for drug disappearance and leaves inactive drug metabolites.
- The drug metabolism mandates infusion of the drug as the main effective mechanism of action; its bolus administration should be done very cautiously since bolus dose has the possibility for severe bradycardia, hypotension, decreased cardiac output, and cardiac arrest.
- Its analgesic dose is 0.05–1 μg/Kg/min, based on ideal body mass.
- Only IV route is recommended; never use intrathecal or epidural routes for its administration due to glycine added to drug combination.
- Remifentanil is the only opioid with no special consideration in patients with either renal or hepatic disease regarding its metabolism.
- A meta-analysis demonstrated that "remifentanil is associated with increased incidence of postoperative shivering compared with alfentanil or fentanyl" (Hoshijima et al. 2016).

17.8.2 Alpha 2 Agonists

α2 Adrenergic agonists can cause analgesia, sedation, and sympatholysis. These agents are primarily known in practice as clonidine (natural) and its synthetic analog, dexmedetomidine which is a pure α2 adrenergic agonist and has a half-life of 2–3 h. They could be administered orally, intrathecally, or intravenously. The mechanism of action in these agents is creation of sedation through stimulation of α2 receptors in the locus coeruleus and creation of analgesia through stimulation of α2 receptors within the locus coeruleus and the spinal cord; also, these agents could enhance the analgesic effects of the opioids via an unknown mechanism of action. Their clinical effects could be classified after systemic administration (antinociception and sedation) and intrathecal administration (only antinociception). There are reports that have mentioned tolerance to these agents after their prolonged administration. When used as sedative for post-CABG patients, their perioperative superior effects may include:

- Increased stability of the hemodynamic parameters and attenuated hemodynamic responses.
- Decreased perioperative myocardial ischemia and cardioprotective effects.
- Decreased need for analgesic agents.
- Treatment of delirium.
- Antiarrhythmic effects.
- Decreased postoperative opioid consumption, pain intensity, and nausea, accompanied with decreased use of analgesics, beta-blockers, antiemetics, epinephrine, and diuretics.
- There might be some protective effects in a number of organs.

However, overdose of these agents could induce excessive postoperative sedation accompanied with postoperative hemodynamic instability, bradycardia, and/or hypotension with bradycardia, at times mandating pharmacologic treatment (Dabbagh 2011; Blaudszun et al. 2012; Moghadam et al. 2012; Jabbary Moghaddam et al. 2013; Zhang et al. 2015b; Cruickshank et al. 2016; Liu et al. 2017a, b).

17.8.3 Nonsteroidal Anti-inflammatory Drugs (NSAIDs)

Having analgesic and anti-inflammatory properties, a number of agents are categorized in this class of analgesics. Their main mechanism of action is blockade of cyclooxygenase (COX) enzyme leading to prostaglandin synthesis inhibition described by Vane in 1971 for the first time. Their analgesic mechanism is theoretically classified as two main groups: traditional NSAIDs inhibiting COX in a nonselective manner and relatively newer class of NSAIDs which inhibit COX-2 in a selective manner. Selective COX-2 inhibitors were produced in order to decrease the unwanted effects of nonselective inhibition of COX-1 by traditional NSAIDs, especially regarding the GI mucosa; however, their merit was not completely fulfilled because of the deep concern of potential unwanted cardiac effects of COX-2 inhibitors. NSAIDs are used frequently in the perioperative period; however, they are used usually in combination with other analgesic methods (mainly in combination with opioids, local anesthetics, or regional techniques) as a multimodal analgesic technique. NSAIDs are clinically effective in suppressing acute postoperative pain; in decreasing the need for postoperative opioid use, an effect named as opioid-sparing effect; and, also, in improving the clinical outcome. If contraindications of NSAIDs are considered logically, accompanied with close observation of their potential side effects, these agents could be used cautiously and safely. Potential contraindications of NSAIDs are elderly people, heart failure, hypovolemic states, cirrhotic patients, renal failure, history of active GI tract disease and peptic ulcer disease, active bleeding diathesis, and pregnant patients (Bell et al. 2006; Langford and Mehta 2006; Derry and Moore 2012; Khan and Fraser 2012; Jalkut 2014; Huang and Sakata 2016):

The most important adverse effects of NSAIDs are as follows:

1. Gastrointestinal complications which could lead to serious and life-threatening hemorrhage, especially in postoperative period of cardiac surgery due to concomitant administration of anticoagulants.
2. Increased risk of bleeding which could be a potential complication in patients receiving neuraxial block for postoperative pain suppression.
3. Acute renal ischemia, especially if administered concomitantly with diuretics, angiotensin-converting enzyme inhibitors “ACE inhibitors,” and/or angiotensin receptor antagonists “ARA”; this drug combination is known as the “triple whammy” (Loboz and Shenfield 2005).

NSAIDs as adjuvant analgesics could reduce the dose of opioids needed for acute pain suppression in postoperative period; the concomitant administration of NSAIDs with opioids helps us to administer them while this method of NSAID use does not create clinically important renal impairments, though they might be able to decrease renal function during the early postoperative period in a transient and insignificant mode; meanwhile, these agents do not boost the risk of postoperative renal failure in cardiac surgery patients would they be prescribed within a logical dose range and avoiding their contraindications (Buvanendran and Kroin 2009; Frampton and Quinlan 2009; Acharya and Dunning 2010; Barletta 2012; Huang and Sakata 2016).

17.8.3.1 Paracetamol (N-Acetyl-P-Aminophenol)

Paracetamol (N-acetyl-p-aminophenol) is one of the most common analgesics used worldwide, mainly acting through central blockade of acute pain pathways and creating mild to moderate analgesia and mild anti-inflammatory effects. Its mechanism is not fully elucidated yet; however, some clinicians consider paracetamol as one of NSAIDs, though it does not have the same mechanism as classic drugs of this category. Its main toxicity could be after large doses to create hepatotoxicity, manifested much earlier in alcoholics. A Cochrane Database Systematic Review has provided "high quality evidence" demonstrating effective analgesia (4 h) in about 36% of patients having acute postoperative pain, after "a single dose of either IV paracetamol or IV propacetamol" (McNicol et al. 2016). However, other studies have claimed that analgesic properties of paracetamol in cardiac surgery patients are not so much considerable. In practice, the drug is recommended as part of a multimodal analgesic regimen (Lahtinen et al. 2002; Pettersson et al. 2005; McDaid et al. 2010; Maund et al. 2011; Tzortzopoulou et al. 2011).

17.8.4 Other Pharmaceutical Agents

Among the pharmaceuticals used for acute pain suppression in cardiac surgery patients, a number of other agents could be mentioned.

17.8.4.1 Ketamine

Ketamine is an intravenous anesthetic, mainly acting through "N-methyl-D-aspartate receptor" blockade; this drug could suppress acute pain effectively by a mechanism completely different from opioids: it acts mainly through dissociative anesthesia, "i.e., a combination of analgesia, hallucination, catalepsy, and some degrees of amnesia"; so, ketamine does not cause respiratory depression as much as opioids and also does not perturb the hemodynamic status as much. However, due to unwanted clinical experience of the patients (known as emergence reactions), it is strongly recommended that ketamine should *not be used solely* unless preceded by an amnestic agent (like one of the benzodiazepine family); otherwise, the patients would have a *very bad experience* from the effects of the drug; however, a number of studies have demonstrated fewer unwanted effects of ketamine when administered as the S(+)-ketamine isomer. Currently, smaller doses of the drug are used as a part of a multimodal analgesic regimen, especially for thoracic incisions, in such a way that the needed amount of other analgesic drugs, especially opioids, are decreased, possibly improving the respiratory function. Ketamine could be used through many different routes including intravenous or intravenous patient-controlled analgesia (IV or IV-PCA). Some studies have claimed an anti-inflammatory effect for ketamine in patients undergoing CPB, possibly through its mechanism of action: NMDA antagonism (Lahtinen et al. 2004; Michelet et al. 2007; Buvanendran and Kroin 2009; Suzuki 2009; Carstensen and Moller 2010; Mathews et al. 2012; Liu et al. 2017a).

17.8.4.2 Magnesium Sulfate ($MgSO_4$)

This ionic compound has gained frequent attention during recent years; its analgesic mechanism is mainly through calcium channel antagonism and NMDA antagonism; however, bolus doses of the drug could lead to asystole, and accumulation of the drug in the blood, "i.e., overdose," could lead to severe afterload reduction and, hence, hypotension. Anti-inflammatory effects of magnesium sulfate in patients undergoing CPB have been observed in a number of studies (Ferasatkish et al. 2008;

Buvanendran and Kroin 2009; Dabbagh et al. 2009, 2010, 2013; Aryana et al. 2014; Duan et al. 2015; Pearce et al. 2015; Fairley et al. 2017).

17.8.4.3 Gabapentin and Pregabalin

This is mainly an anticonvulsant agent belonging to a class of drugs known as "alpha-2-delta receptor modulators," also used for management of chronic pain; its mechanism of action is inhibition of glutamate release through NMDA antagonism. Gabapentin has been used for treatment of acute pain as an adjuvant in the multimodal analgesia regimen, with opioid-sparing effect goal; however, results are still inconclusive (Ucak et al. 2011; Ho et al. 2006; Fabritius et al. 2016). Pregabalin is also an anticonvulsant agent inhibiting the voltage-dependent calcium channel in CNS leading to inhibition of release of a number of agents including glutamate. Its use as an analgesic for acute pain suppression is off-label; though it is one of the agents used in multimodal analgesia regimen (Buvanendran and Kroin 2009; Dauri et al. 2009; Graterol and Linter 2012; Chang et al. 2014; Liu et al. 2017a).

17.8.5 Multimodal Analgesia

Multimodal or "balanced" analgesia is a method of analgesia which considers the multistep nature of pain. In acute pain management, this method involves administration of analgesics throughout the perioperative period; so pain management is performed through administration of more than one single drug (opioids plus non-opioids), or even we can add non-pharmacologic analgesia methods to our list of pharmacologic analgesics. Adjuvant analgesics (i.e., drugs in which their primary effect is not necessarily analgesia) and non-pharmacologic analgesia methods are mainly added to our battery of opioid compounds and the wide range of opioid administration. The main goals of multimodal analgesia are summarized as follows:

- Create additive analgesia from administration of different classes of analgesic methods.
- Decrease the dose of each analgesic modality.
- Experience less unwanted side effects of each drug or non-drug method.
- Counteract pain at different levels, i.e., at the level of CNS, spinal cord, peripheral nerves, wound site, etc.
- Decrease time duration of recovery from surgery (Kehlet and Dahl 1993; Kehlet et al. 2006; Buvanendran and Kroin 2009; Gandhi et al. 2011; Rafiq et al. 2014; Correll 2017; Liu et al. 2017a).

17.8.6 Patient-Controlled Analgesia

During the last decades, patient-controlled analgesia (PCA) has been proposed to replace the conventional method of analgesia prescription, in order to increase the efficacy of analgesic methods. Among its benefits, the following have been proposed:

- Increased patient autonomy
- Decreased time from pain sensation until the first dose of analgesics
- Increased concordance between analgesics and patient demands
- Decreased frequency of opioid complications including nausea and vomiting

There are a vast number of pro and con studies regarding the efficacy of the method. Compared with intramuscular analgesics, PCA is more effective; however, compared with nurse-administered intravenous (IV) analgesia or epidural PCA, it is not yet determined which method is more effective (Boldt et al. 1998; Dolin et al. 2002; Bainbridge et al. 2006; Hansdottir et al. 2006; Hudcova et al. 2006; Mota et al. 2010; McNicol et al. 2015).

In order to have a successful PCA, it is suggested to follow these considerations (Bainbridge et al. 2006; McNicol et al. 2015):

- As a standard, use a baseline analgesic infusion which should be added to PCA in order to prevent unwanted effects of delayed analgesia administration, meanwhile benefiting concomitant effective analgesia.
- Always consider baseline opioid dose; this baseline opioid, added to other analgesics, could increase the efficacy of pain management.
- Beware of respiratory depression which should be always considered as a potential risk.
- Apply a baseline-appropriate PCA dose accompanied with lockout interval, and adjust it for each patient.
- Try to increase patient cooperation as much as possible; insufficient patient cooperation leads to ineffectiveness of PCA; in case of impaired patient cooperation, PCA use should be discouraged.

17.9 Regional Anesthetic Techniques for Acute Pain Suppression in Cardiac Surgeries

There are a number of regional anesthetic techniques used for acute pain suppression in cardiac surgery patients, each having their benefits and drawbacks. These techniques include the following; however, they are not limited just to the following list:

- Infiltration of local anesthetic in wound
- Intercostal nerve block
- Intrapleural infiltration of local anesthetics
- Neuraxial analgesia (paravertebral, intrathecal, thoracic epidural)

17.9.1 Infiltration of Local Anesthetics in Wound

This is an effective method in cardiac surgery patients especially when used as an adjunct to other analgesic methods for controlling acute postoperative pain and administered as parasternal approach or, possibly, directly into the surgical wound; we could control sternotomy-related acute pain and also pain related to chest tubes and thoracic pain. This method has two characteristics in order to be effective for pain control:

- It is better to use this technique as "post-incision infiltration method" of local anesthetic; however, pre-incision local anesthetic infiltration is "equivocal," since acute postoperative pain in cardiac surgery patients is originated mainly from sternotomy.
- It should be used primarily in patients after sternotomy.

Infusion of local anesthetic directly into the surgical wound is another possible method, with tissue necrosis being the most common potential complication; however, cellulitis, infection, and tissue necrosis of the wound are very rare after cardiac surgery. In cardiac surgery patients, it is possible that the use of bilateral catheters for continuous infusion of local anesthetics could be even more effective, when used as a part of multimodal analgesia technique (Dowling et al. 2003; White et al. 2003; Chaney 2005a; McDonald et al. 2005; Kocabas et al. 2008; Buvanendran and Kroin 2009; Eljezi et al. 2012; Kossowsky et al. 2015; Ozturk et al. 2016).

17.9.2 Intercostal Nerve Block

Intercostal nerve block is a simple and efficient method for administration of local anesthetic agents into the intercostal neurovascular bundle(s), which could be an effective adjuvant analgesic method for acute postoperative pain suppression, causing pain temporal blockade; however, it would last between 6 and 12 h unless an indwelling catheter is placed adjacent to the intercostal nerves or repeated injections are needed. The block is better to be performed under direct vision, i.e., before chest closure by the surgeon or after the operation, by injecting the local anesthetics into intercostal nerves through the subcostal approach for each of the nerves. However, prophylactic administration (i.e., before surgical incision) is equivocal. Ropivacaine (0.5–0.75%) or bupivacaine (0.25–0.5%) is often used for this purpose (Barr et al. 2007; Chaudhary et al. 2012; Kossowsky et al. 2015).

17.9.3 Intrapleural Infiltration of Local Anesthetics

This method involves administration of local anesthetics between the visceral and parietal pleura. The main origin of pain is parietal pleura; however, the proposed mechanism of analgesia in this method is diffusion of local anesthetics in the potential space between the two pleural layers leading to diffusion of a very thin layer of local anesthetics distributed between the two pleura layers and, finally, blocking pain, though some studies are controversial regarding its clinical outcome. Local anesthetics may be administered as a single shot or continuous infusion through a catheter. The method has a number of limitations (Chaney 2005a, b; May and Bartram 2007; Ogus et al. 2007; Mansouri et al. 2011; Esme et al. 2012; Ziyaeifard et al. 2014; Yousefshahi et al. 2016):

- Intact anatomy and physiology of the pleural layers.
- If the patient has chest tubes, it may lead to leakage of local anesthetics into chest bottle.
- The lung is not damaged (e.g., after lung surgery).
- There is the possibility for systemic absorption of local anesthetics.

17.9.4 Neuraxial Blocks (Paravertebral, Intrathecal, Thoracic Epidural)

17.9.4.1 Thoracic Paravertebral Block

Thoracic paravertebral block is considered as one of the neuraxial analgesia techniques by some authors; being considered an old technique, it was reappraised just in the last two to three decades used for local anesthetic blockade though the paravertebral spaces, so, to some clinicians, it is not as much familiar as intrathecal and epidural techniques. Paravertebral spaces are located bilaterally, in each side; they are anatomically located lateral to the spine, where the nerve endings pass through them to go from spine to end in their related nerve fibers. Thoracic epidural analgesia is usually considered as the gold standard of care for acute postoperative pain management, namely, in some procedures like thoracic and cardiac surgeries, especially regarding cardiovascular and pulmonary outcomes; however, thoracic paravertebral block could be a good potential alternative when performed appropriately. The interested reader is referred to study the related referenced for the classic approach of Eason and Wyatt in performing thoracic paravertebral block; however, a summary of the technique is described and includes a step-by-step process:

- Placing the patient in sitting position with the spine being curved as a "C" letter or in lateral decubitus position, i.e., "fetal position"
- Using strict aseptic technique
- Finding and localizing the 6th cervical vertebra (C_6)
- Localizing the spinous process at the level of 4th thoracic vertebra (T_4)
- Going 3–6 cm laterally in horizontal direction
- Creating a local wheal by local anesthetics in awake patients
- Inserting the needle in a perpendicular direction
- Reaching the transverse process

- Walking downward and lateral until a sense of "loss of resistance" is reached
- Finally, injecting local anesthetic slowly

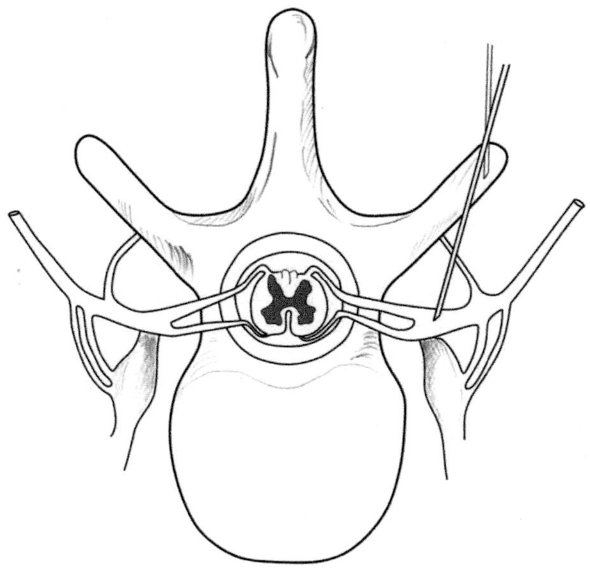

The main benefits of thoracic paravertebral block compared with thoracic epidural could be considered as:

- Being less invasive.
- Very lower risk for epidural hematoma formation.
- Less hemodynamic derangement (albeit some degrees of sympathetic block exists).
- Fewer contraindications.
- Easier technique.
- Lower incidence of complications (especially neurologic complications).
- Fewer reports of postoperative complications like nausea, vomiting, and urinary retention.
- Rare reports of systemic toxicity due to local anesthetics, though very high doses are used in this technique.
- Improved patient outcome especially regarding pulmonary function.
- Nowadays, application of ultrasound leads to increased safety and efficacy features of the block.

Some clinicians believe that bilateral thoracic paravertebral block is not as effective as thoracic epidural analgesia in suppressing acute pain-induced stress response, especially in major procedures like cardiac surgery, while there are others who believe exactly vice versa and consider thoracic paravertebral block as effective as, and even at times more effective than, thoracic epidural analgesia improving clinical outcomes with reduced rate of complications (Eason and Wyatt 1979; Richardson and Sabanathan 1995; Davies et al. 2006; Daly and Myles 2009; Scarci et al. 2010; Thavaneswaran et al. 2010; Richardson et al. 2011; Rawal 2012; Ding et al. 2014; Li and Halaszynski 2015; Okitsu et al. 2016; Yeung et al. 2016; Monico and Quiñónez 2017; Dabbagh 2014).

17.9.4.2 Spinal (Intrathecal) Analgesia

Postoperative analgesia through intrathecal (IT) administration of drugs is a very popular method among clinicians for non-cardiac surgeries of the abdominal and pelvic area and/or lower extremities used for more than 100 years. However, in cardiac surgeries, the idea of IT analgesia was first described in 1980 which included IT morphine administration (Mathews and Abrams 1980). Later, IT administration of local anesthetics was also used which was performed through lumbar interspaces accompanied with downward positioning of the patient (usually after induction of general anesthesia) to deliberately create a high level of spinal block. Theoretically, this method appeared effective, since spinal receptors of pain are located in substantia gelatinosa of Rolando, posterior horn of the spinal cord (Wu et al. 1999; Furue et al. 2004; Fujita and Kumamoto 2006; Ellenberger et al. 2017); hence the drug could attach the receptors with much easier access and higher efficacy than the intravenous route of drug administration of analgesics. Potential benefits of this method would be possibly:

- Improved postoperative analgesia with better quality of pain control
- Fewer postoperative respiratory problems
- Decreased level of postoperative stress response
- Improved clinical outcome

The first studies favored IT morphine usage for cardiac surgery, and even during the recent years, some studies approved it. These studies have usually administered a wide range of IT opioids "from 0.3 to 10 mg IT morphine as single shot" administered just before induction of general anesthesia, just after induction of anesthesia, or even during the early postoperative period; however, further studies have demonstrated that IT opioid for cardiac surgery could not suppress the level of stress response. Also, improved postoperative analgesia and decreased respiratory problems are gained at the expense of unwanted opioid effects in the postoperative period including pruritus, respiratory depression (early or delayed), urinary retention, nausea and vomiting, and delayed extubation. To the above, the fact that shorter-acting opioids are possibly less effective during the postoperative period should be added, shifting the choice for IT opioids to opioid compounds like morphine with a longer time profile in order to have adequate postoperative analgesia which at the same time would result in increased chance for postoperative opioid complications, especially delayed postoperative respiratory depression (which is usually due to delayed or cephalad migration of water-soluble opioids like morphine) and delayed extubation; also, we should add to the above items that the unwanted respiratory depression and delayed extubation are aggravated by concomitant use of other sedatives and anesthetics; besides, some other factors like underlying age could not be neglected; elderly people are at increased risk for unwanted postoperative respiratory depression of IT opioids (Chaney et al. 1997, 1999; Boulanger et al. 2002; Chaney 2005b, 2006, 2009; Dabbagh et al. 2011; Nigro Neto et al. 2014; Li and Halaszynski 2015; Tabatabaie et al. 2015; Xu et al. 2015a; Huang and Sakata 2016; Ellenberger et al. 2017; Hong et al. 2017).

On the other hand, IT administration of local anesthetics in a way to create high spinal levels of block covering the spinal thoracic nerve roots could create a sufficient sensory block to decrease the level of tress response; however, simultaneous widespread sympathetic block associated with this method leads to repeated episodes of hypotension and hemodynamic instability mandating administration of vasopressors and inotropes. Finally, most studies have claimed that benefits of IT local anesthetics could not clearly outweigh its risks. Besides, the effects of IT local anesthetics usually last shorter duration and often disappear or vanish during the early postoperative hours.

Finally, though the risk of neurologic complications (including epidural hematoma) is much lower in spinal technique compared to thoracic epidural technique, it is not negligible and could be as high as 1:1500 up to 1:220.000. Detailed discussion about prevention and management of this complication is presented just in the next pages, and the reader is addressed to refer there (Horlocker et al. 2010; Horlocker 2011b; Leffert et al. 2017).

In summary, creating analgesia through administration of IT opioids or IT local anesthetics in cardiac surgery patients could not improve the clinical outcome sharply and is not usually considered as a main analgesic method in such patients.

17.9.4.3 Thoracic Epidural Analgesia

Thoracic epidural analgesia (TEA) is considered by many as the "gold standard" of care for acute postoperative pain management in adult cardiac surgery mainly for nearly two decades, because of the following features:

- Adequate and qualitative analgesia (both intraoperative and postoperative).
- Efficient suppression of stress response (induced by CPB and the surgery).
- Thoracic sympathectomy which is relatively selective in TEA and does not involve total sympathetic block as seen in total spinal anesthesia.
- Improved myocardial blood flow (mainly due to thoracic sympathetic block which covers cardiac sympathetic nerves, T1–T5) and is claimed to be associated with increased diameter of the coronary arteries (especially the stenotic epicardial coronary arteries).
- Improved left ventricular function due to the previous item.
- Decreased level of myocardial ischemia mainly due to cardiac sympathetic block (T1–T5).
- Cardiac sympathetic blockade (T1–T5) would lead to decreased need for postoperative use of beta-blockers.
- Decreased incidence of cardiac arrhythmias mainly after improved myocardial perfusion status.

- Earlier postoperative extubation time comparable or even earlier than conventional general anesthesia mainly due to decreased need for rescue analgesia in postoperative period.
- Improved postoperative pulmonary function possibly due to decreased level of stress response, improved postoperative analgesia, improved patient ability for deep breathing, and earlier postoperative ambulation.
- The possibility to perform "awake" off-pump coronary bypass surgery or some other percutaneous valve replacements using TEA as the main anesthetic method (Karagoz et al. 2000; Schachner et al. 2003; Campos 2009; Royse 2009; Breivik et al. 2010; Watanabe et al. 2011; Karadeniz et al. 2013; Toda et al. 2013; Bektas and Turan 2015; Paliwal et al. 2016).

However, during the last years, some clinicians have seriously criticized TEA for cardiac surgery and questioned its validity as "gold standard of care" for cardiac surgery. Their reason is mainly the very serious associated risk of "epidural hematoma" which could heavily outweigh the above detailed list of benefits. The issue is that in patients undergoing cardiac surgery receiving very high doses of perioperative anticoagulants, and also under full systemic heparinization, TEA is potentially much more "risky" than all the other surgical patient groups. Based on a variety of studies, the risk of epidural hematoma after TEA for cardiac surgery is widely divergent, ranging from 1:1500 to 1:150,000, though in some patient groups, the risk is "increasing" as much as 1:3000 (upper). Also, during the postoperative period, when trying to normalize the coagulation profile in order to remove the catheter, there is an increased risk of thromboembolic events which should be considered as another potential complication (Chaney et al. 1997, 1999; Schwann and Chaney 2003; Chaney 2005a, b; Chaney and Labovsky 2005; Chaney 2006, 2009; Royse 2009; Breivik et al. 2010; Horlocker et al. 2010; Horlocker 2011b; Svircevic et al. 2011a, b; Rawal 2012; Li and Halaszynski 2015).

Most importantly, clinicians should have sophisticated care accompanied with vigilance and a very high degree of suspicion during early postoperative hours in order to be able to detect new onset epidural hematoma through surgical evacuation in its "golden time" of neurologic recovery. This golden time is good if less than 8 h, partial if between 8–24 h, and poor if no intervention is performed (Neal et al. 2008; Breivik et al. 2010; Horlocker 2011a). Occurrence of epidural hematoma is possible during needle introduction, bolus drug injection, catheter insertion, systemic heparinization period until restoration of coagulation profile, and finally during or after catheter removal; however, we have always to keep in mind that occurrence of epidural hematoma and its neurologic complications is a *catastrophe*.

Based on the 3rd version of the "American Society of Regional Anesthesia and Pain Medicine Evidence-Based Guideline: Regional Anesthesia in the Patient Receiving Antithrombotic or Thrombolytic Therapy" released in 2010 and also the 2009 version of "Nordic guidelines for neuraxial blocks in disturbed haemostasis" released by "the Scandinavian Society of Anaesthesiology and Intensive Care Medicine," the following items could help us prevent potential high-risk patients (Breivik et al. 2010; Horlocker et al. 2010; Horlocker 2011b):

- Underlying hemostatic disorders
- Dose and preoperative "drug-free" interval for anticoagulants
- Any preexisting anatomical disorders and malalignments in the spine, spinal cord, vertebrae, and spinal arteries and vessels
- Elderly
- Technical problems when introducing the epidural needle or the catheter
- Underlying liver or kidney disorders imposing patient to abnormal coagulation profile

Also, according to the 2010 American Society of Regional Anesthesia and Pain Medicine guideline and the 2009 the Scandinavian Society of Anaesthesiology and Intensive Care Medicine, the following recommendations should be kept in mind if there is the possibility of epidural hematoma after neuraxial block:

1. Do not use neuraxial blocks if the patient has a "known underlying coagulopathy" no matter what is the etiology.
2. If the epidural needle tap is traumatic, surgery should be postponed for at least 24 h.
3. Time interval from the end of the epidural technique (including needle tap, drug administration, etc.) until start of systemic heparinization should be at least more than 60 min.
4. The clinicians should adhere strictly to the administration doses of heparin and its reversal agents (try strictly to administer as low as possible doses of heparin which are adjusted for the "shortest duration" for the desired "therapeutic objective").
5. Removing the epidural catheter is permitted only when the coagulation profile tests are resumed to normal values; besides, catheter removal should be followed by strict control of signs and symptoms for any potential epidural hematoma (Neal et al. 2008; Breivik et al. 2010; Horlocker et al. 2010; Horlocker 2011a; b; Leffert et al. 2017).

17.10 Summary

The readers could find a summary of the analgesia methods (pharmacological and non-pharmacological) used for acute and chronic pain management in adult cardiac surgery.

References

Acharya M, Dunning J. Does the use of non-steroidal anti-inflammatory drugs after cardiac surgery increase the risk of renal failure? Interact Cardiovasc Thorac Surg. 2010;11:461–7.

Alzahrani T. Pain relief following thoracic surgical procedures: a literature review of the uncommon techniques. Saudi J Anaesth. 2017;11:327–31.

American Society of Anesthesiologists Task Force on Acute Pain Management. Practice guidelines for acute pain management in the perioperative setting: an updated report by the American

Society of Anesthesiologists Task Force on Acute Pain Management. Anesthesiology. 2012;116:248–73.
Anselmi L, Huynh J, Duraffourd C, Jaramillo I, Vegezzi G, Saccani F, Boschetti E, Brecha NC, De Giorgio R, Sternini C. Activation of mu opioid receptors modulates inflammation in acute experimental colitis. Neurogastroenterol Motil. 2015;27:509–23.
Aryana P, Rajaei S, Bagheri A, Karimi F, Dabbagh A. Acute effect of intravenous Administration of Magnesium Sulfate on serum levels of Interleukin-6 and tumor necrosis factor-alpha in patients undergoing elective coronary bypass graft with cardiopulmonary bypass. Anesth Pain Med. 2014;4:e16316.
Aslan FE, Badir A, Arli SK, Cakmakci H. Patients' experience of pain after cardiac surgery. Contemp Nurse. 2009;34:48–54.
Azzopardi S, Lee G. Health-related quality of life 2 years after coronary artery bypass graft surgery. J Cardiovasc Nurs. 2009;24:232–40.
Bainbridge D, Martin JE, Cheng DC. Patient-controlled versus nurse-controlled analgesia after cardiac surgery—a meta-analysis. Can J Anaesth. 2006;53:492–9.
Barletta JF. Clinical and economic burden of opioid use for postsurgical pain: focus on ventilatory impairment and ileus. Pharmacotherapy. 2012;32:12S–8S.
Barr AM, Tutungi E, Almeida AA. Parasternal intercostal block with ropivacaine for pain management after cardiac surgery: a double-blind, randomized, controlled trial. J Cardiothorac Vasc Anesth. 2007;21:547–53.
Bektas SG, Turan S. Does high thoracic epidural analgesia with levobupivacaine preserve myocardium? A prospective randomized study. Biomed Res Int. 2015;2015:658678.
Bell RF, Dahl JB, Moore RA, Kalso E. Perioperative ketamine for acute postoperative pain. Cochrane Database Syst Rev. 2006:CD004603.
Bigeleisen PE, Goehner N. Novel approaches in pain management in cardiac surgery. Curr Opin Anaesthesiol. 2015;28:89–94.
Blaudszun G, Lysakowski C, Elia N, Tramer MR. Effect of perioperative systemic alpha2 agonists on postoperative morphine consumption and pain intensity: systematic review and meta-analysis of randomized controlled trials. Anesthesiology. 2012;116:1312–22.
Bodnar RJ. Endogenous opiates and behavior: 2011. Peptides. 2012;38(2):463–522.
Boldt J, Thaler E, Lehmann A, Papsdorf M, Isgro F. Pain management in cardiac surgery patients: comparison between standard therapy and patient-controlled analgesia regimen. J Cardiothorac Vasc Anesth. 1998;12:654–8.
Bosilkovska M, Walder B, Besson M, Daali Y, Desmeules J. Analgesics in patients with hepatic impairment: pharmacology and clinical implications. Drugs. 2012;72:1645–69.
Boulanger A, Perreault S, Choiniere M, Prieto I, Lavoie C, Laflamme C. Intrathecal morphine after cardiac surgery. Ann Pharmacother. 2002;36:1337–43.
Breivik H, Bang U, Jalonen J, Vigfusson G, Alahuhta S, Lagerkranser M. Nordic guidelines for neuraxial blocks in disturbed haemostasis from the Scandinavian Society of Anaesthesiology and Intensive Care Medicine. Acta Anaesthesiol Scand. 2010;54:16–41.
Bruce J, Drury N, Poobalan AS, Jeffrey RR, Smith WC, Chambers WA. The prevalence of chronic chest and leg pain following cardiac surgery: a historical cohort study. Pain. 2003;104:265–73.
Buvanendran A, Kroin JS. Multimodal analgesia for controlling acute postoperative pain. Curr Opin Anaesthesiol. 2009;22:588–93.
Camilleri M, Lembo A, Katzka DA. Opioids in gastroenterology: treating adverse effects and creating therapeutic benefits. Clin Gastroenterol Hepatol. 2017;15:1338–49.
Campos JH. Fast track in thoracic anesthesia and surgery. Curr Opin Anaesthesiol. 2009;22:1–3.
Caputo M, Alwair H, Rogers CA, Pike K, Cohen A, Monk C, Tomkins S, Ryder I, Moscariello C, Lucchetti V, Angelini GD. Thoracic epidural anesthesia improves early outcomes in patients undergoing off-pump coronary artery bypass surgery: a prospective, randomized, controlled trial. Anesthesiology. 2011;114:380–90.
Carstensen M, Moller AM. Adding ketamine to morphine for intravenous patient-controlled analgesia for acute postoperative pain: a qualitative review of randomized trials. Br J Anaesth. 2010;104:401–6.

Chaney MA. How important is postoperative pain after cardiac surgery? J Cardiothorac Vasc Anesth. 2005a;19:705–7.

Chaney MA. Cardiac surgery and intrathecal/epidural techniques: at the crossroads? Can J Anaesth. 2005b;52:783–8.

Chaney MA. Intrathecal and epidural anesthesia and analgesia for cardiac surgery. Anesth Analg. 2006;102:45–64.

Chaney MA. Thoracic epidural anaesthesia in cardiac surgery—the current standing. Ann Card Anaesth. 2009;12:1–3.

Chaney MA, Labovsky JK. Thoracic epidural anesthesia and cardiac surgery: balancing postoperative risks associated with hematoma formation and thromboembolic phenomenon. J Cardiothorac Vasc Anesth. 2005;19:768–71.

Chaney MA, Furry PA, Fluder EM, Slogoff S. Intrathecal morphine for coronary artery bypass grafting and early extubation. Anesth Analg. 1997;84:241–8.

Chaney MA, Nikolov MP, Blakeman BP, Bakhos M. Intrathecal morphine for coronary artery bypass graft procedure and early extubation revisited. J Cardiothorac Vasc Anesth. 1999;13:574–8.

Chang CY, Challa CK, Shah J, Eloy JD. Gabapentin in acute postoperative pain management. Biomed Res Int. 2014;2014:631756.

Chaudhary V, Chauhan S, Choudhury M, Kiran U, Vasdev S, Talwar S. Parasternal intercostal block with ropivacaine for postoperative analgesia in pediatric patients undergoing cardiac surgery: a double-blind, randomized, controlled study. J Cardiothorac Vasc Anesth. 2012;26:439–42.

Chen LK, Wang MH, Yang HJ, Fan SZ, Chen SS. Prospective observational pharmacogenetic study of side effects induced by intravenous morphine for postoperative analgesia. Medicine. 2017a;96:e7009.

Chen Y, Qin Y, Li L, Chen J, Zhang X, Xie Y. Morphine can inhibit the growth of breast cancer MCF-7 cells by arresting the cell cycle and inducing apoptosis. Biol Pharm Bull. 2017b;40:1686–92.

Chou R, Gordon DB, de Leon-Casasola OA, Rosenberg JM, Bickler S, Brennan T, Carter T, Cassidy CL, Chittenden EH, Degenhardt E, Griffith S, Manworren R, McCarberg B, Montgomery R, Murphy J, Perkal MF, Suresh S, Sluka K, Strassels S, Thirlby R, Viscusi E, Walco GA, Warner L, Weisman SJ, Wu CL. Management of postoperative pain: a clinical practice guideline from the American Pain Society, the American Society of Regional Anesthesia and Pain Medicine, and the American Society of Anesthesiologists' Committee on Regional Anesthesia, Executive Committee, and Administrative Council. J Pain. 2016;17:131–57.

Correll D. Chronic postoperative pain: recent findings in understanding and management. F1000Res. 2017;6:1054.

Cruickshank M, Henderson L, MacLennan G, Fraser C, Campbell M, Blackwood B, Gordon A, Brazzelli M. Alpha-2 agonists for sedation of mechanically ventilated adults in intensive care units: a systematic review. Health Technol Assess. 2016;20:v–xx, 1–117.

Cuthbert AW. Lubiprostone targets prostanoid EP(4) receptors in ovine airways. Br J Pharmacol. 2011;162:508–20.

Dabbagh A. Clonidine: an old friend newly rediscovered. Anesth Pain. 2011;1:8–9.

Dabbagh A. Postoperative pain management in cardiac surgery. In: Dabbagh A, Esmailian F, Aranki S, editors. Postoperative critical care for cardiac surgical patients. 1st ed. New York: Springer; 2014. p. 257–94.

Dabbagh A, Rajaei S. The role of anesthetic drugs in liver apoptosis. Hepat Mon. 2013;13:e13162.

Dabbagh A, Elyasi H, Razavi SS, Fathi M, Rajaei S. Intravenous magnesium sulfate for postoperative pain in patients undergoing lower limb orthopedic surgery. Acta Anaesthesiol Scand. 2009;53:1088–91.

Dabbagh A, Rajaei S, Shamsolahrar MH. The effect of intravenous magnesium sulfate on acute postoperative bleeding in elective coronary artery bypass surgery. J Perianesth Nurs. 2010;25:290–5.

Dabbagh A, Moghadam SF, Rajaei S, Mansouri Z, Manaheji HS. Can repeated exposure to morphine change the spinal analgesic effects of lidocaine in rats? J Res Med Sci. 2011;16:1361–5.

Dabbagh A, Bastanifar E, Foroughi M, Rajaei S, Keramatinia AA. The effect of intravenous magnesium sulfate on serum levels of N-terminal pro-brain natriuretic peptide (NT pro-BNP) in elective CABG with cardiopulmonary bypass. J Anesth. 2013;27:693–8.
Daly DJ, Myles PS. Update on the role of paravertebral blocks for thoracic surgery: are they worth it? Curr Opin Anaesthesiol. 2009;22:38–43.
Dauri M, Faria S, Gatti A, Celidonio L, Carpenedo R, Sabato AF. Gabapentin and pregabalin for the acute post-operative pain management. A systematic-narrative review of the recent clinical evidences. Curr Drug Targets. 2009;10:716–33.
Davies RG, Myles PS, Graham JM. A comparison of the analgesic efficacy and side-effects of paravertebral vs epidural blockade for thoracotomy—a systematic review and meta-analysis of randomized trials. Br J Anaesth. 2006;96:418–26.
Derry S, Moore RA. Single dose oral celecoxib for acute postoperative pain in adults. Cochrane Database Syst Rev. 2012;3:CD004233.
Dick F, Hristic A, Roost-Krahenbuhl E, Aymard T, Weber A, Tevaearai HT, Carrel TP. Persistent sensitivity disorders at the radial artery and saphenous vein graft harvest sites: a neglected side effect of coronary artery bypass grafting procedures. Eur J Cardiothorac Surg. 2011;40: 221–6.
Ding X, Jin S, Niu X, Ren H, Fu S, Li Q. A comparison of the analgesia efficacy and side effects of paravertebral compared with epidural blockade for thoracotomy: an updated meta-analysis. PLoS One. 2014;9:e96233.
Djafarzadeh S, Vuda M, Takala J, Jakob SM. Effect of remifentanil on mitochondrial oxygen consumption of cultured human hepatocytes. PLoS One. 2012;7:e45195.
Dolin SJ, Cashman JN, Bland JM. Effectiveness of acute postoperative pain management: I. Evidence from published data. Br J Anaesth. 2002;89:409–23.
Dowling R, Thielmeier K, Ghaly A, Barber D, Boice T, Dine A. Improved pain control after cardiac surgery: results of a randomized, double-blind, clinical trial. J Thorac Cardiovasc Surg. 2003;126:1271–8.
Duan L, Zhang CF, Luo WJ, Gao Y, Chen R, Hu GH. Does magnesium-supplemented cardioplegia reduce cardiac injury? A meta-analysis of randomized controlled trials. J Card Surg. 2015;30:338–45.
Eason MJ, Wyatt R. Paravertebral thoracic block-a reappraisal. Anaesthesia. 1979;34:638–42.
Eftekhar-Vaghefi S, Esmaeili-Mahani S, Elyasi L, Abbasnejad M. Involvement of mu opioid receptor signaling in the protective effect of opioid against 6-hydroxydopamine-induced SH-SY5Y human neuroblastoma cells apoptosis. Basic Clin Neurosci. 2015;6:171–8.
Eljezi V, Duale C, Azarnoush K, Skrzypczak Y, Sautou V, Pereira B, Tsokanis I, Schoeffler P. The analgesic effects of a bilateral sternal infusion of ropivacaine after cardiac surgery. Reg Anesth Pain Med. 2012;37:166–74.
Ellenberger C, Sologashvili T, Bhaskaran K, Licker M. Impact of intrathecal morphine analgesia on the incidence of pulmonary complications after cardiac surgery: a single center propensity-matched cohort study. BMC Anesthesiol. 2017;17:109.
Esme H, Apiliogullari B, Duran FM, Yoldas B, Bekci TT. Comparison between intermittent intravenous analgesia and intermittent paravertebral subpleural analgesia for pain relief after thoracotomy. Eur J Cardiothorac Surg. 2012;41:10–3.
Fabritius ML, Geisler A, Petersen PL, Nikolajsen L, Hansen MS, Kontinen V, Hamunen K, Dahl JB, Wetterslev J, Mathiesen O. Gabapentin for post-operative pain management—a systematic review with meta-analyses and trial sequential analyses. Acta Anaesthesiol Scand. 2016;60:1188–208.
Fairley JL, Zhang L, Glassford NJ, Bellomo R. Magnesium status and magnesium therapy in cardiac surgery: a systematic review and meta-analysis focusing on arrhythmia prevention. J Crit Care. 2017;42:69–77.
Ferasatkish R, Dabbagh A, Alavi M, Mollasadeghi G, Hydarpur E, Moghadam AA, Faritus ZS, Totonchi MZ. Effect of magnesium sulfate on extubation time and acute pain in coronary artery bypass surgery. Acta Anaesthesiol Scand. 2008;52:1348–52.

Floettmann E, Bui K, Sostek M, Payza K, Eldon M. Pharmacologic profile of Naloxegol, a peripherally acting micro-opioid receptor antagonist, for the treatment of opioid-induced constipation. J Pharmacol Exp Ther. 2017;361:280–91.

Frampton C, Quinlan J. Evidence for the use of non-steroidal anti-inflammatory drugs for acute pain in the post anaesthesia care unit. J Perioper Pract. 2009;19:418–23.

Fujita T, Kumamoto E. Inhibition by endomorphin-1 and endomorphin-2 of excitatory transmission in adult rat substantia gelatinosa neurons. Neuroscience. 2006;139:1095–105.

Furue H, Katafuchi T, Yoshimura M. Sensory processing and functional reorganization of sensory transmission under pathological conditions in the spinal dorsal horn. Neurosci Res. 2004;48:361–8.

Gallagher R, McKinley S, Dracup K. Post discharge problems in women recovering from coronary artery bypass graft surgery. Aust Crit Care. 2004;17:160–5.

Gandhi K, Heitz JW, Viscusi ER. Challenges in acute pain management. Anesthesiol Clin. 2011;29:291–309.

Geng X, Zhao H, Zhang S, Li J, Tian F, Feng N, Fan R, Jia M, Guo H, Cheng L, Liu J, Chen W, Pei J. Kappa-opioid receptor is involved in the cardioprotection induced by exercise training. PLoS One. 2017;12:e0170463.

George JA, Lin EE, Hanna MN, Murphy JD, Kumar K, Ko PS, Wu CL. The effect of intravenous opioid patient-controlled analgesia with and without background infusion on respiratory depression: a meta-analysis. J Opioid Manag. 2010;6:47–54.

Graterol J, Linter SP. The effects of gabapentin on acute and chronic postoperative pain after coronary artery bypass graft surgery. J Cardiothorac Vasc Anesth. 2012;26:e26; author reply e26.

Griesdale DE, Neufeld J, Dhillon D, Joo J, Sandhu S, Swinton F, Choi PT. Risk factors for urinary retention after hip or knee replacement: a cohort study. Can J Anaesth. 2011;58:1097–104.

Guimaraes-Pereira L. Persistent postoperative pain and the problem of strictly observational research. Pain. 2016;157:1173–4.

Guimaraes-Pereira L, Farinha F, Azevedo L, Abelha F, Castro-Lopes J. Persistent postoperative pain after cardiac surgery: incidence, characterization, associated factors and its impact in quality of life. Eur J Pain. 2016a;20:1433–42.

Guimaraes-Pereira L, Valdoleiros I, Reis P, Abelha F. Evaluating persistent postoperative pain in one tertiary hospital: incidence, quality of life, associated factors, and treatment. Anesth Pain Med. 2016b;6:e36461.

Guimaraes-Pereira L, Reis P, Abelha F, Azevedo LF, Castro-Lopes JM. Persistent postoperative pain after cardiac surgery: a systematic review with meta-analysis regarding incidence and pain intensity. Pain. 2017;158:1869–85.

van Gulik L, Janssen LI, Ahlers SJ, Bruins P, Driessen AH, van Boven WJ, van Dongen EP, Knibbe CA. Risk factors for chronic thoracic pain after cardiac surgery via sternotomy. Eur J Cardiothorac Surg. 2011;40:1309–13.

Gunther T, Dasgupta P, Mann A, Miess E, Kliewer A, Fritzwanker S, Steinborn R, Schulz S. Targeting multiple opioid receptors—improved analgesics with reduced side effects? Br J Pharmacol. 2017.

Guo P, East L, Arthur A. A preoperative education intervention to reduce anxiety and improve recovery among Chinese cardiac patients: a randomized controlled trial. Int J Nurs Stud. 2012;49:129–37.

Hakim SM, Narouze SN. Risk factors for chronic saphenous neuralgia following coronary artery bypass graft surgery utilizing saphenous vein grafts. Pain Pract. 2015;15:720–9.

Hansdottir V, Philip J, Olsen MF, Eduard C, Houltz E, Ricksten SE. Thoracic epidural versus intravenous patient-controlled analgesia after cardiac surgery: a randomized controlled trial on length of hospital stay and patient-perceived quality of recovery. Anesthesiology. 2006;104:142–51.

Ho KY, Gan TJ, Habib AS. Gabapentin and postoperative pain—a systematic review of randomized controlled trials. Pain. 2006;126:91–101.

Holzer P. Non-analgesic effects of opioids: management of opioid-induced constipation by peripheral opioid receptor antagonists: prevention or withdrawal? Curr Pharm Des. 2012;18(37):6010–20.

Hong RA, Gibbons KM, Li GY, Holman A, Voepel-Lewis T. A retrospective comparison of intrathecal morphine and epidural hydromorphone for analgesia following posterior spinal fusion in adolescents with idiopathic scoliosis. Paediatr Anaesth. 2017;27:91–7.

Horlocker TT. Complications of regional anesthesia and acute pain management. Anesthesiol Clin. 2011a;29:257–78.

Horlocker TT. Regional anaesthesia in the patient receiving antithrombotic and antiplatelet therapy. Br J Anaesth. 2011b;107(Suppl 1):i96–106.

Horlocker TT, Wedel DJ, Rowlingson JC, Enneking FK, Kopp SL, Benzon HT, Brown DL, Heit JA, Mulroy MF, Rosenquist RW, Tryba M, Yuan CS. Regional anesthesia in the patient receiving antithrombotic or thrombolytic therapy: American Society of Regional Anesthesia and Pain Medicine Evidence-Based Guidelines (Third Edition). Reg Anesth Pain Med. 2010;35:64–101.

Hoshijima H, Takeuchi R, Kuratani N, Nishizawa S, Denawa Y, Shiga T, Nagasaka H. Incidence of postoperative shivering comparing remifentanil with other opioids: a meta-analysis. J Clin Anesth. 2016;32:300–12.

Huang AP, Sakata RK. Pain after sternotomy—review. Brazilian J Anesthesiol. 2016;66:395–401.

Hudcova J, McNicol E, Quah C, Lau J, Carr DB. Patient controlled opioid analgesia versus conventional opioid analgesia for postoperative pain. Cochrane Database Syst Rev. 2006:CD003348.

Hughes MM, Atayee RS, Best BM, Pesce AJ. Observations on the metabolism of morphine to hydromorphone in pain patients. J Anal Toxicol. 2012;36:250–6.

Ing Lorenzini K, Daali Y, Dayer P, Desmeules J. Pharmacokinetic-pharmacodynamic modelling of opioids in healthy human volunteers. A minireview. Basic Clin Pharmacol Toxicol. 2012;110:219–26.

International Pain Summit of the International Association for the Study of Pain. Declaration of Montreal: declaration that access to pain management is a fundamental human right. J Pain Palliat Care Pharmacother. 2011;25:29–31.

Ishii Y, Iida N, Miyauchi Y, Mackenzie PI, Yamada H. Inhibition of morphine glucuronidation in the liver microsomes of rats and humans by monoterpenoid alcohols. Biol Pharm Bull. 2012;35:1811–7.

Jabbary Moghaddam M, Ommi D, Mirkheshti A, Dabbagh A, Memary E, Sadeghi A, Yaseri M. Effects of clonidine premedication upon postoperative shivering and recovery time in patients with and without opium addiction after elective leg fracture surgeries. Anesth Pain Med. 2013;2:107–10.

Jalkut MK. Ketorolac as an analgesic agent for infants and children after cardiac surgery: safety profile and appropriate patient selection. AACN Adv Crit Care. 2014;25:23–30; quiz 31–22.

Jeleazcov C, Saari TI, Ihmsen H, Schuttler J, Fechner J. Changes in total and unbound concentrations of sufentanil during target controlled infusion for cardiac surgery with cardiopulmonary bypass. Br J Anaesth. 2012;109:698–706.

Karadeniz U, Ozturk B, Yavas S, Biricik D, Saydam GS, Erdemli O, Onan B, Onan IS, Kilickan L, Sanisoglu I. Effects of epidural anesthesia on acute and chronic pain after coronary artery bypass grafting. Biomed Res Int. 2013;28:248–53.

Karagoz HY, Sonmez B, Bakkaloglu B, Kurtoglu M, Erdinc M, Turkeli A, Bayazit K. Coronary artery bypass grafting in the conscious patient without endotracheal general anesthesia. Ann Thorac Surg. 2000;70:91–6.

Kehlet H, Dahl JB. The value of "multimodal" or "balanced analgesia" in postoperative pain treatment. Anesth Analg. 1993;77:1048–56.

Kehlet H, Jensen TS, Woolf CJ. Persistent postsurgical pain: risk factors and prevention. Lancet. 2006;367:1618–25.

Khan M, Fraser A. Cox-2 inhibitors and the risk of cardiovascular thrombotic events. Ir Med J. 2012;105:119–21.

Klockgether-Radke AP. F. W. Serturner and the discovery of morphine. 200 years of pain therapy with opioids. Anasthesiol Intensivmed Notfallmed Schmerzther. 2002;37:244–9.
Kocabas S, Yedicocuklu D, Yuksel E, Uysallar E, Askar F. Infiltration of the sternotomy wound and the mediastinal tube sites with 0.25% levobupivacaine as adjunctive treatment for postoperative pain after cardiac surgery. Eur J Anaesthesiol. 2008;25:842–9.
Komatsu R, Turan AM, Orhan-Sungur M, McGuire J, Radke OC, Apfel CC. Remifentanil for general anaesthesia: a systematic review. Anaesthesia. 2007;62:1266–80.
Kossowsky J, Donado C, Berde CB. Immediate rescue designs in pediatric analgesic trials: a systematic review and meta-analysis. Anesthesiology. 2015;122:150–71.
Kuip EJ, Zandvliet ML, Koolen SL, Mathijssen RH, van der Rijt CC. A review of factors explaining variability in fentanyl pharmacokinetics; focus on implications for cancer patients. Br J Clin Pharmacol. 2017;83:294–313.
Lahtinen P, Kokki H, Hendolin H, Hakala T, Hynynen M. Propacetamol as adjunctive treatment for postoperative pain after cardiac surgery. Anesth Analg. 2002;95:813–9, table of contents.
Lahtinen P, Kokki H, Hakala T, Hynynen M. S(+)-ketamine as an analgesic adjunct reduces opioid consumption after cardiac surgery. Anesth Analg. 2004;99:1295–301; table of contents.
Langford RM, Mehta V. Selective cyclooxygenase inhibition: its role in pain and anaesthesia. Biomed Pharmacother. 2006;60:323–8.
Ledowski T, Stein J, Albus S, MacDonald B. The influence of age and sex on the relationship between heart rate variability, haemodynamic variables and subjective measures of acute post-operative pain. Eur J Anaesthesiol. 2011;28:433–7.
Ledowski T, Reimer M, Chavez V, Kapoor V, Wenk M. Effects of acute postoperative pain on catecholamine plasma levels, hemodynamic parameters, and cardiac autonomic control. Pain. 2012;153:759–64.
Leffert LR, Dubois HM, Butwick AJ, Carvalho B, Houle TT, Landau R. Neuraxial anesthesia in obstetric patients receiving thromboprophylaxis with unfractionated or low-molecular-weight heparin: a systematic review of spinal epidural hematoma. Anesth Analg. 2017;125:223–31.
Leung K. [6-O-methyl-11C]Diprenorphine. 2004a.
Leung K. (20R)-4,5-alpha-Epoxy-17-methyl-3-hydroxy-6-[11C]methoxy-alpha,17-dimethyl-alpha- (2-phenylethyl)-6,14-ethenomorphinan-7-methanol. 2004b.
Li J, Halaszynski T. Neuraxial and peripheral nerve blocks in patients taking anticoagulant or thromboprophylactic drugs: challenges and solutions. Local Reg Anesth. 2015;8:21–32.
Liu SS, Wu CL. Effect of postoperative analgesia on major postoperative complications: a systematic update of the evidence. Anesth Analg. 2007;104:689–702.
Liu H, Ji F, Peng K, Applegate RL 2nd, Fleming N. Sedation after cardiac surgery: is one drug better than another? Anesth Analg. 2017a;124:1061–70.
Liu X, Xie G, Zhang K, Song S, Song F, Jin Y, Fang X. Dexmedetomidine vs propofol sedation reduces delirium in patients after cardiac surgery: a meta-analysis with trial sequential analysis of randomized controlled trials. J Crit Care. 2017b;38:190–6.
Loboz KK, Shenfield GM. Drug combinations and impaired renal function—the 'triple whammy'. Br J Clin Pharmacol. 2005;59:239–43.
Mahler DA. Opioids for refractory dyspnea. Expert Rev Respir Med. 2013;7:123–34; quiz 135.
Mansouri M, Bageri K, Noormohammadi E, Mirmohammadsadegi M, Mirdehgan A, Ahangaran AG. Randomized controlled trial of bilateral intrapleural block in cardiac surgery. Asian Cardiovasc Thorac Ann. 2011;19:133–8.
Mathews ET, Abrams LD. Intrathecal morphine in open heart surgery. Lancet. 1980;2:543.
Mugabure Bujedo B. A clinical approach to neuraxial morphine for the treatment of postoperative pain. Pain Res Treat. 2012;2012:612145.
Mathews TJ, Churchhouse AM, Housden T, Dunning J. Does adding ketamine to morphine patient-controlled analgesia safely improve post-thoracotomy pain? Interact Cardiovasc Thorac Surg. 2012;14:194–9.

Mota FA, Marcolan JF, Pereira MH, Milanez AM, Dallan LA, Diccini S. Comparison study of two different patient-controlled anesthesia regiments after cardiac surgery. Rev Bras Cir Cardiovasc. 2010;25:38–44.

Maund E, McDaid C, Rice S, Wright K, Jenkins B, Woolacott N. Paracetamol and selective and non-selective non-steroidal anti-inflammatory drugs for the reduction in morphine-related side-effects after major surgery: a systematic review. Br J Anaesth. 2011;106:292–7.

May G, Bartram T. Towards evidence based emergency medicine: best BETs from the Manchester Royal Infirmary. The use of intrapleural anaesthetic to reduce the pain of chest drain insertion. Emerg Med J. 2007;24:300–1.

McDaid C, Maund E, Rice S, Wright K, Jenkins B, Woolacott N. Paracetamol and selective and non-selective non-steroidal anti-inflammatory drugs (NSAIDs) for the reduction of morphine-related side effects after major surgery: a systematic review. Health Technol Assess. 2010;14:1–153, iii–iv.

McDonald SB, Jacobsohn E, Kopacz DJ, Desphande S, Helman JD, Salinas F, Hall RA. Parasternal block and local anesthetic infiltration with levobupivacaine after cardiac surgery with desflurane: the effect on postoperative pain, pulmonary function, and tracheal extubation times. Anesth Analg. 2005;100:25–32.

McNicol ED, Ferguson MC, Hudcova J. Patient controlled opioid analgesia versus non-patient controlled opioid analgesia for postoperative pain. Cochrane Database Syst Rev. 2015:CD003348.

McNicol ED, Ferguson MC, Haroutounian S, Carr DB, Schumann R. Single dose intravenous paracetamol or intravenous propacetamol for postoperative pain. Cochrane Database Syst Rev. 2016:CD007126.

Michelet P, Guervilly C, Helaine A, Avaro JP, Blayac D, Gaillat F, Dantin T, Thomas P, Kerbaul F. Adding ketamine to morphine for patient-controlled analgesia after thoracic surgery: influence on morphine consumption, respiratory function, and nocturnal desaturation. Br J Anaesth. 2007;99:396–403.

Moghadam MJ, Ommi D, Mirkheshti A, Shadnoush M, Dabbagh A. The effect of pretreatment with clonidine on propofol consumption in opium abuser and non-abuser patients undergoing elective leg surgery. J Res Med Sci. 2012;17:728–31.

Monico E, Quiñónez Z. Postoperative pain management in patients with congenital heart disease. In: Dabbagh A, Conte AH, Lubin L, editors. Congenital heart disease in pediatric and adult patients: anesthetic and perioperative management. 1st ed. New York: Springer; 2017. p. 871–87.

Neal JM, Bernards CM, Hadzic A, Hebl JR, Hogan QH, Horlocker TT, Lee LA, Rathmell JP, Sorenson EJ, Suresh S, Wedel DJ. ASRA practice advisory on neurologic complications in regional anesthesia and pain medicine. Reg Anesth Pain Med. 2008;33:404–15.

Nigro Neto C, do Amaral JL, Arnoni R, Tardelli MA, Landoni G. Intrathecal sufentanil for coronary artery bypass grafting. Braz J Anesthesiol. 2014;64:73–8.

Oehler B, Mohammadi M, Perpina Viciano C, Hackel D, Hoffmann C, Brack A, Rittner HL. Peripheral interaction of Resolvin D1 and E1 with opioid receptor antagonists for antinociception in inflammatory pain in rats. Front Mol Neurosci. 2017;10:242.

Ogus H, Selimoglu O, Basaran M, Ozcelebi C, Ugurlucan M, Sayin OA, Kafali E, Ogus TN. Effects of intrapleural analgesia on pulmonary function and postoperative pain in patients with chronic obstructive pulmonary disease undergoing coronary artery bypass graft surgery. J Cardiothorac Vasc Anesth. 2007;21:816–9.

van Ojik AL, Jansen PA, Brouwers JR, van Roon EN. Treatment of chronic pain in older people: evidence based choice of strong-acting opioids. Drugs Aging. 2012;29:615–25.

Okitsu K, Iritakenishi T, Iwasaki M, Imada T, Kamibayashi T, Fujino Y. Paravertebral block decreases opioid administration without causing hypotension during transapical transcatheter aortic valve implantation. Heart Vessel. 2016;31:1484–90.

Olofsen E, Boom M, Nieuwenhuijs D, Sarton E, Teppema L, Aarts L, Dahan A. Modeling the non-steady state respiratory effects of remifentanil in awake and propofol-sedated healthy volunteers. Anesthesiology. 2010;112:1382–95.

Owusu Obeng A, Hamadeh I, Smith M. Review of opioid pharmacogenetics and considerations for pain management. Pharmacotherapy. 2017;37:1105–21.
Ozaki N, Ishizaki M, Ghazizadeh M, Yamanaka N. Apoptosis mediates decrease in cellularity during the regression of Arthus reaction in cornea. Br J Ophthalmol. 2001;85:613–8.
Ozturk NK, Baki ED, Kavakli AS, Sahin AS, Ayoglu RU, Karaveli A, Emmiler M, Inanoglu K, Karsli B. Comparison of transcutaneous electrical nerve stimulation and parasternal block for postoperative pain management after cardiac surgery. Pain Res Manag. 2016;2016:4261949.
Paliwal B, Kamal M, Chauhan DS, Purohit A. Off-pump awake coronary artery bypass grafting under high thoracic epidural anesthesia. J Anaesthesiol Clin Pharmacol. 2016;32:261–2.
Papadopoulos N, Hacibaramoglu M, Kati C, Muller D, Floter J, Moritz A. Chronic poststernotomy pain after cardiac surgery: correlation of computed tomography findings on sternal healing with postoperative chest pain. Thorac Cardiovasc Surg. 2013;61(3):202–8.
Pearce A, Lockwood C, Van Den Heuvel C. The use of therapeutic magnesium for neuroprotection during global cerebral ischemia associated with cardiac arrest and cardiac bypass surgery in adults: a systematic review protocol. JBI Database System Rev Implement Rep. 2015;13:3–13.
Pergolizzi JV Jr, LeQuang JA, Berger GK, Raffa RB. The basic pharmacology of opioids informs the opioid discourse about misuse and abuse: a review. Pain Ther. 2017;6:1–16.
Peters ML, Sommer M, de Rijke JM, Kessels F, Heineman E, Patijn J, Marcus MA, Vlaeyen JW, van Kleef M. Somatic and psychologic predictors of long-term unfavorable outcome after surgical intervention. Ann Surg. 2007;245:487–94.
Pettersson PH, Jakobsson J, Owall A. Intravenous acetaminophen reduced the use of opioids compared with oral administration after coronary artery bypass grafting. J Cardiothorac Vasc Anesth. 2005;19:306–9.
Phillips SN, Fernando R, Girard T. Parenteral opioid analgesia: does it still have a role? Best Pract Res Clin Anaesthesiol. 2017;31:3–14.
Plein LM, Rittner HL. Opioids and the immune system—friend or foe. Br J Pharmacol. 2017.
Popping DM, Elia N, Marret E, Remy C, Tramer MR. Protective effects of epidural analgesia on pulmonary complications after abdominal and thoracic surgery: a meta-analysis. Arch Surg. 2008a;143:990–9; discussion 1000.
Popping DM, Zahn PK, Van Aken HK, Dasch B, Boche R, Pogatzki-Zahn EM. Effectiveness and safety of postoperative pain management: a survey of 18 925 consecutive patients between 1998 and 2006 (2nd revision): a database analysis of prospectively raised data. Br J Anaesth. 2008b;101:832–40.
Rachinger-Adam B, Conzen P, Azad SC. Pharmacology of peripheral opioid receptors. Curr Opin Anaesthesiol. 2011;24:408–13.
Rafiq S, Steinbruchel DA, Wanscher MJ, Andersen LW, Navne A, Lilleoer NB, Olsen PS. Multimodal analgesia versus traditional opiate based analgesia after cardiac surgery, a randomized controlled trial. J Cardiothorac Surg. 2014;9:52.
Ravven S, Bader C, Azar A, Rudolph JL. Depressive symptoms after CABG surgery: a meta-analysis. Harv Rev Psychiatry. 2013;21:59–69.
Rawal N. Epidural technique for postoperative pain: gold standard no more? Reg Anesth Pain Med. 2012;37:310–7.
Richardson J, Sabanathan S. Thoracic paravertebral analgesia. Acta Anaesthesiol Scand. 1995;39:1005–15.
Richardson J, Lonnqvist PA, Naja Z. Bilateral thoracic paravertebral block: potential and practice. Br J Anaesth. 2011;106:164–71.
Royse CF. High thoracic epidural anaesthesia for cardiac surgery. Curr Opin Anaesthesiol. 2009;22:84–7.
Saadat H, Ziai SA, Ghanemnia M, Namazi MH, Safi M, Vakili H, Dabbagh A, Gholami O. Opium addiction increases interleukin 1 receptor antagonist (IL-1Ra) in the coronary artery disease patients. PLoS One. 2012;7:e44939.
Sangesland A, Storen C, Vaegter HB. Are preoperative experimental pain assessments correlated with clinical pain outcomes after surgery? A systematic review. Scand J Pain. 2017;15:44–52.

Scarci M, Joshi A, Attia R. In patients undergoing thoracic surgery is paravertebral block as effective as epidural analgesia for pain management? Interact Cardiovasc Thorac Surg. 2010;10:92–6.
Schachner T, Bonatti J, Balogh D, Margreiter J, Mair P, Laufer G, Putz G. Aortic valve replacement in the conscious patient under regional anesthesia without endotracheal intubation. J Thorac Cardiovasc Surg. 2003;125:1526–7.
Schwann NM, Chaney MA. No pain, much gain? J Thorac Cardiovasc Surg. 2003;126:1261–4.
Scott LJ. Fentanyl iontophoretic transdermal system: a review in acute postoperative pain. Clin Drug Investig. 2016;36:321–30.
Servin F. Remifentanil; from pharmacological properties to clinical practice. Adv Exp Med Biol. 2003;523:245–60.
Servin FS. Update on pharmacology of hypnotic drugs. Curr Opin Anaesthesiol. 2008;21:473–7.
Servin FS, Billard V. Remifentanil and other opioids. Handb Exp Pharmacol. 2008:283–311.
Smith TH, Grider JR, Dewey WL, Akbarali HI. Morphine decreases enteric neuron excitability via inhibition of sodium channels. PLoS One. 2012;7:e45251.
Stenman M, Holzmann MJ, Sartipy U. Association between preoperative depression and long-term survival following coronary artery bypass surgery—a systematic review and meta-analysis. Int J Cardiol. 2016;222:462–6.
Stephens RS, Whitman GJ. Postoperative critical care of the adult cardiac surgical patient. Part I: routine postoperative care. Crit Care Med. 2015a;43:1477–97.
Stephens RS, Whitman GJ. Postoperative critical care of the adult cardiac surgical patient. Part II: procedure-specific considerations, management of complications, and quality improvement. Crit Care Med. 2015b;43:1995–2014.
Suzuki M. Role of N-methyl-D-aspartate receptor antagonists in postoperative pain management. Curr Opin Anaesthesiol. 2009;22:618–22.
Svircevic V, Nierich AP, Moons KG, Diephuis JC, Ennema JJ, Brandon Bravo Bruinsma GJ, Kalkman CJ, van Dijk D. Thoracic epidural anesthesia for cardiac surgery: a randomized trial. Anesthesiology. 2011a;114:262–70.
Svircevic V, van Dijk D, Nierich AP, Passier MP, Kalkman CJ, van der Heijden GJ, Bax L. Meta-analysis of thoracic epidural anesthesia versus general anesthesia for cardiac surgery. Anesthesiology. 2011b;114:271–82.
Swartjes M, Mooren RA, Waxman AR, Arout C, Van De Wetering K, Den Hartigh J, Beijnen JH, Kest B, Dahan A. Morphine induces hyperalgesia without involvement of mu-opioid receptor or morphine-3-glucuronide. Mol Med. 2012;18(1):1320–6.
Tabatabaie O, Matin N, Heidari A, Tabatabaie A, Hadaegh A, Yazdanynejad S, Tabatabaie K. Spinal anesthesia reduces postoperative delirium in opium dependent patients undergoing coronary artery bypass grafting. Acta Anaesthesiol Belg. 2015;66:49–54.
Talebi ZPH, Dabbagh A. Cellular and molecular mechanisms in perioperative hepatic protection: a review of current interventions. J Cell Mol Anesth. 2017;2:82–93.
Tanaka K, Kersten JR, Riess ML. Opioid-induced cardioprotection. Curr Pharm Des. 2014;20:5696–705.
Tejada MA, Montilla-Garcia A, Cronin SJ, Cikes D, Sanchez-Fernandez C, Gonzalez-Cano R, Ruiz-Cantero MC, Penninger JM, Vela JM, Baeyens JM, Cobos EJ. Sigma-1 receptors control immune-driven peripheral opioid analgesia during inflammation in mice. Proc Natl Acad Sci U S A. 2017;114:8396–401.
Thavaneswaran P, Rudkin GE, Cooter RD, Moyes DG, Perera CL, Maddern GJ. Brief reports: paravertebral block for anesthesia: a systematic review. Anesth Analg. 2010;110:1740–4.
Toda A, Watanabe G, Matsumoto I, Tomita S, Yamaguchi S, Ohtake H. Monitoring brain oxygen saturation during awake off-pump coronary artery bypass. Asian Cardiovasc Thorac Ann. 2013;21:14–21.
Tzortzopoulou A, McNicol ED, Cepeda MS, Francia MB, Farhat T, Schumann R. Single dose intravenous propacetamol or intravenous paracetamol for postoperative pain. Cochrane Database Syst Rev. 2011:CD007126.
Ucak A, Onan B, Sen H, Selcuk I, Turan A, Yilmaz AT. The effects of gabapentin on acute and chronic postoperative pain after coronary artery bypass graft surgery. J Cardiothorac Vasc Anesth. 2011;25:824–9.

Valdez-Morales E, Guerrero-Alba R, Ochoa-Cortes F, Benson J, Spreadbury I, Hurlbut D, Miranda-Morales M, Lomax AE, Vanner S. Release of endogenous opioids during a chronic IBD model suppresses the excitability of colonic DRG neurons. Neurogastroenterol Motil. 2013;25:39–46.e34.

Vosoughian M, Dabbagh A, Rajaei S, Maftuh H. The duration of spinal anesthesia with 5% lidocaine in chronic opium abusers compared with nonabusers. Anesth Analg. 2007;105:531–3.

Walker SM, Yaksh TL. Review article: neuraxial analgesia in neonates and infants: a review of clinical and preclinical strategies for the development of safety and efficacy data. Anesth Analg. 2012;115:638–62.

Watanabe G, Tomita S, Yamaguchi S, Yashiki N. Awake coronary artery bypass grafting under thoracic epidural anesthesia: great impact on off-pump coronary revascularization and fast-track recovery. Eur J Cardiothorac Surg. 2011;40:788–93.

White PF, Rawal S, Latham P, Markowitz S, Issioui T, Chi L, Dellaria S, Shi C, Morse L, Ing C. Use of a continuous local anesthetic infusion for pain management after median sternotomy. Anesthesiology. 2003;99:918–23.

Whiteside GT, Boulet JM, Walker K. The role of central and peripheral mu opioid receptors in inflammatory pain and edema: a study using morphine and DiPOA ([8-(3,3-diphenylpropyl)-4-oxo-1-phenyl-1,3,8-triaza-spiro[4.5]dec-3-yl]-acetic acid). J Pharmacol Exp Ther. 2005;314:1234–40.

Wolf AR. Effects of regional analgesia on stress responses to pediatric surgery. Paediatr Anaesth. 2012;22:19–24.

Wu SY, Dun SL, Wright MT, Chang JK, Dun NJ. Endomorphin-like immunoreactivity in the rat dorsal horn and inhibition of substantia gelatinosa neurons in vitro. Neuroscience. 1999;89:317–21.

Xie N, Khabbazi S, Nassar ZD, Gregory K, Vithanage T, Anand-Apte B, Cabot PJ, Sturgess D, Shaw PN, Parat MO. Morphine alters the circulating proteolytic profile in mice: functional consequences on cellular migration and invasion. FASEB J. 2017;31(12):5208–16.

Xu JT, Sun L, Lutz BM, Bekker A, Tao YX. Intrathecal rapamycin attenuates morphine-induced analgesic tolerance and hyperalgesia in rats with neuropathic pain. Transl Perioper Pain Med. 2015a;2:27–34.

Xu ZZ, Kim YH, Bang S, Zhang Y, Berta T, Wang F, Oh SB, Ji RR. Inhibition of mechanical allodynia in neuropathic pain by TLR5-mediated A-fiber blockade. Nat Med. 2015b;21:1326–31.

Yamanaka T, Sadikot RT. Opioid effect on lungs. Respirology. 2013;18:255–62.

Yeung JH, Gates S, Naidu BV, Wilson MJ, Gao SF. Paravertebral block versus thoracic epidural for patients undergoing thoracotomy. Cochrane Database Syst Rev. 2016;2:CD009121.

Yousefshahi F, Predescu O, Colizza M, Asenjo JF. Postthoracotomy Ipsilateral shoulder pain: a literature review on characteristics and treatment. Pain Res Manag. 2016;2016:3652726.

Zhang K, Li M, Peng XC, Wang LS, Dong AP, Shen SW, Wang R. The protective effects of Sufentanil pretreatment on rat brains under the state of cardiopulmonary bypass. Iran J Pharm Res. 2015a;14:559–66.

Zhang X, Zhao X, Wang Y. Dexmedetomidine: a review of applications for cardiac surgery during perioperative period. J Anesth. 2015b;29:102–11.

Zhang R, Xu B, Zhang MN, Zhang T, Wang ZL, Zhao G, Zhao GH, Li N, Fang Q, Wang R. Peripheral and central sites of action for anti-allodynic activity induced by the bifunctional opioid/NPFF receptors agonist BN-9 in inflammatory pain model. Eur J Pharmacol. 2017;813:122–9.

Zheng H, Schnabel A, Yahiaoui-Doktor M, Meissner W, Van Aken H, Zahn P, Pogatzki-Zahn E. Age and preoperative pain are major confounders for sex differences in postoperative pain outcome: a prospective database analysis. PLoS One. 2017;12:e0178659.

Ziesenitz VC, Vaughns JD, Koch G, Mikus G, van den Anker J. Pharmacokinetics of fentanyl and its derivatives in children: a comprehensive review. Clin Pharmacokinet. 2018;57(2):125–49.

Ziyaeifard M, Azarfarin R, Golzari SE. A review of current analgesic techniques in cardiac surgery. Is epidural worth it? J Cardiovasc Thorac Res. 2014;6:133–40.

18 Postoperative Considerations of Cardiopulmonary Bypass in Adult Cardiac Surgery

Mahnoosh Foroughi

Abstract

Development of the cardiopulmonary bypass (CPB) technology in the second half of the twentieth century was one of the most important medical advances and has been the main part of cardiac surgery as a routine procedure. Providing a completely motionless, bloodless heart is the main goal of CPB. CPB fulfills the role of the heart (and lungs) by preserving the systemic circulation and gas exchange.

Since the first initial machine, evolution from cross-sectional technique till to minimal extracorporeal circulation continues. The practice of cardiac surgery with CPB is safe and effective (but not perfect). CPB is a non-physiologic state and could cause multi-organ dysfunction. Although it simplifies cardiac surgery, CPB by itself induces a systemic inflammatory response syndrome, mostly due to blood contact with artificial surfaces. It activates complement, leukocyte, coagulation and fibrinolytic cascade, upregulation of proinflammatory cytokines, and production of oxygen free radicals and alters nitric oxide metabolism. Nearly all organs can be affected by these inflammatory mediators. In majority of patients these changes are asymptomatic due to adequate physiologic reserve. With improved knowledge in pathophysiology of CPB effects, efforts led to make new extracorporeal technology with less side effects.

The first section describes the structural parts of CPB. The second section discusses about the CPB effects on vital organs.

Keywords

Cardiopulmonary bypass circuit structures · History · Blood circuit · Cardiotomy Membrane oxygenator · Anticoagulation · Cannulation · Cardioplegia · Heat exchanger · Arterial filter · Minimal invasive extracorporeal circulation

M. Foroughi, M.D.
Cardiovascular Research Center, Shahid Beheshti University of Medical Sciences, Tehran, Iran
e-mail: m_foroughi@sbmu.ac.ir

A. Dabbagh et al. (eds.), *Postoperative Critical Care for Adult Cardiac Surgical Patients*, https://doi.org/10.1007/978-3-319-75747-6_18

Ultrafiltration · Cardiopulmonary bypass-related complications · Inflammation
Hematologic effect · CPB and Kidney · CPB and Lung · CPB and CNS · Off-pump coronary artery bypass

18.1 Cardiopulmonary Bypass Circuit Structure

18.1.1 History

In spite of other fields of surgery, cardiac surgery was suspended for centuries due to lack of knowledge and technology. The lack of its requirements was the cause of this slow and delayed evolution:

1. Inability to preserve systemic circulation and gas exchange independent to heart contraction and lung function, respectively
2. Need to preserve systemic anticoagulation that could be reversed at the end of the operation (insufficient knowledge about blood group types, transfusion, heparin, and protamine)

The introduction of the heart-lung machine in 1953 and development of CPB are among the most important advances in medicine to permit cardiac surgery. It has become a standard part of cardiac operations to make possible the surgical correction of intracardiac diseases, with a good example of competent team working requirement (surgeon, perfusionist and anesthesiologist).

Its development had a prolonged evolution way from concept of extracorporeal circulation (Le Gallois in 1813) to the hopeless Theodor Billroth attitude in 1881 “No surgeon who wished to preserve the respect of his colleagues would ever attempt to suture a wound of the heart” to the first heart surgery using CPB by John Gibbon in 1953, to the present trend of minimal extracorporeal circulation, assist devices, and total artificial hearts.

The CPB machine is an equipment that provides mechanical circulatory function of the heart and lungs. The machine consists of pumps, membrane oxygenator, venous and arterial cannula, tubing, reservoir cardiotomy, and heat exchanger. This section discusses in brief the parts of CPB system for better understanding of issues related to post-cardiac surgery problems (Hessel 2015).

18.1.2 Blood Circuit

In normal condition, blood enters the heart in the right atrium and passes through the right ventricle. The blood leaves the heart into the lungs where carbon dioxide is extracted from the blood and substituted by oxygen. Then the blood is sent back into the left atrium, enters into the left ventricle, and is injected into the aorta where it transfers to the systemic circulation.

The CPB acts nearly the same performance outside of the body. At the beginning of the operation, polyvinyl chloride or silicone tubing is primed by crystalloid solution. Colloid solutions, mannitol, sodium bicarbonate, heparin, and sometimes blood are prime additives. Venous line removes blood by means of gravity or vacuum from right side of the heart and returns it in oxygenated form to the systemic circulation via arterial line by pump. Pump acts like a ventricle. The two most common types are roller and centrifugal pumps.

18.1.2.1 Roller Pump

This pump consists of two rollers placed on the ends of a rotating arm, opposite to each other. The roller rotates and engages the tubing which is then compressed against the pump's housing. It pushes the blood ahead and forward continuous flow is induced (Fig. 18.1). It has occlusive nature and generates shear stress.

The flow rate is determined by the diameter of the tubing and the rotation rate of the rollers (per minute). It is not dependent on preload and afterload changes. The flow rate of 2–2.4 L/m^2/min is sufficient for adequate systemic perfusion, with consideration of patient's temperature. Optimal perfusion targets remain to be in controversy, but it is recommended to preserve mean arterial pressure of 50–70 mmHg, CVP < 5 mmHg, hematocrit more than 20%, and mixed venous saturation > 65% during CPB (Gravlee 2008; Saczkowski et al. 2012).

18.1.2.2 Centrifugal Pump

In plastic housing, a complex of nested cones are coupled magnetically to an electric motor. They rotate rapidly; by creating a pressure gradient between the inlet and outlet of the pump, kinetic energy is transferred to blood resulting in forward blood flow (Fig. 18.2). This pump is used less often than roller pump. The flow rate is dependent on preload and afterload. In spite of roller pump, centrifugal pump is nonocclusive and has less shear stress disturbance.

Some studies have shown that centrifugal pump is associated with less trauma to blood elements and postoperative neurologic complications (Asante-Siaw et al. 2006; Gravlee 2008; Saczkowski et al. 2012).

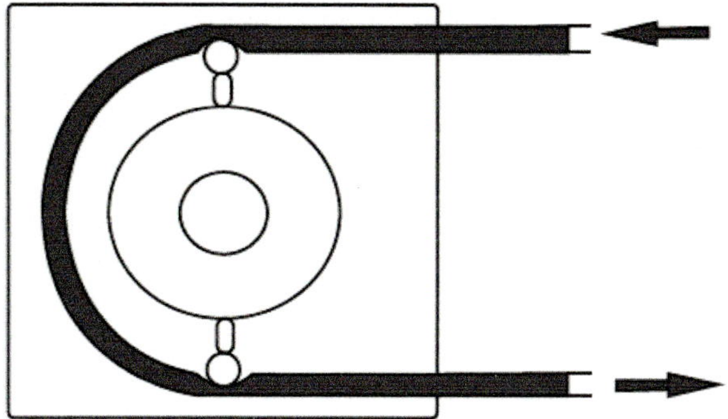

Fig. 18.1 Roller pump (Foroughi 2014)

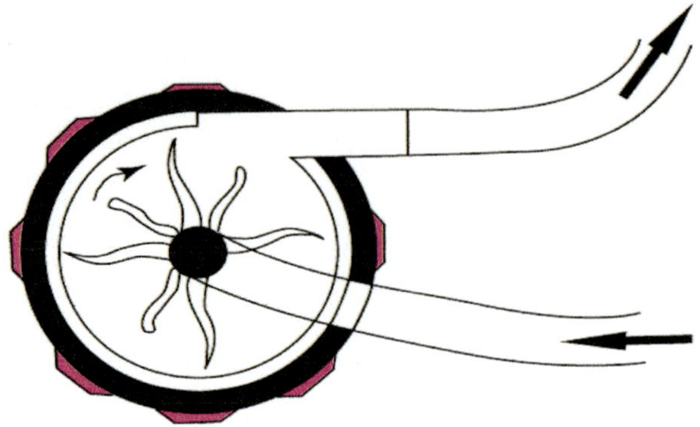

Fig. 18.2 Centrifugal pump

18.1.3 Cardiotomy

A filtered reservoir collects blood drained from the venous circulation. It is for storage, defoaming, and filtration before pumped to oxygenator and arterial circuit. Fluid, blood products, and medication may also be added.

Reservoir design may be open or closed systems. The open system (solid container) has graduated lines that show blood volume in the container. The design is open to atmosphere, allowing blood interface with atmosphere gases. In the closed system, the soft collapsible bag eliminates the air-blood interface. Volume is measured by weight or by changes in radius of the container (Stammers and Trowbridge 2008).

18.1.4 Membrane Oxygenator

Membrane oxygenator is equivalent to lung. A flat sheet of hollow fibers imitates the pulmonary capillary function, by interposing a thin membrane interface between blood and gases, without mixture. Gas flows through the hollow fiber and blood flow is around the fiber. In spite of carbon dioxide, oxygen is not diffusible in plasma well, so the blood is spread very thin to facilitate the transfer of oxygen by increased gradient pressure (Stammers and Trowbridge 2008; Hessel 2015).

18.1.5 Anticoagulation

Adequate anticoagulation is the integral part of CPB to maintain blood fluidity, avoidance of coagulation factor consumption, and thrombosis. Unfractionated heparin is used to achieve adequate systemic anticoagulation, by measuring activated clotting time (ACT) ≥400 s. It remains the absolute choice of anticoagulant drug in cardiac surgery. Heparin is obtained from animal tissues (bovine lung and porcine intestine). It doesn't have anticoagulant properties itself but could potentiate the effects of antithrombin III (AT), a potent endogenous anticoagulant in the body.

Heparin is given in the bolus dose of 2.5–4 mg/kg to aim an ACT of 400–600 s, before aortic and venous cannulation. For adequate anticoagulation state additional heparin is repeated to maintain ACT above 400 s during CPB.

An inadequate response of ACT to high doses of heparin (heparin resistance) may be seen in patients with AT deficiency (such as long preoperative heparin use, liver disease, congenital AT deficiency). This condition is corrected by fresh frozen plasma or recombinant AT administration.

At the end of operation, after CPB weaning heparin is reversed by protamine (isolated from fish sperm) to establish normal hemostasis condition after surgery. There are some ways to determine the protamine dose: protamine titration, fixed dose of protamine (in the ratio of 1–1.5 mg for 100 units of heparin previously administrated), ACT/heparin dose–response curve, and heparin concentration.

Protamine has a mild anticoagulant effect too and inhibits platelet-induced aggregation. Although protamine has a short half-life, care should be taken not to infuse too fast as it can induce systemic hypotension due to systemic vasodilation and pulmonary vasoconstriction.

Heparin rebound, a state of recurrent anticoagulant activity of heparin after adequate protamine administration, contributes to postoperative bleeding. Because not all of heparin is bounded to protamine, some of it binds to other plasma proteins and vascular cells, and reappears in circulation gradually.

Direct thrombin inhibitor is recommended in patients who should not receive heparin such as heparin-induced thrombocytopenic setting (Hessel 2015; Sniecinski and Levy 2015; Rehfeldt and Barbara 2016).

18.1.6 Cannulation

Cannula is made from clear polyvinyl chloride; the oxygenator casing and connections are from polycarbonate. Arterial and venous cannulation sites are influenced by the planned operation. In routine valve and coronary surgeries, the ascending aorta and right atrium are selected. Alternative arterial cannulation sites are the femoral artery, axillary artery, and left ventricular apex. Cannulation site for venous access can be the inferior and superior vena cava, femoral vein, and internal jugular vein (Hessel 2015; Ren et al. 2015).

18.1.7 Cardioplegia

A blood-free and motionless operative field is obtained by potassium-based cardioplegic solution. It causes diastolic electromechanical arrest. In addition to stop electrical and consequently mechanical activation, other main goals are preserving myocardial function and attenuating ischemic-reperfusion injury. Combination of electromechanical arrest and hypothermia reduces oxygen consumption up to 97%. Cardioplegic solution can be categorized according to the type of solution (crystalloid vs. bloody), temperature (cold vs. tepid), infusion type (antegrade into aortic root vs. retrograde through coronary sinus), and infusion interval (continuous vs. intermittent vs. single dose). There is no consensus about optimal choice of cardioplegia (Baikoussis et al. 2015; Gong et al. 2015).

18.1.8 Heat Exchanger

The heat exchanger is used in combination with the oxygenator. This device is typically placed just before the oxygenator, to prevent bubble forming in the blood too. Heat exchanger controls the body temperature through cooling or warming the blood passing the circuit, at the beginning and end of CPB, respectively. In heat exchanger, the blood and water lines are separated by a metallic barrier. As the water temperature is changed, the blood temperature which enters the body circulation and the tissue temperature change. There is a consensus on hypothermic protective effect for organ protection during ischemic period. Hypothermia reduces oxygen consumption and metabolic rate. Even mild hypothermic condition can increase brain tolerance against ischemic injury. However hypothermia is associated with side effects such as induced coagulopathy, free radical generation, metabolic acidosis, and leftward shift of oxygen-hemoglobin dissociation curve. Depending on the type of operation, the patient's temperature may be kept normothermic to less than 20 °C. Monitoring the blood temperature during the operation, and the speed and temperature of rewarming, is mandatory. Rewarming too great or too quickly may make important problems. Hyperthermia during rewarming period is known to increase ischemic damages especially in the brain and kidney (Baikoussis et al. 2015; Hessel 2015).

18.1.9 Arterial Filter

Inclusion of arterial filter in CPB circuit is used to reduce embolic events and improve neurologic outcome after cardiac surgery. Arterial filter with 20–40 μm porous screen holds air bubble, particles of platelet aggregation, and thrombus during CPB (De Somer 2012; DeFoe et al. 2014).

18.1.10 Minimal Invasive Extracorporeal Circulation

Minimal invasive extracorporeal circulation (MiECC) is an alternative option to conventional CPB. It consists of membrane oxygenator, centrifugal pump, short heparin-coated closed circuit, heat exchanger, venous bubble gas detector, and arterial filter. Priming volume is reduced. There is no cardiotomy suction and venous reservoir, and the blood-air interface is limited, while conventional CPB circuit is an open circuit because of blood-air free contact. The shed blood is washed through cell-saving device before return to arterial line.

It seems that these differences lead to attenuation of the adverse effect of conventional CPB: less inflammatory response, reduced hemodilution (less need to blood transfusion), and less changes in hemostasis system. Some studies showed that cardiac surgery with MiECC is associated with less postoperative neurologic deficit, less postoperative bleeding, and improved end-organ protection (Hessel 2015; Anastasiadis et al. 2016; Ganushchak et al. 2016).

18.1.11 Ultrafiltration

At the beginning of CPB, acute hemodilution is an inevitable event, as there is a mixture of patients' blood with crystalloid priming fluid of CPB circuit. Although hemodilution decreases blood viscosity and facilitates tissue perfusion in hypothermic setting, studies have shown that intraoperative hematocrit less than 20% is associated with disturbance in oxygen-carrying capacity, interstitial edema (decreased oncotic pressure) in vital organs, and increased mortality.

Ultrafiltration removes plasma water and low-molecular-weight materials from blood to a filtrate part under hydrostatic pressure through a hollow fiber semipermeable membrane. It reverses excessive hemodilution during pump and need for blood transfusion. It attenuates systemic inflammatory response by removing inflammatory mediators. Several studies have shown improvement in pulmonary compliance and shorter time on mechanical ventilation with ultrafiltration.

There are three types of ultrafiltration. Conventional ultrafiltration is done during CPB and hemoconcentration causes less blood reservoir volume after CPB. If the patient is in stable hemodynamic condition, modified ultrafiltration is performed after CPB weaning to concentrate circulating blood and remaining reservoir volume. Zero-balance ultrafiltration is done after rewarming during CPB. Filtrated volume is replaced by the balanced electrolyte solution. It corrects electrolytes and acid-base balance, and removes inflammatory mediators in the setting of constant blood volume (Wang et al. 2012; Foroughi et al. 2014; Landis et al. 2014).

18.2 Cardiopulmonary Bypass-Related Complications

The practice of cardiac surgery with CPB is safe and effective (but not perfect). CPB is a non-physiologic state and could cause multi-organ dysfunction. In the majority of patients these changes are asymptomatic due to adequate physiologic reserve.

18.2.1 Inflammation

Blood contact with synthetic surface of CPB circuit can promote whole-body systemic inflammatory response that plays an important role in multi-organ failure. Continuous exposure of heparinized blood to artificial surfaces in the perfusion circuit and nonendothelial cells in the wound could activate complement anaphylatoxins, adhesion molecules, proinflammatory cytokines, vasoactive substances, coagulation, and fibrinolytic cascades. In addition, ischemic reperfusion injury (due to aortic clamp, myocardial ischemia, cardioplegic arrest, and declamping), endotoxemia (due to splanchnic hypoperfusion), hypothermia, surgical trauma, bleeding, and blood transfusion may contribute to activation of inflammatory cascade. Accumulation of activated neutrophil is responsible for initiating the release of inflammatory mediators that have negative impact on all organs. The severity of this exaggerated response can range from subclinical state to severe complications (respiratory failure, coagulopathy, arrhythmias, and organ dysfunction).

There are suggested strategies to limit and attenuate inflammatory response, though there is not a consensus regarding their clinical outcome and benefits; these include heparin-coated circuit, steroids, hemofiltration, leukocyte depletion, minimized extracorporeal circulation, aprotinin, complement inhibitors, free radical scavengers, statins, and antioxidants (Landis et al. 2014; Hessel 2015; Zakkar et al. 2015; Ebrahimi et al. 2016).

18.2.2 CPB and Hematologic Effect

All blood elements have been impressed during CPB by different cascades. Close interaction of coagulation and inflammatory system aggregates this effect. Prolonged pump time and influence of biomaterial substances in surface area of CPB have the most effect on the severity of humoral and cellular activation. In coagulation system, reduction in platelet count and function, platelet activation, dilution, and consumption of coagulation factors and increased activity in fibrinolytic field occur. Blood contact with artificial and non-physiologic surfaces of CPB circuit makes intrinsic coagulation pathway activation. Extrinsic coagulation pathway is activated in pericardial blood, which is usually aspirated and returned to pump circulation. In addition to mechanical trauma to red blood cell and increased fragility of cell elements by shear stress force, mixture of patients' blood with priming solution brings to a significant hemodilution in the beginning of CPB.

There are strategies to decrease these responses: heparin-coated CPB circuit, corticosteroids, leukocyte filter, and ultrafiltration (Ranucci 2015; Ebrahimi et al. 2016).

18.2.3 CPB and Kidney

There is no consensus in the definition of acute kidney injury (AKI) after cardiac surgery; its prevalence has been reported between 1 and 30%, according to definitions used for AKI. Postoperative need to renal replacement therapy is a serious complication; it increases patient mortality as much as 50%.

Attention to preventable causes, early detection, and treatment are among the valuable issues for prevention of AKI after cardiac surgery.

After cardiac surgery, only minimal changes of serum creatinine as small as 0.3 mg/dL or 25% increase over baseline could predict adverse prognosis, even it remains in normal range or recovers to baseline. For active management to prevent further progression, there is a narrow period of reversibility shortly after insult. Early detection of AKI is an opportunity to improve clinical outcome. Delay from injury to diagnosis and after established AKI could be an explanation of limited success for AKI treatment.

Kidney function is usually evaluated by serum creatinine and urinary output. But they are poor indicators during acute stage of AKI. Rise in serum creatinine indicates the significant reduction of glomerular filtration rate, but it occurs slowly in 2–3 days after proved injury. It could be changed by nonrenal factors as age, muscle mass, protein intake, fever, trauma, and medication. It is not a specific and sensitive marker during early stages of kidney injury. Multiple studies have suggested that NGAL (neutrophil gelatinase-associated lipocalin) is a sensitive biomarker that shows proximal tubular damage as early as 2 h after the event. It can be used as a reliable biomarker for diagnosis of acute kidney injury in post-cardiac surgery. Other experimental biomarkers of AKI are cystatin C, interleukin18, and kidney injury molecule-1 (KIM-1).

The most important causes of AKI during CPB, which overlap, and consequences of multiple pathways are:

1. Hemodynamic insults (perioperative low cardiac output, hypovolemic state, and vasoconstriction)
2. Ischemic reperfusion injury and release of inflammatory agents
3. Embolic events (both gaseous and particulate)
4. Patient-related predisposing factors (left ventricular dysfunction, emergent surgery, preexisting kidney dysfunction, advanced age, nephrotoxic agents, preoperative anemia, blood transfusion, and need to IABP)

CPB per se is responsible for decreased renal blood flow and GFR due to nonpulsatile flow. Other factors that are related to CPB include duration of CPB time and cross-clamp time, hemolysis, and hemodilution.

1. *Duration of CPB and cross-clamp:* The consequences of prolonged CPB are extension of hypoperfusion time and release of more inflammatory mediators.
2. *Hemolysis:* Hemolysis is the result of prolonged CPB time, cardiotomy suction, overocclusion roller pump, blood exposure to artificial surface, and shear forces.
3. *Hemodilution:* Because of priming solution in CPB tubes, hemodilution is an inevitable event. It is suggested that hemodilution improves regional blood flow (by reduction of blood viscosity) in the setting of hypothermia and hypoperfusion. Although it was thought that improvement in regional blood flow compensates the risk of acute anemia (loss of O_2-carrying capacity of blood), recent studies have expressed that intraoperative hematocrit less than 20% is an independent risk factor for postoperative AKI. Kidneys receive 20% of cardiac

output. Highly metabolic renal medulla has limited reserve and is more sensitive to hemodynamic insults (anemia and hypoperfusion).

Type of operation has an effect on AKI. Among adult cardiac surgeries, coronary artery bypass graft (CABG) has the lowest incidence of AKI, while the combination of CABG and valve surgery is the highest risk factor.

Perioperative hemodynamic optimization is the key to renoprotection. Modifiable factors that reduce the risk of AKI are pulsatile CPB, preserved mean arterial pressure ≥ 60 mmHg (and higher threshold in diabetic and hypertensive patients) during CPB, prevention of excessive hemodilution, shorter duration of CPB, adequate pump flow (to improve O_2 delivery), retrograde autologous priming, decreased prime volume, optimal glucose control, euvolemia, prevention of low cardiac output to preserve adequate renal perfusion pressure, and avoidance of nephrotic agents.

There is no specific therapy to prevent and treat AKI. Several studies have shown that mannitol, dopamine, $NaHCO_3$, N-acetylcysteine, fenoldopam and ultrafiltration have no renal protective effects (Foroughi et al. 2014; Ho et al. 2015; Kramer et al. 2015; Long et al. 2015; Hu et al. 2016)

18.2.4 CPB and Lung

Pulmonary dysfunction and prolonged ventilation after cardiac surgery are well-known problems and important causes of morbidity. It occurs due to combined effects of anesthesia, surgical trauma, and CPB. Its pathophysiology is complex and multifactorial:

1. Inadequate lung perfusion
2. Ischemic-reperfusion injury
3. Change in respiratory mechanics (pleural opening and lack of chest wall integrity)
4. Hyperoxemia
5. Blood product transfusion
6. Blood contact with artificial surfaces of CPB circuit
7. Local and systemic inflammatory reaction

The pulmonary blood flow is stopped during aortic cross-clamp period and the lung perfusion is limited to bronchial arterial system. This ischemic insult can exaggerate the damaging effect of other factors.

Studies have shown that neutrophil accumulation in lung during CPB, its activation, release of chemical mediators, and proteolytic enzymes are in charge of lung injury. In addition to inflammation response, volume overload during CPB plays an important role in accumulation of interstitial fluid in lung too. It was shown that prolonged CPB time, aortic valve surgery, and combined valve/CABG procedures are independent factors of postoperative respiratory failure. The clinical importance of this injury has a range from subclinical atelectasis to ARDS. During CPB there is some degree of lung edema, atelectasis, increased alveolar-arterial oxygen gradient, abnormal gas exchange, increased intrapulmonary shunting, and decreased lung compliance.

There are some therapeutic interventions to prevent or attenuate pulmonary dysfunction, such as off-pump surgery, corticosteroid administration, leukocyte filter, biocompatible circuit, ultrafiltration, continuous ventilation during CPB, maintaining lung perfusion during CPB, pump time reduction, use of MiECC, and modifying ventilator setting from traditional to lung-protective strategies (by lower tidal volume to 6–8 cm^3/kg, FIO_2 below 0.40, higher PEEP to 8–12 cmH_2O, and increased respiratory rate) (Young 2014; Al Jaaly et al. 2015; Lellouche et al. 2015).

18.2.5 CPB and CNS

Neurologic abnormalities including stroke (prolonged or permanent focal neurologic deficit) and postoperative cognitive dysfunction are relatively common problems despite improvement in anesthetic and surgical techniques. Cognitive disorder, a transient decrease in baseline performance, is the most notable complication after adult cardiac surgery (up to 50% of patients during the first week after surgery) by the same mechanisms.

The patient-related factors that predict neurocognitive impairment are:

1. Peripheral vascular disease
2. Diabetes mellitus
3. History of cerebrovascular disease
4. High transfusion requirement
5. Urgent operation
6. Type of surgery (coronary bypass, valvular operation, or aortic arch surgery)
7. Age
8. Postoperative atrial fibrillation

CPB-related mechanisms include:

1. Macro- or microemboli (gas, atheromatous plaque, inorganic and biologic debris from open cardiac procedures)
2. Systemic inflammatory response
3. Perioperative hypoperfusion and low cardiac state
4. Extensive aortic calcification
5. Prolonged CPB time
6. Hemorrhage
7. Cerebral hyperthermia

The majority of strokes are due to embolic event, and watershed component is seen in few patients. The most atheromatous embolic event happens during manipulation of atherosclerotic aorta (cannulation, cross clamp, and declamping). Its consequences are crack or rupture of atherosclerotic plaque leading to debris release, cerebral embolization, and ischemic brain injury. Aortic clamping in the presence of exophytic plaque is contraindicated, and elimination of CPB is recommended in this condition. It is suggested that epiaortic ultrasonography be used to identify atheromatous plaque and help to select the suitable site for aortic cannulation in the diseased ascending aorta. It is more sensitive than digital palpation and transesophageal echocardiography, and gives information about the entire length of the ascending aortic wall. Epiaortic ultrasonography can affect the rate of stroke whenever operative strategies are changed.

Cerebral autoregulatory mechanism is functional during CPB. Blood pressure outside the regulatory range would be associated with adverse outcome.

In patients who have impaired autoregulatory mechanism in cerebral circulation (such as old, diabetic, and hypertensive patients), prolonged period of hypoperfusion is a well-known predisposing factor of ischemic events.

Maintaining higher mean arterial pressure (80–90 mmHg) is recommended in these patients during CPB.

Neurologic monitoring is important during cardiac surgery. Near-infra red spectroscopy can be used to assess cerebral perfusion adequacy during cardiac surgery. Whenever cerebral hypoperfusion is detected, hemodynamic management could be achieved by increased pump flow, increased perfusion pressure, and blood transfusion.

Decrease and increase in temperature of brain (during cooling and rewarming period) happen more quickly than other parts of the body because of the well-perfused state. Rapid rewarming at the end of CPB can lead to cerebral hyperthermia and exacerbated neurologic dysfunction.

During complex aortic arch surgery, neurologic complication is less associated in antegrade cerebral perfusion (through right axillary artery and or right common carotid artreycannulation) than retrograde cerebral perfusion and deep hypothermic circulatory arrest.

Those who experienced stroke during 24 h of CPB had adverse outcome in contrast to late presentation, delayed stroke. The majority of strokes happen after initial normal neurologic recovery of CPB.

Prevention of microemboli is accomplished by the use of membrane oxygenator, prevention of air entering the circuit, and use of a microfilter that will effectively trap microemboli and prevent from reentering the bloodstream (Ganavati et al. 2009; Goto and Maekawa 2014; Ono et al. 2014; Scott et al. 2014; Fraser et al. 2015).

18.2.6 Off-Pump Coronary Artery Bypass

In an attempt to decrease the negative effects of CPB, off-pump coronary artery bypass (OPCAB) on the beating heart was suggested as a solution and less invasive option from the early 1990s.

It is important to balance the advantages/disadvantages of OPCAB vs. CPB. During CPB, activation of physiologic mechanisms (due to blood contact with artificial surfaces of bypass circuit, surgical trauma, and ischemic reperfusion injury) is the cause of systemic inflammatory response, affecting multiple-organ systems. This response is significantly less in OPCAB operations.

Coagulopathy and activation of fibrinolytic cascade attributed largely to CPB do not happen in OPCAB patients. There is less blood loss and transfusion requirement in OPCAB operations. Better preservation of renal function is seen in OPCAB patients by prevention of renal hypopersufion and non-pulsatile flow in CPB state. Even in patients with chronic kidney disease, OPCAB operation is associated with less hospital mortality and need for renal replacement therapy.

There is better myocardial protection and rapid recovery in OPCAB. It offers no aortic cross clamp and cardiac arrest. Using of intracoronary shunt maintains blood flow to distal part of coronary artery during surgery. However, there is no convincing difference with regard to short-term mortality and postoperative MI.

OPCAB patients with preexisting pulmonary disease have better postoperative clinical course. It may be interpreted by more inflammatory reactions in the lung and fluid retention observed with CPB operations. The protective effect of OPCAB in end-organ function and safer outcome profile was shown in reoperative surgeries.

There is no trend for reduction in neurologic complication (embolic stroke and cognitive dysfunction) in OPCAB patients. It may be related to side-biting aortic clamp used for proximal anastomoses and embolization risk from atherosclerotic plaque. To reduce postoperative neurologic events in the presence of diseased ascending aorta, OPCAB with total arterial revascularization (no-touch aortic technique) was described to preclude aortic manipulation.

The concerns about OPCAB are incomplete revascularization, less grafts per patients, suboptimal anastomoses and graft patency, hemodynamic instability during operation, and increased coronary re-intervention. It is a challenging technique, and requires more time and experience with a long learning curve that may compromise long-term patient's outcome.

It is not recommended for small, intramyocardial coronary arteries and moderate aortic or mitral regurgitation. When coronary surgery is indicated in acute coronary syndrome, on-pump beating heart surgery is a more effective option. Decompression of ventricles by CPB reduces myocardial oxygen consumption, while OPCAB surgery prevents global myocardial ischemia by avoiding aortic cross clamp.

Although CABG using CPB is the standard surgical treatment for ischemic heart disease, studies have shown that in experienced hands and in high-volume OPCAB centers the outcome parameters are comparable, effective, and safe as on-pump surgery. It may be acceptable and beneficial in selected moderate- to high-risk patients (Euroscore ≥ 5) (Afilalo et al. 2012; Møller et al. 2012; Sepehripour et al. 2014; Puskas et al. 2015; Kowalewski et al. 2016).

Bibliography

Afilalo J, Rasti M, Ohayon SM, Shimony A, Eisenberg MJ. Off-pump vs. on-pump coronary artery bypass surgery: an updated meta-analysis and meta-regression of randomized trials. Eur Heart J. 2012;33:1257–67.

Al Jaaly E, Zakkar M, Fiorentino F, Angelini GD. Pulmonary protection strategies in cardiac surgery: are we making any progress? Oxidative Med Cell Longev. 2015;2015:416235.

Anastasiadis K, Murkin J, Antonitsis P, Bauer A, Ranucci M, Gygax E, Schaarschmidt J, Fromes Y, Philipp A, Eberle B. Use of minimal invasive extracorporeal circulation in cardiac surgery: principles, definitions and potential benefits. A position paper from the minimal invasive extracorporeal technologies international society (MiECTiS). Interact Cardiovasc Thorac Surg. 2016;22(5):647–62.

Asante-Siaw J, Tyrrell J, Hoschtitzky A, Dunning J. Does the use of a centrifugal pump offer any additional benefit for patients having open heart surgery? Interact Cardiovasc Thorac Surg. 2006;5:128–34.

Baikoussis NG, Papakonstantinou NA, Verra C, Kakouris G, Chounti M, Hountis P, Dedeilias P, Argiriou M. Mechanisms of oxidative stress and myocardial protection during open-heart surgery. Ann Card Anaesth. 2015;18:555.

De Somer F. Evidence-based used, yet still controversial: the arterial filter. J Extra Corpor Technol. 2012;44:P27.

DeFoe GR, Dame NA, Farrell MS, Ross CS, Langner CW, Likosky DS. Embolic activity during in vivo cardiopulmonary bypass. J Extra Corpor Technol. 2014;46:150.

Ebrahimi L, Kheirandish M, Foroughi M. The effect of methylprednisolone treatment on fibrinolysis, the coagulation system, and blood loss in cardiac surgery. Turkish J Med Sci. 2016;46:1645–54.

Foroughi M. Postoperative considerations of cardiopulmonary bypass in adult cardiac surgery. In: Postoperative critical care for cardiac surgical patients. Berlin: Springer; 2014. p. 295–311.

Foroughi M, Argani H, Hassntash S, Hekmat M, Majidi M, Beheshti M, Mehdizadeh B, Yekani B. Lack of renal protection of ultrafiltration during cardiac surgery: a randomized clinical trial. J Cardiovasc Surg. 2014;55:407–13.

Fraser J, Bannon PG, Vallely MP. Neurologic injury and protection in adult cardiac and aortic surgery. J Cardiothorac Vasc Anesth. 2015;29:185–95.

Ganavati A, Foroughi M, Esmaeili S, Hasantash S, Bolourain A, Shahzamani M, Beheshti MM, Hekmat M, Rangbar KT, Aahi E. The relation between post cardiac surgery delirium and intraoperative factors. Iran J Surg. 2009;17(3):16–25.

Ganushchak Y, Körver E, Yamamoto Y, Weerwind P. Versatile minimized system-a step towards safe perfusion. Perfusion. 2016;31:295–9.

Gong B, Ji B, Sun Y, Wang G, Liu J, Zheng Z. Is microplegia really superior to standard blood cardioplegia? The results from a meta-analysis. Perfusion. 2015;30:375–82.

Goto T, Maekawa K. Cerebral dysfunction after coronary artery bypass surgery. J Anesth. 2014;28:242–8.

Gravlee GP. Cardiopulmonary bypass: principles and practice. Philadelphia: Lippincott Williams & Wilkins; 2008.

Hessel EA. History of cardiopulmonary bypass (CPB). Best Pract Res Clin Anaesthesiol. 2015;29:99–111.

Ho J, Tangri N, Komenda P, Kaushal A, Sood M, Brar R, Gill K, Walker S, MacDonald K, Hiebert BM. Urinary, plasma, and serum biomarkers' utility for predicting acute kidney injury associated with cardiac surgery in adults: a meta-analysis. Am J Kidney Dis. 2015;66:993–1005.

Hu J, Chen R, Liu S, Yu X, Zou J, Ding X. Global incidence and outcomes of adult patients with acute kidney injury after cardiac surgery: a systematic review and meta-analysis. J Cardiothorac Vasc Anesth. 2016;30:82–9.

Kowalewski M, Pawliszak W, Malvindi PG, Bokszanski MP, Perlinski D, Raffa GM, Kowalkowska ME, Zaborowska K, Navarese EP, Kolodziejczak M. Off-pump coronary artery bypass grafting improves short-term outcomes in high-risk patients compared with on-pump coronary artery bypass grafting: meta-analysis. J Thorac Cardiovasc Surg. 2016;151:60–77.e58.

Kramer RS, Herron CR, Groom RC, Brown JR. Acute kidney injury subsequent to cardiac surgery. J Extra Corpor Technol. 2015;47:16.

Landis RC, Brown JR, Fitzgerald D, Likosky DS, Shore-Lesserson L, Baker RA, Hammon JW. Attenuating the systemic inflammatory response to adult cardiopulmonary bypass: a critical review of the evidence base. J Extra Corpor Technol. 2014;46:197–211.

Lellouche F, Delorme M, Bussières J, Ouattara A. Perioperative ventilatory strategies in cardiac surgery. Best Pract Res Clin Anaesthesiol. 2015;29:381–95.

Long D, Jenkins E, Griffith K. Perfusionist techniques of reducing acute kidney injury following cardiopulmonary bypass: an evidence-based review. Perfusion. 2015;30:25–32.

Møller CH, Penninga L, Wetterslev J, Steinbrüchel DA, Gluud C. Off-pump versus on-pump coronary artery bypass grafting for ischaemic heart disease. Cochrane Database Syst Rev. 2012;(3):CD007224.

Ono M, Brady K, Easley RB, Brown C, Kraut M, Gottesman RF, Hogue CW. Duration and magnitude of blood pressure below cerebral autoregulation threshold during cardiopulmonary bypass is associated with major morbidity and operative mortality. J Thorac Cardiovasc Surg. 2014;147:483–9.

Puskas JD, Martin J, Cheng DC, Benussi S, Bonatti JO, Diegeler A, Ferdinand FD, Kieser TM, Lamy A, Mack MJ. ISMICS consensus conference and statements of randomized controlled trials of off-pump versus conventional coronary artery bypass surgery. Innovations. 2015;10:219–29.

Ranucci M. Hemostatic and thrombotic issues in cardiac surgery. Semin Thromb Hemost. 2015;41(1):84–90.

Rehfeldt KH, Barbara DW. Cardiopulmonary bypass without heparin. In: Seminars in cardiothoracic and vascular anesthesia. Los Angeles, CA: Sage; 2016. p. 40–51.

Ren Z, Wang Z, Hu R, Wu H, Deng H, Zhou Z, Hu X, Jiang W. Which cannulation (axillary cannulation or femoral cannulation) is better for acute type a aortic dissection repair? A meta-analysis of nine clinical studies. Eur J Cardiothorac Surg. 2015;47:408–15.

Saczkowski R, Maklin M, Mesana T, Boodhwani M, Ruel M. Centrifugal pump and roller pump in adult cardiac surgery: a meta-analysis of randomized controlled trials. Artif Organs. 2012;36:668–76.

Scott DA, Evered LA, Silbert BS. Cardiac surgery, the brain, and inflammation. J Extra Corpor Technol. 2014;46:15–22.

Sepehripour AH, Harling L, Ashrafian H, Casula R, Athanasiou T. Does off-pump coronary revascularization confer superior organ protection in re-operative coronary artery surgery? A meta-analysis of observational studies. J Cardiothorac Surg. 2014;9:115.

Sniecinski RM, Levy JH. Anticoagulation management associated with extracorporeal circulation. Best Pract Res Clin Anaesthesiol. 2015;29:189–202.

Stammers AH, Trowbridge CC. Principles of oxygenator function: Gas exchange, heat transfer, and operation. In: Cardiopulmonary bypass: principles and practice. 2nd ed. Philadelphia: Lippincott Williams & Wilkins; 2008. p. 47–62.

Wang S, Palanzo D, Ündar A. Current ultrafiltration techniques before, during and after pediatric cardiopulmonary bypass procedures. Perfusion. 2012;27:438–46.

Young RW. Prevention of lung injury in cardiac surgery: a review. J Extra Corpor Technol. 2014;46:130–41.

Zakkar M, Ascione R, James A, Angelini G, Suleiman M. Inflammation, oxidative stress and postoperative atrial fibrillation in cardiac surgery. Pharmacol Ther. 2015;154:13–20.

Postoperative Care of Adult Cardiac Transplant Patients

19

Paul A. Perry and Fardad Esmailian

Abstract

Cardiac transplantation remains the definitive therapy for end-stage heart failure. Meticulous postoperative management is essential for optimizing successful outcomes in this relatively complex patient cohort. While the critical care considerations of heart transplant recipients are largely similar to that of other cardiac surgery patients, there exist important transplant-specific factors which require attention.

This chapter provides a concise overview of post-transplant critical care. Key topics include initial evaluation, operative considerations, post-transplant physiology, hemodynamic management, dysrhythmias, immunosuppression, and organ-system based assessment and optimization.

Keywords

Transplant · Immunosuppression · Endomyocardial · Orthotopic heart transplantation · Donor Organ Considerations · Posttransplant monitoring · Primary graft dysfunction · Rhythm disturbances · Coagulopathy · Hemorrhage · Heart and kidney transplantation · Hepatotoxicity · Infection · Outcome

P. A. Perry, M.D. (✉)
University of California, Davis, Davis, CA, USA
e-mail: paperry@ucdavis.edu

F. Esmailian, M.D.
Department of Surgery, Cedars-Sinai Heart Institute, Los Angeles, CA, USA

Heart Transplantation, Cedars-Sinai Heart Institute, Los Angeles, CA, USA

A. Dabbagh et al. (eds.), *Postoperative Critical Care for Adult Cardiac Surgical Patients*, https://doi.org/10.1007/978-3-319-75747-6_19

19.1 Introduction

Heart failure remains the definitive therapy for end-stage heart failure. While the critical care management following heart transplantation is largely similar to that of other cardiac surgical patients, there are many important differences that can drastically affect postoperative management. It is important for critical care providers involved with heart transplantation to have a firm knowledge of these unique characteristics. It is also imperative that all involved practitioners embrace a multidisciplinary "heart-transplant team" approach with frequent and effective communication with other providers to ensure optimal care delivery for this relatively complex patient population (Costanzo et al. 2010). This chapter reviews posttransplant critical care with an emphasis on unique characteristics of heart transplantation relative to other cardiac surgical patients.

19.2 Historical Background

The first successful human heart transplant was performed by Dr. Christiaan Barnard in Cape Town, South Africa, on December 3, 1967 (Barnard 1967). This was followed by the world's first pediatric heart transplant 3 days later at Maimonides Hospital in Brooklyn, New York, by Dr. Adrian Kantrowitz, though the recipient expired just 19 days later. The first adult heart transplant in the United States was accomplished the following month by Dr. Norman Shumway at Stanford University Hospital.

Despite these early pioneering efforts, the extensive challenges and poor outcomes associated with the procedure limited early enthusiasm and adoption. Significant early challenges included surgical technique, methods of donor-organ preservation, predicting immunoreactivity, and managing immunosuppression. Through the 1970s substantial efforts were made, largely by Dr. Shumway and colleagues at Stanford, to refine the procedure. Advances including endomyocardial biopsy, improved surgical technique, and emergence of cyclosporine A had a profound effect on improving outcomes (Caves et al. 1973; Oyer et al. 1983). Thus, by the early 1980s the procedure was well positioned to gain traction with the wider medical community and there was a substantial resurgence in enthusiasm for heart transplantation. Over the ensuing decade there were impressive increases in the number of transplants being performed and the number of centers providing them. Heart transplant volumes eventually leveled out to approximately 3000–4000 implants per year and have stayed relatively constant since that time, largely due to limits in organ availability (Lund et al. 2015).

19.3 Surgical Considerations

19.3.1 Operative Technique

Orthotopic heart transplantation operations are typically performed using either the "bicaval" or "biatrial" technique, with the bicaval method being much more

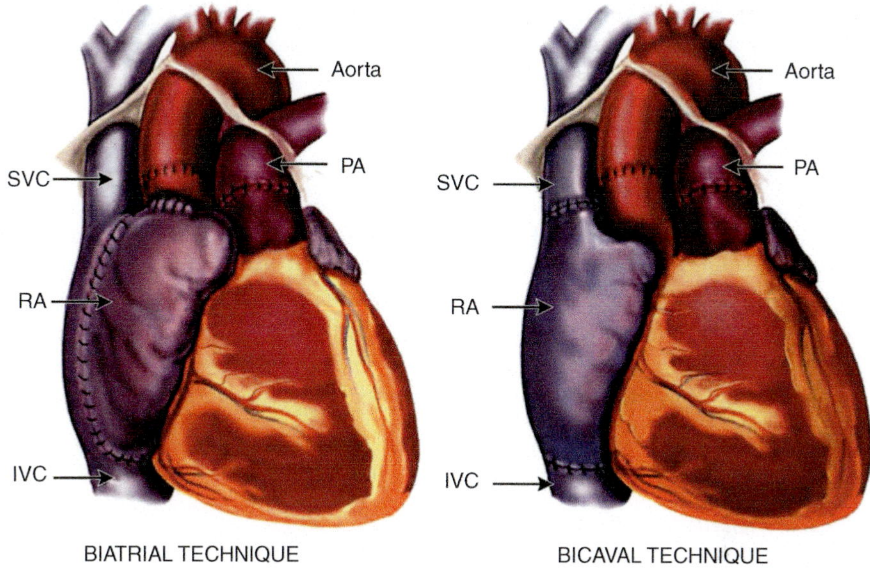

Fig. 19.1 Biatrial and bicaval orthotopic heart transplant. Source: Chen RH, Kadner A, Adams DH. Surgical techniques in heart transplantation. Graft. 1999;2:119–22 (Sage publications)

common in the modern era (Fig. 19.1). The biatrial method was the original operative technique for heart transplantation and was widely utilized in the 1980s. Although the biatrial technique has been largely supplanted by the bicaval it remains useful in certain surgical circumstances (e.g., dense pericardial adhesions that present severe hazard in dissecting out the cavae).

The bicaval technique is associated with less postoperative rhythm disturbances requiring permanent pacemaker and improved survival as compared to biatrial (Davies et al. 2010). With the bicaval technique, the native heart is near-completely excised leaving a cuff of remnant SVC, IVC, aorta, main pulmonary artery, and posterior wall of the left atrium. The donor graft is then sequentially anastomosed (typical order is left atrium, IVC, pulmonary artery, aorta, SVC) with reperfusion of the graft occurring after the aortic anastomosis is completed.

19.3.2 Donor Organ Considerations

Appropriate donor selection is a critical element of pretransplant planning and can have an important impact on the postoperative course as well as long-term outcome. Most heart organ donors have suffered a severe neurologic insult rendering them legally brain-dead, though there is currently a renewed interest in expanding the donor pool with utilization of Deceased by Cardiac Death (DCD) heart donation (Dhital et al. 2017). Prior to a final decision on organ acceptance, potential donor organs undergo thorough evaluation including echocardiography, biomarker monitoring, coronary angiography if indicated, and visual inspection by an experienced procurement surgeon. Pre-donation medical management is typically provided by the medical staff of the Organ Procurement Organization (OPO), often in collaboration with the potential receiving transplant center(s).

Posttransplant function of the organ, both short term and long term, will be influenced by a multitude of factors. The quality of the organ itself may be compromised by ventricular hypertrophy, valvular abnormalities, coronary artery disease, trauma, or other issues (Goodroe et al. 2007). Medical comorbidities of the donor including morbid obesity, end-stage renal disease, and alcohol abuse have been demonstrated to affect graft function (Freimark et al. 1996). Additional considerations for the organ selection team include predicted ischemic times and immune compatibility, both of which have associations with posttransplant performance (Russo et al. 2007).

19.3.3 Intraoperative

It is important for the critical care team to be made aware of any significant intraoperative events or observations that may impact early postoperative resuscitation and management. Examples include rhythm disturbances, coagulopathy, and unusual anatomy. Cold, warm, and total ischemic times may influence early function of the graft and necessary hemodynamic support. Goal hemodynamic parameters based on intraoperative observations of the surgical and anesthesia teams should be communicated, such as observed optimal filling pressures and blood pressure. Such considerations emphasize the importance of a thorough and efficient operating room-to-intensive care unit transfer procedure.

19.4 Operating Room-to-Intensive Care Unit (ICU) Transfer

19.4.1 Transfer Process

The operating room-to-ICU transfer sequence presents an opportunity for multiple complications. The physical move from bed to bed may infer some degree of hemodynamic instability secondary to fluid/pressure shifts and patient discomfort. There exists potential for invasive equipment disruption (e.g., endotracheal tube, intravenous lines) and interruption in medication administration. Upon arrival to the ICU all monitoring systems must be efficiently transferred from the mobile units to those of the ICU to minimize gaps in monitoring. All intravenous infusions must similarly be rapidly transitioned and confirmed to be functional so that there are no interruptions in resuscitative therapy. During this time period it is preferable for key providers such as the intensivist, anesthesia, surgical, and nursing teams to work collaboratively to ensure a safe and efficient transition.

19.4.2 Immediate Postoperative Studies

All heart-transplant patients should receive routine immediate post-cardiac surgery studies. These include laboratory studies (CBC, CMP, coagulation, ABG), 12-lead electrocardiogram (ECG), and chest X-ray (CXR).

19.5 Posttransplant Monitoring

Postoperative monitoring in heart-transplant recipients is similar to other cardiac surgical patients but with a few additional considerations. All patients will receive continuous monitoring of rhythm and blood pressure. Special attention should be given to urine output, temperature, and chest tube output which should be assessed at least hourly. Hemodynamic assessment provided by a pulmonary artery catheter can be of critical value early after transplant. Trends in pulmonary artery pressure, central venous pressure, cardiac output, and systemic vascular resistance can provide essential data to assist in guiding postoperative fluid management and vasoactive infusion support. Serial laboratory studies, EKGs, and CXRs are obtained. One must be aware of the immune-modulating drugs being utilized and how they may affect other organ systems, especially hematologic, neurologic, renal, and hepatic. Posttransplant endomyocardial biopsies are performed routinely, with the first typically occurring around postoperative day 7.

19.6 Posttransplant Physiology

An important consequence of the heart transplantation procedure is the loss of cardiac autonomic nervous system (ANS) regulation. Excision of the donor heart in the procurement operation results in loss of parasympathetic and sympathetic nerve fiber input. This loss of ANS regulation makes the donor heart largely dependent on circulating catecholamines to modulate stress and activity response.

Cardiac output (CO) is determined by heart rate (HR) and stroke volume (SV). During periods of stress a normal heart will rapidly increase CO largely by increasing HR via inputs from the ANS and circulating catecholamines. In denervated hearts, increases in HR are achieved by changes in catecholamine secretion alone and maximum HR takes longer to achieve. Alterations in cardiac output also become more dependent on preload and increased filling volumes result in increased contractility via the Frank-Starling mechanism. Thus, transplanted hearts can be considered "preload dependent" as myocardial stretch becomes a more important determinant of stroke volume and cardiac output in response to stress (Pope et al. 1980).

Cardiac denervation also has important pharmacologic implications. The dependence on catecholamine input experienced by the denervated donor heart results in the cardiac myocytes having increased sensitivity to medications that act on beta-receptors (e.g., beta-blockers) and decreased responsiveness to those that work in the autonomic pathways (e.g., digoxin, atropine).

19.7 Hemodynamics

19.7.1 Inotropic and Vasoactive Support

In the very early postoperative phase the donor myocytes remain somewhat stunned and in need of resuscitation and recovery. Some degree of hemodynamic instability can be expected and thus inotropic support is routinely utilized. The goal is to optimize ventricular function and systemic perfusion, which requires an effective combination of circulating volume and inotropic/vasoactive medications. The specific pharmacologic agents applied posttransplant chosen will vary among practitioners based on experience and clinical need (Table 19.1). Commonly utilized inotropes include continuous infusions of epinephrine, dopamine, dobutamine, isoproterenol, and milrinone.

For those with low SVR the use of vasopressors may be required. Epinephrine, norepinephrine, and phenylephrine all are effective direct alpha-adrenergic agonists. Of note, norepinephrine may also result in increased pulmonary vascular tone which can impact right ventricular function. Vasopressin is also effective in improving postsurgical vasoplegia by increasing vascular tone and fluid retention. Methylene blue can improve SVR in refractory vasoplegia but has shown mixed results on outcomes and is commonly reserved as salvage therapy (Mehaffey et al. 2017).

In some circumstances vasodilation may be required. Decreased pulmonary vascular resistance can improve right ventricular performance. Inhaled agents such as nitric oxide and iloprost can have a profound effect on lowering PAP (Semigran et al. 1994). Phosphodiesterase inhibitors like sildenafil have similar effect on PAP and can be given orally (de Groote et al. 2015). Nitroglycerin and nitroprusside are effective systemic vasodilators for decreasing systemic pressure but can similarly function to decrease pulmonary vascular resistance to augment right ventricular function. Milrinone also dilates the pulmonary vascular bed with the added benefit of increased inotropy; however, some patients are unable to tolerate the decrease in SVR that can be anticipated with milrinone administration.

Table 19.1 Effect of various inotropes and vasopressors on the heart-transplant recipients

Agent	Cardiac output	Cardiac contractility	Chronotropy	Peripheral vascular resistance	Pulmonary vascular resistance	Risk of arrhythmia
Dobutamine	+++	++	++	0	0	+
Dopamine	++	++	++	+	+	+
Epinephrine	+++	+++	++	++	+	++
Isoproterenol	++	+++	+++	–	–	+++
Milrinone	++	++	++	–	–	++
Norepinephrine	+	+	+	+++	++	+
Phenylephrine	0	0	0	+++	0	0
Vasopressin	0	0	0	+++	0	0

19.7.2 Fluids

Heart-transplant patients require precise management of circulating volume. The goal is to deliver adequate filling volumes while carefully avoiding volume overload. As discussed earlier, transplanted hearts are "preload dependent"; however, ventricular overdistension can be catastrophic, particularly in regard to right ventricular function. Accordingly, it is not uncommon for the surgical team to leave the operating room with the patient relatively "dry" to help minimize strain on the newly recovering myocytes. It is imperative that the surgical and intensivist teams be aware of and sensitive to these hemodynamic goals in the early perioperative period which can be well monitored by pulmonary artery catheter values and central venous pressure.

Colloid fluids are often preferred to crystalloid to help minimize resuscitation volumes. Commonly utilized solutions include 5 and 25% albumin solution, as well as blood products. Exact practices regarding hematocrit goals will vary among centers and practitioners and it is important to clarify these goals in the early postoperative phase.

If the patient is showing evidence of volume overload, often manifested as high central venous pressures and/or pulmonary artery diastolic pressures in the setting of worsening cardiac output, rapid intervention is critical. This may include the addition of diuretics, minimization of volume intake (e.g. concentrating intravenous drips), systemic and/or pulmonary artery afterload reduction (e.g. nitric oxide), heightened monitoring of graft function, assessment for cardiac tamponade, and continuous assessment of response to intervention to determine if additional adjuncts are required.

19.7.3 Primary Graft Dysfunction

Primary graft dysfunction (PGD) following heart transplantation is a feared and serious complication. It refers to acute ventricular dysfunction occurring within 24 hours of the transplant operation. It may manifest as left, right, or biventricular failure. It is the most common cause of mortality within the first 30 days of heart transplantation and occurs in about 7% of recipients (Kobashigawa et al. 2014).

PGD is classified as mild, moderate, and severe. Mild and moderate PGD can generally be well managed with inotropes and possibly an Intra-Aortic Balloon Pump (IABP). For cases of severe PGD, mechanical circulatory support with a ventricular assist device (VAD) is often required until such time as the graft has adequately recovered (Kittleson et al. 2011). Ventricular function is optimized by carefully manipulating preload, inotropic support, and afterload. The intraoperative observations by the surgical team can provide insight into optimal hemodynamic parameters as related to ventricular behavior. The pulmonary artery catheter can be critical for optimizing filling pressures and monitoring the hemodynamic response. In cases that require further objective information a bedside echocardiogram can help delineate the functional state of the allograft.

If new-onset PGD is suspected it is imperative for the critical care provider to immediately notify the advanced heart failure team including cardiology and cardiac surgery so that a cohesive management plan can be rapidly implemented. Appropriate and aggressive management of PGD is essential for rescue due to the high potential for rapid decompensation.

19.8 Rhythm Disturbances

The expected rhythm immediately following heart transplantation is normal sinus rhythm (NSR) or sinus tachycardia. Cardiac denervation results in a higher intrinsic rate (typically 90–100 beats per minute) and reduced rate variability. Most transplant surgeons will place atrial and ventricular pacing wires to help manipulate rhythm and heart rate in case of early bradycardia or atrioventricular dyssynchrony.

The most common rhythm disturbance in the early posttransplantation period is sinus bradycardia. This is the result of sinus node dysfunction. While the exact etiology of sinus node dysfunction following heart transplantation is unclear, possible contributing factors include surgical trauma, denervation effect, and ischemia (Bexton et al. 1983). Sinus bradycardia is also more common in patients that have received preoperative amiodarone due to its long half-life and residual affect. Management of bradycardia usually includes temporary atrioventricular pacing to maintain a heart rate of at least 90 bpm (Costanzo et al. 2010). Other commonly used pharmacologic adjuncts include terbutaline, dopamine, isoproterenol, and dobutamine.

It is not unusual for patients to experience transient arrhythmias in the early recovery phase. These are often asymptomatic and well tolerated clinically. Close electrolyte management is important for all cardiac surgery patients and is indicated after heart transplantation as well. Persistent dysrhythmias soon after the transplant procedure should raise concern for acute rejection and trigger an appropriate evaluation by the advanced heart failure team. Tachydysrhythmias are generally managed similar to non-transplant cardiac surgery, but it should be noted that amiodarone is associated with significant interactions with common posttransplant immunosuppressive agents (e.g., tacrolimus) and thus immunosuppressant levels and effect should be closely monitored (Nalli et al. 2006).

19.9 Coagulopathy

All cardiac surgery patients are at risk for postoperative hemorrhage and this risk is often relatively higher for heart-transplant recipients. The technical components of the transplant operation include multiple lengthy suture lines which have potential for significant bleeding. Advanced heart failure is associated with increased renal and hepatic dysfunction which can be deleterious to platelet and clotting factor efficiency. Prior sternotomy, a common entity for heart-transplant recipients, generates extensive mediastinal adhesions which will increase the difficulty of dissection and increase blood loss. Redo sternotomy is also generally associated with longer cardiopulmonary bypass times which can worsen coagulopathy due to increased trauma to the clotting system factors and platelets. These challenges are further exacerbated in patients that present for transplant on durable mechanical circulatory support (e.g., durable LVAD), which is becoming an increasingly larger segment of the recipient population (Moazami et al. 2011). Patients with a durable VAD can be expected to have relatively severe mediastinal adhesions as well as inherent coagulopathy due to relative destruction of high-molecular-weight von Willebrand factor (Crow et al. 2010).

19.9.1 Management of Hemorrhage

All patients will present to the intensive care unit after heart transplantation with mediastinal drainage tubes in place. Some chest tube output in the early postoperative phase is to be expected. Indeed, extremely low tube drainage immediately postoperatively should raise concern for poor tube function which may lead to lack of evacuation of mediastinal fluids and progression to cardiac tamponade. Institutional and provider protocols will vary, but most surgeons are comfortable monitoring chest tube drainage of <100–150 mL/h for the first few hours following the operation. If the drainage volume exceeds this, or if the output does not steadily decrease over time, the surgical team should be immediately notified of the potential for ongoing hemorrhage. When severe postoperative hemorrhage is encountered there should be no hesitation in returning to the operating room for exploration.

In cases of suspected ongoing postoperative hemorrhage adjunctive measures to promote coagulation and stability should be promptly applied. Coagulation studies including International Normalized Ratio (INR), activated partial thromboplastin time (aptt), fibrinogen level, and platelet count are rapidly available and will help guide blood product resuscitation. Thromboelastography (TEG) can provide similar data and help guide management. Hematocrit levels should be checked regularly to ensure that the patient is not developing dangerously severe anemia. It is important to communicate effectively with transfusion services to ensure that adequate products continue to be made available during the resuscitation process.

Normothermia and calcium replacement are essential for appropriate function of the clotting system. While it is critical to maintain adequate systemic perfusion, excess hypertension will have a negative effect on achieving hemostasis. The use of elevated levels of positive end expiratory pressure (PEEP) is employed by some practitioners on the theory of tamponading bleeding via increased intrathoracic pressure (Yildiz et al. 2014). High PEEP can have a deleterious effect on preload, especially in the setting of acute volume loss seen during large-volume hemorrhage.

Other procoagulant adjuncts have been utilized for the treatment of postcardiotomy hemorrhage, often with mixed results. Aminocaproic acid or tranexamic acid is often administered while on cardiopulmonary bypass for their antifibrinolytic effect. These agents have also been employed to combat postoperative hemorrhage (Koul et al. 2012). Recombinant estrogen has a known pro-thrombotic effect which has led some practitioners to use it to attenuate postoperative bleeding (Livio et al. 1986). Similarly, desmopressin (DDAVP), a vasopressin analogue, will increase secretion of von Willebrand factor and factor VII from endothelial cells to assist in hemostasis (Wademan and Galvin 2014). Lastly, the recent emergence of prothrombin complex concentrates (PCC), including factor VII, has provided practitioners with another highly effective medical adjunct to counter hemorrhage. Prior to utilizing such measures in a heart-transplant patient it is imperative for the intensive care unit team to communicate with the transplant surgeon to collaboratively develop a management plan.

19.10 Respiratory

Postoperative respiratory management after heart transplant generally differs little from other cardiac surgical patients. Ventilator weaning strategies should be goal directed based on the clinical circumstance. The ventilator can be an important adjunct in manipulating PA pressure to decrease right ventricular strain of the freshly implanted donor heart, as both hypoxia and hypercapnia can elevate pulmonic vascular resistance. Sufficient oxygen delivery is also important for the recovering myocytes to enhance metabolic function. PEEP is often effective at improving oxygenation but may come at the expense of preload return by increasing intrathoracic pressures. Ventilator-associated pneumonia remains a concern for any ICU patient, but heart-transplant patients are further compromised by necessary immunosuppressive medications.

An important consideration in the respiratory management of heart-transplant recipients concerns the utilization of inhaled pulmonary vasodilators such as nitric oxide and prostacyclin. While these agents are effective at decreasing pulmonary vascular resistance and thus decreasing right ventricular strain, they can pose a challenge to separation from ventilator support as endotracheal intubation is the most effective means of delivery. It is valuable for the critical care team to develop explicit weaning protocols for these agents in order to avoid abrupt cessation or prolonged administration. For instances in which pulmonary artery pressures are particularly improved by inhaled medication consideration can be given to alternative pulmonary vasodilators such as sildenafil to aid in transition off mechanical ventilation (Leuchte et al. 2004).

19.11 Renal

It is not unusual for patients with advanced heart failure necessitating heart transplantation to develop some degree of renal insufficiency preoperatively secondary to low CO and increased venous congestion. Preexisting renal dysfunction must be recognized in the perioperative period and can have significant implications for early management. It is also important to be aware of the nephrotoxic effects of many immunosuppressive agents commonly used in heart transplantation.

19.11.1 Volume Management

As described earlier, newly transplanted hearts are very sensitive to preload and poorly tolerate volume overload. Fluid management must therefore be judicious with the goal of optimizing chamber volumes but avoiding over-resuscitation. This often manifests as a state of relative hypovolemia, which can be detrimental to renal function. While on cardiopulmonary bypass and during the immediate post-pump period most patients will experience high-volume urine output, largely due to osmotic shifts. Additionally, many patients will receive diuretic therapy in the early postoperative period to maintain urine production and/or avoid excess preload volumes. During this time period the intensivist team should pay close attention to urine output as measured by indwelling urinary catheter and serum markers of renal function to help balance the fluid needs of the kidney to that of the cardiac function.

19.11.2 Nephrotoxicity

All heart-transplant recipients require some combination of immunosuppressive therapy. The most commonly utilized regimen includes a calcineurin inhibitor, a glucocorticoid, and an anti-proliferative agent. The nephrotoxic potential of tacrolimus is well described and those receiving it will require close monitoring of serum levels to help prevent renal injury (Randhawa et al. 1997; Nielsen et al. 1994). For cases in which the preexisting renal function is significantly impaired, or in instances of evolving renal insufficiency, careful dose adjustment or utilization of alternative agents (e.g., cyclosporine) may be employed.

19.11.3 Heart and Kidney Transplantation

As many patients with advanced heart failure also develop significant renal dysfunction, it is important to give consideration for dual-organ transplant at the time of initial transplant evaluation. Potential candidates include those with concomitant severe cardiac and renal dysfunction. Combined heart-kidney transplantation was previously performed infrequently; however, improvement in long-term outcomes has led to a steady increase in this procedure (Schaffer et al. 2014). Critical care delivery is largely unaffected by combined heart-kidney transplantation other than increased awareness and monitoring of the renal graft which may include ultrasound and biopsy in collaboration with the renal transplant team.

19.12 Hepatic

Chronic hepatic congestion is commonly associated with long-standing advanced heart failure, especially in relation to severely compromised right ventricular function and tricuspid valve regurgitation. Congestive hepatopathy can result in compromised hepatic synthetic function with deleterious clinical consequence. Despite seemingly normal coagulation parameters these patients may have a functional coagulopathy that increases perioperative bleeding risk. Additionally, alterations in vasoactive agent production can generate vasoplegia (La Villa and Gentilini 2008).

The best way to avoid hepatic insufficiency after heart-transplant is careful preoperative patient selection. Unfortunately, reliable predictors of perioperative hepatic failure are lacking. Standard hepatic assessment tools such as serum studies (e.g., bilirubin, albumin), abdominal ultrasound, and physical exam may raise suspicion for hepatic insufficiency. The use of liver biopsy to help elucidate hepatic dysfunction is often employed; however, the clinical significance of biopsy results for heart transplant remains imprecise and controversial (Louie et al. 2015; Mohan et al. 2016). Overall, it is the duty of the transplant selection committee to carefully consider baseline hepatic function as part of the selection criteria.

For patients that develop hepatic insufficiency soon after heart transplant the focus of care usually remains supportive. It is critical to rule out right ventricular dysfunction of the allograft as a contributing factor. All medications must be carefully reviewed to avoid any agents associated with hepatotoxicity. Expert consultation with a hepatologist may be valuable for optimizing support and guiding management. Hepatic failure following heart transplant is associated with extremely poor outcomes and thus be avoided whenever possible (Hsu et al. 2007).

19.12.1 Hepatotoxicity

Immunosuppressive medications commonly utilized in heart transplantation generally have little adverse effect on hepatic function. However, there are several agents that undergo hepatic metabolism and thus may be affected by hepatic dysfunction. Examples include prednisone, tacrolimus, sirolimus, everolimus, and cyclosporine. Clinical response assessment and/or serum-level monitoring of these medications should be performed when hepatic dysfunction is present.

19.12.2 Heart and Liver Transplantation

For patients deemed to be at too high risk for heart transplant due to liver dysfunction, consideration may be given to heart and liver transplant. These dual-organ operations are relatively of high risk and infrequently performed. Despite these challenges, acceptable outcomes have been reported and continue to be obtained at experienced centers (Cannon et al. 2012). Management of these dual-organ recipients can be particularly challenging for the critical care team and will require a multidisciplinary approach. Combined heart-liver transplant is associated with decreased antibody-mediated rejection and it is hypothesized that the liver confers protection by absorbing donor-specific antibodies.

19.13 Neurologic

Neurologic abnormalities can occur after any cardiac operation. The most common etiology for acute neurologic injury is embolic phenomena related to aortic manipulation. Patients may also suffer hypoxic neurologic insult due to perioperative hypoperfusion, most often related to prolonged periods of hypotension. Heart-transplant operations carry these same risks and may arguably be at increased risk for embolic and hypoperfusion events secondary to the complex nature of many transplant operations, especially in the setting of redo sternotomy. An additional consideration for heart-transplant recipients demonstrating posttransplant neurologic dysfunction is the adverse effects of calcineurin inhibitors (CNIs). Elevated serum levels of tacrolimus can lead to depressed neurologic function including severe obtundation and coma (Bechstein 2000). Anticonvulsants can also alter the metabolism of CNIs.

19.14 Nutrition

Heart-transplant recipients may be somewhat malnourished prior to the transplant operation. For patients with advanced heart failure "cardiac cachexia" can be a persistent and difficult problem as low CO may result in poor nutrient absorption. Following the transplant procedure, nutrition is generally initiated within the first 1–3 days. Enteric feeding is preferential to parenteral supplementation and may require nasogastric tube delivery in those who are unable to meet oral intake goals. Enteral nutrition should include appropriate amounts of protein, vitamins, and electrolytes to optimize postsurgical recovery. Many of the posttransplant medications including glucocorticoids can have significant effects on metabolism and electrolyte balance and thus these should be monitored routinely. In particular, glucose control can be challenging and often requires continuous intravenous insulin infusion in the early postoperative period to meet goal parameters.

19.15 Immune System

19.15.1 Rejection

Cardiac allograft rejection is most common early after transplant, with 80% of episodes occurring within the first 3 months (Kubo et al. 1995). If left unchecked, it is associated with high mortality due to the development of allograft vasculopathy. Early recognition of rejection is critical and it is best assessed with endomyocardial biopsy. Endomyocardial biopsy is a relatively safe procedure with an overall complication rate of less than 6% (From et al. 2011). Some important potential complications include dysrhythmia, tricuspid valve injury, and ventricular perforation with potential cardiac tamponade.

Hyperacute rejection is mediated by preformed antibodies to the allograft in the recipient due to HLA antigen exposure. It is characterized by graft thrombosis and hemorrhage and onset is within minutes to hours of reperfusing the graft. Fortunately this is an extremely rare complication owing to prospective cytotoxic and virtual cross-matching. Acute cellular rejection (ACR) is the most common form of rejection after transplant and is characterized by T-cell-mediated myocardial injury. The majority of ACR occurs within the first 6 months after transplant. Antibody-mediated rejection (AMR) develops when recipient antibodies develop against donor-HLA antigens ultimately resulting in activation of the complement cascade and allograft injury.

Management of cardiac allograft rejection will vary based on the severity and etiology of rejection. Although there are no definitive management protocols for treatment of rejection, therapy will typically include increased glucocorticoids with or without additional immunosuppressive adjuncts (e.g. IV immune globulin, anti-thymocyte globulin) based on the severity of the rejection episode (Uber et al. 2007). In extreme circumstances of rejection causing allograft dysfunction the patient may require temporary mechanical circulatory support while the immune response is attenuated (Listijono et al. 2011). The consequences of cardiac rejection can be severe so it is imperative that a multidisciplinary transplant team collaborate effectively on management for these highly vulnerable patients.

19.15.2 Immunosuppression

Immunosuppressive medications have undergone important transformation since the birth of heart transplant. While programmatic protocols will vary, common practice consists of "triple therapy" with a glucocorticoid, a CNI, and an antiproliferative agent. These agents should be initiated early after the implant procedure, generally within 12 hours.

Recipients usually receive a bolus of high-dose glucocorticoids in the operating room and then are progressively tapered. While glucocorticoids are effective for preventing rejection, common adverse effects include hyperglycemia, poor wound healing, hypertension, hypernatremia, and emotional lability.

Calcineurin inhibitors function by blocking calcium-activated calcineurin, ultimately inhibiting production of interleukin-2 and other inflammatory cytokines. It was largely due to the discovery of the dramatic benefit of cyclosporine A for heart transplantation in the 1970s that outcomes improved sufficiently to permit widespread adoption. Tacrolimus is currently the most widely used CNI based on data demonstrating reduced rates of rejection and adverse effects compared to cyclosporine. Conversely, tacrolimus is associated with increased rates of nephrotoxicity, diabetes mellitus, and neurotoxicity (Taylor et al. 1999).

Antiproliferative agents function by inhibiting DNA synthesis, thus limiting de novo cellular proliferation and decreasing T cell and B cell production. The most commonly used agents include azathioprine and mycophenolate mofetil (MMF). MMF is generally preferred to other antiproliferatives due to reduced adverse effects as well as improved survival and prevention of rejection (Kobashigawa et al. 1998; Hosenpud and Bennett 2001). The most common side effects of MMF include nausea, vomiting, diarrhea, hepatic dysfunction, and pancytopenia.

19.15.3 Infection

Infection is a significant issue in the early posttransplant period, with about 25% of recipients being affected within the first 2 months after transplant (Lund et al. 2014). Bacterial infections predominate in the first few weeks after transplant and are often wound or catheter associated. Perioperative antibiotic prophylaxis protocols will vary among programs but general principles include adequate prophylaxis against skin flora for at least 48 h immediately following surgery and appropriate antiviral prophylaxis against CMV and HSV with valganciclovir or acyclovir.

Although postsurgical infection is a large concern for any cardiac surgery patient, heart-transplant recipients carry the co-founding risk of necessary immunosuppression. Preventive measures against infection include antimicrobial prophylaxis, appropriate vaccination pretransplant, diligent handwashing precautions, and avoiding contact with people suspected to have air-transmissible disease. Clinical signs of infection include fever, dysuria, altered mental status, diarrhea, wound abnormality, and pulmonary infiltrates. Common bacterial, viral, and fungal organisms posttransplant are shown in Table 19.2.

If acute infection is suspected posttransplant intervention should proceed expeditiously. Urine, blood, and sputum cultures are obtained. Surgical wounds must be meticulously inspected. In select cases additional imaging adjuncts such as CT or tagged white blood cell nuclear medicine scans may be useful for elucidating the source of infection. Lumbar punctures are rarely indicated but may be necessary. While such investigations are being pursued it is critical to implement aggressive antimicrobial therapy early with broad-spectrum antibiotics and possibly antivirals/antifungals. There should be a very low threshold to involve an infectious disease specialist early. Culture data should be reviewed daily and trigger appropriate alterations in therapy.

Table 19.2 Common microorganisms affecting heart-transplant recipients

Bacterial	Viral	Fungal
Staphylococci	Cytomegalovirus	Candida
Streptococci	Herpes simplex	Aspergillus
C. difficile	Varicella zoster	
Pseudomonas		
Legionella		
Listeria		
Nocardia		

19.16 Outcomes

Short- and long-term outcomes following heart transplantation are generally favorable, especially given the acuity of most heart-transplant recipients. Overall survival rates are approximately 85% at 1 year, 80% at 3 years, 75% at 5 years, 60% at 10 years, and 20% at 20 years posttransplant (Lund et al. 2014). Of course, individual survival is influenced by several variables including but not limited to recipient comorbidities, quality of the donor heart, and graft-recipient immune compatibility. All centers practicing heart transplantation should observe excellent 30-day mortality rates of at least >90%. In addition to appropriate donor/recipient selection and excellent surgical support, critical care management in the early postoperative period is of tremendous importance in optimizing outcomes for heart-transplant recipients.

References

Barnard CN. A human cardiac transplant: an interim report of a successful operation performed at the Groote Schuur Hospital, Cape Town. S Afr Med J. 1967;41:1271.

Bechstein W. Neurotoxicity of calcineurin inhibitors: impact and clinical management. Transpl Int. 2000;13(5):313–26.

Bexton RS, Nathan AW, Hellestrand KJ, Cory-Pearce R, Spurrell RA, English TA, Camm AJ. Electrophysiological abnormalities in the transplanted human heart. Br Heart J. 1983;50(6):555–63.

Cannon RM, Hughes MG, Jones CM, Eng M, Marvin MR. A review of the United States experience with combined heart-liver transplantation. Transpl Int. 2012;25(12):1223–8.

Caves PK, Stinson EB, Billingham ME, et al. Percutaneous endomyocardial biopsy in human heart recipients. Experience with a new technique. Ann Thorac Surg. 1973;16:325.

Costanzo MR, Dipchand A, Starling R, et al. The International Society of Heart and Lung Transplantation guidelines for the care of heart transplant recipients. J Heart Lung Transplant. 2010;29(8):914–56.

Crow S, Chen D, Milano C, Thomas W, Joyce L, Piacentino V 3rd, Sharma R, Wu J, Arepally G, Bowles D, Rogers J, Villamizar-Ortiz N. Acquired von Willebrand syndrome in continuous-flow ventricular assist device recipients. Ann Thorac Surg. 2010;90(4):1263–9.

Davies RR, Russo MJ, Morgan JA, Sorabella RA, Naka Y, Chen JM. Standard versus bicaval techniques for orthotopic heart transplantation: an analysis of the United Network for Organ Sharing database. J Thorac Cardiovasc Surg. 2010;140(3):700–8.

Dhital KK, Chew HC, Macdonald PS. Donation after circulatory death heart transplantation. Curr Opin Organ Transplant. 2017;22(3):189–1978.

Freimark D, Aleksic I, Trento A, Takkenberg JJ, Valenza M, Admon D, Blanche C, Queral CA, Azen CG, Czer LS. Hearts from donors with chronic alcohol use: a possible risk factor for death after heart transplantation. J Heart Lung Transplant. 1996;15(2):150–9.

From AM, Maleszewski JJ, Rihal CS. Current status of endomyocardial biopsy. Mayo Clin Proc. 2011;86(11):1095–102.

Goodroe R, Bonnema DD, Lunsford S, Anderson P, Ryan-Baille B, Uber W, Ikonomidis J, Crumbley AJ, VanBakel A, Zile MR, Pereira N. Severe left ventricular hypertrophy 1 year after transplant predicts mortality in cardiac transplant recipients. J Heart Lung Transplant. 2007;26(2):145–51.

de Groote P, El Asri C, Fertin M, Goéminne C, Vincentelli A, Robin E, Duva-Pentiah A, Lamblin N. Sildenafil in heart transplant candidates with pulmonary hypertension. Arch Cardiovasc Dis. 2015;108(6–7):375–84.

Hosenpud JD, Bennett LE. Mycophenolate mofetil versus azathioprine in patients surviving the initial cardiac transplant hospitalization: an analysis of the Joint UNOS/ISHLT Thoracic Registry. Transplantation. 2001;72(10):1662–5.
Hsu RB, Lin FY, Chen RJ, Chou NK, Ko WJ, Chi NH, Wang SS, Chu SH. Incidence, risk factors, and prognosis of postoperative hyperbilirubinemia after heart transplantation. Eur J Cardiothorac Surg. 2007;32(6):917–22.
Kittleson MM, Patel JK, Moriguchi JD, Kawano M, Davis S, Hage A, Hamilton MA, Esmailian F, Kobashigawa JA. Heart transplant recipients supported with extracorporeal membrane oxygenation: outcomes from a single-center experience. J Heart Lung Transplant. 2011;30(11):1250–6.
Kobashigawa J, Miller L, Renlund D, Mentzer R, Alderman E, Bourge R, Costanzo M, Eisen H, Dureau G, Ratkovec R, Hummel M, Ipe D, Johnson J, Keogh A, Mamelok R, Mancini D, Smart F, Valantine H. A randomized active-controlled trial of mycophenolate mofetil in heart transplant recipients. Mycophenolate Mofetil Investigators. Transplantation. 1998;66(4):507–15.
Kobashigawa J, Zuckermann A, Macdonald P, et al. Report from a consensus conference on primary graft dysfunction after cardiac transplantation. J Heart Lung Transplant. 2014;33(4):327–40.
Koul A, Ferraris V, Davenport DL, Ramaiah C. The effect of antifibrinolytic prophylaxis on postoperative outcomes in patients undergoing cardiac operations. Int Surg. 2012;97(1):34–42.
Kubo SH, Naftel DC, Mills RM Jr, O'Donnell J, Rodeheffer RJ, Cintron GB, Kenzora JL, Bourge RC, Kirklin JK. Risk factors for late recurrent rejection after heart transplantation: a multiinstitutional, multivariable analysis. Cardiac Transplant Research Database Group. J Heart Lung Transplant. 1995;14(3):409–18.
La Villa G, Gentilini P. Hemodynamic alterations in liver cirrhosis. Mol Asp Med. 2008;29(1–2):112–8.
Leuchte HH, Schwaiblmair M, Baumgartner RA, Neurohr CF, Kolbe T, Behr J. Hemodynamic response to sildenafil, nitric oxide, and iloprost in primary pulmonary hypertension. Chest. 2004;125(2):580–6.
Listijono DR, Watson A, Pye R, Keogh AM, Kotlyar E, Spratt P, Granger E, Dhital K, Jansz P, Macdonald PS, Hayward CS. Usefulness of extracorporeal membrane oxygenation for early cardiac allograft dysfunction. J Heart Lung Transplant. 2011;30(7):783–9.
Livio M, Mannucci PM, Viganò G, Mingardi G, Lombardi R, et al. Conjugated estrogens for the management of bleeding associated with renal failure. N Engl J Med. 1986;315:731–5.
Louie CY, Pham MX, Daugherty TJ, Kambham N, Higgins JP. The liver in heart failure: a biopsy and explant series of the histopathologic and laboratory findings with a particular focus on pre-cardiac transplant evaluation. Mod Pathol. 2015;28(7):932–43.
Lund LH, Edwards LB, Kucheryavaya AY, Benden C, Christie JD, Dipchand AI, Dobbels F, Goldfarb SB, Levvey BJ, Meiser B, Yusen RD, Stehlik J, International Society of Heart and Lung Transplantation. The registry of the International Society for Heart and Lung Transplantation: thirty-first official adult heart transplant report—2014; focus theme: retransplantation. J Heart Lung Transplant. 2014 Oct;33(10):996–1008.
Lund LH, Edwards LB, Ms YK, et al. The Registry of the International Society for Heart and Lung Transplantation: 32nd official adult heart transplantation report—2015. J Heart Lung Transplant. 2015;34(10):1244–54.
Mehaffey JH, Johnston LE, Hawkins RB, Charles EJ, Yarboro L, Kern JA, Ailawadi G, Kron IL, Ghanta RK. Methylene blue for vasoplegic syndrome after cardiac operation: early administration improves survival. Ann Thorac Surg. 2017;104(1):36–41.
Moazami N, Sun B, Feldman D. Stable patients on left ventricular assist device support have a disproportionate advantage: time to re-evaluate the current UNOS policy. J Heart Lung Transplant. 2011;30(9):971–4.
Mohan R, Patel J, Kittleson M, Chang D, Aintablian T, Czer L, Esmailian F, Kobashigawa J. Liver evaluation for heart transplantation: which is better, noninvasive scans or liver biopsy? Am J Transplant. 2016;16(Suppl 3)
Nalli N, Stewart-Teixeira L, Dipchand AI. Amiodarone-sirolimus/tacrolimus interaction in a pediatric heart transplant patient. Pediatr Transplant. 2006;10(6):736–9.

Nielsen FT, Leyssac PP, Kemp E, Starklint H, Dieperink H. Nephrotoxicity of FK-506: a preliminary study on comparative aspects of FK-506 and cyclosporine nephrotoxicity. Transplant Proc. 1994;6:3104–5.

Oyer PE, Stinson EB, Jameison SA, et al. Cyclosporine a in cardiac allografting: a preliminary experience. Transplant Proc. 1983;15:1247.

Pope SE, Stinson EB, Daughters GT, Schroeder JS, Ingels NB Jr, Alderman EL. Exercise response of the denervated heart in long-term cardiac transplant recipients. Am J Cardiol. 1980;46(2):213–8.

Randhawa PS, Starzl TE, Demetris AJ. Tacrolimus (FK506)-associated renal pathology. Adv Anat Pathol. 1997;4(4):265–76.

Russo MJ, Chen JM, Sorabella RA, Martens TP, Garrido M, Davies RR, George I, Cheema FH, Mosca RS, Mital S, Ascheim DD, Argenziano M, Stewart AS, Oz MC, Naka Y. The effect of ischemic time on survival after heart transplantation varies by donor age: an analysis of the United Network for Organ Sharing database. J Thorac Cardiovasc Surg. 2007;133(2):554–9.

Schaffer JM, Chiu P, Singh SK, Oyer PE, Reitz BA, Mallidi HR. Heart and combined heart-kidney transplantation in patients with concomitant renal insufficiency and end-stage heart failure. Am J Transplant. 2014;14(2):384–96.

Semigran MJ, Cockrill BA, Kacmarek R, Thompson BT, Zapol WM, Dec GW, Fifer MA. Hemodynamic effects of inhaled nitric oxide in heart failure. J Am Coll Cardiol. 1994;24(4):982–8.

Taylor DO, Barr ML, Radovancevic B, Renlund DG, Mentzer RM Jr, Smart FW, Tolman DE, Frazier OH, Young JB, VanVeldhuisen P. A randomized, multicenter comparison of tacrolimus and cyclosporine immunosuppressive regimens in cardiac transplantation: decreased hyperlipidemia and hypertension with tacrolimus. J Heart Lung Transplant. 1999;18(4):336–45.

Uber WE, Self SE, Van Bakel AB, Pereira NL. Acute antibody-mediated rejection following heart transplantation. Am J Transplant. 2007;7(9):2064–74.

Wademan BH, Galvin SD. Desmopressin for reducing postoperative blood loss and transfusion requirements following cardiac surgery in adults. Interact Cardiovasc Thorac Surg. 2014;18(3):360–70.

Yildiz Y, Salihoglu E, Celik S, Ugurlucan M, Caglar IM, Turhan-Caglar FN, Isik O. The effect of postoperative positive end-expiratory pressure on postoperative bleeding after off-pump coronary artery bypass grafting. Arch Med Sci. 2014;10(5):933–40.

Postoperative Care of ECMO/Mechanical Circulatory Support

20

Kevin Koomalsingh and Fardad Esmailian

Abstract

The perioperative management of mechanical support patients can be challenging. These patients are plagued by decompensated heart failure resulting in a low output state and, consequently, end organ dysfunction. They are additionaly challenged by immobility and deconditioning and very often require emergent temporary support or elective durable support. This can create for a lengthy, arduous convalescence. A standardized approach to critical care management can help optimize both the short and long term outcomes.

Keywords

Extracorporeal membrane oxygenator · Cardiovascular · Preload · Afterload Contractility · Hepatic congestion · Mesenteric ischemia · Endocrine Hematologic considerations · Infectious considerations

Abbreviations

ACT	Activated clotting time
AKI	Acute kidney injury
AMP	Adenosine monophosphate
ARDS	Acute respiratory distress syndrome
BiVAD	Biventricular assist device

K. Koomalsingh, M.D. (✉)
Department of Cardiothoracic Surgery, University of Washington, Seattle, WA, USA
e-mail: kkoom@uw.edu

F. Esmailian, M.D.
Department of Surgery, Cedars-Sinai Heart Institute, Los Angeles, CA, USA

Heart Transplantation, Cedars-Sinai Heart Institute, Los Angeles, CA, USA

A. Dabbagh et al. (eds.), *Postoperative Critical Care for Adult Cardiac Surgical Patients*, https://doi.org/10.1007/978-3-319-75747-6_20

CABG	Coronary artery bypass grafting
CFLVAD	Continuous flow left ventricular assist device
CI	Cardiac index
CNS	Central nervous system
CO	Cardiac output
COPD	Chronic obstructive pulmonary disease
CPAP	Continuous positive airway pressure
CPB	Cardiopulmonary bypass
CPR	Cardiopulmonary resuscitation
CT	Computed tomography
CVP	Central venous pressure
CXR	Chest X-ray
DVT	Deep venous thrombosis
ECLS	Extracorporeal life support
ECMO	Extracorporeal membrane oxygenation
FiO_2	Fractional inspired oxygen
GI	Gastrointestinal
GIB	Gastrointestinal bleeding
IABP	Intra-aortic balloon pump
ICP	Intra-cranial pressure
ICU	Intensive care unit
iNO	Inhaled nitric oxide
INR	International normalized ratio
IV	Intravenous
LDH	Lactated dehydrogenase
LV	Left ventricle
LVAD	Left ventricular assist device
MAP	Mean arterial pressure
MCS	Mechanical circulatory support
MR	Mitral regurgitation
NMDA	N-methyl-D-aspartate receptor
NSAID	Nonsteroidal anti-inflammatory drugs
OR	Operating room
PA	Pulmonary artery
PAD	Pulmonary artery diastole
PEEP	Peak end-expiratory pressure
PI	Pulsatility index
PPI	Proton pump inhibitor
PTT	Partial prothrombin time
RA	Right atrium
RASS	Richmond Agitation Sedation Scale
RHF	Right heart failure
RR	Respiratory rate
RV	Right ventricle
RVAD	Right ventricular assist device

SaO_2	Oxygen saturation
SIMV	Synchronized intermittent mechanical ventilation
SVO_2	Mixed venous saturation
TAH	Total artificial heart
TEE	Trans-esophageal echocardiogram
TRALI	Transfusion-related acute lung injury
TTE	Transthoracic echocardiogram
UGIB	Upper gastrointestinal bleeding
V/Q	Ventilation/perfusion
VA ECMO	Veno-arterial extra corporeal membrane oxygenation
VAD	Ventricular assist device
VT	Ventricular tachycardia
WBC	White blood cell

20.1 Introduction

The perioperative management of mechanical support patients can be challenging. These patients are plagued by decompensated heart failure resulting in a low output state and, consequently, end-organ dysfunction. Furthermore, they are often deconditioned and immobile due to their recent decline. The triggers for intervention can be acute or chronic with patients needing either emergent temporary support such as ECMO or elective durable support. In either scenario, a standardized approach to patient management can help optimize short- and long-term outcomes.

20.2 Neurologic

Upon arrival to the intensive care unit, most patients will be intubated and under the effects of cardiac anesthesia. This typically includes an induction agent, an anxiolytic, an amnestic, an inhaled anesthetic, a neuromuscular blocker, and an analgesic (Bojar 2011). Most of these agents will have lingering effects for hours after arrival to the cardiac surgery ICU. The specific combination of drugs used is a multifactorial decision but usually tailored for an extubation plan. Patients who are deemed early extubation (i.e., temporary devices) are more likely to receive shorter-acting agents such as sevoflurane for an inhaled anesthetic, propofol for sedation, and remifentanil for analgesia. Those with an open chest or who will likely require several days of mechanical ventilation (i.e., urgent or high-risk durable devices) are more likely to receive isoflurane as an inhaled anesthetic and long-acting sedatives and analgesics such as versed (midazolam) and fentanyl, respectively. Midazolam's half-life is over 10 h and can delay extubation for days. Propofol tends to have a cardio-depressant effect and delayed clearance; thus, its use is minimized in the heart failure population. The adverse effects can persist for days depending on dosing, duration, hepatic or renal insufficiency, and the patient's body habitus (Barr

Table 20.1 Commonly used sedatives

Sedatives		
Drug	Infusion	Comments
Dexmedetomidine	0.2–0.7 μg/kg/h	Good anxiolytic; Delayed clearance with hepatic/renal insufficiency
Midazolam	0.5–20 mg/h	Unpredictable drug clearance
Propofol	10–75 μg/kg/min	Hypotension

et al. 2001). Morphine, due to histamine release, can cause a vasodilatory effect and precipitate severe hypotension. A handy alternative is dexmedetomidine. It provides excellent analgesia and sympatholytic coverage without any sedating effects. Additionally, it can be used safely after extubation. See Table 20.1 for additional drug profiles.

Adequate sedation and analgesia must be provided in the early postoperative period to minimize untoward perturbation of hemodynamics. Patients can become agitated, anxious, combative, develop ventilator dyssynchrony, etc. The net effect is increased afterload of both the pulmonic and systemic circulations. This can impose significant harm on mechanical circulatory support devices and native ventricular function. Devices are afterload sensitive; thus, flow decreases when vascular resistance increases. This applies to both right- and left-sided devices when faced with either high pulmonary or systemic vascular resistance. Perhaps more worrisome is compromised RV function due to high pulmonary arterial pressure in patients with a left ventricular assist device. RV failure in this population carries about a 30% mortality rate (Kirklin et al. 2014; Kirklin et al. 2015). Hence, adequate analgesia and sedation are of paramount importance in the initial perioperative period.

The stress response, akin to the "fight-or-flight response," causes modifications in a number of body systems including the hematopoietic, inflammatory, metabolic, and neurohormonal systems. Collectively, the effects can be disruptive for a critically ill perioperative patient. It can precipitate bleeding, a catabolic state, immunosuppression, and poor wound healing. Hence, acute postoperative pain management not only prevents undesirable hemodynamic conditions, it can potentially neutralize neuroendocrine, hematologic, and immunologic mediators, which may decrease overall morbidity (Peters et al. 2007; Caputo et al. 2011).

During the pre-extubation stage, adequate analgesic coverage is imperative. See Table 20.2. However, this must be balanced against the untoward effects of sedation and preservation of a functional respiratory drive. Options include an intravenous infusion or bolus, a thoracic epidural, a regional block (intercostal, intrapleural, or paravertebral), a local infusion, or simply *per oris*. Many strategies have been attempted with varying degrees of success. For example, the On-Q system, which delivers a continuous suprasternal infusion of bupivacaine, has demonstrated efficacy for reducing pain (Gommers and Bakker 2008; Sessler and Varney 2008), but the uptake has been less than enthusiastic. A multimodal approach utilizing various pharmacologic classes of medications is another popular strategy. It respects the multidimensional nature of acute pain management. Balancing opiates with

Table 20.2 Commonly used analgesics

Analgesics		
Drug	Dosing	Organs affected
Fentanyl	0.7–10 μg/kg/h	CNS, Respiratory, CVS, GI, GU
Hydromorphone	7–15 μg/kg/h	As above
Morphine	0.07–0.5 mg/kg/h	As above; Histamine release
Ketorolac	15–30 mg IV/IM q6h × 5 days	GI, Renal

Table 20.3 Ramsay scale

Ramsay scale	
1	Agitated
2	Cooperative
3	Responds to verbal commands
4	Responds to light stimulation
5	Responds to deep stimulation
6	Comatose

Table 20.4 Richmond agitation-sedation scale (RASS)

Richmond Agitation Sedation Scale (RASS)	
+4	Combative
+3	Harm to self
+2	Restless, ventilator dyssynchrony
+1	Anxious
0	Calm
-1	Awakens to voice
-2	Light sedation
-3	Moderate sedation
-4	Deep sedation
-5	Comatose

non-opiate analgesic such as acetaminophen, NSAIDs (Toradol, indomethacin), and NMDA antagonists (gabapentin, pregabalin) can be synergistic, decrease individual requirement, and minimize undesirable side effects (Buvanendran and Kroin 2009; Gandhi et al. 2011). Toradol should be used cautiously in the elderly and those with renal insufficiency. It should also be limited to less than 5 days. Gabapentin is being investigated in the perioperative period and is demonstrating a promising track record (Ucak et al. 2011).

The caveat to polypharmacy in this population is the group's high-risk status. Many have pre-existing organ dysfunction, especially liver congestion (from RHF) and kidney injury (from cardiorenal syndrome). Pharmacokinetics can be significantly altered and must be factored into the equation. Fortunately, objective assessment has emerged as a gold standard for evaluating and reevaluating neurologic status postoperatively. Several grading systems are commonly utilized. See Tables 20.3 and 20.4. This permits dose titration to an effect (e.g., RASS-2) and promotes individualized therapy (Jacobi et al. 2002, Vender et al. 2004).

Emergence from anesthesia remains an important milestone. The reality of a neurologic injury, given the risk profile of this population is a significant concern.

Many patients have cardiogenic shock or low output syndrome resulting in a low flow state prior to anesthesia induction. In patients with a prior neurologic event, the blood-brain barrier might already be compromised, thereby heightening the risk of a repeat injury during the operative period (Redmond et al. 1996). Additionally, some patients may have sustained a preoperative cardiac arrest with variable downtimes. Others may have developed a ventricular thrombus from a low flow state with risk of embolization during surgical manipulation. These are just some of the more commonly encountered scenarios, but the threat of injury in this population is high and should not be overlooked.

There are two major types of postoperative CNS injury. Type 1 includes stroke, encephalopathy, and coma. Type 2 includes memory or cognitive impairment (Newman et al. 2001a; Marasco et al. 2008). Type 1 is less common but carries a significant risk of mortality. Patients are prone to developing a perioperative stroke for the following: if they've had a prior stroke or other neurologic injury; if they are older in age; if they had multiple comorbidities, low ejection fraction, emergency surgery or redo-sternotomy, long CPB time, high transfusion requirement, LV thrombus, and aortic calcification; or if they have perioperative hypotension. An overwhelming majority are thromboembolic in nature, thus aortic manipulation is a significant culprit. Some authors have proposed preventative measures as screening carotid ultrasounds, preoperative statins, epi-aortic scanning, minimizing attempts at cross-clamping, avoiding use of pump suckers, and performing circulatory arrest if a porcelain aorta is encountered (Zibgone et al. 2006; Rosenberger et al. 2008; Bojar 2011). These are reasonable suggestions with a favorable risk to benefit ratio and should be executed when feasible. Cerebral oximetry can provide useful intraoperative feedback. Maneuvers to improve brain saturations include increased pump flow, increased MAP, increased hemoglobin, and increased $PaCO_2$ (for cerebral autoregulation). Patients who develop a perioperative stroke will manifest a focal deficit. Presentation can be early or delayed. Cross-sectional imaging with computed tomography is usually diagnostic. About 30% of perioperative infarcts will be hemorrhagic, thus complicating device anticoagulation management (Filsoufi et al. 2008a). The goal however is to decrease ICP by maintaining a higher MAP, forced diuresis, and early steroid administration. If feasible the addition of an antiplatelet agent and systemic heparin can be beneficial. Early rehabilitation is strongly encouraged. Unfortunately, long-term mortality remains high in this population due to progressive debilitation (Salazar et al. 2001; Dacey et al. 2005). Type 2 CNS injury is neurocognitive decline. This is the more prevalent of the two but still underdiagnosed. The exact etiology is unclear but may be related to cardiopulmonary bypass and a compromise blood-brain barrier. Symptoms can appear early or late. Early decline is likely from intraoperative micro-embolization and/or hypoperfusion. Late decline is likely due to underlying cerebrovascular disease. Patients will present with a deterioration of intellectual function and impaired memory. Prevention is best, with close attention to intraoperative care. Management, once recognized, is supportive. Many of these patients will survive well beyond discharge but neurologic subtleties persist. This was seen by Newman et al. in 2001 as 42% of CABG patients demonstrated a degree of cognitive impairment at 5 years (Newman et al. 2001b). This is unlikely attributable to solely a history of surgery but more so, progressive cerebrovascular disease.

20.3 Respiratory

Patients will arrive to the ICU intubated and under the effects of cardiac anesthesia. Seldom are patients extubated in the operating room. This may be possible for lower-risk patients (INTERMACS 2–3) undergoing urgent (as opposed to emergent) temporary mechanical support such as an axillary IABP or an axillary Impella 5.0. Both generally require a surgical cut down for vascular access so patients will customarily receive general anesthesia. Depending on the degree of cardiogenic shock and overall intraoperative hemodynamic status, they may still be considered a candidate for OR extubation. This is advantageous in terms of early ambulation and overall recovery.

More commonly, INTERMACS 2–3 patients should be extubated within the first 12 h after ICU arrival. Standard respiratory system management includes volume-controlled ventilation at an FiO_2 100%, tidal volume of 6–8 cm^3/kg, and PEEP of 5 cmH_2O. This will ensure efficient gas exchange and minimize the work of breathing. Naturally, settings should be individualized based on a patient's respiratory demands. Obese patients with a heavy chest wall may need slightly higher tidal volumes and/or PEEP. COPD patients may need longer expiration times to prevent "auto-PEEP." Those with violated pleural spaces and significant atelectasis may need additional recruitment maneuvers. Nevertheless, "resting" the respiratory system is extremely critical, while other common postoperative hurdles are being assessed and managed, such as hypothermia, acid-base disturbances, electrolyte disturbances, arrhythmias, preload status, myocardial contractility, and altered systemic vascular resistance. Most patients will have a pulmonary artery catheter thus PA pressures, CI and SVO_2 should be closely monitored. It is imperative to maintain baseline PA pressures with aggressive ventilator management. This will minimize unnecessary RV strain from the increased afterload. For patients whom are able to initiate spontaneous breaths, the SIMV setting can be utilized with a pressure support of 5–8 cmH_2O. The bedside monitor will display a continuous pulse oximetry reading. The FiO_2 should be continually adjusted to maintain a $SaO_2 > 93–95\%$ and/or a $PaO_2 > 70–80$ mmHg. Arterial blood gases should be checked 15–30 min after arrival and then as needed to ensure adequate oxygenation, ventilation, and neutralization of any acid-base disturbance. A CXR is integral for evaluation of vascular catheters and endotracheal tube position, the pleural spaces, the lung parenchyma, the mediastinal width, and most importantly device cannula(e) position. It is not uncommon to experience cannula malposition after transportation from the operating room to the ICU. Device flows needs to be assessed. If needed, subtle manipulations can be done at the bedside with CXR or echocardiographic assistance. For significant malposition, a return trip to the operating room is prudent for fluoroscopic repositioning.

General anesthesia and the operative details are significant culprits for postoperative V/Q mismatch and intrapulmonary shunting. Cessation of the respiratory system with conversion to mechanical ventilation causes inherent atelectasis. A sternotomy (mini or full) or thoracotomy will inevitably result in postoperative splinting and altered ventilatory dynamics (Toraman et al. 2005; Lena et al. 2008). Violation of the pleural spaces induces pleural effusions and contributes to compressive atelectasis. Furthermore, chest tubes can result in significant discomfort causing further V/Q mismatch (Reis et al. 2002). To reiterate, integral patient care management includes early ambulation and adequate postoperative analgesia to facilitate deep breathing. Cardiopulmonary bypass results in fluid overload, hemodilution, and a lowered oncotic pressure (Mora et al. 1996; Yende and Wunderlink 2002). It also manifests a systemic inflammatory response that creates additional lung injury. The net effect is increased extravascular water and pulmonary edema. Thus, as soon as volume resuscitation is completed, diuresis is vital to facilitate adequate gas exchange and extubation. Transfusion of blood and products introduces microemboli and pro-inflammatory mediators that can also affect the pulmonary microcirculation and increase pulmonary morbidity (Constantinides et al. 2006; Hemmerling et al. 2008a, b). The most feared complication of course being TRALI and furthermore ARDS. Lastly, as with all open mediastinal procedures, the phrenic nerves must be identified, if within the surgical field, and preserved. Caution must also be exercised with indirect contact, such as traction and thermal injury. Phrenic nerve palsy can be an unforgiving complication and contribute to significant morbidity.

Once stabilization has been reached, patients can begin assessment for ventilator weaning. This involves a global assessment.

1. Neurologically—they should be awake, appropriate, and following commands; temperature should be near normal (>36 °C).
2. Respiratory—$PaO_2/FiO_2 > 150$ and $PCO_2 < 45$ cmH_2O.
3. Cardiovascular—stable rhythm and MAP (>65 mmHg) and a CI >2.2 L/min/m^2.
4. Renal—adequate diuresis or plans for renal replacement therapy.
5. Heme—minimal chest tube drainage.

Perhaps the most crucial element is the PA pressure. As a patient's ventilatory drive returns and normalizes, they can develop patient-ventilator dyssynchrony or impaired mechanics which can result in turbulent PA pressures, endangering the right ventricle. Thoughtful decisions should be made regarding anxiolytics, sedation, analgesics, inotropes, and pulmonary vasodilators prior to initiating a wean or expeditiously, during the weaning process. Again, RV function should be at the forefront with the focus being to minimize insult. Patients demonstrating any concerning sign should remain intubated and reassessed after improvement. This can include neurologic: somnolence or agitation; respiratory: hypoxia, hypercarbia, or excessive tachypnea; or cardiovascular: arrhythmia or sudden changes in hemodynamics.

Once things are aligned for weaning, the patient is assessed for extubation. They must be awake and appropriate. Ventilation is switched to CPAP with an $FiO_2 < 50\%$

and a pressure support of 10–15 cmH_2O. A spontaneous breathing trial should be performed. Appropriate ventilatory mechanics include a negative inspiratory force >25 cmH_2O, a tidal volume > 5 mL/kg, a vital capacity >10–15 mL/kg, and a RR <24 breaths/min. Arterial blood gases should demonstrate a $PaO_2 > 70$ cmH_2O, a $PCO_2 < 45$ cmH_2O, and a pH of 7.35–7.45. Post-extubation care is equally important, as RV failure can ensue with even subtle respiratory compromise or delayed intervention. Again, caution and vigilance should be exercised with difficult airway patients, as delays in re-intervention can be catastrophic. Pulse oximetry is closely monitored. Supplemental oxygen should be provided and escalated to maintain a $SaO_2 > 93$–95%. Pain control is vital to minimize splitting. Aggressive pulmonary toilet should be enforced. This includes using an incentive spirometer 10–20×/h and doing deep breathing exercises. Some studies have demonstrated a lack of benefit of incentive spirometry with regards to postoperative pulmonary complications (Overend et al. 2001; Westerdahl et al. 2003; Freitas et al. 2007). However, it remains a staple of quality postoperative care. Chest physiotherapy is recommended for select patients, those with underlying pulmonary disease, borderline pulmonary function, or copious secretions (Pasquina et al. 2003). Bronchodilators should be limited to those with bronchospasm. Patients should continue to receive adequate diuresis if they have significant third spacing, assessed by clinical exam and daily weights. Antibiotics should be broadened from surgical prophylaxis to sepsis prophylaxis if any concern of pulmonary infection. Perhaps most importantly is early mobilization. Patients should be transitioned to an upright position as soon as possible. This can include a cardiac chair or simply out of bed to chair. Ambulation should commence once medically safe. This is undoubtedly the most effective therapy for pulmonary toilet. In fact, some ICUs have protocols for walking with PA catheters and ECMO circuits (non-femoral cannulation) to champion early ambulation (Lehr et al. 2015). As many patients on mechanical support require heparinization, chemical DVT prophylaxis is usually bypassed, but mechanical prophylaxis should be utilized unless contraindicated. Finally, swallowing should be carefully monitored as aspiration risks are high after prolonged intubation periods. If any concern, obtain a formal swallow evaluation which may include a videoscopic assessment.

Despite the optimism of an uncomplicated extubation and a streamlined recovery, respiratory complications are common. See Fig. 20.1. Most heart failure patients receiving temporary or durable support are critically ill and are typically INTERMACS stage 1–2. Many have significant underlying cardiopulmonary comorbidities (COPD, smoking history, severe MR, obesity, renal insufficiency, or even restrictive lung disease from recurrent pleural effusions); are hospitalized with decompensated heart failure, on inotropes; and are minimally ambulatory. Some are even intubated in the critical care unit. Therefore, their preoperative reserve is diminished at best. Prolonged intubation can be anticipated. Some cases can be physiologically challenging thus delaying ventilator wean and extubation. There can be hemodynamic lability, ongoing ventricular tachyarrhythmias, excessive third spacing with persistent pulmonary edema, intrinsic pulmonary disease, pulmonary infection, poor gas exchange, or even neurologic injury. Acute lung injury is

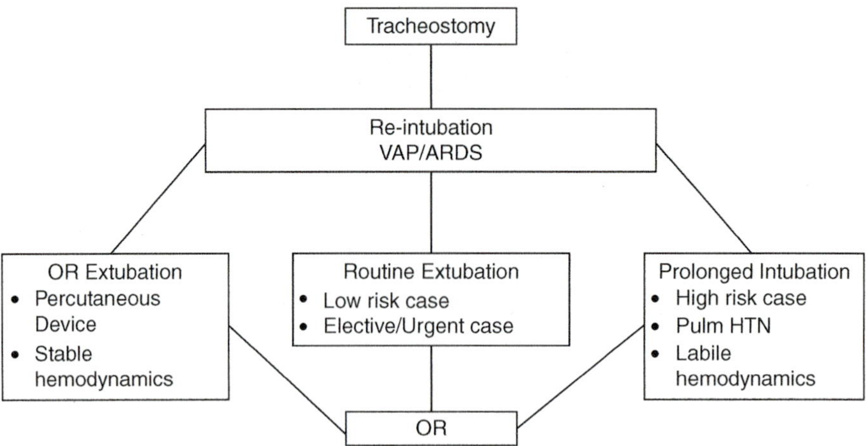

Fig. 20.1 Progression to respiratory failure requiring tracheostomy

characterized by bilateral infiltrates and a P/F ratio of 200-300 and can be a common finding in a postoperative MCS patient. This can be due to the aforementioned reasons as well as inadequate O_2 delivery, excessive oxygen utilization due to poor perfusion, pulmonary issues (atelectasis, pulmonary edema, pneumonia, worsening underlying lung disease, transfusion-related lung injury, pneumothorax, or pleural effusions), metabolic derangements, or even adverse pharmacologic effects (Bojar 2011). Management is supportive until gas exchange improves and weaning can be commenced. This includes maximal ventilatory support with recruitment maneuvers, pleural drains, aggressive diuresis, inotropic and vasopressor support, and especially, nutritional support. Mechanical support with veno-veno ECMO remains a viable option and should be considered sooner than later, depending on nature of injury and likelihood of recovery. Unfortunately, those with acute lung injury have higher complication rates, including multi-organ system dysfunction which can carry a mortality rate up to 30% (Filsoufi et al. 2008b).

In a small percentage of patients, respiratory insufficiency persists to a chronic phase. The timing of this is variable but generally considered when >5 days of mechanical support is needed. The etiology again can be due to persistent hypoxia (from either a circulatory issue or a pulmonary issue), persistent hypercarbia (due to an imbalance between ventilation capacity and demand), or worsening ARDS. Patients who stumble along this path are usually not candidates for ECLS due to their lower likelihood of recovery. Management is supportive. An appropriate mode of ventilation and setting should be chosen to adhere to lung protective strategies. Patients should receive appropriate sedation to minimize dyssynchrony and discomfort. The hemodynamic status should be optimized with inotropes and pressors to ensure adequate tissue perfusion. Nutrition should be minimally interrupted. But most importantly, the respiratory system should be properly cared for. As such, antibiotics, diuretics, pleural drainage procedures, atraumatic suctioning, and toilet bronchoscopies become critical maintenance therapies to help curb injury and promote recovery (Bojar 2011). Chronic patient care issues as avoidance of decubitus ulcers, muscle strengthening exercises, and stress ulcer prophylaxis are also of utmost importance. The critical question becomes tracheostomy timing. Most sternotomy patients will be deferred for 2–3 weeks as to minimize the risk of a deep sternal wound infection, though this association is still debatable (Trouillet et al. 2009; Ngaage et al. 2008; Byhahn et al. 2000; Curtis et al. 2001; Force et al. 2005). Non-sternotomy patients can be considered for tracheostomy if ventilatory support is needed beyond 7 days. Of note, caution should be exercised with all interventional procedures as risk for bleeding is high due to systemic anticoagulation for device management and the inherent quantitative and qualitative clotting dysfunction that occurs in the MCS population. Heparin should be turned off for 4–6 h and factors and platelets corrected to an appropriate level, prior to intervention. Bleeding is exacerbated in this population and can be difficult to control thus increasing the risk of morbidity and mortality. Prudent judgment is key.

20.4 Cardiovascular

20.4.1 Intro

Patients undergoing mechanical support generally have a low output state and decompensated heart failure. They've usually failed maximal medical management and are starting to demonstrate worsening end-organ dysfunction. The components of CO have become compromised. See Fig. 20.2. Assuming the proper patient, device, and timing were chosen, the intraoperative course can significantly reverse the deleterious effects from decompensated heart failure. Frequently, inotropic support can be reduced. Renal function typically improves, and the overall hemodynamics stabilize. The particulars do vary from device to device and whether support is a uni- vs. biventricular configuration. Regardless, the goal is circulatory support and reversibility of end-organ injury.

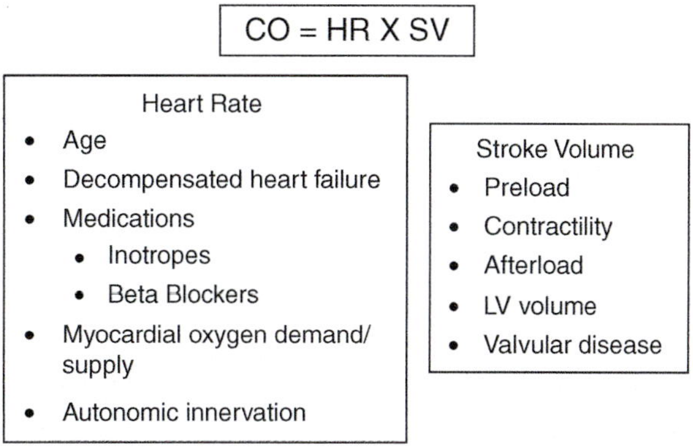

CO = HR X SV

Heart Rate

- Age
- Decompensated heart failure
- Medications
  - Inotropes
  - Beta Blockers
- Myocardial oxygen demand/supply
- Autonomic innervation

Stroke Volume

- Preload
- Contractility
- Afterload
- LV volume
- Valvular disease

Fig. 20.2 Determinants of cardiac output

20.4.2 Rate and Rhythm

A normal rate and rhythm is always the goal, as it minimizes myocardial oxygen demand and facilitates ventricular unloading. Unfortunately, impediments exist—a catecholamine requirement, an overloaded cavity, an ongoing myocardial ischemia, a pre-existing arrhythmia, a valvular regurgitation, a cannula position, as well as non-cardiac etiologies—all contributing to persistent arrhythmias. The most common rhythm disturbance in this population is tachyarrhythmias—both supraventricular and ventricular. The initial response should be electrical cardioversion for rhythm stabilization. However, most heart failure patients will already have an implantable defibrillator that may detect and shock prior to any planned intervention. Defibrillators can be interrogated to review rhythm and treatment activity; sensitivities can be adjusted for more tailored therapy. Pacing functions can also be activated to manage bradyarrhythmias and certain tachyarrhythmias (atrial fibrillation and atrial flutter) as with overdrive pacing. Common things are common though, so an astute investigation for an electrolyte, respiratory or metabolic imbalance should be ruled out or corrected. Mechanical triggers should be checked for and adjusted—endotracheal tubes, PA catheter, chest tubes, and cannula position. A PA catheter that is too deep in the RV can trigger ventricular tachyarrhythmias. Infrequent but an anteriorly placed mediastinal chest tube can compress the RV free wall after chest closure and trigger arrhythmias once suction is applied. A malpositioned temporary support device can certainly be a culprit for ectopy. Subtle adjustments can be done at the bedside, but a return trip to the operating room with image guidance should be arranged, if needed. Repositioning a durable device is not commonly performed but maneuvers as adjusting pump speeds and volume loading may alleviate any mechanical friction. Persistent VT in a postoperative durable LVAD patient with underlying ICM can be due to ongoing ischemia. Such patients may require ablative therapy depending on severity as revascularization is not usually feasible. Correctable ischemia should be identified and treated (kinked or occluded graft). The real danger of persistent VT though is the negative impact on the unsupported ventricle. The most common scenario being an LVAD patient (temporary or durable) with persistent VT who runs the risk of compromised RV function, decreased LVAD flow, and inevitably RVF. Less common but certainly lethal would be an RVAD patient who develops persistent VT, as LV ejection and systemic perfusion could cease with development of flash pulmonary edema. Patients on ECMO may develop refractory ventricular tachyarrhythmia from LV distention. In such cases, LV decompression with an additional cannula or temporary support device (e.g., Impella CP) is prudent to offload the LV and prevent further insult. Finally, miscellaneous causes should be sought out and treated—fever, hypothermia, patient discomfort, septic foci, etc. Most arrhythmias can be tempered with pharmacologic means while a search is ongoing. Most commonly this involves the utilization of an amiodarone infusion and, rarely, propafenone for supraventricular arrhythmias and a lidocaine infusion with or without amiodarone for ventricular tachyarrhythmias. The entire spectrum of class I–IV agents, common after routine cardiac surgery, is infrequently a viable option with this population due to the negative inotropy inherent with many of the agents as well as their side effect profile. Occasionally, conversion to oral formulations (amiodarone, sotalol, digoxin, mexiletine) is needed for maintenance therapy, but the underlying etiology should be sought out and corrected, if possible.

20.4.3 Preload

CVP, though a crude hemodynamic parameter, is a staple for postoperative fluid management. Although there is value in looking at the PAD pressure to ascertain LV preload, the more commonly utilized parameter is CVP. The variability with PAD due to respiratory perturbations lends reluctance to placing too much emphasis on this value. Furthermore, a PA catheter is not feasible when a right-sided device or venous cannulae are utilized. The astute surgeon needs to gauge what CVP range represents the ideal filling pressure for each individual patient. This can vary significantly from patient to patient, based on underlying pathophysiology and the specific device used. The assessment is done intraoperatively by examining the heart, either directly in the field or on echocardiogram, in parallel with device flows, ventricular unloading, and overall hemodynamics. Loading conditions are carefully assessed as speed alterations are made while keeping a critical eye on ventricular compliance and function, hemodynamics, and overall perfusion. Once a steady state is reached, the ideal filling pressures are noted and passed along to the intensive care unit team to facilitate postoperative management. Euvolemia for most LVAD patients (temporary or durable) falls between a CVP 10–15 mmHg and a PAD 15–20 mmHg. The situation is a bit more challenging for right-sided devices and when a venous drainage cannula is present. A normal or high CVP is less reliable, but a low CVP usually indicates hypovolemia. The crucial parameter will be device flow. When flow rates are decreased or the ECMO circuit is "chattering," volume loading is likely needed. However, cannula position should be ascertained to ensure adequate positioning as a cause for flow disturbance.

Patients undergoing chest closure are particularly vulnerable for hemodynamic fluxes. Ventricular unloading can predominate requiring volume resuscitation. Tamponade physiology can prevail with or without bleeding. Sternotomy closure can impair contractility and RV filling by direct compression, thus limiting forward flow and resulting in an elevated CVP. This is especially common in hypervolemic patients who have significant third spacing and prominent myocardial edema. The most prudent thing in these situations is to leave the chest open and to consider leaving a spacer in between the sternal edges as tamponade is still possible in open-chested cases. Bleeding within a closed space can result in venous inflow compression and tamponade. Re-exploration should not be delayed because significant ventricular dysfunction can ensue.

It is not uncommon after initiation of mechanical support for volume resuscitation to be needed. Although patients tend to be fluid overloaded, their intravascular volume status may be limited requiring fluid boluses, which is typical for capillary leak. Ventricular unloading can be surprisingly rapid and urine production excessive, requiring continuous volume replacement until a steady state is reached. Loses can be ongoing, as with puncture site bleeding, an expanding retroperitoneal hematoma, or chest wall bleeding from aggressive CPR, requiring blood and blood products. Vasodilatory shock can ensue from postoperative rewarming to post-CPB inflammatory mediators, both requiring volume loading and afterload support. The focus should remain on device flow and hemodynamic status. For patients with total cardiac replacement, such as with a total artificial heart, haptic feedback is continuously provided, the fill volume of each ventricle. A low fill volume and downward-sloping waveform usually signify that additional volume is needed.

At the other end of the spectrum is ventricular over distention from overzealous resuscitation or flow. This can position the unsupported ventricle too far rightward along the Starling curve resulting in failure. Overdistention increases wall tension and myocardial oxygen demand and decreases the trans-myocardial gradient, resulting in impaired coronary blood flow (Bojar 2011). The imbalance results in depressed contractility. Prompt recognition is key to reverse the potentially deleterious effects of myofiber overstretching. An echocardiogram should be obtained to evaluate ventricular size and function, and inotropes should be adjusted to stabilize flow and hemodynamic parameters. Low LVAD flow with an elevated CVP and normal PA pressure is a red flag for RV overdistention and RVF. Alternatively, aggressive RVAD flow with a low MAP and new pulmonary edema signifies excessive forward flow and LVF.

CVP becomes an important hemodynamic parameter for managing mechanical support devices in the perioperative period. Although there is merit in the exact numerical value, it needs to be interpreted with the context of device type, a patient's underlying physiology, and other pertinent variables.

20.4.4 Pulmonary Afterload

Pulmonary vascular resistance is the net result of left heart dysfunction, pre-existing pulmonary disease, and superimposed perioperative pulmonary insults, as infection, interstitial edema, or pleural space issues. Microcirculatory constriction from various stimuli either new or old increases shunting and decreases pulmonary runoff. This increased RV afterload can be detrimental to RV function. In fact, RV failure post-LVAD implantation carries about a 25% mortality rate. The RV is responsible for forward flow to the left side. Thus a distended, poorly contractile RV, combined with high PA pressures and an under-filled LV, is a grave situation. Immediate intervention, perhaps with mechanical support, is vital. See Fig. 20.3.

For patients supported with an LVAD, it is important to create an environment conducive for optimal RV function. Preoperative pulmonary function testing and resting PA pressures need careful attention. Patients considered having moderate to high PA pressures need proper surgical planning. A threshold should be established for mechanical support. Intraoperatively, the optimal combination of preload, contractility, and afterload needs to be configured. As previously mentioned the RV should be volume loaded to the point of maximal contractility without causing

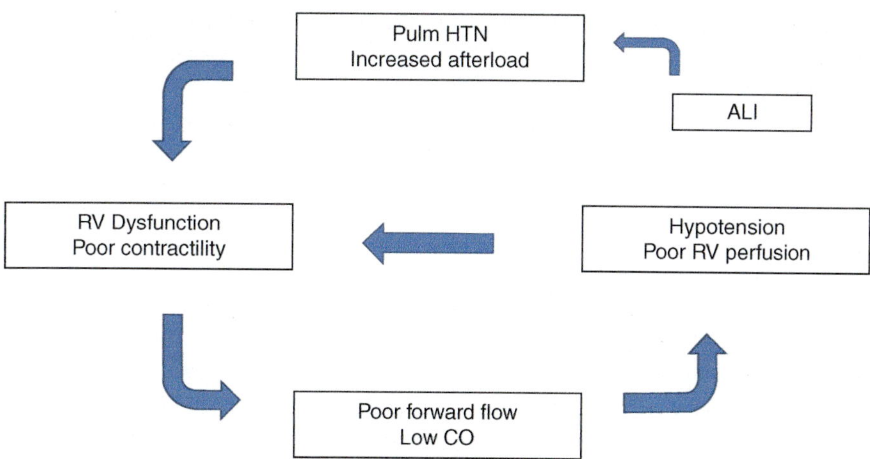

Fig. 20.3 Vicious cycle of RVF

overstretching or dysfunction. Inotropes should be adjusted to maintain a thermodilution CI > 2.2 L/min/m^2 and VAD flows >2.2CI L/min/m^2. Pulmonary afterload should be carefully managed with pulmonary vasodilators. This may include inotropes with dilator properties (milrinone or dobutamine), a synthetic natriuretic peptide (nesiritide), nitro-dilators (nitroglycerin and nitroprusside), or direct pulmonary dilators (inhaled nitric oxide, intravenous epoprostenol or inhaled iloprost). Inhaled nitric oxide has a desirable profile. It decreases pulmonary vascular resistance, improves RV function, and exerts minimal systemic effects. The limitations include high costs, a cumbersome setup, and a rebound phenomenon during weaning. Epoprostenol is a potent intravenous dilator and so affects both the pulmonic and systemic vascular trees. Its major limitation is hemodynamic instability. Iloprost, like iNO, is an inhaled formulary; thus, the effects are concentrated on the pulmonary circulation with little systemic effects. Its lower cost and ease of use increases the appeal, but the uptake has been less than enthusiastic. Studies comparing the various dilators have been mixed. In any case, most institutions will have their inherent biases, which also deserve merit.

Patients supported with an RVAD also need carefully regulated pulmonary vascular pressures. Since most devices are afterload sensitive, flow will be impaired once pulmonary resistance increases. This situation can potentially be fatal. If forward flow ceases, the LV will be under-filled and systemic pressures can drop precipitously. Thus, maintaining adequate flows and pulmonary vascular resistance is vital.

20.4.5 Systemic Afterload

The same concept applies to systemic afterload and LVADs. As systemic vascular resistance increases, LVAD flows decrease. Depending on the contribution from the native ventricle, this can have grave physiologic effects. Additionally, lower flow can result in less ventricular decompression, septal shift, and impairment of the unsupported ventricle. It can also result in stasis increasing the risk of thrombogenicity (Bennett and Adatya 2015). A common scenario is peripheral vasoconstriction after cardiopulmonary bypass and cross-clamping. The net effect is increased systemic vascular resistance and higher MAPs. As patients rewarm, runoff increases and the vascular resistance decreases. Nevertheless, maintaining a tightly controlled afterload range is key for proper LVAD function. Typically, the MAP is kept between 70 and 85 mmHg. Studies have demonstrated higher hemorrhagic stroke rates in MCS patients with a MAP>85 mmHg; thus, it is advantageous to have afterload reducers and dilators available during the perioperative period. This may include nitroprusside and/or nitroglycerin, respectively. Nitroprusside should be a first-line agent as it works on the arterial tree, whereas nitroglycerin will veno-dilate and alter loading condition. Alternatively, inotropes can be down titrated, but this is a less preferable solution as many cases have borderline contractility.

Alternatively, low systemic vascular resistance should be supported to ensure adequate perfusion pressures. A goal MAP 70–85 mmHg should be targeted. Patients will commonly develop vasoplegic shock and may require one or more vasopressors to stabilize the blood pressure. Most commonly, vasopressin is used first, then norepinephrine, and lastly, phenylephrine. Methylene blue has also demonstrated utility in cases of profound shock. It inhibits guanylate cyclase activation by nitric oxide, therefore lowering circulating GMP, a local vasodilator, and raising the blood pressure.

20.4.6 Contractility

Almost every patient supported with a mechanical support device will be placed on a cocktail of inotropes. The rare exceptions are total cardiac replacement, intolerance due to arrhythmias, and situations where myocardial recovery is futile. However, myocardial contractility and optimization are the usual goals. Central to inotrope selection is an understanding of mechanism of actions and side effect profiles. See Table 20.5.

Epinephrine, dobutamine, and/or dopamine will often be used first. Epinephrine is a common first-line agent. It has excellent inotropic and chronotropic effects mostly from its beta-1 properties. At low concentrations it can exert beta-2 effects,

Table 20.5 Effects of common inotropes

Inotropes				
Drug	HR	CO	SVR	PVR
Epinephrine	↑↑	↑	↑	↑
Dobutamine	↑↑	↑	↓	↓
Dopamine	↑↑	↑	↔	↔
Milrinone	↑	↑	↓	↓

and at high concentrations its vasoconstrictor properties predominate. A typical infusion is between 1 and 6 μg/min. Dobutamine also has a strong beta-1 effect making it a good inotrope. The systemic effects are unclear, but reports have shown decrease systemic vascular resistance (Romson et al. 1999). Additional benefits include augmentation of coronary blood flow, thus balancing out myocardial oxygen supply and demand (Fowler et al. 1984) and lowered pulmonary vascular resistance, thereby improving RV function. It typically runs between 5 and 20 μg/kg/min. Dopamine, like epinephrine, has dose-dependent effects. At low doses (<5 μg/kg/min), it has a dopaminergic effect as various receptors are activated, resulting in diuresis, inotropy, chronotropy, and vasoconstriction. The effects are generally mild. The renal benefits, however, remain controversial (Lassnigg et al. 2000; Woo et al. 2002). At moderate doses (5–10 μg/kg/min), the beta-1 effects predominate. At high doses (>10 μg/kg/min), the alpha vasoconstrictor effects predominate. Milrinone is a favored choice for cases of RV dysfunction and high pulmonary vascular resistance. It is a phosphodiesterase inhibitor which increases cyclic AMP levels. This induces smooth muscle relaxation, manifesting as reduced filling pressures and reduced pulmonic and systemic vascular resistance. Limitations of milrinone are its long half-life (~2 h) and systemic effects. In a majority of cases, when used, the blood pressure is often supported with a vasopressor.

Myocardial preservation is essential. Contractility helps unload the ventricles and adds pulsatility to the circulation. The contribution may be mild at best, but its trophic effects are beneficial. For durable device cases, myocardial viability is essential for survival to transplantation or survival overall (for destination cases). For cases of temporary support, myocardial preservation can be monumental in helping to parse out bridging decisions.

LVF in the MCS population has variable significance depending on degree of dysfunction and type of support employed. As previously mentioned, maintaining inotropic support for LV contractility and emptying is a beneficial strategy. Infusions should be titrated as the clinical course unfolds. For patients supported with a left-sided device, overt LVF is not too worrisome, assuming the device continues to function well and the cavity remains decompressed. When device flows become compromised though, the situation escalates. The ventricle can quickly distend causing septal shift and RV dysfunction. Pulmonary edema can rapidly ensue. The device will either need to be switched out or the patient supported via alternate means—pharmacologic and/or mechanical. Prompt decision-making and prevention of additional organ injury are key goals. For patients with a right-sided device who develop LVF, this can be catastrophic and even fatal. Continued forward flow will overstretch the LV, deteriorating function even more while flooding the lungs at the same time. Ejection can cease and the patient arrests. Response times are absolutely critical because even a delayed response of a few minutes can be irreversible. The safest bailout in these situations is conversion to VA ECMO. Patients on VA ECMO who develop worsening LVF and lose pulsatility need assessment of LV distention. If present, the cavity should be vented either surgically or percutaneously.

Vigilance for detecting and ruling out cardiac tamponade should always remain at the forefront for hemodynamic disturbances. It can occur at any time in the post-operative period, not just early on. Prompt recognition, assessment, and intervention are key. Generally, patients will have hypotension, altered device flows or parameters, and elevated filling pressures. The presentation in most cases will be subtle, thereby increasing the diagnostic complexity. Echocardiographic assessment can help identify right-sided compression. Immediate exploration and decompression should follow.

Mechanical failure is a universally feared complication of this form of therapy. Fortunately, it rarely happens without warning signs. LVADs display power readings and waveforms that can be monitored for impending failure. The TAH displays pressure and flow waveforms that translate similar information. The Impella devices monitor purge flow and pressure which can serve as a warning sign. Lastly, ECMO, TandemHeart and CentriMag will demonstrate a buildup of fibrin and clot prior to requiring a change out. Device failure from pump thrombosis and cannula obstruction is uncommon but should remain on the differential. Thrombus can form anywhere along the LVAD circuit. Thrombus can also transit into the circuit from the heart or peripheral circulation. Clot propagation can ultimately obstruct flow. Additionally, the inflow cannula can suck down on the septum causing acute occlusion. This can happen with significant septal motion or improper cannula placement. The outflow cannula can become kinked or externally compressed resulting in occlusion. The common pathway is low device flow and altered hemodynamics. The device will need to be interrogated to help ascertain the likelihood of a mechanical issue. An echocardiogram should be obtained to check ventricular size and response to speed changes. A CT angiogram should follow to look for filling defects. Biomarkers as LDH and plasma-free hemoglobin should be checked to help formalize a diagnosis. The hemodynamics should be supported, while decision about thrombolytic therapy, temporary mechanical support, and device exchange is mapped out.

Perhaps the more commonly feared scenario is acute or acute-on-chronic RVF for patients supported with an LVAD. Unlike the progressive nature of LVF, RV function varies depending on the local milieu. Certainly patients with chronic biventricular failure should not receive uni-ventricular support. But for the overwhelming majority, RV assessment and reassessment are a continuous focus in the perioperative period. Favorable conditions include optimal preload, contractility, and afterload. CVP should be targeted for adequate filling. Inotropes should be titrated to maintain sufficient forward flow. Strategies to decrease pulmonary vascular resistance and RV afterload should be employed and closely titrated. Finally, VAD flows, LV size, and septal position should be frequently surveyed to ensure optimal ventricular interdependence. A rise in CVP with normal PAP and low VAD flows are a red flag for RV failure. Hemodynamic and laboratory derangements can be insidious, progressive, or acute depending on local conditions. A prompt echocardiographic assessment with either TEE or TTE can be instrumental as medical maneuvers to optimize preload, contractility, and afterload are undertaken. Echocardiographic parameters include RV size, contractility, septal position, excursion of the tricuspid annulus, and tricuspid regurgitation (Kapur and Jumean 2014; Korabathina et al. 2012). Consideration for mechanical support should also be given.

20.4.7 Special Considerations

IABPs offer the least amount of hemodynamic support, but they provide a critical function. They augment coronary perfusion by increasing diastolic flow. These devices have the longest proven "track record." They are mostly inserted percutaneously in the femoral artery. Patients requiring longer-term support though, as in status IA patients, can have it placed in the axillary artery via a surgical cutdown, so they can remain ambulatory (Russo et al. 2012). The device will usually remain in place until time of transplant. Complications are minimal but two noteworthy points are malposition and ischemic limb. Insertion into the axillary artery can be directly, with a sheath or indirectly, with a graft. The arm should be monitored for signs of ischemia or neuropathy. During day-to-day care, the CXRs should be reviewed to confirm device position. Occasionally the balloon flips on itself and the tip ends up in the ascending aorta or head vessels. This can happen when the arch anatomy is tortuous and too much inherent torque is stored in the catheter. Once discovered, it usually warrants a return trip to the operating room for device repositioning or exchange. Transplant may not occur for several weeks, thus increasing the complexity of device removal. If inserted with a sheath, the entire assembly is removed and the puncture site closed by tying off the original purse-string suture. Purging the puncture site, to flush out any possible thrombus, is possible but only if appropriate vascular control is obtained and is generally not very effective, the longer the interval from surgery. If inserted with a graft, the device is removed and the graft can be back bled and suctioned completely. Proper proximal and distal control must be maintained. The graft is then trimmed and secured. This blind sac can be a nidus for clot formation with the potential of distal embolization. Embolization can also occur at any point during device removal. Thus, arm pulses and perfusion should be monitored carefully. Having radial arterial lines on both arms can help identify an early discrepancy.

VA ECMO is usually performed in an urgent or emergent manner. Cannulation is typically peripheral and percutaneous. Occasionally it is done as an open insertion. Ongoing bleeding from the surgical cut down site tends to be a cumbersome problem. Bleeding can also ensue after percutaneous placement if multiple sticks were attempted. Occasionally this can surmount into a sizable, expanding hematoma with hemodynamic consequences requiring surgical cut down and vascular repair. Limb ischemia can be another devastating injury. Patients with small vessels can have limited antegrade flow around the femoral arterial cannula and risk ischemia. Bedside assessment with cutaneous oximetry, Doppler signals, and palpation is vital. Placement of a distal perfusion cannula is warranted if not already present but occasionally, access is difficult, or flow remains suboptimal. Some patients may have been cannulated at an outside facility and have been supported for days without a distal perfusion cannula before being transferred to your institution. Those with a threatened limb may end up getting a fasciotomy and, in severe cases, an amputation. The VA ECMO configuration offers biventricular support. The critical focus should be LV contractility and size. In some patients, left-sided venous return can be significant and distend the LV. A poorly contractile or fibrillating LV will quickly overdistend and result in pulmonary edema. Should this occur, a vent is required to unload the heart.

The Impella is an increasingly utilized temporary support device. Several models exist to meet a spectrum of needs. The smaller devices are mostly placed percutaneously via the femoral artery or vein. The Impella 5.0 is usually placed with a surgical cutdown. It's an axial flow device with the pump built into the catheter. The inlet sits in the LV and the outlet in the ascending aorta. Common postoperative issues include malposition, puncture site bleeding, hemolysis, and limb ischemia. Most repositioning can be done at the bedside with echo guidance, but at times a return trip to the operating room is required. Axillary insertion is similar to the IABP technique mentioned above; thus, neurovascular monitoring is essential. Vascular or cardiac injury is possible during insertion. Echocardiography should be utilized to assess for new pericardial fluid. Limb ischemia is uncommon during insertion but an unrecognized vascular injury as dissection can occur which can lead to downstream occlusion. Hemolysis tends to be more common with the lower flow devices, presumably due to a smaller blood channel. Diagnosis and management are described elsewhere in this chapter. Puncture site bleeding from percutaneous placement can usually be controlled with a purse-string suture, but occasionally operative exploration is needed for vascular repair. Patients with deep femoral vessels are at risk of the sheath retracting out of the vessel causing major bleeding from the arteriotomy site. Operative exploration is usually needed for vascular control and placement of a purse-string suture. More commonly is leg ischemia from poor antegrade flow around a percutaneous device. Prompt open removal, femoral thrombectomy, and device relocation, if support is needed, are warranted. Device removal (Impella 5.0) can also risk limb ischemia from acute embolic occlusion. Removal and monitoring techniques as previously mentioned are utilized. The Impella 5.0 has demonstrated great versatility for the spectrum of heart failure (Bansal et al. 2016). It can serve as a bridge to decision, transplant, durable device, or recovery. Patients can be weaned off inotropes and be completely ambulatory. If the Impella fails, it needs to be pulled back into the ascending aorta immediately. Retrograde flow will continue and cause LV distention. Depending on LV function, the device can be removed all together or replaced.

The Tandem products permit secure cannulation. The Tandem RVAD parks the ProTek Duo outflow cannula into the main PA and the inflow into the RA. The cannula remains fixed so migration is a relative nonissue. Access is limited to the RIJ vein. The cannula sizes are typically 29Fr or 31Fr, so fairly large. Insertion can result in central venous or cardiac injury. Thus an awareness for bleeding or tamponade should be maintained. Scanning for a pericardial effusion is not unreasonable. Despite the large cannula size, cerebral drainage is rarely an issue, but it should be monitored. Cannula replacement is not straightforward and should be done with extreme caution. Maximum flow with the Tandem pump is ~4.5 L, which may be insufficient for some patients. An oxygenator can easily be spliced in for conversion to ECMO, if needed. Finally, the tubing and cannula should be monitored for fibrin and clot buildup. When significant accumulation occurs, the circuit should be changed. A significant advantage of this configuration is the ability to mobilize the patient. The TandemHeart LVAD configuration places a drainage cannula trans-septally, into the left atrium, and returns blood to the femoral artery. Unlike the Tandem RVAD, patients with this setup are not able to mobilize. Concerns and other constraints are previously mentioned.

There is a growing awareness and familiarity with CFLVADs as they are being increasingly utilized for long-term therapy. The critical components of perioperative management are outlined throughout the chapter. There are presently three major devices routinely used: HeartMate II, HeartMate III, and HeartWare (Fig. 20.4). These are all implantable, durable pumps. HeartMate II requires a pre-peritoneal pump pocket, a source for additional morbidity. HeartMate III and HeartWare are placed intra-pericardially, permitting a non-sternotomy approach. There are major engineering differences between the three. HeartMate II is an axial pump. HeartMate III is a magnetically levitated centrifugal pump. HeartWare is a hydro-magnetically levitated centrifugal pump. The most crucial management issue in the perioperative period will be device flow, specifically, low flow. The overall clinical picture will need close assessment including hemodynamics, contractility, fluid balances, and relevant pre- and intraoperative details. Each device will also display parameters that will aid in the troubleshooting. HeartMate II and III use a pulsatility index. This gauges left ventricular contractility. A high PI signifies room for speed increase and a low PI speed decrease. These generalities must be taken in clinical context. HeartWare displays a continuous waveform tracing that contains sensitive hemodynamic data. Waveform analysis includes evaluation of waveform regularity, peaks, troughs, amplitude, and width. Details of this analysis are beyond the scope of this chapter. Generally speaking and similar to PI, a high amplitude signifies room for a speed increase, and low amplitude signifies a speed decrease.

A BiVAD can be planned or unplanned. Support can be with either temporary or durable devices. Many iterations are possible: Tandem/Impella, Impella/Impella, Tandem/Tandem, Impella/Tandem, CentriMag/CentriMag, CFLVAD/CFLVAD, CFLVAD + Tandem, Impella or CentriMag, etc. Implantation and perioperative concerns are the same as previously mentioned. The most crucial management issue is vigilant flow monitoring. RVAD flow must remain less than LVAD flow, to prevent pulmonary edema. The greater the native left ventricular contribution, the less critical this becomes.

TAH is a viable bridging solution for patients with clear biventricular failure. Unlike the aforementioned devices, this involves total cardiac replacement (Fig. 20.4). The ventricles are excised leaving a 1–2 cm cuff on each atrium. A "quick connect" is sutured to each atrial cuff, the ventricles are attached, and the outflow grafts are sutured to the aorta and pulmonary artery. The range of intra- and postoperative complications is extensive and discussed throughout this chapter. Perhaps the most crucial observation with this device is identifying early

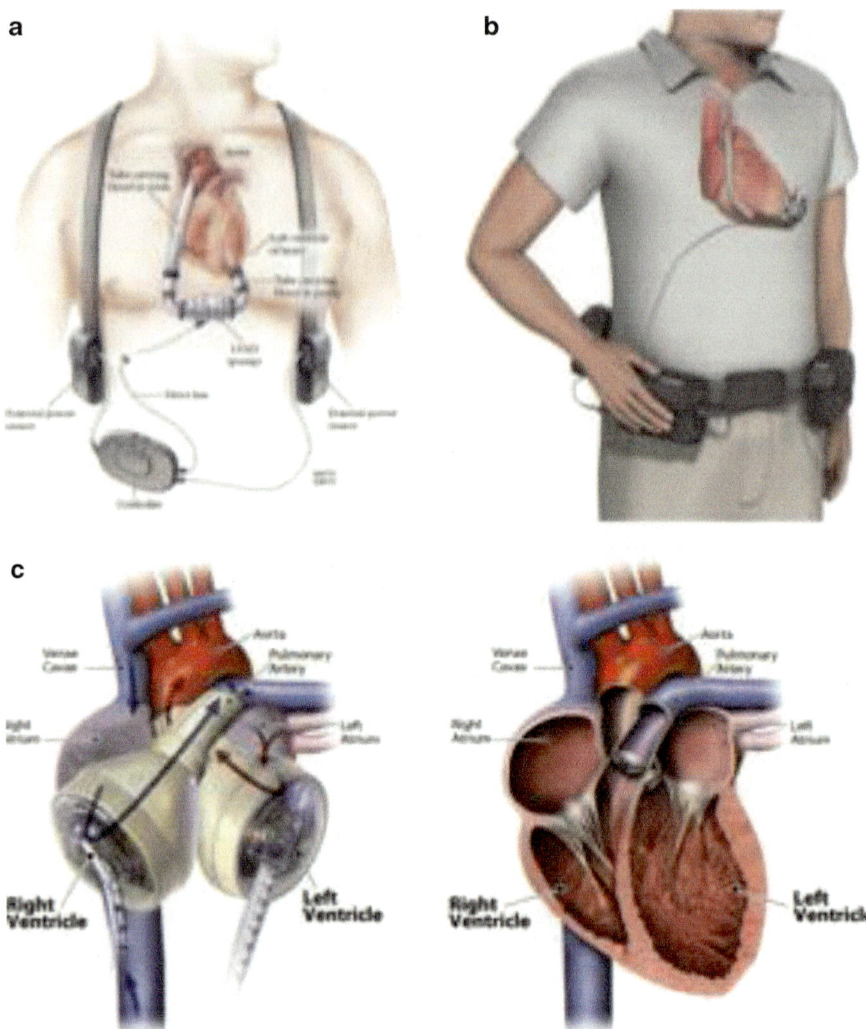

Fig. 20.4 (**a**) HeartMate II continuous flow axial pump (Thoratec Corp.). (**b**) HeartWare continuous flow centrifugal pump (HeartWare Inc.). (**c**) TAH pulsatile pump (Syncardia Systems, Inc.). (**d**) Normal heart for comparison. Reproduced with permission from Sen et al. Critical Care (2016) 20:153. Images were not altered. Creative Commons Attribution 4.0 International License (http://creativecommons.org/licenses/by/4.0/)

tamponade. This may present as a dampening of the RV fill curve. The console provides continuous pressure and flow tracings. Ventricular filling volume and flow measurements will also be displayed. These will fluctuate with loading conditions and afterload, but the trends should be analyzed. Daily CXRs should be reviewed for inspection of pericardial fluid. As fluid accumulates there will be loss of the radiolucent space created by the device membrane.

20.5 Renal

It is well known that perioperative renal dysfunction is a major determinant of both short- and long-term morbidity after cardiac surgery (Cooper et al. 2006; Hillis et al. 2006; Brown et al. 2008; Mehta et al. 2008; Gibson et al. 2008; Najafi et al. 2009). Unlike general adult cardiac cases, mechanical circulatory support patients have a more complicated picture. Typically, they have advanced decompensated heart failure and, in many case, underlying cardiorenal syndrome. In-house patients will already be receiving diuretic therapy and many will also be on low-dose inotropes. Reserves are questionable, at best. With such a delicate physiologic environment, creatinine becomes a marker for end-organ perfusion and subsequent intervention.

Many decompensated heart failure patients fall along one of three trajectories: bridge to transplantation, destination therapy, or maximal medical management. Those exhibiting signs of worsening end-organ function, as a rising creatinine, rise to the forefront of the decision-making trees. Usage of MCS as a bridge to decision, bridge to transplant, bridge to durable device, bridge to palliation, or even bridge to recovery becomes a priority issue. The next layer aims to narrow the spectrum and determine which specific device should be utilized—temporary or permanent. In cases of questionable candidacy for definitive treatments as transplantation and durable device, a temporary device is often utilized. In many instances, this acts as a filter for further interventions. Patients with borderline renal function, who may not be a candidate for dual organ listing (heart-kidney), may receive support with a temporary device to enable reassessment. Alternatively, transplant candidates with a short waiting time but in a low output state and rising creatinine may also be candidates for temporary support as it can enable bridge to transplantation. On the other hand, transplant candidates with a long wait time and decompensated heart failure with a rising creatinine may be routed straight to a durable device. The process can be fluid but does call on a multidisciplinary approach.

Those patients receiving mechanical support, urgently or electively, tend to have a positive response to end-organ perfusion. Achievement of full flow, with a CI > 2.2 L/min/m^2, renal perfusion improves significantly as seeing by copious urine output. The effect can be immediate, seen intraoperatively or delayed, several days later in the ICU. Patients assuming this trajectory usually show a recovery of acute kidney injury and an ability to wean down inotropes and diuretics (Coffin et al. 2015). The fate of emergent cases is somewhat less predictable. These patients are further along their disease curve. They typically have worsened end-organ function, may have sustained a cardiac arrest, and are likely receiving a delayed intervention. Restoration of a CI > 2.2 L/min/m^2 may not immediately suffice. These patients are often best served with early renal replacement therapy. Patients on ECMO can have the dialysis unit connected directly to the ECLS circuit. Those with other forms of mechanical support will need a vascular access catheter. Initiating early renal replacement therapy can be advantageous in terms of volume management, metabolic derangements, and drug clearance; however, drawbacks include quiescence of the native kidneys and limited mobility. Rehabilitative efforts will be delayed until conversion to intermittent hemofiltration and vascular catheters have been relocated from the groin.

In some patients mechanical support can directly impair renal function. Shearing forces can result in blood trauma and cell lysis. Cellular by-products as iron and hemosiderin deposit within renal tubules, decreasing glomerular filtration and precipitate renal failure (Qian et al. 2010). Risk factors for hemolysis include device engineering, low flow rates, and tissue abutment. On bedside assessment, urine quality can change to "coke" colored, the overall output will decrease, and serum biomarkers will be elevated. These include creatinine, lactate dehydrogenase, and plasma-free hemoglobin. Clinically, patients will manifest signs of renal failure. Management includes initiation of renal replacement therapy, device removal, or decommissioning and protection from further renal injury. The all-comer data for renal recovery post-acute tubular necrosis is ~40–50% at 1 year (Bojar 2011), but this figure may be too generous for a high-risk group as the MCS population.

Patients manifesting milder forms of AKI should be managed per routine. Maneuvers to optimize device flow, minimize flow disturbance, improve cardiac output, augment renal function, and protect against further injury are general guidelines (Bojar 2011). Development of oliguria should prompt immediate assessment of intravascular volume and perfusion pressures. A low CVP should be fluid challenged. A high CVP should receive additional diuresis. Contractility and afterload should be assessed for titration of inotropes and pressors. Of note, renal dysfunction can be the red herring for RV failure; thus, prompt assessment and intervention are imperative. Caution should be exercised with high-dose vasopressors as this will intensify renal vasoconstriction and further impair function. Diuretics should be uptitrated rapidly to avoid anuria. Care providers should be vigilant to avoid any nephrotoxic insults. Institution of timely renal replacement therapy should supersede an exhaustive medical management strategy. Finally, an understanding of any preexisting renal dysfunction and intraoperative variables can help formulate a short- and mid-term strategy. A patient's recent history and operative records need close review. Risk factors as chronic renal insufficiency, prolonged low cardiac output period, high-dose pressors, long bypass time, and/or intraoperative hypotension can significantly impact renal recovery.

20.6 Gastrointestinal

20.6.1 Hepatic Congestion

Most patients undergoing urgent or emergent mechanical support have advanced decompensated heart failure thus, are volume overloaded, and have systemic venous hypertension. Venous congestion can impair organ function, especially the brain, kidneys, and liver. Hepatic congestion can be a "silent killer." It is often more virulent than it appears. Patients will have near normal hepatic biomarkers, i.e., transaminases, bilirubin, prothrombin time, and platelet count. Ultrasound and cross-sectional imaging may not reveal any signs of cirrhosis or decompensation.

Mechanical support gets instituted at the appropriate time. But an insult occurs, potentially subclinical, either pre-, intra-, or postoperative, causing a sharp elevation of hepatic biomarkers. This derangement can then amplify to unprecedented levels. Management is supportive as maneuvers to offload the venous circulation are already in play. Depending on hepatic reserve, this can be a fatal event. The challenge is identifying which patients are at risk for this unfortunate progression. Similarly, coagulopathic bleeding can emerge intraoperatively, despite near normal laboratory values. This situation, although morbid, is more controllable as it can be remedied by surgical hemostasis and transfusion of blood and products. It is possible that chronic hepatic congestion is the root cause but the challenge remains in identifying who the at-risk patients are (Jung et al. 2016).

20.6.2 Mesenteric Ischemia

Most patients with vascular occlusive disease are excluded from advanced heart failure therapies. Nevertheless, mesenteric ischemia is still possible. Patients with a left-sided support device can easily develop a thromboembolic complication and selectively embolize to the mesenteric circulation. Thrombogenic surfaces include the oxygenator, tubing, inflow or outflow cannula, or even the motor. Alternatively, it can result from low splanchnic perfusion, either due to low device flow or a low mean arterial pressure (Sen et al. 2016). Patients will present with worsening hypotension, a refractory metabolic acidosis, and rising lactic acidosis. Clinical signs may manifest as abdominal distention or abdominal compartment syndrome. Management is supportive. Utility is questionable so many patients may not receive an abdominal CT scan. A select few may undergo abdominal exploration, but a minority of these will demonstrate a reversible pathology. Prognosis is nearly uniformly fatal.

20.7 GIB

GIBs are perhaps one of the most commonly encountered complications overall with a reported incidence of 20–40% in the durable device population (Morgan et al. 2012). Most present-day devices have a continuous flow configuration. Experience with this type of blood flow pattern has shown maladaptive responses in the gastrointestinal tract such as enlarged submucosal venous plexuses and arteriovenous malformations. This increases the risks of bleeding significantly. Patients are also prone to developing an acquired von Willebrand deficiency, which also predisposes to bleeding (Meyer et al. 2010). These pathophysiologic changes are uncommon in the immediate postoperative period though. More common are iatrogenic injuries and peptic ulcer disease. All patients end up needing an enteral tube for some period of time. Best case scenario, an orogastric tube is inserted in the operating room and removed a short while later at extubation. More commonly though, patients require enteral access for ongoing nutrition or gastric decompression. Despite attempts to minimize morbidity, discontinuation of anticoagulation, correction of coagulation and platelet count abnormalities, and atraumatic techniques, iatrogenic injuries still occur. This results in cumbersome oropharyngeal and/or gastrointestinal bleeding which invariably requires resuscitation, transfusions, and additional interventional procedures. The net effect is heightened morbidity and mortality. Another common postoperative scenario is unprovoked UGIB. Peptic ulcer disease is the usual culprit. The pathophysiology is unclear but it can rapidly become symptomatic. Fortunately, most patients respond well to medical and interventional therapy, but again, morbidity and mortality are increased in this delicate population. GI prophylaxis with PPIs is crucial and included in most electronic order sets. Octreotide has also demonstrated some utility for these types of bleeds (Rennyson et al. 2013; Coutance et al. 2014).

20.8 Endocrine

20.8.1 Glucose

It is well known that perioperative hyperglycemia is associated with increased morbidity and mortality. The stress response, adverse drug effects, hyperalimentation, and/or a developing infection can all contribute to an altered glucose response (Quattara et al. 2005; Swenne et al. 2005; Gandhi et al. 2005; Rassias 2006; Jones et al. 2008). Elevated blood glucose levels may result in fluid imbalance, impaired wound healing, cardiac rhythm disturbances, respiratory or renal complications, and infections. Target glucose level should be <180 mg/dL. Lower thresholds have not been shown to be any more advantageous (Gandhi et al. 2007; Chan et al. 2009). If needed, utilization of an insulin infusion should not be delayed. Strict glycemic control has proven benefit in both the diabetic and nondiabetic populations (Furnary et al. 2003; Carr et al. 2005; Schmeltz et al. 2007).

20.8.2 Adrenal

Adrenal insufficiency is a rare complication after cardiac surgery. It should be entertained in cases of refractory hypotension. A cosyntropin stimulation test can be done for diagnosis. But if clinical suspicion is present, treatment should be initiated with hydrocortisone IV 100 mg every 8 h (Bojar 2011).

20.8.3 Thyroid

Hypothyroidism is generally well tolerated but only in some patients. Those with ischemic disease may have myocardial oxygen supply/demand imbalance with thyroid replacement therapy. Some patients may have postcardiotomy lethargy and ventricular dysfunction, requiring thyroid replacement therapy and inotropes.

20.9 Hematology

Bleeding in the MCS population is the "Achilles' heel" of this form of therapy. Patients can have predisposing factors as an underlying coagulopathy (diagnosed or undiagnosed), be on blood thinning agents (antiplatelet agents, Xa inhibitors, Coumadin, etc.), and have hepatic congestion, cardiac cirrhosis, or other risk factors. An undervalued morbidity is the physiologic reserve of the patient and the gravity of the present illness. In-house patients with a low output state, end-organ dysfunction, limited mobility, and poor nutrition are likely to demonstrate poor surgical hemostasis. However, the variables can be somewhat controlled for by operative timing and planning. Medications can be held for safe intervals. Preoperative transfusions and treatments to bolster the hematopoietic system can also be employed. Nutritional and rehabilitative efforts continued. A hematology consultation can also be obtained for additional suggestions. Since most cases aren't elective, adequate preoperative preparations can be a challenge.

The intraoperative course can certainly affect postoperative bleeding tendencies. An antifibrinolytic agent is usually given before cardiopulmonary bypass. This functions to diminish fibrinolysis after heparin reversal. Failure to adopt this routine can increase surgical bleeding. The duration of cardiopulmonary bypass will inversely affect hemostasis. Longer pump times translates into more cellular trauma and more circulating cytokines. Both contribute to a quantitative and qualitative derangement of platelets and clotting factors. The net effect is poor clotting.

Another significant factor is core body temperature. It's well known that hypothermia impairs the normal clotting cascade. Patients undergoing surgical implantation of a durable or temporary assist device, without any other concomitant procedures are usually kept normothermic. Patients requiring aortic clamping are typically cooled to at least moderate hypothermia. They are then rewarmed, prior to discontinuation of CPB. Maintaining a stable body temperature during the final portion of the operation can be challenging. Convective losses from the open sternotomy, surgical bleeding, transfusion of blood and products, and low perfusion pressures can all contribute to "temperature afterdrop" (Mora et al. 1996; Jones and Roy 1999). Therefore, the time in the operating room after coming off bypass can be extremely crucial. Attention must be paid toward good surgical hemostasis, minimizing transfusions, maintaining a normal body temperature, and minimizing the duration of time that the chest is open.

Closing "wet" can leave behind a coagulopathic milieu. This can serve as a nidus for ongoing bleeding. As commonly seen on "takebacks," no focal bleeding is identified, but removal of residual blood and clot from the mediastinum tends to cease further blood loss. As such, surgical judgment is key. But meticulous behaviors and practices can translate into improved outcomes.

Upon arrival in the intensive care unit, many of the same clinical parameters will be continually reassessed. Core body temperature will be closely watched, and maneuvers will be employed to facilitate rewarming. The most effective therapy is the cutaneous forced-air warming device (Bair Hugger, Arizant) (Pathi et al. 1996; Grocott et al. 2004; Forbes et al. 2009). Additional strategies include warm fluids, blood products, blankets, and room temperature. Together, this helps to warm the extremities, which will keep the core temperature steady. Laboratory values will be followed, and coagulopathies will be corrected pending ongoing losses. The hemoglobin should be kept around 8–9. This will maintain an adequate oxygen supply. When losses are significant though, blood should be given at a reasonable pace to keep up with the ongoing losses. The quantity and quality of the chest tube drainage will be closely scrutinized. Initial drainage of >200 cm^3 bloody fluid during the first hour will warrant additional transfusions. The lack of improvement after another 1–2 h should prompt re-exploration. Vigilance must be exercised in this setting. A decrement of chest tube drainage may not imply hemostasis but instead a clotted, nonfunctional chest tube. Bleeding can persist into the closed mediastinal space and cause cardiac tamponade.

Once adequate hemostasis has been achieved, the next hurdle is anticoagulation. This may start on day 0 for the temporary devices or day 1 for the durable devices. All devices require heparin, either through the device or systemically. The durable devices will require an antiplatelet agent and conversion to Coumadin. The durable devices usually target an INR 2–3. The temporary devices target a PTT 1.5–2× normal and ECMO usually targets an ACT 150–170. Patients who develop heparin-induced thrombocytopenia will require conversion to a direct thrombin inhibitor, as argatroban. Experience with alternate agents in the MCS population is limited but has been used successfully. Although maintaining adequate anticoagulation is essential for proper device function, complications are inevitable. Bleeding can erupt from anywhere—the surgical field or access site, intracerebral, the gastrointestinal tract, urologic, retroperitoneal, or even soft tissue. Bleeding episodes can run the gamut of the severity spectrum. They can be isolated and self-limiting or they can precipitate hemorrhagic shock and result in death. Each episode may warrant cessation of anticoagulation therapy, reversal of coagulopathy, and blood and product resuscitation. For life-threatening bleeding, recombinant factors can be considered but run the risk of the circuit clotting. One of the subtleties about bleeding is the interruption of anticoagulation therapy. It is unknown what impact, if any, this has on long-term device durability, but it can certainly truncate the lifespan of short-term devices. The Impella can abruptly stop. ECMO, TandemHeart, and CentriMag will start to demonstrate increased fibrin and clot buildup, as warning signs. Circuit changes and device exchanges are common solutions for temporary devices. Durable devices may require fibrinolytic treatment and a pump exchange. Fortunately, pump thrombosis with durable devices is mostly a long-term complication; thus, each patient receives a personalized approach to anticoagulation (Petricevic et al. 2015).

20.10 Infectious Disease

Due to local microbiology resistances, most institutions will have a perioperative antibiotic prophylaxis protocol that aims to cover typical skin flora. Modifications are incorporated based on certain variables such as in-house patient versus someone coming from home, open chest vs. closed chest, and drug allergies. They are typically continued for 24–48 h from initial surgery.

Some patients have antecedent infections prior to device implant. The most common is catheter-related bloodstream infections from vascular access catheters. Once recognized, treatment is initiated, and the patient is deferred from surgery until cleared from an infectious standpoint. They must be afebrile and have a normal WBC count and negative blood cultures. Unfortunately, many gray areas exist, and feedback from an infectious disease specialist is usually warranted to help determine the safety of proceeding. Sometimes a leukocytosis persists, while other parameters have been neutralized. Sometimes, a patient's hemodynamic stability changes, prompting risks to benefits discussion about proceeding with surgery. Sometimes an infectious agent remains dormant, requiring long-term suppression. Continuing therapy after surgery is vital in many of these scenarios. Ongoing consultation from the infectious disease experts is a crucial contribution.

More common is development of a new infection. This can occur in up to 50% of this population. The usual culprits are bloodstream infection, urinary tract infection, pneumonia, and surgical site infections. Most ICUs have comprehensive infection prevention protocols to prevent cross-contamination and minimize iatrogenic risks. Additionally, there are national campaigns aimed at reducing rates of ventilator-associated pneumonias and catheter-related bloodstream infections. They promote bundles of care that are adopted by most ICU healthcare professionals (Juknevicius et al. 2012). The goal, however, should always be prevention. Unfortunately, this is a sick population with significant comorbidities who undergo life-saving interventions. Thus, they remain at the highest risk for postoperative morbidity. Vigilance should be exercised for early detection and treatment and appropriate resuscitation and hemodynamic support. Lines should be removed and/or replaced. Good pulmonary hygiene should take place. Surgical site infections should be aggressively managed with early drainage and debridement, when indicated. Many patients are significantly deconditioned and at high risk for poor wound healing, so resilience can be a common sentiment. Hemodynamic support with volume, inotropes, and vasopressors should be instituted without delay. Durable devices are specifically at risk for pump pocket infections and driveline infections. Fortunately, these tend to occur outside of the perioperative period.

References

Bansal A, Bhama JK, Patel R, Desai S, Mandras SA, Patel H, Collins T, Reilly JP, Ventura HO, Parrino PE. Using the minimally invasive Impella 5.0 via the right subclavian artery cutdown for acute on chronic decompensated heart failure as a bridge to decision. Ochsner J. 2016;16(3):210–6.

Barr J, Egan TD, Sandoval NF, et al. Propofol dosing regimens for ICU sedation based upon an integrated pharmacokinetic-pharmacodynamic model. Anesthesiology. 2001;95:324–33.

Bennett MK, Adatya S. Blood pressure management in mechanical circulatory support. J Thorac Dis. 2015;7(12):2125–8.

Bojar RM. Manual of perioperative care in adult cardiac surgery. 5th ed. West Sussex: Wiley-Blackwell; 2011.
Brown JR, Cochran RP, MacKenzie TA, et al. Long-term survival after cardiac surgery is predicted by estimated glomerular filtration rate. Ann Thorac Surg. 2008;86:4–11.
Buvanendran A, Kroin JS. Multimodal analgesia for controlling acute postoperative pain. Curr Opin Anesthesiol. 2009;22:588–93.
Byhahn C, Rinne T, Halbig S, et al. Early percutaneous tracheostomy after median sternotomy. J Thorac Cardiovasc Surg. 2000;120:329–34.
Caputo M, Alwair H, Rogers CA, Pike K, Cohen A, Monk C, Tomkins S, Ryder I, Moscariello C, Lucchetti V, Angelini GD. Thoracic epidural anesthesia improves early outcomes in patients undergoing off-pump coronary artery bypass surgery: a prospective, randomized, controlled trial. Anesthesiology. 2011;114:380–90.
Carr JM, Selke FW, Fey M, et al. Implementing tight glucose control after coronary artery bypass surgery. Ann Thorac Surg. 2005;80:902–9.
Chan RP, Galas FR, Hajjar LA, et al. Intensive perioperative glucose control does not improve outcomes of patients submitted to open-heart surgery: a randomized control trial. Clinics. 2009;64:51–60.
Coffin ST, Waguespack DR, Haglund NA, Maltais S, Dwyer J, Keebler ME. Cardiorenal Med. 2015;5(1):48–60.
Constantinides VA, Tekkis PP, Fazil A, et al. Fast-track failure after cardiac surgery: development of a prediction model. Crit Care Med. 2006;34:2875–82.
Cooper WA, O'Brien SM, Thourani VH, et al. Impact of renal dysfunction on outcomes of coronary artery bypass surgery: results from the Society of Thoracic Surgeons National Adult Cardiac database. Circulation. 2006;113:1063–70.
Coutance G, Saplacan V, Belin A, Repesse Y, Buklas D, Massetti M. Octreotide for recurrent intestinal bleeding due to ventricular assist device. Asian Cardiovasc Thorac Ann. 2014;22(3):350–2.
Curtis JJ, Clark NC, McKenney CA, et al. Tracheostomy: a risk factor for mediastinitis after cardiac operation. Ann Thorac Surg. 2001;72:731–4.
Dacey LJ, Likosky DS, Leavitt BJ, et al. Perioperative stroke and long-term survival after coronary bypass graft surgery. Ann Thorac Surg. 2005;79:532–7.
Filsoufi F, Rahmanian PB, Castillo JG, Bronster D, Adams DH. Incidence, imaging, analysis, and early and late outcomes of stroke after cardiac valve operation. Am J Cardiol. 2008a;101:1472–8.
Filsoufi F, Rahmanian PB, Castillo JG, Chikwe J, Adams DH. Logistic risk model predicting postoperative respiratory failure in patients undergoing valve surgery. Eur J Cardiothorac Surg. 2008b;34:953–9.
Forbes SS, Eskicioglu C, Nathens AB, et al. Evidence-based guidelines for prevention of perioperative hypothermia. J Am Coll Surg. 2009;209:492–503.
Force SD, Miller DL, Peterson R, et al. Incidence of deep sternal wound infections after tracheostomy in cardiac surgery patients. Ann Thorac Surg. 2005;80:618–22.
Fowler MB, Alderman EL, Oesterle SN, et al. Dobutamine and dopamine after cardiac surgery: greater augmentation of myocardial blood flow with dobutamine. Circulation. 1984;70(Suppl I):I103–11.
Freitas ER, Soares BG, Cardoso JR, Atallah AN. Incentive spirometry for preventing pulmonary complications after coronary artery bypass graft. Cochrane Database Syst Rev. 2007;3:CD004466.
Furnary AP, Gao G, Grunkemeier GL, et al. Continuous insulin infusion reduces mortality in patients with diabetes undergoing coronary artery bypass grafting. J Thorac Cardiovasc Surg. 2003;125:1007–21.
Gandhi GY, Nuttall GA, Abel MD, et al. Intraoperative hyperglycemia and perioperative outcomes in cardiac surgery patients. Mayo Clin Proc. 2005;80:862–6.
Gandhi GY, Nuttall GA, Abel MD, et al. Intensive intraoperative insulin therapy verses conventional glucose management during cardiac surgery: a randomized trial. Ann Intern Med. 2007;146:233–43.

Gandhi K, Heitz JW, Viscusi ER. Challenges in acute pain management. Anesthesiol Clin. 2011;29:291–309.

Gibson PH, Croal BL, Cuthbertson BH, et al. The relationship between renal function and outcome from heart valve surgery. Am Heart J. 2008;156:893–9.

Gommers D, Bakker J. Medications for analgesia and sedation in the intensive care unit: an overview. Crit Care. 2008;12(Suppl 3):S4.

Grocott HP, Mathew JP, Carver EH, et al. A randomized controlled trial of the Artic Sun Temperature Management System verses conventional methods for preventing hypothermia during off-pump cardiac surgery. Anesth Analg. 2004;98:298–302.

Hemmerling T, Olivier JR, Le N, Prieto I, Bracco D. Myocardial protection by isoflurane vs sevoflurane in ultra-fast-track anesthesia for off-pump aortocoronary bypass grafting. Eur J Anesthesiol. 2008a;25:230–6.

Hemmerling T, Russo G, Bracco D. Neuromuscular blockade in cardiac surgery: an update for clinicians. Ann Card Anesth. 2008b;11:80–90.

Hillis GS, Croal BL, Buchan KG, et al. Renal function and outcome from coronary artery bypass grafting: impact on mortality after a 2.3 year follow-up. Circulation. 2006;113:1056–62.

Jacobi J, et al. Clinical practice guidelines for the sustained use of sedatives and analgesics in the critically ill adult. Task force of the American College of Critical Care Medicine (ACCM), of the Society of Critical Care Medicine (SCCM), American Society of Heath System Pharmacists (ASHP), American College of Chest Physicians. Crit Care Med. 2002;30(1):119.

Jones T, Roy RC. Should patients be normothermic in the immediate post-operative period? Ann Thorac Surg. 1999;68:1454–5.

Jones KW, Can AS, Mitchell JH, et al. Hyperglycemia predicts mortality after CABG: postoperative hyperglycemia predicts dramatic increase in mortality after coronary artery bypass graft surgery. J Diabetes Complicat. 2008;22:365–70.

Juknevicius G, Balakumar E, Gratrix A. Implementation of evidence-based care bundles in the ICU. Crit Care. 2012;16(Suppl 1):P524.

Jung C, Kelm M, Westenfeld R. Liver function during mechanical circulatory support: from witness to rognostic determinant. Crit Care. 2016;20:134.

Kapur NK, Jumean MF. Management of continuous flow left ventricular assist device patients in the Cardiac Catheterization Laboratory. Cath Lab Digest. 2014;22

Kirklin JK, Naftel DC, Pagani FD, Kormos RL, Stevenson LW, Blume ED, et al. Sixth INTERMACS annual report: a 10,000-patient database. J Heart Lung Transplant. 2014;33(6):555–64.

Kirklin JK, Naftel DC, Pagani FD, Kormos RL, Stevenson LW, Blume ED, et al. Seventh INTERMACS annual report: a 15,000-patient database. J Heart Lung Transplant. 2015;34(12):1495–504.

Korabathina R, Heffernan KS, Paruchuri V, Patel AR, Mudd JO, Prutkin JM, Orr NM, Weintraub A, Kimmelstiel CD, Kapur NK. The pulmonary artery pulsatility index identifies severe right ventricular dysfunction in acute inferior myocardial infarction. Catheter Cardiovasc Interv. 2012;80(4):593–600.

Lassnigg A, Donner E, Grubhofer G, Presterl E, Druml W, Hiesmayr M. Lack of renoprotective ffects of dopamine and furosemide during cardiac surgery. J Am Soc Nephrol. 2000;11:97–104.

Lehr CJ, Zaas DW, Cheifetz IM, Turner DA. Ambulatory extracorporeal membrane oxygenation as a bridge to lung transplantation: walking while waiting. Chest. 2015;147(5):1213–8.

Lena P, Balarac N, Lena D, et al. Fast-track anesthesia with remifentanil and spinal analgesia for cardiac surgery: the effect on pain control and quality of recovery. J Cardiothorac Vasc Anesth. 2008;22:536–42.

Marasco SF, Sharwood LN, Abramson MJ. No improvement in neurocognitive outcomes after off-pump verses on-pump coronary revascularization: a meta-analysis. Eur J Cardiothorac Surg. 2008;33:961–70.

Mehta RH, Hafley GE, Gibson CM, et al. Influence of preoperative renal dysfunction on one-year bypass graft patency and two-year outcomes in patients undergoing coronary artery bypass surgery. J Thorac Cardiovasc Surg. 2008;136:1149–55.

Meyer AL, Malehsa D, Bara C, Budde U, Slaughter MS, Haverich A, Strueber M. Acquired von Willebrand syndrome in patients with an axial flow left ventricular assist device. Circ Heart Fail. 2010;3(6):675–81.
Mora CT, Henson MB, Weintraub WS, et al. The effect of temperature management during cardiopulmonary bypass on neurologic and neuropsychologic outcomes in patients undergoing coronary revascularization. J Thorac Cardiovasc Surg. 1996;112:514–22.
Morgan JA, Paone G, Nemeh HW, Henry SE, Patel R, Vavra J, Williams CT, Lanfear DE, Tita C, Brewer RJ. Gastrointestinal bleeding with the HeartMate II left ventricular assist device. J Heart Lung Transplant. 2012;31(7):715–8.
Najafi M, Goodarzynejad H, Karimi A, et al. Is preoperative creatinine a reliable indicator of outcome in patients undergoing coronary artery bypass surgery. J Thorac Cardiovasc Surg. 2009;137:304–8.
Newman MF, Grocott HP, Mathew JP, White WD, Landolfo K, Reves JG, Laskowitz DT, Mark DB, Blumenthal JA. Report of the substudy assessing the impact of neurocognitive function on quality of life 5 years after cardiac surgery. Stroke. 2001a;32:2874–81.
Newman MF, Kirschner JL, Phillips-Bute B, et al. Longitudinal assessment of neurocognitive function after coronary artery bypass surgery. NEJM. 2001b;344:395–402.
Ngaage DL, Cale AR, Griffin S, Guvendik L, Cowen ME. Is post-sternotomy percutaneous dilation tracheostomy a predictor for sternal wound infections? Eur J Cardiothorac Surg. 2008;33:1076–81.
Overend TJ, Anderson CM, Lucy SD, Bhatia C, Jonsson BI, Timmermans C. The effect of incentive spirometry on postoperative pulmonary complications. A systematic review. Chest. 2001;120:971–8.
Pasquina P, Tramer MR, Walder B. Prophylactic respiratory physiotherapy after cardiac surgery: systematic review. BMJ. 2003;327:1379–81.
Pathi V, Berg GA, Morrison J, Cramp G, McLaren D, Faichney A. The benefits of active rewarming after cardiac operations: a randomized prospective trial. J Thorac Cardiovasc Surg. 1996;111:637–41.
Peters ML, Sommer M, de Rijke JM, Kessels F, Heineman E, Patijn J, Marcus MA, Vlaeyen JW, van Kleef M. Somatic and psychologic predictors of long term unfavorable outcome after surgical intervention. Ann Surg. 2007;245:487–94.
Petricevic M, Milicic D, Boban M, Mihaljevic MZ, Baricevic Z, Kolic K, Dolic K, Konosic L, Kopjar T, Biocina B. Bleeding and thrombotic events in patients undergoing mechanical circulatory support: a review of the literature. Thorac Cardiovasc Surg. 2015;63(8):636–46.
Qian Q, Nath KA, Wu Y, Daoud TM, Sethi S. Hemolysis and kidney failure. Am J Kidney Dis. 2010;56(4):780–4.
Quattara A, Lecomte P, Le Manach Y, et al. Poor intraoperative blood glucose control is associated with worsened hospital outcome after cardiac surgery in diabetic patients. Anesthesiology. 2005;103:687–94.
Rassias AJ. Intraoperative management of hyperglycemia in the cardiac surgical patient. Semin Thorac Cardiovasc Surg. 2006;18:330–8.
Redmond JM, Greene PS, Goldsborough MA, et al. Neurologic injury in cardiac surgical patients with a history of stroke. Ann Thorac Surg. 1996;61:42–7.
Reis J, Mota JC, Ponce P, Costa-Pereira A, Guerreiro M. Early extubation does not increase complication rates after coronary artery bypass surgery with cardiopulmonary bypass. Eur J Cardiothorac Surg. 2002;21:1026–30.
Rennyson SL, Shah KB, Tang DG, Kasirajan V, Pedram S, Cahoon W, Malhotra R. Octreotide for left ventricular assist device-related gastrointestinal hemorrhage: can we stop the bleeding? ASAIO J. 2013;59(4):450–1.
Romson JL, Leung JM, Bellows WH, et al. Effects of dobutamine on hemodynamics and left ventricular performance after cardiopulmonary bypass in cardiac surgical patients. Anesthesiology. 1999;91:1318–28.
Rosenberger P, Shernan SK, Loffler M, et al. The influence of epiaortic ultrasonography on intraoperative surgical management in 6051 cardiac surgical patients. Ann Thorac Surg. 2008;78:2028–32.

Russo MJ, Jeevanandam V, Stepney J, Merlo A, Johnson EM, Malyala R, Raman J. Intra-aortic balloon pump inserted through the subclavian artery: a minimally invasive eapproach to mechanical support in the ambulatory end stage heart failure patient. J Thorac Cardiovasc Surg. 2012;144(4):951–5.

Salazar JD, Wityk RJ, Grega MA, et al. Stroke after cardiac surgery: short and long-term outcomes. Ann Thorac Surg. 2001;72:1195–202.

Schmeltz LR, DeSantis AJ, Thiyagarajan V, et al. Reduction of surgical mortality and morbidity in diabetic patients undergoing cardiac surgery with a combined intravenous and subcutaneous insulin glucose management strategy. Diabetes Care. 2007;30:823–8.

Sen A, Larson JS, Kashani KB, Libricz SL, Patel BM, Guru PK, Alwardt CM, Pajaro O, Farmer JC. Mechanical circulatory assist devices: a primer for critical care and emergency physicians. Crit Care. 2016;20:153.

Sessler CN, Varney K. Patient-focused sedation and analgesia in the ICU. Chest. 2008;133:552–65.

Swenne CL, Lindholm C, Borowiec J, Schnell AE, Carlsson M. Peri-operative glucose control and development of surgical wound infections in patients undergoing coronary artery bypass graft. J Hosp Infect. 2005;61:201–12.

Toraman F, Evrenkaya S, Yuce M, Goksel O, Karabulut H, Alhan C. Fast-track recovery in noncoronary cardiac surgery patients. Heart Surg Forum. 2005;8:E61–4.

Trouillet JL, Combes A, Vaissier E, et al. Prolonged mechanical ventilation after cardiac surgery: outcome and predictors. J Thorac Cardiovasc Surg. 2009;138:948–53.

Ucak A, Onan B, Sen H, Selcuk I, Turan A, Yilmaz AT. The effects of gabapentin on acute and chronic postoperative pain after coronary artery bypass graft surgery. J Cardiothorac Vasc Anesth. 2011;25:824–9.

Vender JS, Szokol JW, Murphy GS, et al. Sedation, analgesia and neuromuscular blockade in sepsis: an evidence-based review. Crit Care Med. 2004;32(suppl):S554–61.

Westerdahl E, Lindmark B, Eriksson T, Hedenstierna G, Tenling A. The immediate effects of deep breathing exercises on atelectasis and oxygenation after cardiac surgery. Scand Cardiovasc J. 2003;37:363–7.

Woo EB, Tang AT, el-Gamel A, et al. Dopamine therapy for patients at risk of renal dysfunction following cardiac surgery: fact or fiction? Eur J Cardiothorac Surg. 2002;22:106–11.

Yende S, Wunderlink R. Causes of prolonged mechanical ventilation after coronary artery bypass surgery. Chest. 2002;122:245–52.

Zibgone B, Rauber E, Gatti G, et al. The impact of epiaortic ultrasonographic scanning on the risk of perioperative stroke. Eur J Cardiothorac Surg. 2006;29:720–8.

Postoperative Safety in Adult Cardiac Surgery Intensive Care Unit

21

Alice Chan and Fardad Esmailian

Abstract

Patient safety is stated as the fundamental principle of good patient care (*Summary of the evidence on patient safety: implications for research*, WHO, Geneva, 2008). Nearly half (45%) of the adverse events in the Critical Care Safety Study were deemed preventable (Shostek, J Ambul Care Manage 30: 105–113, 2007). Patient safety incidents lead to unnecessary suffering and are a major cause of prolonged hospital stays. Human error is stated as the most common cause of patient safety incidents. Ensuring patient safety is becoming increasingly important for cardiac surgery intensive care unit practitioners. The cardiac surgery intensive care unit is particularly prone to medical errors because of the complexity of the patients, interdependence of the practitioners, and dependence on team functioning. Approaches related to high-reliability organizations (HRO) such as aviation have been applied in health care to prevent incidents and to ensure the delivery of proper care (Riley, J Nurs Manag 17: 238–246, 2009). Measurements of patient safety culture, teamwork, and continuous improvement and organizational learning, including team training with the use of simulation (Wilson et al., Qual Saf Health Care 14: 303–309, 2005), are all HRO approaches (Evidence scan: high reliability organizations, The Health Foundation, London, 2011) recommended as initiatives to improve quality and patient safety in health care. A culture of safety is created through changes in health personnel's safety perspective and work behaviors, and human resource professionals are an essential contributor to this development. Human patient simulation-based

A. Chan, R.N., M.N., C.N.S., C.C.R.N. (✉)
Cedars-Sinai Medical Center, Los Angeles, CA, USA
e-mail: Alice.Chan@cshs.org

F. Esmailian, M.D.
Department of Surgery, Cedars-Sinai Heart Institute, Los Angeles, CA, USA

Heart Transplantation, Cedars-Sinai Heart Institute, Los Angeles, CA, USA

A. Dabbagh et al. (eds.), *Postoperative Critical Care for Adult Cardiac Surgical Patients*, https://doi.org/10.1007/978-3-319-75747-6_21

training is a recommended method to make health-care professionals aware of the importance of teamwork and the aspects of team performance (*Crossing the Quality Chasm: A New Health System for the Twenty-First Century*, National Academy Press, Washington, DC, 2001). Team training program based on crew resource management can be used to improve efficiency, morale, and patient safety in health care (West et al., J Nurs Adm 42: 15–20, 2012). Several important factors play a role in fostering patient safety in the postoperative adult cardiac surgery intensive care unit environments, such as a patient safety culture, better communication, team performance, and team training strategies as initiatives for building patient safety within the adult cardiac surgery intensive care unit.

Keywords
Patient safety · Culture · Communication systems · Handoff protocol · Daily multidisciplinary patient-centered round · Team performance · TeamSTEPPS · Crew resource management (CRM) · Simulation

21.1 Promote Patient Safety Culture

Culture can be defined as the set of shared values and beliefs that interact with an organization's structure practices and control systems to reduce behavior norms (Reason 1998). The WHO (2008 and 2009) has confirmed that focusing on culture is one of the most important areas for the improvement of patient safety in hospitals today. The safety culture in health care is an aspect of the wider culture of an organization (Sammer et al. 2010; The Health Foundation London 2011). The properties of a patient safety culture were identified as leadership, teamwork, evidence-based practice, open communication, learning from mistakes, errors recognized as system failures simultaneously holding individuals accountable for their actions, and lastly, patient-centered care. According to Flatten (Wachter and Pronovost 2009), teamwork, communication, and how to handle incidents are particularly important for patient safety in the cardiac surgery ICU. The quality movement in medicine has prompted a shift, from a "name, shame, blame" approach to medical errors into one in which each error is regarded as an opportunity to prevent future patient harms (Edmondson 1999, 2004). Patient safety experts note that improvement initiatives are more successful in environments in which a culture of safety exists. A culture of safety flourishes in an ICU environment in which clinicians and frontline staff feel they are part of a team and understand how to exchange patient information and other information in a meaningful and respectful way. A starting point for improving safety culture in the ICU is to conduct an assessment of the current culture (or climate) in the critical care unit or units to determine whether and how it affects patient care. Measurements of patient safety culture are limited due to the capability to define the measurable components of a culture (Cooper 2000). However, a request for a relatively low-cost and easy-to-use assessment of patient safety culture resulted

Table 21.1 Examples of questions in patient safety culture survey

	Unfavorable	Netural	Favorable
We are actively doing things to improve patient safety			
When one area in this unit gets really busy, others help out			
The culture of this clinical area makes it easy to learn from the mistakes of others			
Staff worry that mistakes that they make are kept in their personnel file			
When an event is reported, it feels like the person is being written up, not the problem			
When one area in this unit gets really busy, others help out			
People support one another in this unit			
After we make changes to improve patient safety, we evaluate their effectiveness			
Hospital management provides a work climate that promotes patient safety.			
The actions of hospital management show that patient safety is a top priority			
Hospital management seems interested in patient safety only after an adverse event happens			
We are informed about errors that happen in this unit			
Hospital units work well together to provide the best care for patients			
Good communication flow exist up the chain of command regarding patient safety issues			
When a lot of work needs to be done quickly, we work together as a team to get the work done			

in support of patient safety climate questionnaires (Nieva and Sorra 2003). Safety climate is described as the measurable component of safety culture, which is regarded as surface features (Flin et al. 2000) and measures aspects of the units that affect patient safety, as well as attitudes of clinicians and staff members. Such aspects include perceptions of leadership's commitment to patient safety, the degree to which teamwork and open communication prevail, and attitudes about nonpunitive responses to errors. An important characteristic of safety culture assessment instrument is whether they take a managerial or staff perspective or combine elements of both. Examples of the statements used to assess safety culture are shown in Table 21.1.

Safety culture assessments are useful tools for measuring organizational conditions that lead to adverse events and patient harm in health-care organizations. Safety culture assessments can have multiple purposes: (1) diagnosis of safety culture and raising awareness, (2) evaluation of patient safety interventions and tracking change over time, (3) internal and external benchmarking, and (4) fulfillment of regulatory or other requirements (Guldenmund 2000). Safety culture assessment should be viewed as the starting point from which action planning begins and patient safety changes emerge. Promotion of patient safety culture can best be conceptualized as a constellation of interventions rooted in principles of leadership, teamwork, and behavior change rather than a specific process, team, or technology. Patient safety experts note that improvement initiatives are more successful in environments in which a culture of safety exists. A culture of safety flourishes in a cardiac surgery ICU environment in which clinicians and frontline staff feel they are part of a team and understand how to exchange patient information and other information in a meaningful and respectful way (Riely 2009; Haynes et al. 2011). Strategies to promote a culture of patient safety may include a single intervention or several interventions combined into a multifaceted approach or series (Morello et al. 2013). Executive walk-round is an interventional strategy that engages organizational leadership directly with frontline care providers. Senior leaders visit frontline patient care areas with the goal of observing and discussing current or potential threats to patient safety, as well as supporting frontline staff in addressing such threats (Frankel et al. 2008; Thomas et al. 2005). Walk-rounds aim to show leadership commitment to safety, foster trust and psychological safety, and provide support for frontline providers to proactively address threats to patient safety (Frankel et al. 2008). Improvement strategies that combine several intervention techniques have also been used to promote safety culture. For example, the Comprehensive Unit-Based Safety Program (CUSP) is a multifaceted strategy for culture change that pairs adaptive interventions (such as continuous learning strategies or team training) with technical interventions (such as translation and use of best available evidence-based clinical care algorithms/bundles, i.e., CLASI, CAUTI, VAP) to improve patient safety and quality (Pronovost et al. 2006; Romig et al. 2010). Standardization of processes has been shown to improve quality and reduce costs in a number of fields. Standardization of practice seems particularly well suited to operations such as CABG, where patients are fairly homogeneous, the operative procedure well scripted, and the postoperative course relatively predictable (Shahian et al. 2007). All patients undergoing cardiac surgery are likely to benefit from standardized management protocols (Sinuff et al. 2013; Shake et al. 2013). Standardizing systems or using clinical pathway guidelines improves quality in a variety of arenas and prevent errors (Shostek 2007). For example, cardiac surgical ICUs have order sets for sedation, analgesia, and delirium that are more consistent with guidelines and include shorter ventilator times than hospitals with lower-quality order sets (Dale et al. 2013). Whether using ventilator-acquired pneumonia "bundles," instituting hemoglobin concentration as a trigger for transfusion, or standardizing extubation protocols to improve early extubation, eliminating the variability innate to individual caregivers, can markedly improve performance (Fitch et al. 2014; Kilic and Whitman 2014). Safety culture is foundational to efforts to improve patient safety and may respond positively to intervention. Bundling multiple interventions or tools is a common strategy to improve safety culture. Low-quality heterogeneous evidence derived primarily from pre-post evaluations suggests that bundled, multicomponent interventions can improve clinician and staff perceptions of safety culture (Tiessen 2008; Saladino et al. 2013). Organizations should consider incorporating these elements into efforts to promote safety culture but also robustly evaluate such efforts across multiple outcomes. Future research should also consider the thorough investigation of safety culture as a cross-cutting contextual factor that can moderate the effectiveness of other patient safety practices (Flin et al. 2006).

21.2 Improving Communication Systems

The importance of developing and maintaining a culture of safety is common to all high-risk industries, including commercial aviation, military, and health care. This concept is based on studies of organizations that consistently minimize adverse events despite carrying out intrinsically complex and hazardous tasks (Patient Safety Primer 2016). Common to these organizations is an emphasis on open communication, a commitment to safety, and an atmosphere in which near misses can be analyzed in a blame-free environment to prevent catastrophic failure (Wiegmann et al. 2009). A review of reports from the Joint Commission reveals that communication failures were implicated at the root of over 70% of sentinel events (Joint Commission Resources 2017). The contributing factor that the nurses had selected was communication issues with physicians, which was one of the two most highly contributing factors. The growing body of literature on safety and error prevention reveals that ineffective or insufficient communication among team members is a significant contributing factor to adverse events. In the acute care setting, communication failures lead to increases in patient harm, the length of stay and resource use, as well as more intense caregiver dissatisfaction (Zwarenstein and Reeves 2002; Sexton et al. 2000). Effective communication among health-care professionals is challenging due to a number of interrelated dynamics, such as care providers often having their own disciplinary view of what the patient needs, with each provider prioritizing the activities in which he or she acts independently (Zwarenstein and Reeves 2002). Health care is complex and unpredictable, with professionals from a variety of disciplines involved in providing care at various times throughout the day, often dispersed over several locations, creating spatial gaps with limited opportunities for regular synchronous interaction (Zwarenstein and Reeves 2002). To develop and implement a handoff protocol and daily multidisciplinary patient-centered rounds using a daily goals sheet are two comprehensive team communication strategies.

21.2.1 Handoff Protocol

Patient handoffs following surgery have often been characterized by poor teamwork, unclear procedures, unstructured processes, and distractions (Segall et al. 2012). A particularly vulnerable time for the critically ill patient is the handoff of care, particularly in the transfer from the cardiothoracic operating room to the cardiac surgery intensive care unit. This period is characterized by the presence of multiple providers, partial disruption in the exhaustive monitoring of hemodynamics, and possible transition of drug infusion and delivery and represents a time

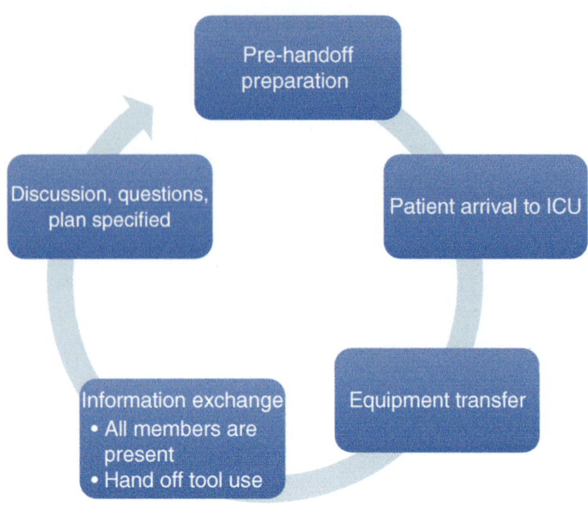

Fig. 21.1 Handoff process

during which clear communication of events in the operating room is imperative. The operating room to cardiac surgery intensive care unit handoff has the potential for communication breakdown and lapses in attention (Chen et al. 2011; Pothier et al. 2005). In 2006, the Joint Commission recognized the importance of handoff communication in ensuring patient safety and designated improved patient handoffs as a National Patient Safety Goal. Processes to ensure structured, safe handoffs were designated among the required Hospital Provision of Care, Treatment, and Services standards in 2010 (Kaufman et al. 2013). Checklists, handoff tools, and handoff protocols have been touted as improving communication among multidisciplinary teams and have become the foundation of many quality improvement initiatives in the medical and nonmedical world. The handoff protocols detail in that it specified who would be present at handoff, the order in which information was communicated, and it required a period for questions and clarifications and included a clear way to conclude the handoff (Petrovic et al. 2012). Handoff protocols (Fig. 21.1) and the standardized handoff tool (Fig. 21.2), from the operating room to the cardiac surgery intensive unit, have been shown to reduce communication errors, decrease patient identification errors, and promote efficiency. These improvements focused on leadership, task allocation, rhythm, standardized processes, checklists, awareness, anticipation, and communication (Kaufman et al. 2013).

21.2.2 Daily Multidisciplinary Patient-Centered Round

Communication failure has been cited as a preventable cause of patient harm (Donchin et al. 1995; Leape et al. 1991). Multidisciplinary rounds provide a common platform for all individuals involved in patient care to communicate, offer their expertise, and contribute to patient management and well-being (Burger 2007). Rounds are focused on open and collaborative communication, decision-making,

CSICU Handoff Assist Information Aid

Date: / / | Time: : | Reporting Attending: | Reporting Fellow/resident

PATIENT Name: Age:

Diagnosis: Allergies:

SURGERY Procedure:

CPB Duration : Circ Arrest Duration :

VENT SETTINGS Difficult intubation? YES NO ET size ETT depth

Tidal Vol | Fi02 | Rate

PEEP | INO | MODE Assist Control | Pressure control

Rapid Extubation YES NO

LINES & DRAINS LOCATION

- Peripheral
- Arterial
- Central
- LA
- RA
- PA Cath
- Foley Cath
- Chest Tube
- IABP
- Gastric Tube
- >

FLUIDS

Designated Donor Blood YES NO

Kiosk Blood YES NO

Crystalloid/Colloid	Given
PRBC	Given
FFP	Given
Platelets	Given
CRYO	Given
Cell Saver	Given
Total Urine Output	

PACING # LOCATION

- Atrial
- Ventricular
- Permanent

Pacemaker: Rate

Pacing: VENTRICULAR ATRIAL AV SEQ

DRIPS

Epinephrine	mcg/min
DoPAmine	mcg/kg/min
Milrinone	mcg/kg/min
DoBUTamine	mcg/kg/min
Nitroglycerin	mcg/min
Nipride	mcg/kg/min
Propofol	mcg/kg/min
Norepi	
Vasopressin	units/min
Insulin Drip	units/hr
Diuretic Drip	BUMEX LASIX
>	
>	

Last Hct		Last K	
Last ABG		Last Glucose	

REVERSAL? YES NO

	TIME	DOSE
Last antibiotic	:	

ANESTHESIA STOP TIME :
TRANSFER OF RESPONSIBILITY
MUST BE COMPLETED

18-24 hr post op Glucose compliance period FROM : AM / PM TO : AM / PM

MECHANICAL CIRCULATORY SUPPORT

Heartware	Flow l/m	Speed rpm	Power w
Heartmate II	Flow l/m	Speed rpm	Power w
TAH	Beat Rate Pressure	Cardiac Output Vacuum	Fill Volume
Centrimag	Flow l/m	Speed rpm	Cannulation site
ECMO	TYPE: A/V V/V	Flows	Cannulation site
Impella	Flow l/m	P-level	Cannulation site
OTHER			

ECHO FINDINGS

LV Normal
Depressed: MILD MODERATE SEVERE

RV Normal
Depressed: MILD MODERATE SEVERE

OTHER /NOTES

NOTES & OTHER INFORMATION
(dysrthymia, difficulty ventilation, unusual reaction anesthesia, bleeding, etc)

POST-OP ORDERS ENTERED? YES NO

GOALS FOR NEXT 24 HRs

PARAMETER	TARGET	NOTES
SBP		
MAP		
CI/CO		
PA mean		

FAMILY CONTACT

Name:

Relationship:

NOT PART OF THE MEDICAL RECORD PLEASE DISCARD AFTER 24 HOURS

Fig. 21.2 Sample of handoff tool from OR to ICU

information sharing, care planning, patient safety issues, cost and quality of care issues, setting daily goals of care, and communicating with patients and/or family members as they are able. Information shared during rounds was supplemented by communication at shift changes between the incoming and the outgoing care providers (Burger 2007; Pierson 2010). Effective communication among health-care providers in the intensive care unit is particularly imperative. The medical care team, with the help of patients and families, must perform specific tasks or work, obtain tests, make diagnoses, implement treatments, remove tubes and catheters, prevent complications, and manage pain so that the patients can progress beyond the intensive care unit or hospital. The care team must understand the goals of care, including the tasks to be performed, the care plan, and the communication plan to manage this work. A daily goal sheet is an interdisciplinary communication tool that serves as a simple way of clarifying work goals among providers (Halm 2008). It provides the means for the care team and the patient/family to define the goals of the day explicitly. The form is typically completed during patient rounds, signed by the fellow or attending physician, and given to the patient's nurse. The care team—physicians, nurses, RTs, and pharmacists—provide input and review the goals of the day (Fig. 21.3).

Another tool that is used in patient rounds is a guideline (Fig. 21.4) that include prompts for the identification of key quality of care elements and post-op assessment to cue a discussion among team members about any considerations that need to be addressed with interventions (Vats et al. 2011; Stone Jr et al. 2011).

Scripting-focused questions during patient rounds can be key in building relationships among participants. Simple yes or no questions often become routine and don't offer much in the way of discussion. Instead of asking yes or no questions, consider more open-ended questions that elicit contemplation and participation by the group. Scripting the questions, even writing them on the goal sheet or using a log that contains thought-provoking questions, requires staff to think about "why" or "when" a task or intervention is appropriate (Lamba et al. 2014; Kim et al. 2010). For examples, see the following:

- Compliance with Ventilator Bundle
  - Sedation vacation: When is the sedation vacation scheduled?
  - Readiness to wean: Has this patient been assessed for readiness to wean? What needs to happen for this patient to be extubated?
- Weaning on drips: Why is the patient still on drip? What needs to happen to get the patient off the drips?
- Central line or urinary catheter: Why is the central line in? What needs to happen to get the urinary catheter or central line removed for this patient?
- Transfer the patient out of the intensive care unit: What needs to happen so the patient can be transferred?

Inviting families to participate in rounds can be powerful as families have a unique perspective on the needs of patients. Before inviting families to participate, ensure that the process of multidisciplinary rounds is consistent and

Weight _____ Kg
Height _____ cm
Allergies ____________________

Date of Surgery: ____ /____ /_______
Start time of Huddle:
End time of Huddle:

<Patient Label>

Antibiotic ____________ Dose Amount ________ ReDose Frequency ________

Surgical Team: Surgeon: ______ 1st Asst: ______	**Goal**	**Post Huddle** Findings:
(1) The planned procedure		
(2) The surgical approach	☐ Sternotomy ☐ Thoracotomy ☐ R ☐ L ☐ Other____	
(3) Concerns from the surgical team		Post-op concerns:
(4) Surgical objectives/Goals		
(5) Blood Conservation plan		Pacing wires ☐ A ☐ V ☐ Paced ______ Rhythm____
		Chest tubes: ☐ Med___ ☐ Pleural___ ☐ PD catheter
Anesthesiology Team:		Post-op Anesthesia issues:
Aneshesiologist: __________	Induction ☐ Benzo ☐ Fen ☐ MSO ☐ Dex ☐ Other____	PCA ☐ NCA ☐ Other:
Fellow Name: __________	Inhalation agent ☐ Y ☐ N _____	
(1) Anesthesia approach/objectives	Maintence ☐ Fen ☐ Dex ☐ MSO ☐ Other_____	IV fluid Pre-bypass______ Total IV fluid______
(2) Airway		Tube size _____ Issues ______
(3) Access plan	Presently in ________ Issues in past________	IVs ☐ ________ PICC ☐ Locaction ______
a. Venous	☐ Yes ☐ No	Central Line location_____ ☐ RAs ☐ Other
b. Arterial	☐ Yes ☐ No	Aline Location _______
(4) Inotropic Need	Mil____ Epi____ Dop___ Other____	Mil____ Epi____ Calcium____ Vaso____ Other____
(5) Blood Conservation plan		Blood use ☐ PRBCs_____ cc
(6) Temperture	☐ Tympanic ☐ Naso ☐ Rectal ☐ Bladder ☐ Other____	FFP ☐ Cryo ☐ Plat ☐ FFP ☐ Factor VIIa ☐ ____
Perfusion: Perfusionist______ 2nd______		Post-op Concerns:
	☐ Amicar ☐ Transamic Acid ☐ Steriods_______	
(1) Planned approach/Objectives/Issues	Circuit ☐ 3/16 x 1/4 ☐ 1/4 x 1/4 ☐ 1/4 x 3/8 ☐ 3/8 x 3/8	AoX _____ CPB_____ Circ arrest time_____
a. Cooling	Temp _____	Temp: Low _____ Off Bypass_____ Post MUF____
b. Flow	Target flow____	Flow_____ Lowest cerebral sats____
(2) Cannulation	Artrerial _____ Venous ☐Single ☐Bicaval	Average cerebral sats_____ Average MvO _____
(3) Target hematocrit on bypass	Starting Hct_____ Calculated Hct on bypass_____	Lactates #1_____ #2_____ #3_____ #4_____
(4) Blood Conservation strategies		Lowest Hct_____ ANH ☐ _____ cc
a. RAP/VAP/ANH	RAP ☐ VAP ☐ ANH ☐	Comments: RAP ☐ VAP ☐
b. Ultrafiltration	☐ Yes ☐ No	Ultra ☐ Volume _____ cc
c. MUF	☐ Yes ☐ No Target Hct post-MUF ___	MUF ☐ Volume _____ cc Hct Pre___ Post____
TEE/Imaging - Cardiology		Findings:
Nursing Issues:		Last ABG: time____ / / / /
Equipment Ready: Bovie, lights, Pulse Ox		Last Lactate: time____
C-arm need, 3D System, Video Routing, Other Equipment, Implants		Bed spot____ Temp now______
Specimens: Pathology/Research	Path ☐______ Research ☐ ______	**Post-op Plan:**
Patient Disposition	☐ CTICU ☐ PACU ☐ Floor ☐ Other__________	
Staffing Concerns		
Visitors		
Surgical Operating Plan (SOP) Form CTS-001 (Rev 8/2011) **Room Color:**		

☐ Scanned into EPIC Progress Note ______

Signatures of Huddle Participants

Pre Post

Anesthesia Team

Surgical Team

Perfusion Team

Nursing Team

Fig. 21.3 Sample of team huddle tool

structured. It is necessary to have a conversation with family members prior to joining rounds, an orientation that introduces them to the focus, routine, and expectations of the rounding process. Posting the times, dates, and patients included in rounds can be valuable for both families and team members. For example, post a sign the day before scheduled rounds that says, "Rounds with

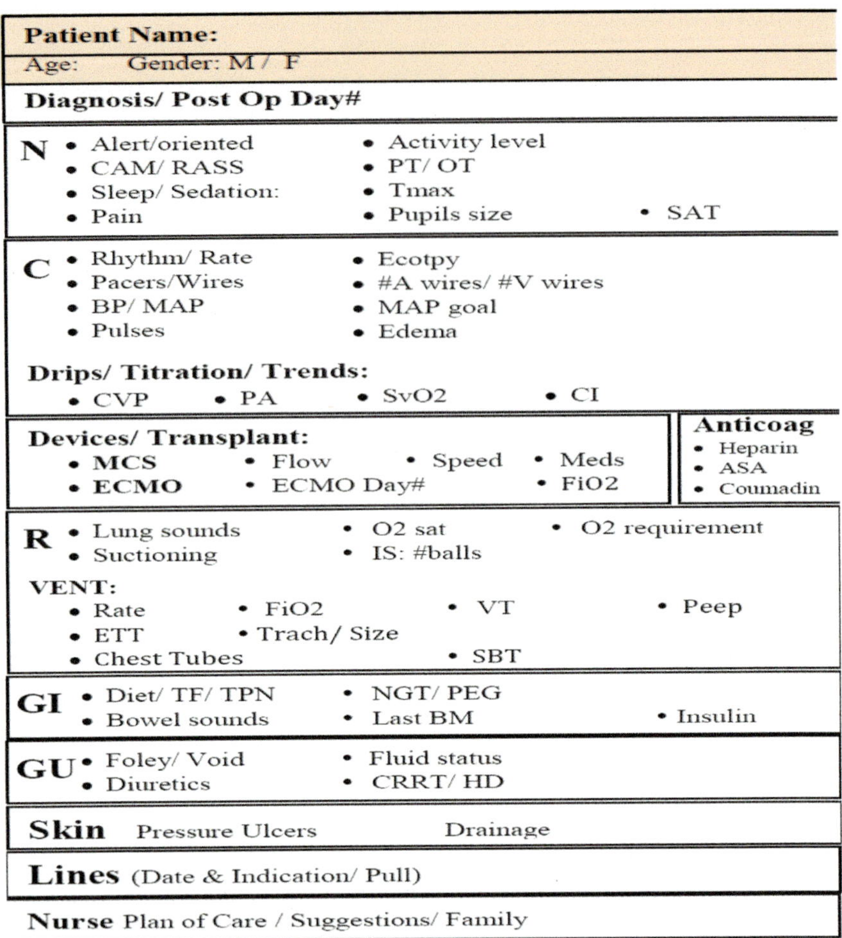

Patient Name:

Age: Gender: M / F

Diagnosis/ Post Op Day#

N
- Alert/oriented
- CAM/ RASS
- Sleep/ Sedation:
- Pain
- Activity level
- PT/ OT
- Tmax
- Pupils size
- SAT

C
- Rhythm/ Rate
- Pacers/Wires
- BP/ MAP
- Pulses
- Ecotpy
- #A wires/ #V wires
- MAP goal
- Edema

Drips/ Titration/ Trends:
- CVP
- PA
- SvO2
- CI

Devices/ Transplant:
- **MCS**
- Flow
- Speed
- Meds
- **ECMO**
- ECMO Day#
- FiO2

Anticoag
- Heparin
- ASA
- Coumadin

R
- Lung sounds
- Suctioning
- O2 sat
- IS: #balls
- O2 requirement

VENT:
- Rate
- FiO2
- VT
- Peep
- ETT
- Trach/ Size
- Chest Tubes
- SBT

GI
- Diet/ TF/ TPN
- Bowel sounds
- NGT/ PEG
- Last BM
- Insulin

GU
- Foley/ Void
- Diuretics
- Fluid status
- CRRT/ HD

Skin Pressure Ulcers Drainage

Lines (Date & Indication/ Pull)

Nurse Plan of Care / Suggestions/ Family

Attending/ Fellow/ NP/ Resident

Overnight Events:

Labs:

X-rays/ Radiology/ Tests:
- Review current studies:
- Pending results:
- Order tests

Meds (start/ stop)

Antibiotics

Transplant meds:

Plan of Care / Suggestions/ Family

Bedside Team Assessment of Patient
- Update white board
- Document & Update family

Fig. 21.4 Sample of rounding script

Nursing, Nurse Practitioner, physician, Pharmacy tomorrow at 8 AM. Family members are invited to attend." When rounds begin, start with a brief introduction to the patient and family member, state the purpose of rounds, and encourage their participation as a necessary part of the process. Family members may have input into the care of the patient both during the hospital stay and at transfer and will appreciate seeing the care team work together to focus on the patient. Posting daily goals in patient rooms may also prompt questions from family members who may not have joined rounds; these are great opportunities to involve the family in conversation about patient care goals at any time of the day. Engaging patients and families in multidisciplinary rounds has many benefits, especially with regard to communication with providers, being part of the care team, and active decision-making (Cypress 2012; Rosen et al. 2009).

21.3 Team Performance

The nature of work has changed. Organizations now face increased competition and collaboration within and across organizational, geographical, and temporal boundaries; a need to engage a demographically heterogeneous workforce; a need to deal with advancements in information technology; a need to promote safety; and a need to foster enduring customer relations (Noe 2002; Pfeffer and Sutton 2000; Tannenbaum 2002). One response to these changes has been the use of work teams as a preferred performance management technique. Both governmental agencies and private industry are increasingly relying on work teams as a preferred performance arrangement to fulfill their visions, execute their complex missions, and accomplish their goals (Salas et al. 2004). Many areas of acute care medicine have a low error tolerance and demand high levels of cognitive and technical performance. Growing evidence suggests that further improvements in patient outcomes depend on measuring and improving system factors, in particular, effective team skills. Teamwork concerns the communication and coordination processes that are required to bring together the individual knowledge, skills, and attitudes in the service of a common and valued team goal (Baker et al. 2005). Individual surgical team members are highly specialized and have their own functional taskwork (e.g., intensivist, nursing, surgeon, and perfusion) yet come together as a team toward the common goal of treating the patient. Interventions focusing on teamwork have shown a relationship with improved teamwork and a safety climate. The role of effective teamwork in accomplishing complex tasks is well accepted in many domains. Similarly, there is good evidence that improved outcomes in cardiac care depend on effective team performance (Sorbero et al. 2008). The cardiac surgical intensive care unit (ICU) is a complex, high-risk, and stressful setting, and it can potentially gain from adopting and integrating the principles and techniques used to train team skills such as Team Strategies and Tools to Enhance Performance and Patient Safety (TeamSTEPPS), crew resource management (CRM), and simulation-based team training. The evidence demonstrates that multidisciplinary

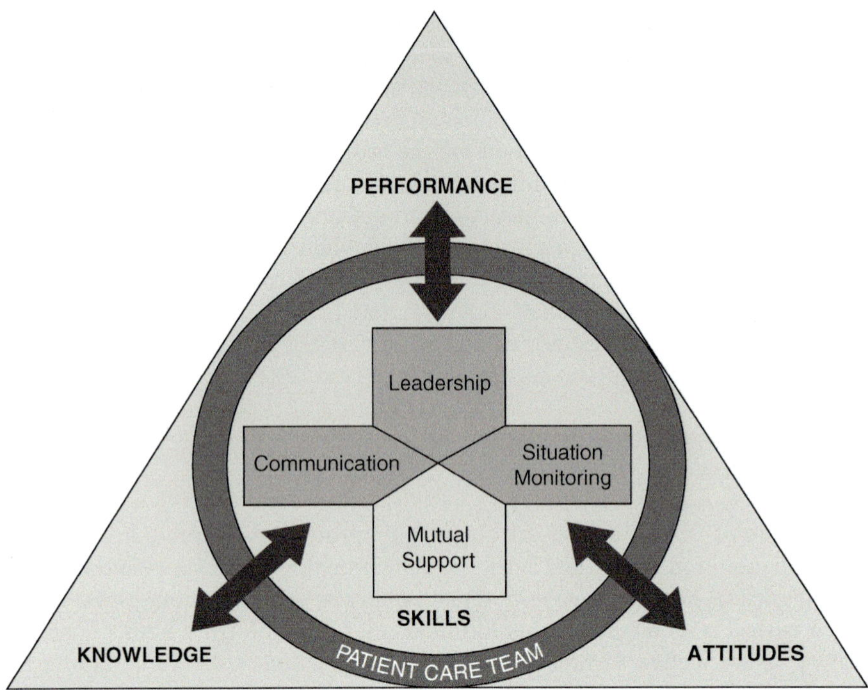

Fig. 21.5 The TeamSTEPPS triangle logo, demonstrating basic concepts related to teamwork training (obtained from AHRQ, TeamSTEPPS: National Implementation, 2011, about the TeamSTEPPS Logo)

team training minimizes poor outcomes by perfecting the elusive teamwork skills and communication (Leonard et al. 2004).

21.3.1 TeamsSTEPPS

TeamSTEPPS is an evidence-based framework to optimize team performance across the health-care delivery system. The core of the TeamSTEPPS framework is comprised of four skills: leadership, situation monitoring, mutual support, and communication. These skills must interplay with the team competency outcomes: knowledge, attitudes, and performance (Fig. 21.5) (Coburn and Croll 2011).

21.3.1.1 Leadership

There are two types of leaders: (1) designated and (2) situational. In effective teams, any member of the team with the skills to best manage the situation can assume the leadership role. An effective team leader organizes the team; articulates clear goals; makes decisions through collective input of members; empowers members to speak up and challenge, when appropriate; actively promotes and facilitates good teamwork; and skillfully resolves conflict (Coburn and Croll 2011).

21.3.1.2 Situation Monitoring

Situation monitoring, or STEP, is the process of continually scanning and assessing what's going on around you to maintain situation awareness (STEP stands for Status of the patient, Team members, Environment, Progress toward goal) (Baker et al. 2010). Situation awareness is knowing what is going on around you and knowing the conditions that affect your work. Shared mental models result from each team member maintaining his or her situation awareness and sharing relevant facts with the entire team. Doing so helps ensure that everyone on the team is on the same page (Barach and Weinger 2007). Cross-monitoring is an error reduction strategy that involves monitoring actions of other team members, providing a safety net for the team, ensuring mistakes or oversights are caught quickly and easily, and watching each other's back (Baker et al. 2010; Barach and Weinger 2007).

21.3.1.3 Mutual Support

Task assistance is one form of mutual support in which team members:

Protect each other from work overload situations.

Place all offers and requests for assistance in the context of patient safety.

Foster a climate where it is expected that assistance will be actively sought and offered.

21.3.1.4 Communication

Effective communication is complete, clear, brief, and timely.

SBARQ is a technique for communicating critical information, concerning a patient's condition, which requires immediate attention and action and is especially important during a handoff (Leonard et al. 2004).

> Situation—What is going on with the patient? Background—What is the clinical background or context? Assessment—What do I think the problem is? Recommendation and Request—What would I do to correct it? Questions—An opportunity to ask or answer any questions.

21.3.2 Crew Resource Management (CRM)

Error reduction and increased patient safety continue to be the focus of teamwork-based training programs. Many health-care organizations are adopting the CRM training from aviation as a patient safety initiative based on strong face validity (France et al. 2005; West et al. 2012). It can be challenging to assemble teams in the cardiac surgical ICU that work together long enough to achieve effectiveness over time. Often, depending on the discipline, clinical responsibilities rotate among attending staff, and medical residents spend limited time in the ICU. Because patient comorbidities in the cardiac surgical ICU are extremely complex, and human factor performance may limit clinicians' recognition of rapidly evolving problems, it is crucial for clinicians to have standardized communication tools and environments that proactively support effective communication. Health care has turned to other complex, high-risk industries for strategies to reduce errors and accident rates and to improve teamwork. In aviation, crew resource management (CRM) is a communication methodology used to train flight crews in critical communication and decision-making, stress management, and team building that can be an effective strategy in enhancing teamwork and lowering risks (Sexton et al. 2000; Helmreich et al. 1999). Structured communication tools with standardized language and procedures that replace hierarchical relationships with mutual decision-making have been adopted in the aviation industry to assist practitioners in daily decision-making (Helmreich et al. 1999). The goal of CRM is to organize members of a team to think and act as a team with the common goal of safety (Salas et al. 2007). CRM teaches team communication and highlights errors in a simulated setting in the hope of avoiding the same error in a real-life setting involving humans. It teaches that all members of a team are vital and that if a team member at any level believes that something is not being done appropriately or in the best interest of the team or other people who have put their trust in the team, then that member must speak up (Hunt et al. 2007). Health-care professionals need to recognize their own limitations, cognitive errors, and stressors such as fatigue that can degrade their performance and contribute to errors and mistakes (Helmreich et al. 1999). Recognizing these limitations and eliminating certain behaviors to reduce errors are part of the CRM training. Key concept emphasized in crew resource management training included the following (Baker et al. 2005; France et al. 2005; Helmreich et al. 1999; Doucette 2006):

- Managing fatigue and workload; stress management
- Creating and managing a team
- Recognizing adverse situations
- Cross-checking and communicating; assertiveness
- Developing and applying shared mental modes for decision-making
- Situational awareness
- Giving and receiving performance feedback

The CRM strategies of team training have been shown to improve the operation of flight crews and the safety of air travel significantly. These same strategies have been applied widely in operating rooms and intensive care units. Despite the interest and research, no studies have shown that CRM training can improve teamwork and quality of care (Baker et al. 2010; Salas et al. 2006). Therefore, it is hoped that improved teamwork and communication will improve patient outcomes and safety, but more research is needed.

21.3.3 Simulation

Simulation-based training is growing in recognition as an instructional strategy incorporating adult learning theory, real-time clinical situations, and video debriefing to allow teams an opportunity to improve their knowledge, to practice skills, and to gain expertise while evaluating their performance (Eppich et al. 2008; Yaeger and Arafeh 2008; Wilson et al. 2005). In fact, actual surgical resuscitations such as massive bleeding, air embolism, and acute tamponade are not optimal training opportunities, because patient care takes precedence over teaching. Meaningful learning occurs after events when there is time to reflect and review events of the care and examine what worked well and what could have been improved. Moreover, many cardiac surgical emergencies occur in an uncontrolled environment and under time pressure constraints. Societal and regulatory pressures will increasingly limit the use of real patients, especially critically ill ones, for hands-on clinical training that can be quite limited, even in a busy medical center (Gaba 2000). High-fidelity simulation provides opportunities to learn and practice desired responses to uncommon events or types of injuries and can also help to capture the complexity of teamwork in a real-world setting and provide opportunities for health-care professionals to grow and learn together. Heath care has entered a new era that has seen several shifts in basic assumptions, regarding the route to effectivity in a healthy and safe work environment, especially in the critical care areas (Barach et al. 2000; Hammond et al. 2002). Two of these assumptions are that (1) teamwork is a critical component of a safe health-care system and (2) simulation-based team training (SBTT) is a critical component in implementing effective teamwork training that is highly transferable to the daily clinical environment (Rosen et al. 2009; Salas et al. 2008; Weaver et al. 2010). The Institute of Medicine (IOM) suggests the use of simulation exercises to enhance teamwork as one of the mechanisms for improving patient safety (Committee on Quality of Health Care 2000; IOM 2001). The success of simulation programs is based on carefully designed clinical scenarios (Table 21.2) that are aligned with the needs of the learner and on skillfully led debriefings (Halamek 2008).

Simulation can provide a replication of the cardiac surgical intensive care unit (CSICU), equipped with the technology and the models of equipment that will be encountered, as well as the complex scenarios that require successful team interactions. Technical or procedural, cognitive, and behavioral skills can also be simulated, allowing for teamwork and competency checks. Leadership skills during emergent situations can be enhanced through the use of role simulation for improving communication skills in relation to discussions about medical care.

Open-chest resuscitation is a high-risk and uncommon event. Health-care providers caring for postoperative cardiac surgery patients may have limited opportunities to participate in extensive resuscitation efforts and to maintain their competency. Providing cardiac practitioners the opportunity to participate in simulation-based resuscitation training allows them to maintain competency in a safe and controlled environment. Through the use of simulation, team training methods provide teams with the opportunity to rehearse team components as well as learn technical skills and build trust (Thomas et al. 2007).

There are a number of factors that affect the effectiveness of team training:

- Training protocol: How is training achieved? What methods are used to impart knowledge? How are practice and feedback incorporated into training?
- Trainer skill: Is the individual who is in charge of leading the training and providing feedback adequately trained?

Table 21.2 Sample of simulation scenario

Scenario synopsis	
Title: High chest tube output	Setup time: 10 min
Diagnosis: *Cardiac Tamponade* with clotted chest tubes	Scenario time: 50 min
Target Audience: Nurses, NP, Physician	Debrief time: 30 min
Prerequisite knowledge and skills:	
Case stem and background information for learner	
Patient is s/p PVR. He was admitted to the unit 4 h ago. Chest tube output has been around 130 ml/h with HR 80 s, BP 100/40 (65), and he's intubated. You continue to tend to your acute patient	
Patient demographics	
Name: Brown	**Gender:** M
Age: 17	
Height: 162.6	**Weight:** 52 kg
Chief complaint: post-op bleeding	
Scenario events summary	
Sequence of events:	
1. RN enters the room performing proper hand hygiene	
2. Patient is 4 h post op PVR. Currently VSS with chest tube output 130 ml/h.	
3. Upon assessment, CT output is now 5 ml/h, HR increased to 130 s, with BP 80/60(70), CVP 18	
4. RN performs assessment mid hears muffled (diminished) heart sounds and feels weak pulses	
5. RM Notifies MD using SBAR mid calls for help →	
6. MD at bedside to perform still ECHO	
7. Confirmation of tamponade	
8. RN needs to prepare for open chest procedure	
9. RN calls for: Crash Cart, Bovie, Surgical Cart, Head Lamp	
10. RN call to notify AOD, OR team and Security for closing unit during procedure	
Observable actions/checklist	
1. Assessment of chest tubes	
2. Physical assessment of patient	
3. Calling for MD using SBAR	
4. Calls for help down the hallway	
5. Calls for proper equipment after ECHO confirmation of tamponade	
Debriefing questions	
1. Could anything have been done to prevent the tamponade?	
2. What about the family?	
3. Chain of command Consider MD privileges, who can actually open the chest?	
4. Delegation	
Take home points	
1. Be aware of the details of preps i.e. surgical cart, bovie, crash cart, push line, suction	
2. Recognize s/s of a cardiac tamponade	
3. Consider 2:1 staffing ratio for procedure	

Table 21.2 (continued)

Scenario events table			
Event name	Patient vitals	Learner actions/triggers	Instructor cues/operator notes
Baseline	ECG: *NSR* HR: *85* BP: *100/40* T: *36.8* SpO2: *100%* RR: *12* etCO2: *36* CVP: *8* Chest Tube output: *130* Labs, imaging studies: *WNL*		
Chest tube output suddenly drops off	ECG: *ST* HR: *130* BP: *80/60(70)* T: *36.4* SpO2: 88% RR: *22* etCO2: *42* CVP: *18* Chest Tube output: *5* Labs, imaging studies: *ECHO*	• Assess pt. what should you observe? • Check CT output	Should hear muffled (diminished) heart sounds, weak or absent pulses
		• Notify MD and get help • Consider ordering for stat CXR or ECHO • Preparation for open chest procedure • Inform family member	Are there clots in the CT? Did you milk/strip them?

- Practice medium and method: How is practice carried out? What simulation environment is used (i.e., mannequin, video)? How much practice is given?
- Training intensity: Is it more effective to conduct training over a short time period (e.g., 1–2 days) or to conduct training over a longer time period (e.g., 3–4 h per week for several weeks)?

Teams make fewer mistakes than do individuals, especially when each team member knows his or her responsibilities as well as those of the other team members. However, simply bringing individuals together to perform a specified task does not automatically ensure that they will function as a team (Mohr et al. 2005). Cardiac teamwork depends on a willingness of clinicians from diverse backgrounds to cooperate in varied clinical settings (i.e., clinic, operating room, intensive care unit, catheterization laboratory, etc.) toward a shared goal, communicate, work together effectively, and improve. To achieve high reliability and consistent performance, each team member must be able to (a) anticipate the needs of the others; (b) adjust to each other's actions to the changing environment; (c) monitor each other's activities and distribute workload dynamically; and (d) have a shared understanding of accepted processes and how events and actions should proceed (shared mental model) (Baker et al. 2006; Aveling et al. 2013).

Currently, it is difficult to suggest that one type of team training is superior to another and that studies are needed in this area. Although some empirical studies show positive outcome after team training, there is little to suggest that these programs and processes actually improve patient safety and outcome. Studies to prove the positive impact of simulation team training on patient outcome may be difficult to perform, but medical team training, based on crew resource management principles, is here to stay.

References

Aveling E-L, McCulloch P, Dixon-Woods M. A qualitative study comparing experiences of the surgical safety checklist in hospitals in high-income and low-income countries. BMJ Open. 2013;3:e003039.

Baker DP, Gustafson S, Beaubien JM, Salas E, Barach P. Medical team training programs in health care. Rockville: Agency for Healthcare Research and Quality; 2005. p. 253–67.

Baker D, Salas E, Barach P, Battles J, King H. The relation between teamwork and patient safety. In: Carayon P, editor. Handbook of human factors and ergonomics in health care and patient safety. Mahawah: Lawrence Erlbaum Associates Inc.; 2006. p. 259–71.

Baker DP, Amodeo AM, Krokos KJ, Slonim A, Herrera H. Assessing teamwork attitudes in healthcare: development of the TeamSTEPPS teamwork attitudes questionnaire. Qual Saf Health Care. 2010;19:e49.

Barach P, Weinger MB. Trauma team performance. In: Wilson WC, Grande CM, Hoyt DB, editors. Emergency resuscitation, perioperative anesthesia, surgical management. New York: Informa HealthCare; 2007. p. 101–14.

Barach P, Fromson J, Kamar R. Ethical and professional concerns of simulation in professional assessment and education. Am J Anesth. 2000;12:228–31.

Burger C. Multidisciplinary rounds: a method to improve quality and safety in critically ill patients. Northeast Florida Med. 2007;58(3):16–9.

Chen JG, Wright MC, Smith PB, Jaggers J, Mistry KP. Adaptation of a postoperative handoff communication process for children with heart disease: a quantitative study. Am J Med Qual. 2011;26(5):380–6.

Coburn AF, Croll ZT. Improving hospital patient safety through teamwork: the use of TeamSTEPPS in critical access hospitals. 2011.

Cooper MD. Towards a model of safety culture. Safety Sci. 2000;36(2):111–36.

Cypress BS. Family presence on rounds: a systematic review of literature. Dimens Crit Care Nurs. 2012;31(1):53–64.

Dale CR, Bryson CL, Fan VS, et al. A greater analgesia, sedation, delirium order set quality score is associated with a decreased duration of mechanical ventilation in cardiovascular surgery patients. Crit Care Med. 2013;41:2610–7.

Donchin Y, Gopher D, Olin M, Badihi Y, Biesky M, Sprung CL, et al. A look into the nature and causes of human errors in the intensive care unit. Crit Care Med. 1995;23(2):294–300.

Doucette JN. View from the cockpit: what the airline industry can teach us about patient safety. Nursing. 2006;36(11):50–3.

Edmondson A. Psychological safety and learning behavior in work teams. Adm Sci Q. 1999;44:350–83.

Edmondson AC. Learning from failure in health care: frequent opportunities, pervasive barriers. Qual Saf Health Care. 2004;13:ii3–9.

Eppich WJ, Brannen M, Hunt EA. Team training: implications for emergency and critical care pediatrics. Curr Opin Pediatr. 2008;20(3):255–60.

Fitch ZW, Debesa O, Ohkuma R, et al. A protocol-driven approach to early extubation after heart surgery. J Thorac Cardioasc Surg. 2014;147:2610–7.

Flin R, Mearns K, O'Connor P, Bryden R. Measuring safety climate: identifying the common features. Saf Sci. 2000;34(1–3):177–92.

Flin R, Burns C, Mearns K, Yule S, Robertson EM. Measuring safety climate in health care. Qual Saf Health Care. 2006;15:109–15.

France DJ, Stiles R, Gaffney FA, et al. Home study program: crew resource management training-clinicians reactions and attitudes. AORN J. 2005;82(2):213–24.

Frankel A, Grillo SP, Pittman M, Thomas EJ, Horowitz L, Page M, et al. Revealing and resolving patient safety defects: the impact of leadership Walk-Rounds on frontline caregiver assessments of patient safety. Health Serv Res. 2008;43:2050–66.

Gaba DM. Human work environment and anesthesia simulators. In: Miller RD, editor. Anesthesia. 5th ed. New York: Churchill-Livingstone; 2000. p. 2613–68.

Guldenmund FW. The nature of safety culture: a review of theory and research. Saf Sci. 2000;34:215–57.

Halamek LP. The simulated delivery-room environment as the future modality for acquiring and maintaining skills in fetal and neonatal resuscitation. Semin Fetal Neonatal Med. 2008;13(6):448–53.

Halm MA. Daily goals worksheets and other checklists: are our critical care units safer? Am J Crit Care. 2008;17(6):577–80.

Hammond J, Bermann M, Chen B, Kushins L. Incorporation of a computerized human patient simulator in critical care training: a preliminary report. J Trauma. 2002;53:1064–7.

Haynes AB, Weiser TG, Berry WR, Lipsitz SR, Breizat AH, Dellinger EP, et al. Safe Surgery Saves Lives Study Group, Changes in safety attitude and relationship to decreased postoperative morbidity and mortality following implementation of a checklist-based surgical safety intervention. BMJ Qual Saf. 2011;20:102–7.

Helmreich RL, Merritt AC, Wilhelm JA. The evolution of crew resource management training in commercial aviation. Int J Aviat Psychol. 1999;9(1):19–32.

Hunt EA, Shilkofski NA, Stavroudis TA, Nelson KL. Simulation: translation to improved team performance. Anesthesiol Clin. 2007;25(2):301–19.

IOM. Crossing the quality chasm: a new health system for the 21st century. Washington, DC: National Academy Press; 2001.

Joint Commission Resources. Comprehensive accreditation manual for hospitals: the official handbook. Oak Brook, IL: Joint Commission Resources; 2017.

Kaufman J, Twite M, Barrett C, Peyton C, Koehler J, Rannie M, Kahn MG, Schofield S, Ing RJ, Jaggers J, Hyman D, da Cruz EM. A handoff protocol from the cardiovascular operating room to cardiac ICU is associated with improvements in care beyond the immediate postoperative period. Jt Comm J Qual Patient Saf. 2013;39:306–11.

Kilic A, Whitman JG. Blood transfusions in cardiac surgery: indications risks, and conservation strategies. Ann Thorac Surg. 2014;97:726–34.

Kim MM, Barnato AE, Angus DC, Fleisher LF, Kahn JM. The effect of multidisciplinary care teams on intensive care unit mortality. Arch Intern Med. 2010;170(4):369–76.

Lamba AR, Linn K, Fletcher KE. Identifying patient safety problems during team rounds: an ethnographic study. BMJ Qual Saf. 2014;23(8):667–9.

Leape LL, Brennan TA, Laird N, Lawthers AG, Localio AR, Barnes BA, et al. The nature of adverse events in hospitalized patients. Results of the Harvard Medical Practice Study II. N Engl J Med. 1991;324(6):377–84.

Leonard M, Graham S, Bonacum D. The human factor: the critical importance of effective teamwork and communication in providing safe care. Qual Saf Health Care. 2004;13(Suppl.1):i85–90.

Mohr JJ, Batalden PB, Barach P. Inquiring into the quality and safety of care in the academic clinical microsystem. In: McLaughlin K, Kaluzny A, editors. Continuous quality improvement in health care. 3rd ed. New York: Aspen; 2005. p. 407–23.

Morello RT, Lowthian JA, Barker AL, McGinnes R, Dunt D, Brand C. Strategies for improving patient safety culture in hospitals: a systematic review. BMJ Qual Saf. 2013;22(1):11–8.

Nieva VF, Sorra J. Safety culture assessment: a tool for improving patient safety in healthcare organizations. Qual Saf Health Care. 2003;12(Suppl):12–23.

Noe RA. Employee training and development. Boston: McGraw-Hill; 2002.

Patient Safety Primer: safety culture. https://psnet.ahrq.gov/primers/primer/5/safety-culture. 2016. November 8.

Petrovic MA, Aboumatar H, Baumgartner WA, et al. Pilot implementation of a perioperative protocol to guide operating room-to-intensive care unit patient handoffs. J Cardiothorac Vasc Anesth. 2012;26:11–6.

Pfeffer JS, Sutton R. The knowing-doing gap: how smart companies turn knowledge into action. Boston: Harvard Business School Press; 2000.

Pierson DJ. Daily multidisciplinary ICU rounds improve patient outcomes. Chicago, IL: AHC Media—Continuing Medical Education Publishing; 2010. p. 1–2.
Pothier D, Monteiro P, Mooktiar M, Shaw A. Pilot study to show the loss of important data in nursing handover. Br J Nurs. 2005;12(20):1090–3.
Pronovost P, Needham D, Berenholtz S, Sinopoli D, Chu H, Cosgrove S, et al. An intervention to decrease catheter-related bloodstream infections in the ICU. N Engl J Med. 2006;355:2725–32.
Reason J. Achieving a safe culture: theory and practice. Work Stress. 1998;12:293–306.
Riley W. High reliability and implications for nursing leaders. J Nurs Manag. 2009;17(2):238–46.
Romig M, Goeschel C, Pronovost P, Berenholtz SM. Integrating CUSP and TRIP to improve patient safety. Hosp Pract. 2010;38:114–21.
Rosen SE, Bochkoris M, Hannon MJ, Kwoh CK. Family-centered multidisciplinary rounds enhance the team approach in pediatrics. Pediatrics. 2009;123(4):e603–8.
Saladino L, Pickett LC, Frush K, Mall A, Champagne MT. Evaluation of a nurse-led safety program in a critical care unit. J Nurs Care Qual. 2013;28(2):139–46.
Salas E, Stagl KC, Burke CS. 25 years of team effectiveness in organizations: research themes and emerging needs. In: Cooper CL, Robertson IT, editors. International review of industrial and organizational psychology. New York: Wiley; 2004. p. 47–9.
Salas E, Wilson KA, Burke CS, Wightman DC. Does crew resource management training work? An update, an extension, and some critical needs. Hum Factors. 2006;48(2):392–412.
Salas E, Wilson KA, Murphy CE. What crew resource management training will not do for patient safety: unless…. J Patient Saf. 2007;3(2):62–4.
Salas E, DizGranados D, Weaver SJ, King H. Does team training work? Principles for health care. Acad Emerg Med. 2008;15:1002–9.
Sammer CE, Lykens K, Singh KP, Mains DA, Lackan NA. What is patient safety culture? A review of the literature. J Nurs Scholarsh. 2010;42(2):156–65.
Segall N, Bonifacio AS, Schroeder RA, et al. Can we make postoperative patient handovers safer? A systematic review of the literature. Anesth Analg. 2012;115: 102–15.
Sexton JB, Thomas EJ, Helmreich RL. Error, stress, and teamwork in medicine and aviation: cross sectional surveys. BMJ. 2000;320(7237):745–9.
Shahian DM, Edwards FH, Ferraris VA, et al. Society of Thoracic Surgeons Quality Measurement Task Force: Quality measurement in adult cardiac surgery: Part 1-Conceptual framework and measure selection. Ann Thorac Surg. 2007;83:S3–12.
Shake JG, Pronovost PJ, Whitman GJ. Cardiac surgical ICU care: eliminating “preventable” complications. J Card Surg. 2013;28:406–13.
Shostek K. Developing a culture of safety in ambulatory care settings. J Ambul Care Manage. 2007;30(2):105–13.
Sinuff T, Muscedere J, Adhikari NK, Stelfox HT, Dodek P, Heyland DK, Rubenfeld GD, Cook DJ, Pinto R, Manoharan V, Currie J, Cahill N, Friedrich JO, Amaral A, Piquette D, Scales DC, Dhanani S, Garland A, KRITICAL Working Group, the Canadian Critical Care Trials Group, and the Canadian Critical Care Society. Knowledge translation interventions for critically ill patients: a systematic review. Crit Care Med. 2013;41:2627–40.
Sorbero ME et al. Outcome measures for effective teamwork in inpatient care. 2008.
Stone ME Jr, Snetman D, O’Neill A, Cucuzzo J, Lindner J, Ahmad S, Teperman S. Daily multidisciplinary rounds to implement the ventilator bundle decreases ventilator-associated pneumonia in trauma patients but does it affect outcome? Surg Infect. 2011;12(5):373–8.
Tannenbaum S. A strategic view of organizational training and learning. In: Kraiger K, editor. Creating, implementing, and managing effective training and development. San Francisco: Jossey-Bass; 2002. p. 10–52.
The Health Foundation. Evidence scan: high reliability organisations. London: The Health Foundation; 2011.
Thomas EJ, Taggart B, Crandell S, et al. Teaching teamwork during the neonatal resuscitation program: a randomized trial. J Perinatol. 2007;27(7):409–14.
Thomas EJ, Sexton JB, Neilands TB, Frankel A, Helmreich RL. The effect of executive walk rounds on nurse safety climate attitudes: a randomized trial of clinical units. BMC Health Serv Res. 2005;5:28.

Tiessen B. On the journey to a culture of patient safety. Health Q. 2008;11:58–63.

Vats A, Goin KH, Villarreal MC, Yilmaz T, Fortenberry JD, Keskinocak P. The impact of lean rounding process in a pediatric intensive care unit. Crit Care Med. 2011;40(2):607–17.

Wachter RM, Pronovost PJ. Balancing "no blame" with accountability in patient safety. N Engl J Med. 2009;361:1401–6.

Weaver SJ, Lyons R, DiazGranados D, Rosen MA, Salas E, Odlesby J, et al. The anatomy of health care team training and the state of practice: a critical review. Acad Med. 2010;85:1746–60.

West P, Sculli G, Fore A, Okam N, Dunlap C, Neily J, Mills P. Improving patient safety and optimizing nursing teamwork using Crew Resource Management techniques. J Nurs Adm. 2012;42(1):15–20.

WHO. Summary of the evidence on patient safety: implications for research. Geneva: WHO; 2008.

WHO. Patient safety research. Geneva: WHO; 2009.

Wiegmann DA, Zhang H, von Thaden TL, Sharma G, Gibbons AM. Safety culture: an integrative review. Int J Aviation Psych. 2009;14:117–34.

Wilson KA, Burke CS, Priest HA, Salas E. Promoting health care safety through training high reliability teams. Qual Saf Health Care. 2005;14(4):303–9.

Yaeger KA, Arafeh JM. Making the move from traditional neonatal education to simulation-based training. J Perinat Neonatal Nurs. 2008;22(2):154–8.

Zwarenstein M, Reeves S. Working together but apart: barriers and routes to nurse-physician collaboration. Jt Comm J Qual Improv. 2002;28:242–7.

Nutrition Support in Postoperative Cardiac of Adult Cardiac Surgery Patients

22

Abdolreza Norouzy and Mehdi Shadnoush

Abstract

Malnutrition is a major morbidity and mortality risk factor in patients undergoing cardiac surgery. Also the risk of malnutrition in post cardiac surgery ICU is estimated be more than 50% of admitted cases. Strategies to combat malnutrition in these patients should be included by routine screening of nutritional status prior to surgery and conditioning nutritional therapy in malnourished patients before surgery. Applying ERAS (Early Recovery After Surgery) protocols in order to optimizing timing of the pre-surgical fasting and re-starting feeding after surgery would be an important step in medical nutrition therapy in cardiac surgery patients. Our aim is to reduce both these timings. Recent scientific evidences have been showing the importance of providing extra micronutrients in this group of patients. Making sure to achieve the growth mile stones in pediatric patients is another issue we should take into consideration in nutritional management of cardiac surgery patients.

Keywords

Malnutrition in cardiac surgery patients · Nutritional status screening · Medical nutrition therapy and nutritional support protocols · Medical nutrition therapy in pediatrics cardiac surgery

A. Norouzy, M.D., Ph.D. (✉)
Department of Nutrition, School of Medicine, Mashhad University of Medical Sciences, Mashhad, Iran
e-mail: NorouzyA@mums.ac.ir

M. Shadnoush, M.D., Ph.D
Department of Clinical Nutrition, School of Nutrition Sciences and Food Technology, Shahid Beheshti University of Medical Sciences, Tehran, Iran

A. Dabbagh et al. (eds.), *Postoperative Critical Care for Adult Cardiac Surgical Patients*, https://doi.org/10.1007/978-3-319-75747-6_22

22.1 Malnutrition in Cardiac Surgery Patients

Malnutrition is a major risk factor in patients undergoing cardiac surgery. Preoperative fasting state, post-acute ischemic fasting state, insulin resistance, nutrient deficiency due to prolonged hypoxic state, and compromised immune function are main causes of nutritional deficiency and malnutrition in patients going under cardiac surgery (Jakob and Stanga 2010). Malnutrition has severe consequences in patients' postoperative recovery. In surgical postoperative ICU patients, cardiac surgery is associated with highest rate of iatrogenic malnutrition (Drover et al. 2010). Energy and protein insufficiency is very high in post-cardiac surgical patients in a way that patients receive around 50% of amount of calorie and protein prescribed for them (Rahman et al. 2016). Another nutritional major risk factor for postoperative cardiac surgery patients is old age. In general, aging is associated with increased risk of malnutrition. On average more than 60% of patients undergoing cardiac surgery are above age of 65 year old (Population Statistics 2005). Comorbidities such as left ventricular failure, chronic renal failure, chronic obstructive pulmonary disease (COPD), peripheral vascular disease, mesenteric thrombotic disease, cerebrovascular disease, and swallowing disorders occur more common in elderly. These conditions have profound effect on nutritional status of elderly and have more pressing impact on nutritional status postoperatively (Ljungqvist and Søreide 2003; Bengmark et al. 2001). Length of stay in ICU is another risk factor for malnutrition. In recent clinical trial on 787 patients in ICU, postoperative cardiac surgery patients who stay in the ICU for 3 or more days are at high risk for inadequate nutrition therapy (Rahman et al. 2017). Cardiac surgery causes a chain of pathophysiological events. These events include release of stress hormones and inflammatory substances. These substances have major effect on body metabolism such as glycogenolysis, lipolysis, and proteolysis.

22.2 Nutritional Status Screening

Screening high-risk patients for malnutrition before operation is very important to set up goals for postoperative critical care. Several scores have been developed and standardized for nutritional risk stratification preoperatively. The Malnutrition Universal Screening Tool (MUST), Subjective Global Assessment (SGA) of Malnutrition, the Mini Nutritional Assessment (MNA) are popular and validated tools (Braga et al. 2009). Recently a more specific nutritional screening tool for cardiac surgery patients has been developed by Johns Hopkins Hospital: the Johns Hopkins Hospital Nutrition Support (JHH NS) score. Scores range from 0 to 36. Each 1-point increase in the JHH NS score is associated with a 20% increase in the risk of requiring nutritional support (Ohkuma et al. 2017). Another appropriate consideration for all critically ill patients at high risk of malnutrition, the Nutrition Risk in Critically Ill (NUTRIC) score, was developed to calculate nutrition risk in ICU patients (Heyland et al. 2011).

22.3 Medical Nutrition Therapy and Nutritional Support Protocols

Severely nutritionally compromised patients should receive perioperative nutritional therapy of longer duration. In order to optimize the malnourished patient, short-term (7–10 days) nutritional conditioning has to be considered (Weimann et al. 2017).

Postsurgical patients commonly receive clear fluid for the day after surgery. Fasting can induce thirst, stress, insulin resistance, and nutrient deficiency (Anthony 2008). A series of orders that put together to minimize stress and maximize the return of function have been developed under Enhanced Recovery after Surgery (ERAS) protocols. These protocols include pre- and postoperative recommendations including IV fluids, sedation, analgesia, nutritional support, and mobilization. Pre- and post-nutritional support protocols have been developed for various conditions such as gastrectomy, colonic surgeries, hysterectomy, and pelvic surgery (Weimann et al. 2017).

Nutritional support for patients undergoing cardiac surgery should be started before surgery. The main goals of perioperative nutritional support are to minimize negative protein balance by avoiding starvation, with the purpose of maintaining muscle, immune, and cognitive function, and to enhance postoperative recovery (Braga et al. 2009). Nutritional support can be included as oral, enteral, parenteral, and a combination of these methods. It is important to notice that hyperalimentation easily can occur due to overfeeding by one source of nutrient, e.g., carbohydrates. So providing a balanced macronutrient regimen is very important in any nutritional support (Simpson and Doig 2005).

There is a strong consensus in using oral and enteral nutrition (EN) in pre- and postoperative surgical patients. Following cardiac surgery, critically ill patients are frequently on vasopressor treatment because of an inflammatory response syndrome, vasoplegia, and/or postoperative low-output syndrome due to myocardial stunning (Stoppe et al. 2017). The need for vasopressor support further results in marked changes in energy expenditure and frequent intolerance to oral feeding, leading to significant energy/protein deficits and increased risk of malnutrition (Stoppe et al. 2017). Parenteral nutrition should be given until enteral function returns. The most important situations where enteral nutrition is contraindicated are intestinal failure, intestinal obstruction, malabsorption, multiple fistulas with high output, intestinal ischemia, hemodynamically unstable patients on large doses of inotropes and/or vasopressors, and severe shock (Stoppe et al. 2017; Weimann et al. 2006). In a large multicenter observational study, Khalid et al. showed that vasopressor- and mechanical ventilation-dependent patients had a significant survival when EN feeding was commenced in early 48 h after ICU admission, compared to those after 48 h admission to ICU (Khalid et al. 2010). This finding was more significant in sickest patients. A group of controversial patients are those on extracorporeal life support systems (ECLSs). In a study by Ferrie et al., all patients on ECLS were fed by enteral nutrition. This did not affect the time to reach the full nutritional tolerance or rate goal (Ferrie et al. 2013). These findings are in contrast with older guidelines which prohibits oral or EN in moderately impaired hemodynamically patients (Venkateswaran et al. 2002).

Setting up an appropriate time to start oral, enteral, parenteral, or mixed feeding in cardiac surgery patients is an important factor in outcome of both nutritional and surgical prognosis. According to the latest consensus of International Multidisciplinary Expert Group on Nutrition in Cardiac Surgery, the following time windows may be of particular relevance (Stoppe et al. 2017):

- Preoperative: at least 2–7 day before surgery
- Early preoperative: ≤24 h before surgery
- Early postoperative: ≤24 h after ICU admission
- Postoperative: >24 h after ICU admission

Using any abovementioned tools for malnutrition screening is practical for patients who have been hospitalized for few days. However, nearly half of the patients are undergoing cardiac surgery, are based on outpatient department, and are hospitalized maximum 24 h before operation.

Using pharmaco-nutrients such as arginine; glutamine; omega 3 fatty acids; vitamin A, C, D, and E; coenzyme Q10; magnesium; lipoic acid; and selenium has shown some promising results in improved oxidative-antioxidative balance status, reduced myocardial damage, and shorter length of stay in hospital (Leong et al. 2010). However, due to small sample sizes and nonhomogeneous patient populations, this needs further scientific evidences (Weimann et al. 2017).

Recent guideline of European Society for Parenteral and Enteral Nutrition (ESPEN) describes nutritional support in surgical patients including critical and noncritical with combining various recommendations from ERAS to other guidelines. These recommendations have been summarized in Table 22.1 (Weimann et al. 2017).

As per mentioned previously, providing energy and protein requirement for adults post-cardiac surgery that have been admitted to ICU has a great importance. The gold standard to calculate the energy requirement is using indirect calorimetry. However, using this method may not be applicable in all ICUs. There are other ways such as using standard formula, e.g., Harris-Benedict plus the severity of the stress level to calculate the energy needs. To calculate the protein needs, use standard 1.1 g/kg/day up to 1.5 g/kg/day depending on nutritional status, fluid excretion, and inflammation degree.

22.4 Medical Nutrition Therapy in Pediatric Cardiac Surgery

Nutritional support in infants and children with congenital heart diseases has slightly different approach compared to adult. Due to daily growth, they have high-energy requirements, poor intake, and compromised digestion and absorption of nutrients in the gut and are frequently malnourished. Delivering adequate nutrition is challenging and may be difficult due to fluid limitations, feeding intolerance, gut

Table 22.1 ESPEN guideline: clinical nutrition in surgery (related recommendations) (Weimann et al. 2017)

	Recommendation	Grade of recommendation/ degree of consensus
Recommendation 1	Patients shall drink clear fluids until 2 h before operation	A—97%
Recommendation 2	Preoperative carbohydrate treatment the night before and 2 h before operation should be administered	A/B—100%
Recommendation 3	Oral nutritional intake shall be continued after surgery without interruption	A—90%
Recommendation 4	Oral intake to be adapted according to individual tolerance and type of surgery with special attention to elderly	GPP—100%
Recommendationn5	Oral intake, including clear liquids, shall be initiated within hours after surgery in most patients	A—100%
Recommendation 6	Assess nutritional status before and after major surgery	GPP—100%
Recommendation 7	Perioperative nutritional therapy is indicated in patients with malnutrition and those at risk or those unable to eat for more than 5 days perioperatively or those cannot maintain above 50% of recommended intake for more than 7 days. Preferable use of EN or oral nutritional supplements (ONS)	GPP/A—100%
Recommendation 8	If more than 50% of intake cannot be maintained by EN or ONS for 7 days, adding parenteral nutrition to the treatment is recommended	B—100%
Recommendation 10	Using all-in-one or pharmacy-prepared PN products is preferable to multi-bottle system	GPP—100%
Recommendation 11	PN glutamine is recommended in exclusively fed PN patients	B—76%
Recommendation 12	PN omega 3 fatty acids are recommended in exclusively fed PN patients	B—97%
Recommendation 13	Peri- or at least postoperative administration of ONS enriched with immunonutrients should be given in malnourished patients	B/0—89%
Recommendation 14	Patients with severe malnutrition should receive nutritional therapy, and operation should be delayed. A period of 7–14 days may be appropriate	A/0—95%
Recommendation 15	Whenever feasible, the oral/enteral nutrition shall be preferred	A/0—100% agreement
Recommendation 16	When patients do not meet their energy needs from normal food, it is recommended to encourage to take ONS during preoperative period irrespective of nutritional status	GPP—86% agreement

(continued)

Table 22.1 (continued)

	Recommendation	Grade of recommendation/ degree of consensus
Recommendation 17	Preoperatively, ONS shall be given to all malnourished cancer, high-risk patients undergoing abdominal surgery and elderly with sarcopenia	A—97% agreement
Recommendation 18	Immune-modulating ONS including arginine, omega 3 fatty acids, and nucleotides can be administered 5–7 days preoperatively	GPP—64%
Recommendation 19	Preoperative EN/ONS should be administered prior to hospitalization to avoid unnecessary hospitalization	0/GPP—64%
Recommendation 20	Preoperative PN shall be administered in patients with malnutrition or severe nutritional risk where energy requirement cannot be adequately met by EN. A period of 7–14 days is recommended	A/0—100%
Recommendation 21	Early EN (within 24 h) shall be initiated in patients in whom early oral nutrition cannot be started or inadequate (less than 50% requirement) for more than 7 days. Special risk groups are major head, neck and GI surgery for cancer, severe trauma, obvious malnutrition	A/GPP—100%
Recommendation 22	For EN, a standardized whole-protein formula is recommended. The use of kitchen-made (blenderized) diets for tube feeding is not recommended	GPP—94%
Recommendation 23	With special regard to malnourished patients, placement of a nasojejunal tube or needle catheter jejunostomy is recommended after major upper GI and pancreatic surgery	B—95%
Recommendation 24	If tube is indicated, it should be started within 24 h after surgery	A—91%
Recommendation 25	Start EN feeding with a low flow rate (e.g., 10–20 mL/h), and increase carefully to targeted level 5–7 days	GPP—85%
Recommendation 26	If long-term EN (>4 weeks) is necessary, consider percutaneous endoscopic gastrostomy (PEG)	GPP—94%
Recommendation 27	Regular assessment of nutritional status during stay in hospital and postdischarge nutritional counselling is recommended	GPP—97%
Recommendation 28	Malnutrition is a major factor influencing outcomes after transplantation; EN or ONS is advised	GPP—100%
Recommendation 29	Regular assessment of nutritional status and qualified dietary counselling in pretransplant patients is advised	GPP—100%
Recommendation 30	Recommendations for living donor and recipients are not different from those with major surgery	GPP—98%
Recommendation 31	After heart, lung, liver, pancreas, and kidney transplantation, early intake of normal food or EN is recommended within 24 h	GPP—100%

Table 22.2 Energy requirement in pediatrics (Koletzko et al. 2005; Mirtall et al. 2004)

	1 month–1 year	1–7 years	7–12 years	>12 years
Calorie requirement (kcal/kg/day)	85–105	75–90	50–75	30–50

Table 22.3 Protein requirement in pediatrics (Koletzko et al. 2005; Mirtall et al. 2004)

	0 month–2 years	2–13 years	13–18 years
Protein requirement (g/kg/day)	2–3	1.5–2.0	1.5

hypoperfusion secondary to low cardiac output and heart failure, hypoxemia, or ductal-dependent blood supply (Vichayavilas et al. 2013). Consequently, calculation of energy and protein needs for infants and children undergoing cardiac surgery is crucial. Resting energy expenditure (REE) has been utilized to determine a patient's minimum caloric requirement in the immediate postoperative period following cardiac surgery (Koletzko et al. 2005). An infant should initially receive 55–60 kcal/kg/day during the acute postoperative phase in order to meet their basal energy requirements. As infants are recovering and becoming more active, it is recommended that the caloric content of their nutrition be advanced to a goal of 90–100 kcal/kg/day (Mirtall et al. 2004). The minimum caloric and protein requirements of patients beyond the newborn period vary depending on age (Tables 22.2 and 22.3) (Koletzko et al. 2005; Mirtall et al. 2004).

22.5 Summary

Nutritional support plays a critical role in cardiac postoperative care. Due to the nature of cardiovascular diseases' need to surgery and also the high-risk group of patients, there are robust evidences on effect of proper medical nutrition therapy on outcome and survival of patients undergoing cardiac surgery.

References

Anthony PS. Nutrition screening tools for hospitalized patients. Nutr Clin Pract. 2008;23:373–82.

Bengmark S, Andersson S, Mangiante G. Uninterrupted perioperative enteral nutrition. Clin Nutr. 2001;20(1):11–9.

Braga M, Ljungqvist O, Soeters P, Fearon K, Weimann A, Bozzetti F. ESPEN guidelines on parenteral nutrition: surgery. Clin Nutr. 2009;28:378–86.

Drover JW, Cahill NE, Kutsogiannis J, Pagliarello G, Wischmeyer P, Wang M, et al. Nutrition therapy for the critically ill surgical patient: we need to do better! JPEN. 2010;34:644–52.

Ferrie S, Herkes R, Forrest P. Nutrition support during extracorporeal membrane oxygenation (ECMO) in adults: a retrospective audit of 86 patients. Intensive Care Med. 2013;39:1989–94.

Heyland DK, Dhaliwal R, Jiang X, Day AG. Identifying critically ill patients who benefit the most from nutrition therapy: the development and initial validation of a novel risk assessment tool. Crit Care. 2011;15:R268.

Jakob SM, Stanga Z. Perioperative metabolic changes in patients undergoing cardiac surgery. Nutrition. 2010;26:349–53.

Khalid I, Doshi P, DiGiovine B. Early enteral nutrition and outcomes of critically ill patients treated with vasopressors and mechanical ventilation. Am J Crit Care. 2010;19:261–8.

Koletzko B, Goulet O, Hunt J, Krohn K, Shamir R. Guidelines on paediatric parenteral nutrition of the European Society of Paediatric Gastroenterology, Hepatology and Nutrition (ESPGHAN) and the European Society for Clinical Nutrition and Metabolism (ESPEN), supported by the European Society of Paediatric Research (ESPR). J Pediatr Gastroenterol Nutr. 2005;41(S2):1–87.

Leong J-Y, van der Merwe J, Pepe S, Bailey M, Perkins A, Lymbury R, et al. Perioperative metabolic therapy improves redox status and outcomes in cardiac surgery patients: a randomised trial. Heart Lung Circ. 2010;19:584–91.

Ljungqvist O, Søreide E. Preoperative fasting. Br J Surg. 2003;90(4):400–6.

Mirtall J, Canada T, Johnson D, Kumpf V, Peterson C, Sacks G. Safe practices for parenteral nutrition. J Parenter Enter Nutr. 2004;28(6):S39–70.

Ohkuma RE, Crawford TC, Brown PM, Grimm JC, Magruder JT, Kilic A, Suarez-Pierre A, Snyder S, Wood JD, Schneider E, Sussman MS, Whitman GJ. A novel risk score to predict the need for nutrition support after cardiac surgery. Ann Thorac Surg. 2017;18:30425–3.

Population Statistics 2005, Part 3. Official Statistics of Sweden, Statistics Sweden 2006.

Rahman A, Hasan RM, Agarwala R, Martin C, Day AG, Heyland DK. Identifying critically-ill patients who will benefit most from nutritional therapy: further validation of the "modified NUTRIC" nutritional risk assessment tool. Clin Nutr. 2016;35:158–62.

Rahman A, Agarwala R, Martin C, Nagpal D, Teitelbaum M, Heyland DK. Nutrition therapy in critically ill patients following cardiac surgery: defining and improving practice. JPEN. 2017;41(7):1188–94.

Simpson F, Doig GS. Parenteral vs. enteral nutrition in the critically ill patient: a meta-analysis of trials using the intention to treat principle. Intensive Care Med. 2005;31:12–23.

Stoppe C, Goetzenich A, Whitmann G, Ohkuma R, Brown T, Hatzakorzian R, Kristof A, Meybohm P, Mechanick J, Evans A, Yeh D, McDonald B, Choudrakis M, Jones P, Barton R, Tripathi R, Elke G, Liakopoulos O, Agarwala R, Lomivorotov V, Marx G, Benstoem C, Lemieux M, Heyland DK. Role of nutrition support in adult cardiac surgery: a consensus statement from an international multidisciplinary expert group on nutrition in cardiac surgery. Crit Care. 2017;21:131.

Venkateswaran RV, Charman SC, Goddard M, Large SR. Lethal mesenteric ischaemia after cardiopulmonary bypass: a common complication? Eur J Cardiothorac Surg. 2002;22:534–8.

Vichayavilas PE, Skillman HE, Krebs NF. Nutrition in congenital heart disease: challenges, guidelines and nutritional support. Paed Congen Cardiol Card Surg Inten Care. 2013;169:3201–12.

Weimann A, Braga M, Harsanyi L, Laviano A, Ljungqvist O, Soeters P, et al. ESPEN guidelines on enteral nutrition: surgery including organ transplantation. Clin Nutr. 2006;25:224–44.

Weimann A, Braga M, Carli F, Higashiguchi T, Hubner M, Klek S, Laviano A, Ljungqvist O, Lobo DN, Martindale R. ESPEN guideline: clinical nutrition in surgery. Clin Nutr. 2017;36:623–50.

Index

A. Dabbagh et al. (eds.), *Postoperative Critical Care for Adult Cardiac Surgical Patients*, https://doi.org/10.1007/978-3-319-75747-6

D

E